Transcultural Concepts in Nursing Care

4th Edition

Margaret M. Andrews, PhD, RN, CTN
Chairperson and Professor
Department of Nursing
Nazareth College of Rochester
Rochester, New York

Joyceen S. Boyle, PhD, RN, FAAN, CTN
Professor and Associate Dean for Faculty Practice
    and Community Programs
School of Nursing
Medical College of Georgia
Augusta, Georgia

CANADIAN EDITOR
Tracy Jean Carr, BN, MSc, PhD(c)
Assistant Professor of Nursing
University of New Brunswick
Saint John, New Brunswick, Canada

LIPPINCOTT WILLIAMS & WILKINS
A **Wolters Kluwer** Company
Philadelphia • Baltimore • New York • London
Buenos Aires • Hong Kong • Sydney • Tokyo

Acquisitions Editor: Margaret Zuccarini
Developmental Editor: Danielle DiPalma
Senior Editorial Coordinator: Helen Kogut
Production Editor: Diane Griffith
Senior Production Manager: Helen Ewan
Managing Editor/Production: Erika Kors

Art Director: Carolyn O'Brien
Design: Jonel Sofian
Manufacturing Manager: William Alberti
Indexer: Greystone Indexing
Compositor: Lippincott Williams & Wilkins
Printer: Maple/Binghampton

4th Edition

9 8 7 6

Library of Congress Cataloging-in-Publication Data
Andrews, Margaret M.
    Transcultural concepts in nursing care/Margaret M. Andrews, Joyceen S. Boyle; Canadian editor, Tracy Jean Carr.–4th ed.
        p. cm
    Includes bibliographical references and index.
    ISBN13: 978-0-7817-3680-0 (alk. paper)
    ISBN 0-7817-3680-3 (alk. paper)
        1. Transcultural nursing. 2. Nursing–Social aspects. 3. Nursing–Cross-cultural studies.
    I. Boyle, Joyceen S. II. Title.
RT86.54 .A53 2003
362.1'73–dc21
                                                                                        2002072496

Care has been taken to confirm the accuracy of the information presented and to describe generally accepted practices. However, the authors, editors, and publisher are not responsible for errors or omissions or for any consequences from application of the information in this book and make no warranty, express or implied, with respect to the content of the publication.

The authors, editors, and publisher have exerted every effort to ensure that drug selection and dosage set forth in this text are in accordance with the current recommendations and practice at the time of publication. However, in view of ongoing research, changes in government regulations, and the constant flow of information relating to drug therapy and drug reactions, the reader is urged to check the package insert for each drug for any change in indications and dosage and for added warnings and precautions. This is particularly important when the recommended agent is a new or infrequently employed drug.

Some drugs and medical devices presented in this publication have Food and Drug Administration (FDA) clearance for limited use in restricted research settings. It is the responsibility of the health care provider to ascertain the FDA status of each drug or device planned for use in his or her clinical practice.

Contributors

Patricia A. Hanson, PhD, RN-C
Associate Professor and Director, Gerontological
   Nurse Practitioner Program
Nazareth College of Rochester
Rochester, New York

Kathryn Hopkins Kavanagh, PhD
Professor
University of Maryland, Baltimore County
   and Towson University
Towson, Maryland

Jana Lauderdale, PhD, MS, RN
Department Head, Family Nursing
Louisiana State University Health Science Center
School of Nursing
New Orleans, Louisiana

Patti A. Ludwig-Beymer, PhD, RN, CTN
Administrative Director of Education and
   Research
Edward Hospital and Health Services
801 South Washington Street
Naperville, Illinois

Margaret A. McKenna, PhD, MPH, MN
Assistant Professor
University of Washington
Seattle, Washington

Dula F. Pacquiao, EdD, RN, CTN
Professor of Nursing
Director, Transcultural Nursing Institute
Coordinator, Graduate Program in Nursing
College of Physical, Applied, and Health Sciences
Kean University
Union, New Jersey

REVIEWERS

Tracy Carr, RN, MSc, PhD (C)
Assistant Professor
Department of Nursing
University of New Brunswick
Saint John, New Brunswick
Canada

Valerie D. George, PhD, RN
Associate Professor
Department of Nursing
Cleveland State University
Cleveland, Ohio

Mary T. Parana, RN, MS, CRNP
Assistant Professor of Nursing
University of Pittsburgh at Bradford
Bradford, Pennsylvania

Kathleen D. Pickrell, RN, MSN
Associate Professor and Chair,
   Associate Degree Nursing Program
Indiana State University
Terre Haute, Indiana

Wanda Wadman, RN, BAAN, MN
Nurse Educator
Centre for Nursing Studies
St. John's, Newfoundland
Canada

Priscilla Ziegler, RN, ND, MSN
Assistant Professor
Seattle Pacific University
School of Health Sciences
Seattle, Washington

Foreword

The 21st Century has found nurses and other health professionals scurrying to learn about different and unknown cultures of the world. The tragic events of September 11, 2001 in the United States, along with other horrible destructive and violent acts worldwide, have hastened people to understand the "why" of such events and to promote justice and peace. This need, however, was anticipated in the mid-1950s when I foresaw that nurses and other health professionals should become educated and competent to function with people of diverse cultures. Today, the transcultural nursing discipline has been established, and is imperative to care for immigrants, refugees, and people of many different cultural backgrounds.

This Fourth Edition by Drs. Andrews and Boyle is an important and major contribution to transcultural nursing. This book is updated to help many nurses in different clinical contexts become knowledgeable and competent in the practice of transcultural nursing. Nothing is more rewarding and encouraging than to see former students become dynamic leaders who advance knowledge in their areas of expertise and transmit such insights to future generations of students. Drs. Andrews and Boyle have been these active leaders, teachers, and researchers who have helped to shape the world of transcultural nursing over the past several decades. They are committed leaders who want to make transcultural nursing a meaningful and useful reality for nurses. Their leadership, demonstrated in community nursing, consultation, education, research, and administration, is well known and reflected in this new edition.

Most assuredly, the Fourth Edition reflects the authors' creative work to refine, explicate, and expand transcultural nursing knowledge and practices throughout the life cycle and in different clinical and community settings. Several chapters have been expanded to show the integration of transcultural nursing concepts and principles into all areas of nursing. Some new content on nutrition, ethics, and administrative organizations has been interwoven and made explicit in this new edition. Most encouraging has been the use of the theory of Culture Care Diversity and Universality as a philosophical, theoretical, and practical guide to help nurses discover ways to provide competent, safe, and meaningful care to clients of similar and diverse cultures. The Sunrise Enabler, with the theoretical tenets of the theory of the three creative new modes of transcultural decision or action on care, is valued and demonstrated in this book.

This edition reflects the authors' scholarly ability to draw upon past historical developments in transcultural nursing and especially important concepts, principles, and research findings. This book reveals the sound cumulative growth of transcultural nursing knowledge over the past 4 decades since my first book, *Nursing and Anthropology*, was published in 1970, and followed by other definitive transcultural nursing publications in 1978, 1995, and 2000.

Moreover, the content in this book clearly reveals the authors' knowledge and experiences in different cultural contexts. Building upon and advancing transcultural nursing knowledge shows scholarly work and publication integrity. A valuable and special feature of this book is the incorporation of comparative cultural care practices in community and clinical settings using ethical values and research findings.

In general, the readers will find this Fourth Edition extremely helpful as they teach and mentor undergraduate students in transcultural nursing courses and clinical–community settings. This book is also valuable as a stepping-stone for students to pursue graduate study in transcultural nursing as it provides a sound and broad foundation for transcultural nursing. This book complements the new and comprehensive Leininger-McFarland transcultural nursing book as students pursue further theoretical, clinical, and research graduate education. Drs. Andrews and Boyle are to be highly commended for their diligent and creative work to update and expand transcultural nursing knowledge and practices in this recent edition. It is an important publication to advance transcultural nursing and to guide students in providing culturally competent, safe, and meaningful care to people of diverse cultures.

Madeline M. Leininger, Ph.D., L.H.D., D.S., R.N., C.T.N., F.A.A.N., FRCNA
Founder and Leader of Transcultural Nursing and
Human Care Theory and Research

Professor Emeritus of Nursing, Wayne State University (Detroit)
and University of Nebraska (Omaha)

Transcultural Global Nursing Consultant and Lecturer
Residing in Omaha, Nebraska

Preface

In the mid-1950s the nurse-anthropologist Dr. Madeleine M. Leininger envisioned *transcultural nursing* as a formal area of study and practice for nurses. Since that time, there has been a major cultural care movement, and transcultural nursing's influence has spread to many nations around the world. During the past 5 decades, transcultural nursing has gradually changed nursing practice, education, research, administration, and consultation as well as contemporary society itself. Transcultural nursing has influenced other health-related disciplines, including medicine, pharmacy, physical therapy, occupational therapy, and many other fields. *Culturally competent* care is now an expected standard of care for individuals, families, groups, and communities in health care settings, and many state and national accrediting bodies include criteria related to the cultural needs of patients.

Our major contribution to transcultural nursing is a synthesis of transcultural theories, models, and research studies compiled into a comprehensive text. Our primary goals are to advance the use of transcultural knowledge in nursing practice and to develop *cultural competence*. While we hope that every reader will draw his or her own conclusions, we believe that we have made a significant contribution to incorporating cultural knowledge in nursing care and providing a state-of-the-art text on this exciting nursing specialty called *transcultural nursing*.

Initially published in 1989, *Transcultural Concepts in Nursing Care* began as a collegial effort among faculty and doctoral students at the University of Utah College of Nursing to help us expand and clarify our view of transcultural nursing. Because many of the contributors had strong clinical backgrounds and an interest in solving practice problems, we wanted a book that would apply transcultural nursing concepts to clinical practice. In particular, we wanted a text that undergraduate students would find interesting, challenging, and, above all, helpful in providing culturally competent nursing care for patients from diverse backgrounds. We have a strong commitment to theory development in nursing that helped us develop an evidence-based theoretical framework for transcultural nursing practice. In the fourth edition, we have many of the same contributors, but have been pleased to have other transcultural nursing experts from various parts of the United States and Canada join us.

Many contributors teach in baccalaureate, masters, and/or doctoral programs. Over the years we have explored ways to creatively and effectively teach our students how to apply transcultural concepts to practice, with the goal of developing their knowledge and skill in providing culturally competent and culturally congruent nursing care. The Commission on Collegiate Nursing Education, the National League for Nursing, most state boards of nursing, and other accrediting and certification bodies require or strongly encourage the inclusion of cultural aspects of care in nursing curricula. This underscores the importance of the purpose, goal, and objectives for *Transcultural Concepts in Nursing Care:*

Purpose: To contribute to the development of theoretically based transcultural nursing and the advancement of transcultural nursing practice.

Goal: To increase the delivery of culturally competent care to individuals, families, groups, communities, and institutions.

Objectives:
1. To apply a transcultural nursing framework to guide nursing practice in diverse health care settings across the lifespan.
2. To analyze major concerns and issues encountered by nurses in providing transcultural nursing care to individuals, families, groups, communities, and institutions.
3. To expand the theoretical basis for using concepts from the natural and behavioral sciences and from the humanities in order to provide culturally competent and culturally congruent nursing care.

We believe that cultural assessment skills, combined with the nurse's critical thinking ability, will provide the necessary knowledge on which to base transcultural nursing care. Using this approach, we are convinced that nurses will be able to provide culturally competent and contextually meaningful care for clients—individuals, families, groups, communities, and institutions.

Given that nurses are likely to encounter people from literally hundreds of different cultures, we believe this approach is more effective than simply memorizing the esoteric health beliefs and practices of a litany of different groups. Thus, we believe that nurses must acquire the knowledge and skills needed to assess and care for clients from virtually any and all cultural groups that they encounter throughout their professional careers.

We would like to comment on the extensive progress that has been made in nursing education, practice, and research in terms of cultural awareness, sensitivity, and competence during the past decade. Although there remains much work to be done, we are pleased that many clinicians, educators, researchers, administrators, and consultants have, with increasing frequency, integrated transcultural nursing concepts into their respective areas of expertise. Similarly, the authors of nursing and health care textbooks and other publications often integrate transcultural nursing into their work or invite certified transcultural nurses do so. While we are pleased with this trend, we also recognize that there remains a need for a comprehensive text that provides nurses with the theoretical foundations for transcultural nursing, develops competence in cultural assessment, and systematically applies transcultural concepts across the lifespan. We also believe that there are contemporary health care issues, problems, and challenges that warrant critical analysis, thus making a text such as *Transcultural Concepts in Nursing Care* a useful adjunct to general and specialty nursing texts.

In light of the development of this book through three editions, it is not surprising to discover that the fourth edition of *Transcultural Concepts in Nursing Care* strongly reflects the current challenges faced by nurses who are practicing in a changing clinical environment. Overall, the authors and contributors share a commitment to:

- Foster the development and maintenance of a disciplinary knowledge base and expertise in culturally competent care.
- Synthesize existing theoretical and research knowledge regarding nursing care of different ethnic/minority, marginalized, and disenfranchised populations.
- Create an interdisciplinary knowledge base that reflects heterogeneous health care practices within various cultural groups.
- Identify, describe, and examine methods, theories, and frameworks appropriate for developing knowledge that will improve health and nursing care to minority, marginalized, and disenfranchised populations.

• RECOGNIZING INDIVIDUAL DIFFERENCES AND ACCULTURATION

When considering transcultural issues, nurses and other health care professionals are, with increasing frequency, referring to the federally defined population categories (i.e., White, Black, Hispanic, Asian/Pacific Islander, and American Indian/Alaska Native). The creation of these defined population categories by the United States and Canadian governments has had a tremendous impact on our conceptualization of the various groups that constitute our society. The unique characteristics and individual differences of the five cultural groups have often been ignored, along with the impact acculturation has had on these groups. The outcome is reminiscent of the melting pot metaphor, only now we have five pots instead of one!

We believe that it is tremendously important to recognize the myriad of health-related beliefs and practices that exist within the population categories. For example, the differences are rarely recognized among people who identify themselves as Hispanic/Latino: this group includes people from Puerto Rico, Mexico, Spain, Guatemala, or "Little Havana" in Miami, who may have some similarities but who also may have distinct cultural differences.

We would like to comment briefly on the terms *minority* and *ethnic minorities*. These terms are perceived to be offensive by some because they connote inferiority and marginalization. Although we have used these terms occasionally, we prefer to make reference to a specific subculture or culture whenever possible. We refer to categorizations according to race, ethnicity, religion, or a combination, such as ethnoreligion (e.g., Amish), but we make every effort to avoid using any label in a pejorative way. We do believe, however, that the concepts or terms *minority* or *ethnicity* are limiting not only for those to whom the label may be applied, but also for nursing theory and practice.

• CRITICAL THINKING LINKED TO DELIVERING CULTURALLY COMPETENT CARE

We believe that cultural assessment skills, combined with the nurse's critical thinking ability, will provide the necessary knowledge on which to base transcultural nursing care. Using this approach, we are convinced that nurses will be able to provide culturally competent and contextually meaningful care for clients from a wide variety of cultural backgrounds, rather than simply memorizing the esoteric health beliefs and practices of any specific cultural group. We believe that nurses must acquire the skills needed to assess clients from virtually any and all groups that they encounter throughout their professional careers.

• NEW TO THE FOURTH EDITION

All content in this edition has been reviewed and updated to capture the nature of the changing health care delivery system and to explain how nurses and other health care providers can use culturally competent skills to improve the care of clients, families, groups, and communities.

Emphasis on Clinical Application

Clinical Application has been emphasized by integrating current evidence-based practice throughout the text and expanding content related to cultural assessment.

New Chapters

At the recommendation of Developmental Editor Danielle DiPalma, Part One, Historical and Theoretical Foundations of Transcultural Nursing, which contains the first four chapters, has been reorganized and revised extensively to make the content more readable and succinct. We have added a new chapter on cultural competence in health care organizations (Chapter 9), which has been written by Dr. Patti Ludwig-Beymer, Vice President for Medical Education and Research at Advocate Health Care, Chicago, Illinois. Dr. Dula Pacquaio, a faculty member at Kean University School of Nursing and President of the Transcultural Nursing Society, has provided a fresh perspective on cultural competence in ethical decision-making. Because there are many excellent texts on nutrition, we decided to eliminate the chapter on nutrition in favor of integrating key nutrition concepts into selected chapters, as we deemed appropriate to developing cultural competence. Although both authors have extensive international health and nursing experience, at the publisher's recommendation, we have decided not to include a separate chapter on international nursing. Rather, we have integrated global perspectives into the text, with a special emphasis on transcultural nursing from a Canadian perspective. Canadian Editor Tracy Carr, a nursing faculty member at the University of New Brunswick-Saint John, has reviewed each chapter in the text from a Canadian vantage point and has contributed significantly to the overall Canadian content contained in the fourth edition. We thank Tracy for her contribution to this edition.

Chapter Pedagogy

Learning Activities

All of the chapters include review questions as well as learning activities to promote critical thinking. In addition, each chapter includes chapter objectives and key terms to help readers understand the purpose and intent of the content they will be reading.

Evidence-based Practice

Current research studies related to the content of the chapter are presented as Evidence-based Practice boxes. We have included a section in each box describing appropriate clinical applications derived from the research.

Case Studies Based on Actual Experiences

Case studies based on the authors' actual clinical experiences and research findings are presented to make conceptual linkages and to illustrate how concepts are applied in health care settings. (Authors' note: The case studies use pseudonyms to protect the confidentiality and anonymity of the authors' clients and research subjects.)

Text Organization

Part One: Historical and Theoretical Foundations of Transcultural Nursing

The first section focuses on the historical and theoretical aspects of transcultural nursing. The development of a transcultural nursing framework that includes concepts from the natural and behavioral sciences is described as it applies to nursing practice. Because nursing perspectives are used to organize the content of *Transcultural Concepts in Nursing Care*, the reader will not find a chapter purporting to describe the nursing care of a specific cultural group. Instead, the nursing needs of culturally diverse groups are used to illustrate cultural concepts used in nursing care. Chapter 1 provides an overview of the historical and theoretical foundations of transcultural nursing and Chapter 2 introduces key concepts associated with cultural competence. In Chapter 3, we discuss the domains of cultural knowledge that are important in cultural assessment and describe how this cultural information can be incorporated into all aspects of nursing care. Chapter 4 provides a summary of the major cultural belief systems embraced by people of the world with special emphasis on their health-related and culturally-based values, attitudes, beliefs, and practices.

Part Two: A Developmental Approach to Transcultural Nursing

Chapters 5–8 use a developmental framework to discuss transcultural concepts across the lifespan. The care of childbearing women and their families, children, adolescents, middle-aged adults, and the elderly is examined, and information about various cultural groups is used to illustrate common transcultural nursing issues, trends, and problems.

Part Three: Nursing in Multicultural Health Care Settings

In the third section of the text, Chapters 9 to 12, we examine cultural competence in health care organizations and we explore the components of cultural competence in mental health and in family and community health care settings. We also examine cultural diversity in the health care workforce and analyze this diversity from the perspectives of multiple disciplines. The clinical application of concepts throughout this section uses situations commonly encountered by nurses and describes how transcultural nursing principles can be applied in diverse settings. The chapters in this section are intended to illustrate the application of transcultural nursing knowledge to nursing practice.

Part Four: Contemporary Challenges in Transcultural Nursing

In the fourth section of the text, Chapters 13 to 15, we look at selected contemporary issues and challenges that face nursing and health care. In Chapter 13, we critically examine the fourth vital sign—pain—from a transcultural perspective, building on the extensive body of research on transcultural aspects of pain. In Chapter 14, we review the major religious traditions of North America and the interrelationships among religion, culture, and nursing. Recognizing the plethora of moral and ethical challenges in contemporary health care, *Transcultural Concepts in Nursing Care* includes a thought-provoking Chapter 15, Cultural Competence in Ethical Decision-Making. This chapter provides a framework for analyzing moral and ethical dilemmas and examines from a transcultural perspective, contemporary ethical issues faced by nurses.

• A FINAL NOTE

We are pleased that several members of the original group who wrote the first edition of *Transcultural Concepts in Nursing Care* are still with us and that colleagues who helped us with the second and third editions are continuing to contribute. New contributors have been welcomed, and we are especially pleased that, in the fourth edition, we have been able to better examine transcultural nursing from a Canadian perspective. The significant submissions from all of our contributors have enriched this fourth edition, both in scope and content.

Margaret M. Andrews, PhD, RN, CTN
Joyceen S. Boyle, PhD, RN, FAAN, CTN

Acknowledgments

We gratefully acknowledge the assistance of our families, friends, and colleagues in making this book possible. We also appreciate the help of the many nursing faculty members, practitioners, and students who have offered their comments and suggestions. In this new edition, we have attempted to address transcultural nursing from a Canadian perspective when it seemed appropriate to do so, and we thank our Canadian Editor, Tracy Carr, for her extensive contributions.

We are indebted to the many individuals who allowed us to take photographs of them, including members of our families and our friends. Particular appreciation is extended to Dr. Patti Ludwig-Beymer, Dr. Margaret A. McKenna, Dr. Kathleen Kavanagh, Dr. M. Katherine Maeve, Dr. Kenneth Weiss, Henry J. Andrews, Jr., and Teresa Cooper, all of whom provided special photographs for us. We also extend our thanks to Kawkab Shishani for allowing us to use a photo of her taken shortly after September 11, 2001 and for her healing words about enhancing cross-cultural communication and breaking down the barriers that divide people from different cultures.

A special word of thanks to Margaret Zuccarini, Senior Acquisitions Editor, Danielle DiPalma, Senior Developmental Editor, and Helen Kogut, Senior Editorial Coordinator, who have supported and encouraged us throughout this project. We are grateful to the Lippincott Williams & Wilkins Production Staff, especially Helen Ewan, Production Manager, Diane Griffith, Production Editor, and Carolyn O'Brien, Designer, for assistance with editing and design and for their careful attention to details during the final stages of production.

We acknowledge and thank our secretaries, Ginny T. Quinn and Lisa M. Carrier, for their help in preparing this manuscript. Their contributions were invaluable. Without their expertise and skill, this project would not have been possible.

We wish to express gratitude to our mothers, Virginia Andrews and Joyce Spencer, and to our fathers (now deceased), Henry J. Andrews, Sr. and Harold Spencer, for teaching us to respect and value differences in people. Thanks also to Henry, Marilyn, Michael, Peter, and Suzanne Andrews and John Boyle for their interest and support over the years. We are also grateful for the support of our friends, too numerous to list by name, who often stopped by our offices, e-mailed, or phoned to express their interest.

Lastly, once again we would like to thank each other for a friendship that has withstood the test of time (and now four editions of this book). We started with sharpened pencils and yellow legal pads with our first edition and have progressed to e-mail, computers, and fax machines. Through it all, we have found our professional endeavors in transcultural nursing and the friends we have made to be both satisfying and rewarding.

Contents

1

Historical and Theoretical Foundations of Transcultural Nursing

CHAPTER 1

Theoretical Foundations of Transcultural Nursing

Margaret M. Andrews

KEY TERMS

Anthropology
Culture-specific nursing care
Culture-universal nursing care
Cultural competence
Cultural congruence

Culturally congruent care
Diversity
Ethnocentric
Leininger's sunrise model

Leininger's theory of culture
   care diversity and universality
Panethnic minority groups
Transcultural nursing

OBJECTIVES

1. Examine the historical origins of transcultural nursing with special emphasis on its roots in anthropology.
2. Critically analyze the need for transcultural nursing in contemporary society.
3. Critically analyze prevailing nursing paradigms and nursing theories from a transcultural nursing perspective.
4. Identify resources available in transcultural nursing and health care.

The term **transcultural nursing** is sometimes used interchangeably with *cross-cultural, intercultural,* or *multicultural* nursing. In analyzing the Latin derivations of the prefixes associated with these terms, you will notice that *trans* means *across, inter* means *between,* and *multi* means *many.* Given these derivations, it is understandable that various words have been used with similar connotative meaning (Andrews, 1992; Andrews 1995b). Some people have used the term *ethnic nursing care* (Orque, Bloch, & Monrroy, 1983) or have referred to caring for *people of color* (Branch & Paxton, 1976).

Approximately 30 years ago, nurse-anthropologists debated the conceptual differences between transcultural and cross-cultural nursing, and debate has continued (Brink, 1999; Lipson, 1999). We have chosen to use *transcultural nursing* in this book in recognition of the historical and theoretical contributions of Dr. Madeleine M. Leininger, a nurse-anthropologist who, in the mid-

1950s, envisioned transcultural nursing as a formal area of study and practice for nurses and coined the term *transcultural nursing* (Andrews & Boyle, 1997; Leininger, 1995; Leininger, 1999; Leininger & McFarland, 2002). In her classic work, *Nursing and Anthropology: Two Worlds to Blend,* Dr. Leininger notes that "the fields of anthropology and nursing must be interdigitated so that each field will profit from the contribution of the other.... It is apparent that if these two fields were sharing their special knowledge and experiences, both would undoubtedly see new pathways in thinking and research" (Leininger, 1970).

As the name implies, transcultural nursing goes across cultural boundaries in a search for the essence of nursing. Transcultural nursing is the blending of anthropology and nursing in both theory and practice (Daugherty & Tripp-Reimer, 1985; Lipson & Bauwens, 1988; McKenna, 1984; Osborne, 1969). Anthropology refers to the study of humans and humankind, including their origins, behavior, social relationships, physical and mental characteristics, customs, and development through time and in all places in the world. Recognizing that nursing is an art and a science, transcultural nursing enables us to view our profession from a cultural perspective. Transcultural nursing is not just for immigrants, people of color, or members of the federally defined **panethnic minority groups**, i.e., Blacks, Hispanics, Asians/Pacific Islanders, and American Indians/Alaska Natives. Everyone has a cultural heritage, including nurses, patients, and other members of the health care team (Andrews & Boyle, 1997).

Transcultural nursing is a specialty within nursing focused on the comparative study and analysis of different cultures and subcultures. These groups are examined with respect to their caring behavior; nursing care; and health-illness values, beliefs, and patterns of behavior. The goal of transcultural nursing is to develop a scientific and humanistic body of knowledge in order to provide **culture-specific** and **culture-universal nursing care** practices. *Culture-specific* refers to particular values, beliefs, and patterns of behavior that tend to be special or unique to a group and that do not tend to be shared with members of other cultures. *Culture-universal* refers to the commonly shared values, norms of behavior, and life patterns that are similarly held among cultures about human behavior and lifestyles (Leininger, 1978, 1991, 1995; Leininger & McFarland, 2002).

Transcultural nursing requires sophisticated assessment and analytic skills and the ability to plan, design, implement, and evaluate nursing care for individuals, families, groups, and communities representing various cultures. You must also be able to apply knowledge related to the culture of organizations, institutions, and agencies, especially those concerned with health and nursing.

• THE IMPORTANCE OF TRANSCULTURAL NURSING

Leininger (1995) cites eight factors that influenced her to establish transcultural nursing:

1. There was a marked increase in the migration of people within and between countries worldwide. Transcultural nursing is needed because of the growing diversity that characterizes our national and global populations. In its broadest sense, **diversity** refers to differences in race, ethnicity, national origin, religion, age, gender, sexual orientation, ability/disability, social and economic status or class, education, and related attributes of groups of people in society.
2. There has been a rise in multicultural identities, with people expecting their cultural beliefs, values, and lifeways to be understood and respected by nurses and other health care providers.
3. The increased use of health care technology sometimes conflicts with cultural values of clients, such as Amish prohibitions against using certain apnea monitors, IV pumps, and other such health care technologic devices in the home.
4. Worldwide, there are cultural conflicts, clashes, and violence that have an impact health care as more cultures interact with one another.
5. There is an increase in the number of people traveling and working in many different parts of the world.
6. There is an increase in legal suits resulting from cultural conflict, negligence, ignorance, and imposition of health care practices.
7. There has been a rise in feminism and gender issues, with new demands on health care systems to meet the needs of women and children.
8. There has been an increased demand for community and culturally based health care services in diverse environmental contexts.

Let's examine a few clinical examples of ways in which transcultural nursing can be used in the care of people with diverse backgrounds. Transcultural nursing enables nurses to communicate more effectively with clients from diverse cultural and linguistic backgrounds and to assist those with mental health problems. Transcultural nursing enables nurses to more accurately assess the cultural expression of pain and to provide culturally appropriate interventions to prevent or alleviate discomfort. Last, incidents have been reported in which parents have been arrested for child abuse because culturally based child-rearing practices were poorly understood. Transcultural nursing is a vehicle for assessing the parent-child relationship and for encouraging forms of parental discipline that promote the health and well-being of children and prevent physical or emotional harm (Andrews, 1992, 1995b; Flaskerud, 2000; Leininger, 1997; Leininger & McFarland, 2002; Mahoney & Engebretson, 2000).

Throughout this book, we shall examine various ways in which transcultural nursing facilitates nurses' knowledge and skill in caring for people from diverse backgrounds. Although much of the emphasis will be on diversity, we shall also explore the universal attributes that we have in common with other members of the human race, such as the need for food, sleep, shelter, safety, and human interaction. Let us now examine some key developments in transcultural nursing from a historical perspective.

• HISTORY OF TRANSCULTURAL NURSING

In the 1950s, Dr. Madeleine M. Leininger noted cultural differences between patients and nurses while working with emotionally disturbed children. This clinical experience led her in 1954 to study cultural differences in the perceptions of care, and in 1965 she earned a doctorate in cultural anthropology from the University of Washington (Leininger, 1995; Reynolds & Leininger, 1993). Leininger recognized that one of anthropology's most important contributions to nursing was the realization that health and illness states are strongly influenced by culture. Table 1-1 gives a summary of Dr. Leininger's contributions to the development of transcultural nursing.

To help develop, test, and organize the emerging body of knowledge in transcultural nursing, it is necessary to have a specific conceptual framework from which various theoretical statements can emerge. **Leininger's Sunrise Model** Figure 1-1 is based on the concept of cultural care and shows three major nursing modalities that guide nursing judgments and activities to provide **culturally congruent care**—that is, care that is beneficial and meaningful to the people being served (Leininger, 1991, 1995; Leininger & McFarland, 2002).

Leininger's Theory of Culture Care Diversity and Universality focuses on describing, explaining, and predicting nursing similarities and differences focused primarily on human care and caring in human cultures. Leininger uses worldview, social structure, language, ethnohistory, environmental context, and the generic (folk) and professional systems to provide a comprehensive and holistic view of influences in culture care and well-being. The three modes of nursing decisions and actions—culture care preservation and/or maintenance, culture care accommodation and/or negotiation, and culture care repatterning and/or restructuring—are presented to demonstrate ways to provide culturally congruent nursing care (Leininger, 1991, 1995; Leininger & McFarland, 2002). Among the strengths of Leininger's theory is its flexibility for use with individuals, families, groups, communities, and institutions in diverse health systems. Leininger's Sunrise Model depicts components of the Theory of Cultural Care Diversity and Universality, and it provides a visual schematic representation of the key components of the theory and the interrelationships among its parts. As the world of nursing and health care has become increasingly multicultural, the theory's relevance has increased as well.

• CRITICAL ANALYSIS OF TRANSCULTURAL NURSING

Transcultural nursing has been criticized for its definitional, theoretical, and practical limitations.

Major Criticisms

Let us begin by examining the criticism that transcultural nursing contains ambiguous terminology and lacks clarity in describing key concepts

TABLE 1–1	CONTRIBUTIONS OF MADELEINE LEININGER TO THE DEVELOPMENT OF TRANSCULTURAL NURSING

DATE	ACHIEVEMENT AND CONTRIBUTION
1954	Dr. Madeleine Leininger noticed and studied the cultural differences in the perception of care
1965	Leininger earned a doctorate in cultural anthropology (U. of Washington)
1965–69	Leininger offered first courses and telelectures offered in transcultural nursing (U. of Colorado School of Nursing) Established first PhD nurse-scientist program combining anthropology and nursing (U. of Colorado School of Nursing)
1973	First academic department in transcultural nursing established (U. of Washington School of Nursing)
1974	Transcultural Nursing Society established as the official organization of transcultural nursing
1978	First advanced degree programs (Master's and Doctoral) established (U. of Utah School of Nursing)
1988	Transcultural Nursing Society initiated certification examinations: Certified Transcultural Nurse (CTN)
1989	Journal of Transcultural Nursing (JTN) first published as official publication of the Transcultural Nursing Society; Dr. Madeleine Leininger is founding editor. Goal of the JTN is to disseminate transcultural ideas, theories, research findings, and/or practice experiences
1991	Dr. Leininger published *Culture Care Diversity and Universality: A Theory of Nursing* in which she outlined her theory (Culture Care Diversity and Universality and the Sunrise Model) and its research applications
1995	Dr. Leininger published *Transcultural Nursing: Concepts Theories, Research and Practices* (2nd edition)
2002	Dr. Leininger (with co-author Dr. Marilyn McFarland) published *Transcultural Nursing: Concepts, Theories, Research, and Practices* (3rd edition)

(Habayeb, 1995; Mulholland, 1995). For example, nurses have struggled to achieve clarity in concepts such as cultural awareness, cultural sensitivity, **cultural competence**, and **cultural congruence**. Color, religion, and geographic location are most often used to narrowly define culture and highlight cultural diversity, which is often portrayed as a minority/majority issue. Discrepancies in definition arise when one fails to recognize that every person has a cultural heritage. Talabere (1996) suggests that *cultural diversity* is itself an **ethnocentric** term because it focuses on "how different the other person is from me" rather than "how different I am from the other." In using the term *cultural diversity,* the white panethnic group is frequently viewed as the norm against which the differences in everyone else (ethnocentrically referred to as nonwhites) are measured or compared.

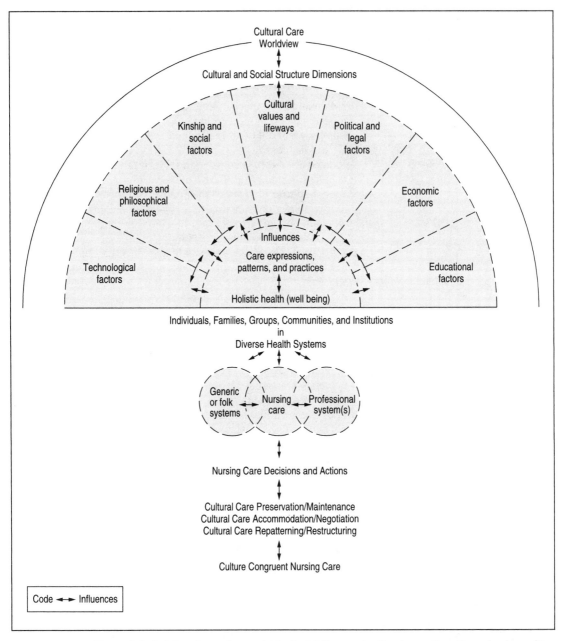

Figure 1–1. Leininger's sunrise model to depict theory of cultural care diversity and universality. (Reprinted by permission from Leininger, M. M. [1991]. *Culture Care Diversity and Universality: A Theory of Nursing.* New York National League for Nursing Press, 1991:43.)

Another criticism of transcultural nursing models is their failure to recognize the relationship between knowledge and power, and their inattention to the complexities associated with prejudice, discrimination, and racism (c.f. Gustafson, 1999; Price & Cortis, 2000). Although Leininger and other transcultural nurses address the need to consider the political, economic, and social dimensions in their theoretical formulations, transcultural nursing has been criticized for doing too little to encourage nurses to be actively involved in setting political, economic, and social policy agendas.

Culley (1996) criticizes transcultural nursing for failing to recognize the power relations that exist between groups. When clients from traditionally underrepresented groups fail to behave as a nurse expects, the behavior is sometimes referred to as *noncompliant,* a term with a negative connotation that is sometimes used synonymously with *different, deviant, abnormal,* or *pathologic.* Problems are thought to be generated by customs or traditions deemed by the nurse to be "inappropriate," a judgment that may be the result of personal bias, lack of knowledge concerning the cultural context in which these customs are practiced, the nurse's inexperience, or other factors. As a result, complex sociocultural phenomena are often reduced to overgeneralized stereotypes. For example, some North American nurses are critical of the role of women in traditional African and Middle Eastern cultures. In concentrating on culturally determined gender issues, you might ignore or minimize the significance of power, inequality, and racism as embedded in structures or institutions (Gustafson, 1999; Price & Cortis, 2000), factors that fundamentally affect the health of cultural groups and their members' access to quality health care. The same criticism might be applied to nursing's failure to address other forms of bias, prejudice, discrimination, and social injustice.

Finally, transcultural nursing has been criticized for embracing models based on the assumption that understanding one's own culture and the culture of others creates tolerance and respect for people from diverse backgrounds. It has become apparent that the mere awareness of one's own culture and that of others is insufficient for the alleviation and potential eradication of prejudice, bigotry, racial, ethnic or cultural conflicts, discrimination, or ethnic violence. Rather, nursing students, nurses, and other health care providers must have positive experiences with members of other cultures and learn to value genuinely the contributions all cultures make to our multicultural society.

Response to Criticisms

In the remainder of this book, we, the authors, will attempt to address these criticisms of transcultural nursing through our approach to topics. It should be noted, however, that many of the issues raised by critics have deeply rooted historical, socioeconomic, religious, cultural, and political origins. Because the nursing profession is a microcosm of society, it mirrors the biases and prejudices found in the larger social order. It is unrealistic to expect that transcultural nursing can reverse all the inequalities cited by the critics. It is realistic, however, to expect more definitional, conceptual, and theoretical clarity. It also is realistic to expect nurses to become increasingly active in setting political, economic, and social policy agendas at the local, state/provincial, national, and international levels.

For example, you can empower yourself and your profession by running for elected offices; supporting candidates with health-related agendas congruent with your own; voting for candidates from diverse cultural backgrounds; using print, broadcast, and web-based media to influence public opinion; and joining professional organizations or unions that employ professional lobbyists to represent them. You have the power to confront prejudice and discrimination by refusing to tolerate ethnic jokes and other expressions of prejudice in health care or educational settings. You can use peer pressure to change culturally insensitive or offensive behavior by others. You can also work with others to ensure that medical and surgical procedures, health-related appointments, and schedules are congruent with the religious and cultural calendars of clients, staff, and students.

Nurse educators can examine admission and recruitment policies, curricula, pedagogy, academic calendars, and teaching strategies from a transcultural nursing perspective. Nurse researchers need to ensure that diversity is represented in the population studied, that appropriate translation and interpretation have been used for non–English-speaking informants or subjects, and that research instruments are appropriate for use with diverse populations. Finally, nurses in key administrative positions can critically assess the organizational climate and culture for its encouragement of diversity, examine the organization's administrative hierarchy for the presence of diversity in leadership positions, evaluate its commitment to culturally sensitive and appropriate personnel policies, and foster an openness to different perspectives on leadership and management. The examples cited are intended to be illustrative, not exhaustive.

A variety of organizations, professional publications, and electronic resources (Andrews, 1995a; Mahon, 1997) support the development of transcultural nursing and health. Table 1-2 provides some basic information on selected resources.

Appendix A provides the names, addresses, phone numbers, and Internet and e-mail addresses for selected professional organizations that are concerned with the cultural aspects of care or with the issues of nurses from particular cultural groups.

SUMMARY

In this introductory chapter, we have examined the historical origins of transcultural nursing as a blending of two fields: anthropology and nursing. Founded by the nurse-anthropologist Dr. Madeleine M. Leininger, transcultural nursing has provided a theoretical foundation to guide nurses in the provision of culturally congruent and competent care for individual clients

TABLE 1–2	SELECTED RESOURCES FOR TRANSCULTURAL NURSING	

PROFESSIONAL RESOURCES	DESCRIPTION	DESCRIPTION AND PURPOSE
Professional Organizations	Council on Nursing and Anthropology Association (CONAA) (1968)	Organization for nurse-anthropologists, transcultural nurses, and anthropologists Purpose: promotes interdisciplinary research exchange
	Transcultural Nursing Society (TNS) (1974)	Organization of transcultural nurses Purpose: to promote transcultural nursing knowledge and competencies globally through education, research, consultation, and clinical services
	Council on Cultural Diversity of the American Nurses' Association (1978)	ANA Council of transcultural nurses Purpose: to focus on diversity issues in clinical practice
	International Association of Human Caring (1987)	Organization of qualitative researchers, some of whom are nurses Purpose: to explore the cultural similarities and differences in expressions of human care
	Committee on Cultural Diversity	Committee established by the American Academy of Nursing Purpose: to develop guidelines for culturally competent nursing
Refereed Printed Materials on Transcultural Nursing and Health	*Journal of Transcultural Nursing*	Only publication focused on transcultural nursing theory, research methods, consultation, teaching, and clinical community practices
	Journal of Multicultural Nursing and Health (MNCNH)	Interdisciplinary; addresses multiculturalism in nursing education and/or health
	Journal of Cultural Diversity	Focuses on cultural diversity theory and principles from a variety of perspectives
	Association of Black Nursing Faculty Journal (ABNF)	Documents the distinct nature and health care needs of the black patient
	International Nursing Review	Both published by the International Council of Nurses
	International Journal of Nursing Studies	

(continued)

TABLE 1-2 *(Continued)*		
PROFESSIONAL RESOURCES	**DESCRIPTION**	**DESCRIPTION AND PURPOSE**
Nonrefereed Print Materials	*Minority Nurse Newsletter*	Examines minority issues affecting patient care and nursing education
	Closing the Gap (newsletter)	Published by the Federal Office of Minority Health; focuses on federal interventions aimed at improving the health of panethnic groups
	IHS Primary Care Provider (newsletter)	Published by the Federal Indian Health Service; free to nursing and medical students and health care providers.
Electronic Resources	www.tcns.org	Official web site for the Transcultural Nursing Society, provides information about membership in the organization, conferences, regional workshops, transcultural nursing certification, and the *Journal of Transcultural Nursing;* useful links to other web sites of relevance to transcultural nursing.

and patients of all ages, families, groups, and communities. Transcultural nursing also enables nurses to examine the cultural dimensions of health and nursing organizations, institutions, and agencies. Leininger's Theory of Culture Care Diversity and Universality and her Sunrise Model were introduced. Finally, selected resources in transcultural nursing and health care were identified.

REVIEW QUESTIONS

1. Conceived in the early 1950s by the nurse-anthropologist Dr. Madeleine M. Leininger, the term *transcultural nursing* was coined in 1970 with her seminal work, *Nursing and Anthropology: Two Worlds to Blend.* Define *transcultural nursing* in your own words.
2. Summarize the historical development of transcultural nursing since its founding by Dr. Madeleine Leininger.
3. Review the limitations of transcultural nursing cited by critics. What can be done to address the criticisms?
4. Identify electronic and print resources in transcultural nursing and health.

CRITICAL THINKING ACTIVITIES

1. Visit the Transcultural Nursing Society's official web site (*www.tcns.org*).
   a. Briefly summarize the information you found at the web site.
   b. Critically evaluate the strengths and limitations of the information source and data available.
   c. What clinical relevance does the electronic information on transcultural nursing have for you as a nurse?
   d. Visit links to other related web sites on transcultural nursing.
2. Using the Cumulative Index to Nursing and Allied Health Literature (CINAHL), enter the words *transcultural nursing* and search for references cited during the past year. How many references are identified? What are the subcategories under which you can narrow your search? If you want information about a specific cultural, ethnic, or minority group, what key words will help you to narrow the search? Consult a reference librarian for assistance if you need help.

• References

Andrews, M. M. (1992). Cultural perspectives on nursing in the 21st century. *Journal of Professional Nursing, 8*(1), 1–9.

Andrews, M. M. (1995a). Guide to searching on-line for information on transcultural nursing and health. *Journal of Transcultural Nursing, 7*(1), 36–40.

Andrews, M. M. (1995b). Transcultural nursing: Transforming the curriculum. *Journal of Transcultural Nursing, 6*(2), 4–9.

Andrews, M. M., & Boyle, J. S. (1997). Competence in transcultural nursing care. *American Journal of Nursing, 97*(8), 16AAA–16DDD.

Branch, M. F., & Paxton, P. P. (Eds.). (1976). *Providing safe nursing care for ethnic people of color*. New York: Appleton-Century-Crofts.

Brink, P.J. (1999). Transcultural versus cross-cultural. *Journal of Transcultural Nursing, 10*(1), 6.

Culley, L. (1996). A critique of multiculturalism in health care: The challenge for nursing education. *Journal of Advanced Nursing, 23*, 564–570.

Dougherty, M. C., & Tripp-Reimer, T. (1985). The interface of nursing and anthropology. *Annual Review of Anthropology, 14*, 219–241.

Flaskerud, J. H. (2000). Ethnicity, culture and neuropsychiatry. *Issues in Mental Health Nursing, 21*(5), 5–29.

Gustafson, D. L. (1999). Toward inclusionary practices in the education of nurses: A critique of transcultural nursing theory. *The Alberta Journal of Educational Research, 45*(4), 468–470.

Habayeb, G. L. (1995). Cultural diversity: A nursing concept not yet reliably defined. *Nursing Outlook, 43*(5), 224–227.

Kavanaugh, K., & Kennedy, P. (1992). *Promoting cultural diversity*. Newbury Park, NJ: Sage.

Leininger, M. (1970). *Nursing and anthropology: Two worlds to blend*. New York: John Wiley & Sons.

Leininger, M. (1978). *Transcultural nursing: Concepts, theories and practices*. New York: John Wiley & Sons.

Leininger, M. (1991). *Culture care diversity and universality: A theory of nursing*. New York: National League for Nursing.

Leininger, M. (1995). *Transcultural nursing: Concepts, theories, research and practices*. New York: McGraw-Hill.

Leininger, M. M. (1997). Future directions in transcultural nursing in the 21st century. *International Nursing Review, 44*(1), 19–23.

Leininger, M. M. (1999). What is transcultural nursing and culturally competent care? *Journal of Transcultural Nursing, 10*(1), 9.

Leininger, M. M., & McFarland, M. R. (2002). *Transcultural nursing: Concepts, theories and practices*. New York: McGraw-Hill.

Lipson, J. G. (1999). Cross-cultural nursing: The cultural perspective. *Journal of Transcultural Nursing, 10*(1), 7.

Lipson, J., & Bauwens, E. (1988). Uses of anthropology in nursing. *Practicing Anthropology, 10*, 4–5.

Mahon, P. Y. (1997). Transcultural nursing: A source guide. *Journal of Nursing Staff Development, 13*(4), 218–222.

Mahoney, J. S., & Engebretson, J. (2000). The interface of anthropology and nursing guiding culturally competent care in psychiatric nursing. *Archives of Psychiatric Nursing, 14*(4), 183–190.

McKenna, M. (1984). Anthropology and nursing: The interaction between two fields of inquiry. *Western Journal of Nursing Research, 6*(4), 423–431.

Mulholland, J. (1995). Nursing humanism and transcultural theory: The "bracketing out" of reality. *Journal of Advanced Nursing, 22,* 442–449.

Orque, M. S., Bloch, B., & Monrroy, L. S. (1983). *Ethnic nursing care.* St. Louis: C. V. Mosby.

Osborne, O. (1969). Anthropology and nursing: Some common traditions and interests. *Nursing Research, 18*(3), 251–255.

Price, K. M., & Cortis, J. D. (2000). The way forward for transcultural nursing. *Nurse Education Today, 20*(3), 233–243.

Reynolds, C. L., & Leininger, M. (1993). *Madeleine Leininger: Cultural care diversity and universality theory.* Newbury Park: Sage.

Talabere, L. R. (1996). Meeting the challenge of culture care in nursing: Diversity, sensitivity, and congruence. *Journal of Cultural Diversity, 3*(2), 53–61.

CHAPTER 2

Culturally Competent Nursing Care

Margaret M. Andrews

KEY TERMS

Collateral relationships
Cross-cultural communication
Cultural code
Cultural competence
Cultural congruent care
Cultural self-assessment

Distance
Environmental context
Eye contact
Lineal relationships
Linguistic competence
Nonverbal communication

Proxemics
Sick role behavior
Silence
Space
Touch

OBJECTIVES

1. Analyze the complex integration of knowledge, attitudes, and skills needed for cultural competence.
2. Explore cross-cultural communication as the foundation for the provision of culturally competent nursing care.
3. Identify strategies for promoting effective cross-cultural communication in multicultural health care settings.

In the examination of **cultural competence**, several perspectives are worth considering because the concept refers to a complex integration of knowledge, attitudes, and skills that enhance cross-cultural communication and appropriate/effective interactions with others (American Academy of Nursing, 1992, 1993). Cultural competence has been defined as a process, as opposed to an end point, in which the nurse continuously strives to work effectively within the cultural context of an individual, family, or community from a diverse cultural background (Andrews & Boyle, 1997; Campinha-Bacote, 1995, 1999, 2000; Campinha-Bacote & Munoz, 2001; Meleis, 1999; Smith, 1998; Wells, 2000). Summarized in Evidenced-Based Practice Box 2-1 are findings from a study of Mexican Americans' perceptions of culturally competent care.

In addition to cultural competence, some experts have noted the considerable impact that **linguistic competence** by health care providers has on

EVIDENCE-BASED PRACTICE 2–1
Mexican Americans' Perceptions of Culturally Competent Care

The purpose of this study was to identify culturally competent concepts from the perspective of Mexican Americans. Cultural competence was defined as a set of academic and interpersonal skills that allow individuals to increase their understanding and appreciation of cultural differences and similarities within, among, and between groups. Focus group interviews with 22 Mexican-American nurses and Mexican-American lay recipients of health care were used to explore the participants' subjective perceptions regarding indicators of culturally competent care. For the Mexican-American registered nurses, the influence of culture predominated despite nursing professional experience and knowledge of Western biomedicine. The predominance of themes emphasizing respect, caring, understanding, and patience in health care encounters support the critical importance of personal processes of health care with Mexican Americans.

Clinical Applications

The most significant contributions of this study to nursing are a comparison of Mexican-American registered nurses' and Mexican-American health care recipients' perceptions of culturally competent care and the identification of the critical importance of culturally based patterns of social behavior to Mexican Americans' perceptions of culturally competent care. First, this study contributes to knowledge development by documenting the impact of nurses' culture, education, income, and level of acculturation on their perceptions of culturally competent care. Second, communication is frequently identified as the first challenge when human interactions involve diversity. When nurses are bilingual, there is a perception of cultural competence. Themes relating to the concepts of family obligation and spirituality are representative of the pervasive nature of these cultural values among nurses and lay recipients of health care. Mexican Americans expect *personalisms* and *respeto* (respect) from health care providers. For example, patients expect a handshake in greeting, and not offering this is considered rude.

The nurses' familiarity with cultural aspects of health care and accommodation of sociodemographic factors in health care planning and delivery were cited as pertinent to the respondents' access and acceptance of health care. Data indicate that an incongruent health care experience is characterized by system barriers, discounting (failure to acknowledge the client's perception), and blaming.

Reprinted with permission from Warda, M. R. (2000). Mexican Americans' perceptions of culturally competent care. *Western Journal of Nursing Research, 22*(2), 203-224.

clients' access and response to health care services. *Cultural and linguistic competence* refers to an ability by health care providers and health care organizations to understand and effectively respond to the cultural and linguistic needs brought by clients to the health care encounter. Summarized in Box 2-1 are the recommended standards for culturally and linguistically appropriate health care services proposed by the Office of Minority Health (1999).

Instead of using the term *cultural competence*, Leininger (1991, 1995, 1999; Leininger & McFarland, 2002) prefers **culturally congruent care**, which she

BOX 2–1	**OFFICE OF MINORITY HEALTH STANDARDS FOR CULTURALLY AND LINGUISTICALLY APPROPRIATE HEALTH CARE BY HEALTH CARE ORGANIZATIONS**

- Promote and support attitudes, behaviors, knowledge, and skills necessary for staff to work respectfully and effectively with patients and each other in a culturally diverse work environment
- Have a comprehensive management strategy, including strategic goals, plans, policies, procedures, and designated staff responsible for implementation
- Utilize formal mechanisms of community and consumer involvement in the development and execution of service delivery
- Develop and implement a strategy to recruit, retain, and promote qualified diverse and culturally competent administrative, clinical, and support staff who are trained to address the needs of racial and ethnic communities
- Require and arrange for ongoing education and training for administrative, clinical, and support staff in culturally and linguistically competent delivery of service
- Provide all clients having limited English proficiency with access to bilingual interpretation services
- Provide oral and written notices, including translated signage at key points of entry, to clients in their primary language, informing them of their right to receive interpreter services
- Translate and make available signage and commonly used written patient educational materials in the predominant language(s) in the service area
- Ensure that interpreters and bilingual staff can demonstrate bilingual proficiency and receive training that includes the skills and ethics of interpreting
- Ensure that the clients' primary spoken language and self-identified race/ethnicity are included in the health care organization's information system
- Use a variety of methods to collect and utilize accurate demographic, cultural, epidemiological, and clinical outcome data for racial and ethnic groups and become informed about the ethnic/cultural needs, resources, and assets of the surrounding community
- Undertake ongoing organizational self-assessments of cultural and linguistic competence and measure for access, satisfaction, quality, and outcome using internal audits and performance improvement programs
- Develop structures and procedures to address cross-cultural ethical and legal issues in health care delivery and complaints or grievances by patients and staff about unfair, culturally insensitive, or discriminatory treatment, or difficulty in accessing services, or denial of services
- Prepare an annual progress report documenting progress in implementing these standards, including information on programs, staffing, and resources

Source: Office of Minority Health (1999). Assuring cultural competence in health care: Recommendations for national standards and an outcomes-focused research agenda. Department of Health and Human Services, U.S. Public Health Service. Washington, D.C. *www.omhre.gov/clas/ds.htm*

defines as the provision of care that is meaningful and fits with cultural beliefs and lifeways. Leininger's definition of culturally congruent care is holistic and focuses on the complex interrelationship of lifeways, religion, kinship, politics, law, education, technology, language, environmental context, and worldview—all factors that contribute to culturally congruent care.

Because you may encounter clients from literally hundreds of different cultures in your professional career and clients of mixed cultural heritage, it is virtually impossible to know about the culturally based, health-related beliefs and practices of them all. It is, however, possible to master the knowledge and skills associated with cultural assessment and learn about *some* of the cultural dimensions of care for clients representing the groups most frequently encountered. In-depth knowledge of several cultures is often a reasonable goal if you live in a large urban center characterized by a high degree of diversity.

• CULTURAL SELF-ASSESSMENT

Before you can provide culturally competent care for people from diverse backgrounds, it's important to engage in a **cultural self-assessment**. When interacting with clients from various cultural backgrounds, you must be aware of your own cultural values, attitudes, beliefs, and practices. To gain insight into the way that you relate to various groups of people in society, describe your level of response to the groups identified in Box 2-2.

Through self-assessment, it is possible to gain insights into the health-related values, attitudes, beliefs, and practices that have been transmitted to you by your own family. These insights also enable you to overcome ethnocentric tendencies and cultural stereotypes, which are vehicles for perpetuating prejudice and discrimination against members of certain groups.

After you have engaged in a cultural self-assessment, it is possible to conduct a cultural assessment of others.

• CULTURAL ASSESSMENT

The author believes that cultural assessment is the foundation for culturally competent and culturally congruent nursing care. Appendix A contains the Andrews/Boyle Transcultural Assessment Guide, an instrument that is intended to help you to ask key questions during your assessment interview. Please refer to Chapter 3, Cultural Competence in the Health History and Physical Examination, for a complete discussion of cultural assessment.

• SKILLS NEEDED FOR CULTURAL COMPETENCE

Cultural competence implies that you have developed certain psychomotor or behavioral skills. Box 2-3 contains selected examples of these skills, and others will be presented throughout the text. It should be noted that the

BOX 2–2	**HOW DO YOU RELATE TO VARIOUS GROUPS OF PEOPLE IN THE SOCIETY?**

Described below are different levels of response you might have toward a person.

Levels of Response

1. *Greet:* I feel I can *greet* this person warmly and welcome him or her sincerely.

2. *Accept:* I feel I can honestly *accept* this person as he or she is and be comfortable enough to listen to his or her problems.

3. *Help:* I feel I would genuinely try to *help* this person with his or her problems as they might relate to or arise from the label-stereotype given to him or her.

4. *Background:* I feel I have the *background* of knowledge and/or experience to be able to help this person.

5. *Advocate:* I feel I could honestly be an *advocate* for this person.

The following is a list of individuals. Read down the list and place a checkmark next to anyone you would *not* "greet" or would hesitate to "greet." Then move to response level 2, "accept," and follow the same procedure. Try to respond honestly, not as you think might be socially or professionally desirable. Your answers are only for your personal use in clarifying your initial reactions to different people.

			Level of Response		
	1	2	3	4	5
Individual	Greet	Accept	Help	Background	Advocate
Ethnic/racial					
1. Haitian American	☐	☐	☐	☐	☐
6. Mexican American	☐	☐	☐	☐	☐
11. Native American	☐	☐	☐	☐	☐
16. Vietnamese American	☐	☐	☐	☐	☐
21. Black American	☐	☐	☐	☐	☐
26. White Anglo-Saxon	☐	☐	☐	☐	☐
Social issues/problems					
2. Child abuser	☐	☐	☐	☐	☐
7. IV drug user	☐	☐	☐	☐	☐
12. Prostitute	☐	☐	☐	☐	☐
17. Gay/lesbian	☐	☐	☐	☐	☐
22. Unmarried expectant teenager	☐	☐	☐	☐	☐
27. Alcoholic	☐	☐	☐	☐	☐
Religious					
3. Jew	☐	☐	☐	☐	☐
8. Catholic	☐	☐	☐	☐	☐
13. Jehovah's Witness	☐	☐	☐	☐	☐
18. Atheist	☐	☐	☐	☐	☐
23. Protestant	☐	☐	☐	☐	☐
28. Amish person	☐	☐	☐	☐	☐

(continued)

BOX 2–2	HOW DO YOU RELATE TO VARIOUS GROUPS OF PEOPLE IN THE SOCIETY? (Continued)

Level of Response

	1 Greet	2 Accept	3 Help	4 Background	5 Advocate
Physically/mentally handicapped					
4. Person with hemophilia	☐	☐	☐	☐	☐
9. Senile elderly person	☐	☐	☐	☐	☐
14. Cerebral palsied person	☐	☐	☐	☐	☐
19. Person with AIDS	☐	☐	☐	☐	☐
24. Amputee	☐	☐	☐	☐	☐
29. Person with cancer	☐	☐	☐	☐	☐
Political					
5. Neo-Nazi	☐	☐	☐	☐	☐
10. Teamster Union member	☐	☐	☐	☐	☐
15. ERA proponent	☐	☐	☐	☐	☐
20. Communist	☐	☐	☐	☐	☐
25. Ku Klux Klansman	☐	☐	☐	☐	☐
30. Nuclear armament proponent	☐	☐	☐	☐	☐

Level of Response

Individual	1 Greet	2 Accept	3 Help	4 Background	5 Advocate
1. Haitian	☐	☐	☐	☐	☐
2. Child abuser	☐	☐	☐	☐	☐
3. Jew	☐	☐	☐	☐	☐
4. Person with hemophilia	☐	☐	☐	☐	☐
5. Neo-Nazi	☐	☐	☐	☐	☐
6. Mexican American	☐	☐	☐	☐	☐
7. IV drug user	☐	☐	☐	☐	☐
8. Catholic	☐	☐	☐	☐	☐
9. Senile, elderly person	☐	☐	☐	☐	☐
10. Teamster Union member	☐	☐	☐	☐	☐
11. Native American	☐	☐	☐	☐	☐
12. Prostitute	☐	☐	☐	☐	☐
13. Jehovah's Witness	☐	☐	☐	☐	☐
14. Cerebral palsied person	☐	☐	☐	☐	☐
15. ERA proponent	☐	☐	☐	☐	☐
16. Vietnamese American	☐	☐	☐	☐	☐
17. Gay/lesbian	☐	☐	☐	☐	☐
18. Atheist	☐	☐	☐	☐	☐
19. Person with AIDS	☐	☐	☐	☐	☐

(continued)

BOX 2–2	**HOW DO YOU RELATE TO VARIOUS GROUPS OF PEOPLE IN THE SOCIETY? (Continued)**

Level of Response

	1 Greet	2 Accept	3 Help	4 Background	5 Advocate
20. Communist	☐	☐	☐	☐	☐
21. Black American	☐	☐	☐	☐	☐
22. Unmarried expectant teenager	☐	☐	☐	☐	☐
23. Protestant	☐	☐	☐	☐	☐
24. Amputee	☐	☐	☐	☐	☐
25. Ku Klux Klansman	☐	☐	☐	☐	☐
26. White Anglo-Saxon	☐	☐	☐	☐	☐
27. Alcoholic	☐	☐	☐	☐	☐
28. Amish person	☐	☐	☐	☐	☐
29. Person with cancer	☐	☐	☐	☐	☐
30. Nuclear armament proponent	☐	☐	☐	☐	☐

Scoring Guide: The previous activity may help you anticipate difficulty in working with some clients at various levels. The 30 types of individuals can be grouped into 5 categories: ethnic/racial, social issues/problems, religious, physically/mentally handicapped, and political. Transfer your checkmarks to the following form. If you have a concentration of checks within a specific category of individuals or at specific levels, this may indicate a conflict that could hinder you from rendering effective professional help.

Reproduced with permission of the Association for the Care of Children's Health, 7910 Woodmont Avenue, Suite 300, Bethesda, MD 20814, from E. Randall-David (1989). *Strategies for Working with Culturally Diverse Communities and Clients*, pp. 7–9.

mastery of some skills, such as the assessment of cyanosis in people with darkly pigmented skin, may be critical for a patient's survival. Other skills may be helpful in promoting hygiene or comfort, but they do not have such dire consequences. Because communication is a skill foundational to all nursing interactions, the remainder of this chapter will focus on this important topic.

• CROSS-CULTURAL COMMUNICATION

Communication is an organized, patterned system of behavior that regulates and makes possible all nurse-client interactions. It is the exchange of messages and the creation of meaning. Because communication and culture are acquired simultaneously, they are integrally linked. In effective communication there is mutual understanding of the meaning attached to the messages.

BOX 2–3	**SELECTED EXAMPLES OF PSYCHOMOTOR SKILLS USEFUL IN TRANSCULTURAL NURSING**

Assessment

- Techniques for assessing biocultural variations in health and illness, e.g., assessing cyanosis, jaundice, anemia, and related clinical manifestations of disease in darkly pigmented clients; differentiating between mongolian spots and ecchymoses (bruises)
- Measurement of head circumference and fontanelles in infants using techniques not in violation of taboos for selected cultural groups
- Growth and development monitoring for children of Asian heritage, using culturally appropriate growth grids
- Cultural modification of the Denver II and other developmental tests used for children
- Conducting culturally appropriate obstetric and gynecologic examinations of women from various cultural backgrounds

Communication

- Speaking and writing the language(s) used by clients
- Using alternative methods of communicating with non–English-speaking clients and families when no interpreter is available (e.g., pantomime)

Hygiene

- Skin care for clients of various racial/ethnic backgrounds
- Hair care for clients of various ethnic/racial backgrounds, e.g., care of African-American clients' hair

Activities of Daily Living

- Assisting Chinese-American clients to regain use of chopsticks as part of rehabilitation regimen after a stroke
- Assisting paralyzed Amish client with dressing when buttons and pins are used
- Assisting West African client who uses "chewing stick" with oral hygiene

Religion

- Emergency baptism and anointing of the sick for Catholics
- Care before and after ritual circumcision by *mohel* (performed 8 days after the birth of a male Jewish infant)

Barriers to communication include differences in language, worldview, and values. It is estimated that up to 90% of all difficulties in nurse-client interactions have resulted from miscommunication.

To begin the discussion on **cross-cultural communication**, it is necessary to examine the ways in which people from various cultural backgrounds communicate with one another. In addition to oral and written communication, messages are conveyed nonverbally through gestures, body movements, posture, tone of voice, and facial expressions (Figure 2-1). Frequently

Figure 2–1. Effective cross-cultural communiction is vital to the establishment of a strong nurse-patient relationship. It is important to understand both verbal and non verbal cues when communicating with people from various cultural backgrounds. (© Copyright B. Proud)

overlooked is the context in which communication occurs. The **environmental context** imparts its own message and is influenced by the setting, the purposes of the communication, and the perceptions of the nurse and client concerning time, space, distance, touch, modesty, and other factors. For example, let us imagine you know that a Mexican-American patient is extremely anxious about having a mammogram. After the procedure, you intend to send an empathetic, caring message by remarking, "It's all over, *Señora* Garcia." *Señora* Garcia bursts into tears because she believes she has been diagnosed with terminal breast cancer. Needless to say, even communication between individuals having the same cultural background may be fraught with pitfalls. When you communicate with others from cultural backgrounds unlike your own and with those for whom English is a second language, the probability of miscommunication increases significantly. In promoting effective cross-cultural communication, you should avoid technical jargon, slang, colloquial expressions, abbreviations, and excessive use of medical terminology.

Lipson and Steiger (1996) suggest affective, cognitive, and behavioral strategies for effective cross-cultural communication. In the affective domain, they suggest respect for, appreciation of, and comfort with cultural differences; enjoyment of learning through cultural exchange; ability to observe behavior without judging; awareness of one's own cultural values and biases; and belief in cultural relativity: that there are many acceptable cultural ways. In the cognitive domain, they emphasize knowledge about different cultures, ability to recognize when there is a cultural explanation for an interpersonal problem, understanding that meanings can differ for others, and understanding the sociopolitical system with respect to its treatment of minorities. In the behavioral domain (communication skills), they advocate flexibility in verbal and nonverbal communication style, ability to speak slowly and clearly without excessive slang, ability to encourage others to express themselves, ability to communicate sincere interest and empathy, patience, and ability to observe and intervene when there is misunderstanding.

Important factors to consider for cross-cultural communication include communication with family members and significant others; space, distance, and intimacy; nonverbal communication; language; and sick role behaviors (Figure 2–2).

Figure 2–2. Conceptual model for understanding cultural influences on nurse-patient interactions.

Communication with Family Members and Significant Others

Knowledge of a client's family and kinship structure helps you to ascertain the values, decision-making patterns, and overall communication within the household. It is necessary to identify the significant others whom clients perceive to be important in their care and who may be responsible for decision making that affects their health care. For example, for many clients, *familism*—which emphasizes interdependence over independence, affiliation over confrontation, and cooperation over competition—may dictate that important decisions affecting the client be made by the family, not the individual alone. When you work with clients from cultural groups that value cohesion, interdependence, and collectivism, you may perceive the family as being overly involved and usurping the autonomy of the client. Clients are likely to perceive the involvement with family as a source of mutual support, security, and fulfillment.

The family is the basic social unit in which children are raised and learn culturally based values, beliefs, and practices about health and illnesses. The essence of *family* consists of living together as a unit. Relationships that may seem obvious sometimes warrant further exploration when the nurse interacts with clients from culturally diverse backgrounds. For example, most European Americans define siblings as two persons with either the same mother, the same father, the same mother and father, or the same adoptive parents. In some Asian cultures, a sibling relationship is defined as any infants breast-fed by the same woman. In other cultures, certain kinship patterns, such as maternal first cousins, are defined as sibling relationships. In some African cultures, anyone from the same village may be called brother or sister.

Members of some ethnoreligious groups (e.g., Roman Catholics of Italian, Polish, Spanish, or Mexican descent) recognize relationships such as *godmother* or *godfather* in which an individual who is not the biologic parent promises to assist with the moral or spiritual development of an infant and agrees to care for the child in the event of parental death. The godparent makes these promises during the religious ceremony of baptism.

In communicating with the parent or parent surrogate of infants and children, it is important to identify the primary provider of care and the key decision maker who acts on behalf of the child. In some instances, this person may not be the biologic parent. Among some Hispanic groups, for example, female members of the nuclear or extended family such as sisters and aunts are primary providers of care for infants and children. In some African-American families, the grandmother may be the decision maker and primary caretaker of children. To provide culturally congruent care, you must be certain that you are effectively communicating with the appropriate decision maker(s).

When making health-related decisions, some members of culturally diverse backgrounds in which **lineal relationships** predominate may seek assistance from other members of the family. It is sometimes culturally expected that a relative (e.g., parent, grandparent, eldest son, or eldest brother) will make decisions about important health-related matters. For example, in many Asian cultures, it is the obligation and duty of the eldest son to assume primary responsibility for his aging parents and to make health care decisions for them. If **collateral relationships** are valued, decisions about the client may be interrelated with the impact of illness on the entire family or group. For example, among the Amish, the entire community is affected by the illness of a member because the community pays for health care from a common fund, members join together to meet the needs of both the sick person and his or her family throughout the illness, and the roles of dozens of people in the community are likely to be affected by the illness of a single member. The *individual values orientation* concerning relationships is predominant among the dominant cultural majority in North America. Although members of the nuclear family may participate to varying degrees, decision making about health and illness is often an individual matter.

Cultural Perspectives on Intimacy

Interactions between you and your client are influenced by the degree of intimacy desired, which may range from very formal interactions to close personal relationships. For example, some clients of Asian origin expect you and other health care providers to be authoritarian, directive, and detached. In seeking health care, some clients of Chinese descent may expect you to know intuitively what is wrong with them, and you may actually lose some credibility by asking a fairly standard interview question such as "What brings you here?" The Asian-American patient may be thinking, "Don't you know why I'm here? You're supposed to be the one with all the answers." The reserved interpersonal behavior characteristics of many Asian Americans may leave you with the impression that the client agrees with or understands your explanation. Nodding or smiling by Asians may simply reflect their cultural value for interpersonal harmony, not agreement with what you have said. The emphasis on social harmony among Asian-North American clients may prevent the full expression of concerns or feelings.

In Thai culture, a high value is placed on *kreengcaj*, or awareness and anticipation of the feelings of others by kindness and the avoidance of interpersonal conflict. By obtaining validation of assumptions, you may distinguish between genuine concurrent and socially compliant client responses aimed at maintaining harmony. This may be accomplished by inviting the client to respond frankly to suggestions or by giving the client "permission" to disagree.

By contrast, Appalachian clients often have close family interaction patterns that lead them to expect close personal relationships with health care providers. The Appalachian client may evaluate your effectiveness on the basis of interpersonal skills rather than professional competencies. Some Appalachian clients may be uncomfortable with the impersonal orientation of most health care institutions.

Among some Hispanic groups, such as Mexican Americans and Cuban Americans, *simpatia* and *personalismo* should be considered. *Simpatia* refers to the need for smooth or harmonious interpersonal relationships, characterized by courtesy, respect, and the absence of critical or confrontational behavior. The concept of *personalismo* emphasizes intimate personal relationships. Persons of Latin American or Mediterranean origins often expect a high degree of intimacy and may attempt to involve you in their family system by expecting you to participate in personal activities and social functions. These individuals may come to expect personal favors that extend beyond the scope of what you believe to be professional practice, and they may feel it is their privilege to contact you at home during any time of the day or night for care. If your cultural value system emphasizes a high level of personal privacy, you may choose to give clients the agency's phone number and address rather than disclose information about your personal residence.

Because initial impressions are so important in all human relationships, cross-cultural considerations concerning introductions warrant a few brief remarks. To ensure that a mutually respectful relationship is established, you should introduce yourself and indicate to the client how you prefer to be called: by first name, last name, and/or title. You should elicit the same information from the client because this enables you to address the person in a manner that is culturally appropriate.

Nonverbal Communication

Because **nonverbal communication** patterns vary widely across cultures, nurses must be alert for cues that convey cultural differences in the use of silence, eye contact, touch, space, distance, and facial expressions. Cultural influences on appropriate communication between individuals of different genders also need to be considered.

Silence

Wide cultural variation exists in the interpretation of **silence**. Some individuals find silence extremely uncomfortable and make every effort to fill conversational lags with words. By contrast, many Native North Americans consider silence essential to understanding and respecting the other person. A pause following your question signifies that what has been asked is important enough to be given thoughtful consideration. In traditional Chinese and Japanese cultures, silence may mean that the speaker wishes the listener to consider the content of what has been said before continuing. Other cultural meanings of silence may be found. English persons and Arabs may use silence out of respect for another's privacy, whereas French, Spanish, and Russian persons may interpret it as a sign of agreement. Asian cultures often use silence to demonstrate respect for elders. Among some African Americans, silence is used in response to what is perceived as an inappropriate question.

Eye Contact

The use of **eye contact** is among the most culturally variable nonverbal behaviors that clients use to communicate with you. Although most nurses have been taught to maintain eye contact when speaking with clients, individuals from culturally diverse backgrounds may attribute other culturally based meanings to this behavior. Asian, Native North American, Indochinese, Arab, and Appalachian clients may consider direct eye contact impolite or aggressive, and they may avert their own eyes when talking with you. Native North Americans often stare at the floor during conversations—a culturally appropriate behavior indicating that the listener is paying close attention to the speaker. Some African Americans use *oculistics* (eye rolling) in response to what is perceived to be an inappropriate question. Among Hispanic clients, respect dictates appropriate deferential behavior in the form of downcast eyes toward others on the basis of age, sex, social position, economic status, and position of authority. Elders expect respect from younger individuals, adults from children, men from women, teachers from students, and employers from employees. In the nurse-client relationship with Hispanic clients, eye contact is expected of you but will not necessarily be reciprocated by the client.

In some cultures, including Arab, Latino, and African-American groups, *modesty for both women and men* is interrelated with eye contact. Muslim-Arab women achieve modesty, in part, by avoiding eye contact with males (except for one's husband) and keeping the eyes downcast when encountering members of the opposite sex in public situations. In many cultures, the only woman who smiles and establishes eye contact with men in public is a prostitute. Hasidic Jewish males also have culturally based norms concerning eye contact with females: you may observe a man avoiding direct eye contact and turning his head in the opposite direction when walking past or speaking to a woman. The preceding examples are intended to be illustrative, not exhaustive.

Touch

You are urged to give careful consideration to issues concerning **touch**. While we recognize the often-reported benefits in establishing rapport with clients through touch, including the promotion of healing through therapeutic touch, physical contact with clients conveys various meanings cross-culturally. In many Arab and Hispanic cultures, male health care providers may be prohibited from touching or examining part or all of the female body. Adolescent girls may prefer female health care providers or may refuse to be examined by a male. You should be aware that the client's significant others also may exert pressure by enforcing these culturally meaningful norms in the health care setting.

In some cultures, there are strict norms related to touching children. Many Asians believe that touching the head is a sign of disrespect because it is thought to be the source of a person's strength. You need to be aware that patting a child on the head or examining the fontanelles of a Southeast Asian infant should be avoided or done only with parental permission. Whenever possible, you should explore alternative ways to express affection or to obtain information necessary for assessment of the client's condition. For example, you might ask the mother to hold the child on her lap while you observe for other manifestations of increased intracranial pressure or signs of premature fontanelle closure. You might also try placing your hand over the mother's while asking for a description of what she feels.

Space and Distance

The concepts of **space** and **distance** are significant in cross-cultural communication. The perception of appropriate distance zones varies widely among cultural groups. Although there are individual variations in spatial requirements, people of the same culture tend to act in similar ways. For example, if you are of European North American heritage, you may find yourself backing away from clients of Hispanic, East Indian, or Middle Eastern origins who seem to invade your personal space with annoying regularity. Such behavior by these clients is probably an attempt to bring you closer into the space that is comfortable to them. Although you may be uncomfortable with close physical proximity to these clients, they are perplexed by *your* distancing behavior and may perceive you as aloof and unfriendly.

Because individuals are usually not consciously aware of their personal space requirements, they frequently have difficulty understanding a different cultural pattern. For example, sitting in close proximity to another person may be perceived by one client as an expression of warmth and friendliness but by another as a threatening invasion of personal space. According to Watson (1980), Americans, Canadians, and British require the most personal space, whereas Latin Americans, Japanese, and Arabs need the least.

In the early 1960s, Edward T. Hall pioneered the study of **proxemics**, which focuses on how people in various cultures relate to their physical space. Although there are intercultural variations, the intimate distance in interpersonal interactions ranges from 0 to 18 inches. At this distance, people experience visual detail and each other's odor, heat, and touch. Personal distance varies from 1.5 to 4 feet, the usual space within which communication between friends and acquaintances occurs. Nurses frequently interact with clients in the intimate or personal distance zones. Social distance refers to 4 to 12 feet, whereas anything greater than 12 is considered public distance (Hall, 1963).

Sex and Gender

Nonverbal behaviors are culturally very significant, and failure to adhere to the **cultural code** (set of rules or norms of behavior used by a cultural group to guide behavior and to interpret situations) is viewed as a serious transgression. Violating norms related to appropriate male-female relationships among various cultures may jeopardize your therapeutic relationship with clients and their families. Among Arab Americans, you may find that adult males avoid being alone with members of the opposite sex (except for their wives) and are generally accompanied by one or more male companions when interacting with females. The presence of the companion(s) conveys that the purpose of the interaction is honorable and that no sexual impropriety will occur. Some women of Middle Eastern origin do not shake hands with men, nor do men and women touch each other outside the marital relationship. Given that clients who have recently immigrated are in various stages of assimilation, traditional customs such as these may or may not be practiced. If in doubt, you should ask the client or observe the client's behaviors, preferably at the time of admission.

A brief comment about same-sex relationships is warranted. In some cultures, it is considered an acceptable expression of friendship and affection to openly and publicly hold hands with or embrace members of the same sex without any sexual connotation being associated with the behavior. For example, you may note that although a Nigerian-American woman may not demonstrate overt affection for her husband or other male family members, she will hold hands with female relatives and friends while walking or talking with them. You may find that clients display similar behaviors toward you, and you should feel free to discuss cultural differences and similarities openly with the client. The discussion should include how each person feels about the cultural practice and exploration of mutually acceptable—and unacceptable—avenues for communicating.

Language

In the United States, nearly 45 million people aged 5 five years or older speak a language other than English at home (U.S. Census Bureau, 2000). Summarized in Table 2-1 are the numbers of Americans who speak other languages and who report that they have difficulty speaking English well. One of the greatest challenges in cross-cultural communication occurs when you and your client speak different languages. After assessing the language skills of non–English-speaking clients, you may find yourself in one of two situations: either struggling to communicate effectively through an interpreter or communicating effectively when there is no interpreter.

Interviewing the non–English-speaking person requires a bilingual interpreter for full communication. Even a person from another culture or country who has a basic command of English (someone for whom English is a second language) may need an interpreter when faced with the anxiety-provoking situation of entering a hospital, encountering a strange symptom, or discussing a sensitive topic such as birth control or gynecologic or urologic concerns. Ideally, a trained medical interpreter should be used. This person knows interpreting techniques, has a health care background, and understands patients' rights. The trained interpreter is also knowledgeable about cultural beliefs and health practices. This person can help you to bridge the cultural gap and can give advice concerning the cultural appropriateness of your recommendations.

TABLE 2–1	CENSUS 2000 SUMMARY OF LANGUAGES SPOKEN AT HOME	
LANGUAGE SPOKEN AT HOME		**Estimate**
POPULATION 5 YEARS OLD AND OVER		254,746,174
English only		209,860,377
Language other than English		44,885,797
Speak English less than "very well"		19,492,832
Spanish		26,745,067
Speak English less than "very well"		12,463,516
Other Indo-European languages		9,479,670
Speak English less than "very well"		3,103,665
Asian and Pacific Islander languages		6,864,461
Speak English less than "very well"		3,395,653
Other languages		1,796,599
Speak English less than "very well"		529,998

Adapted from: United States Census Bureau (2000). Census 2000 Supplementary Survey. *www.factfinder.census.gov*

Although you will be in charge of the focus and flow of the interview, the interpreter should be viewed as an important member of the health care team. It is tempting to ask a relative, a friend, or even another client to interpret because this person is readily available and likely is anxious to help. However, this violates confidentiality for the client, who may not want personal information shared. Furthermore, the friend or relative, though fluent in ordinary language usage, is likely to be unfamiliar with medical terminology, hospital or clinic procedures, and health care ethics.

Whenever possible, work with a bilingual member of the health care team. In ideal circumstances, you should ask the interpreter to meet the client beforehand to establish rapport and to obtain basic descriptive information about the client such as age, occupation, educational level, and attitude toward health care. This eases the interpreter into the relationship and allows the client to talk about aspects of his or her life that are relatively nonthreatening.

When using an interpreter, you should expect that the interaction with the client will require more time than is needed in the care of English-speaking clients. It will be necessary to organize nursing care so that the most important interactions or procedures are accomplished first before any of the parties (including yourself) becomes fatigued.

Both you and the client should speak only a sentence or two and then allow the interpreter time to translate. You should use simple language, not medical jargon that the interpreter must simplify before it can be translated. Summary translation—allowing a person to speak in his or her native language, then having an interpreter summarize what was said—goes faster and is useful for teaching relatively simple health techniques with which the interpreter is already familiar. Be alert for nonverbal cues as the client talks; they can give valuable data. A skilled interpreter also will note nonverbal messages and pass them on to you.

Summarized in Box 2-4 are suggestions for the selection and use of an interpreter and for overcoming language barriers when an interpreter is unavailable. Although the use of an interpreter is the ideal, you will need a strategy for promoting effective communication when none is present.

Sick Role Behaviors

If you find yourself feeling uncomfortable because a client is asking too many questions, assuming a defensive posture, or otherwise showing discomfort, it might be appropriate to pause for a moment to examine the source of the conflict from a transcultural perspective. During illness, culturally acceptable **sick role behavior** may range from aggressive, demanding behavior to silent passivity. Researchers have found that complaining, demanding behavior during illness is often rewarded with attention among Jewish and Italian groups. Because Asian and Native North American patients are likely to be quiet and compliant during illness, they may not receive the attention they need. Children are socialized into culturally acceptable sick role behaviors at an early age.

| BOX 2–4 | **OVERCOMING LANGUAGE BARRIERS** |

Use of an Interpreter

- Before locating an interpreter, be sure that the language the client speaks at home is known, since it may be different from the language spoken publicly (e.g., French is sometimes spoken by well-educated and upper-class members of certain Asian or Middle Eastern cultures).
- Avoid interpreters from a rival tribe, state, region, or nation (e.g., a Palestinian who knows Hebrew may not be the best interpreter for a Jewish client).
- Be aware of gender differences between interpreter and client. In general, same gender is preferred.
- Be aware of age differences between interpreter and client. In general, an older, more mature interpreter is preferred to a younger, less experienced one.
- Be aware of socioeconomic differences between interpreter and client.
- Ask the interpreter to translate as closely to verbatim as possible.
- An interpreter who is not a relative may seek compensation for services rendered.

Recommendations for Institutions

- Maintain a computerized list of interpreters who may be contacted as needed.
- Network with area hospitals, colleges, universities, and other organizations that may serve as resources.
- Utilize the translation services provided by telephone companies (e.g., American Telephone and Telegraph Company).

What to Do When There Is No Interpreter

- Be polite and formal.
- Greet the person using the last or complete name. Gesture to yourself and say your name. Offer a handshake or nod. Smile.
- Proceed in an unhurried manner. Pay attention to any effort by the patient or family to communicate.

(continued)

Clients of Asian heritage may provide you with the answers that they think are expected. This behavior is consistent with the dominant cultural value for harmonious relationships with others. Thus, you should attempt to phrase questions or statements in a neutral manner that avoids foreshadowing an expected response.

SUMMARY

In this chapter we have explored culturally competent and culturally congruent nursing care as well as the importance of linguistic competence. We have discussed cultural self-assessment and encouraged you to gain insights into your own attitudes and beliefs about different ethnic, religious, and social groups.

Most of the chapter focused on the complex, multifaceted topic of cross-cultural communication, including aspects of verbal and nonverbal communi-

BOX 2–4	OVERCOMING LANGUAGE BARRIERS (Continued)

- Speak in a low, moderate voice. Avoid talking loudly. Remember that there is a tendency to raise the volume and pitch of your voice when the listener appears not to understand. The listener may perceive that the nurse is shouting and/or angry.
- Use any words known in the patient's language. This indicates that the nurse is aware of and respects the client's culture.
- Use simple words, such as *pain* instead of *discomfort.* Avoid medical jargon, idioms, and slang. Avoid using contractions. Use nouns repeatedly instead of pronouns. Example: Do *not* say, "He has been taking his medicine, hasn't he?" Do say, "Does Juan take medicine?"
- Pantomime words and simple actions while verbalizing them.
- Give instructions in the proper sequence. Example: Do *not* say, "Before you rinse the bottle, sterilize it." Do say, "First, wash the bottle. Second, rinse the bottle."
- Discuss one topic at a time. Avoid using conjunctions. Example: Do *not* say, "Are you cold and in pain?" Do say, "Are you cold [while pantomiming]?" Are you in pain?"
- Validate whether the client understands by having him or her repeat instructions, demonstrate the procedure, or act out the meaning.
- Write out several short sentences in English, and determine the person's ability to read them.
- Try a third language. Many Indo-Chinese speak French. Europeans often know three or four languages. Try Latin words or phrases, if the nurse is familiar with that language.
- Ask who among the client's family and friends could serve as an interpreter.
- Obtain phrase books from a library or bookstore, make or purchase flash cards, contact hospitals for a list of interpreters, and use both formal and informal networking to locate a suitable interpreter.

Adapted from M. Andrews (1995). Transcultural considerations: in health assessment. In C. Jarvis, *Physical Examination and Health Assessment* (p. 75). Philadelphia: W.B. Saunders. Reprinted by permission.

cation that enable nurses to provide culturally competent and culturally congruent nursing care.

R E V I E W   Q U E S T I O N S

1. Summarize the key standards for culturally and linguistically competent health care recommended by the Office of Minority Health, U.S. Department of Health and Human Services.
2. Critically examine the strategies for promoting effective cross-cultural communication between nurses and clients. Identify actions that you can take to overcome communication barriers when caring for non–English-speaking clients.
3. What are the major languages spoken in households in the United States and Canada?

CRITICAL THINKING ACTIVITIES

1. After critically analyzing the definitions of cultural competence presented in the chapter, craft a definition of the term in your own words.
2. To provide culturally competent nursing care, you should engage in a cultural self-assessment. Answer the questions in Box 2-2, How Do You Relate to Various Groups of People in the Society?, and score your answers using the guide provided. What did you learn about yourself? How would you learn more about the background of those groups mentioned, including information about their health-related beliefs and practices? What resources might you use in your search for information?
3. After identifying someone for whom English is a second language, ask the person what he or she believes (a) promotes effective communication and (b) sets up barriers to effective communication. What has the person found to be the most challenging in communicating health-related needs to physicians, nurses, and other health care providers?
4. Interview a nurse with experience in caring for clients whose primary language is not English. What challenges in communicating with these clients does the nurse report? What strategies does the nurse use to promote effective cross-cultural communication? How effective does the nurse believe these strategies have been in the care of these clients?

• References

American Academy of Nursing (1993). *Promoting cultural competence in and through nursing education.* Subpanel on Cultural Competence in Nursing Education, American Academy of Nursing: New York.

American Academy of Nursing (1992). AAN expert panel report: Culturally competent health care. *Nursing Outlook, 40,* 277–283.

Andrews, M. M., & Boyle, J. S. (1997). Competence in transcultural nursing care. *American Journal of Nursing,* 98(8), 16AAA–16DDD.

Campinha-Bacote, J. (1995). Cultural competence: A critical factor in nursing research. In J. Campinha-Bacote. *Readings in transcultural health care (pp. 117–121).* Wyoming, OH: Transcultural C.A.R.E. Associates.

Campinha-Bacote, J. (1999). A model and instrument for addressing cultural competence in health care. *Journal of Nursing Education,* 38(5), 203–207.

Campinha-Bacote, J. (2000) A model of practice to address cultural competent health care in the home. *Home Care Provider,* 5(6), 213–219.

Campinha-Bacote, J., & Munoz, C. (2001). A guiding framework for delivering culturally competent services in case management. *The Case Manager,* 12(2), 48–52.

Hall, E. (1963). Proxemics: The study of man's spatial relationships. In I. Gladstone (Ed.). *Man's image in medicine and anthropology (pp. 109–120).* New York: International University Press.

Leininger, M. M. (1991). *Culture care diversity and universality: A theory of nursing.* New York: National League for Nursing Press.

Leininger, M. M. (1995). *Transcultural nursing: Concepts, theories, research and practices.* New York: McGraw-Hill.

Leininger, M. M. (1999). What is transcultural nursing and culturally competent care? *Journal of Transcultural Nursing,* 10(1), 9.

Leininger, M .M., & McFarland, M. R. (2002). *Transcultural nursing: Concepts, theories, research and practices.* New York: McGraw-Hill.

Lipson, J. G., & Steiger, N. J. (1996). *Self-care nursing in a multicultural context.* Thousand Oaks, CA: Sage.

Meleis, A. I. (1999). Culturally competent care. *Journal of Transcultural Nursing,* 10(1), 12.

United States Census Bureau (2000). *2000 census of population and housing.* Washington, DC: U.S. Government Printing Office. *www.census.gov*

Office of Minority Health (1999). *Assuring cultural competence in health care: Recommendations for national standards and an outcomes-focused research agenda.*

Washington, DC: Department of Health and Human Services, U.S. Public Health Service. *www.omhrc. gov/clas/ds.htm*

Smith, L. S. (1998). Concept analysis: Cultural competence. *Journal of Cultural Diversity, 5*(1), 4–10.

Watson, O. M. (1980). *Proxemic behavior: A cross cultural study.* The Hague, Netherlands: Mouton Press.

Wells, M. I. (2000). Beyond cultural competence: A model for individual and institutional cultural development. *Journal of Community Health Nursing 17*(4), 189–199.

CHAPTER 3

Cultural Competence in the Health History and Physical Examination

Margaret M. Andrews

KEY TERMS

Biocultural variations
Clinical decision making
Cultural assessment
Cultural care accommodation
  and/or negotiation
Cultural care repatterning
  and/or restructuring
Cultural preservation and/or
  maintenance

Culture-bound syndrome
Cyanosis
Ecchymotic lesions
Erythema
Ethnohistory
Evaluation
Jaundice
Leukoedema
Mongolian spots

Nursing actions
Oral hyperpigmentation
Pallor
Petechiae
Plant-derived medications
Transcultural Nursing
  Assessment Guide

OBJECTIVES

1. Explore the process and content needed for the comprehensive cultural assessment of individuals, families, and groups from diverse cultures.
2. Identify biocultural variations in health and illness for individuals, families, and groups from diverse cultures.
3. Discuss biocultural variations in common laboratory tests.
4. Critically review transcultural perspectives in the health history and physical examination.
5. Examine cultural factors that influence clinical decision making, nursing actions, and evaluation.

Cultural **assessment**, or *culturologic nursing assessment,* refers to a systematic, comprehensive examination of individuals, groups, and communities regarding their health-related cultural beliefs, values, and practices. The goal of cultural assessment is to determine the explicit nursing and health care needs of people and to intervene in ways that are culturally congruent and meaningful (cf. Leininger, 1995; Leininger & McFarland, 2002). Because they deal with cultural values, belief systems, and lifeways, cultural assessments tend to be broad and comprehensive, although it is possible to focus on a smaller segment (Andrews and Boyle, 1997). Cultural assessment consists of both *process* and *content. Process* refers to your approach to the client, consideration of verbal and nonverbal communication, and the sequence and order in which data are gathered. The *content* of the cultural assessment consists of the actual data categories in which information about clients is gathered.

This chapter will be divided into two major sections: (1) transcultural perspectives on the health history and (2) transcultural perspectives on the physical examination. Ideally, the cultural assessment should be integrated into the overall assessment of the client, family, group, and/or community. It is usually impractical to expect that nurses will have the time to conduct a separate cultural assessment, so questions aimed at the gathering of cultural data should be integrated into the overall assessment.

In Appendix B you will find the Andrews and Boyle **Transcultural Nursing Assessment Guide**. The major categories in this guide include cultural affiliation(s), values orientation, health-related beliefs and practices, nutrition, socioeconomic considerations, organizations providing cultural support, education, religion, cultural aspects of disease incidence, biocultural variations, and developmental considerations across the life span.

• TRANSCULTURAL PERSPECTIVES ON THE HEALTH HISTORY

The purpose of the health history is to gather *subjective data*—a term that refers to things that people say about themselves. The health history provides a comprehensive overview of a client's past and present health, and it examines the manner in which the person interacts with the environment. The health history enables the nurse to assess health strengths, including cultural beliefs and practices that might influence the nurse's ability to provide culturally competent nursing care. The history is combined with the *objective data* from the physical examination and the laboratory results to form a diagnosis about the health status of a person (Jarvis, 2000).

For the well client, the history is used to assess lifestyle, which includes activity, exercise, diet, and related personal choices that enable you to identify potential risk factors for disease. For the ill client, the health history includes a chronologic record of the health problem(s). For both well and ill clients, the health history is a screening tool for abnormal symptoms, health problems, and concerns. The health history also provides you with valuable information about the coping strategies used previously by clients (Jarvis, 2000).

In many health care settings, the client is expected to fill out a printed history form or checklist. From a transcultural perspective, this approach has both positive and negative aspects. On the positive side, this approach provides the client with ample time to recall details such as relevant family history and the dates of health-related events such as surgical procedures and illnesses. It is expedient for nurses because it takes less time to review a form than to elicit the information in a face-to-face or telephone interview.

However, this approach has limitations. First, the form is likely to be in English. Those whose primary language is not English might find the form difficult or impossible to complete accurately. Although some health care facilities provide forms translated into Spanish, French, or other languages known to be spoken by relatively large numbers of people who use the facility, it is costly to translate forms into multiple languages. In some instances, the literal translation of medical terms isn't possible. In other instances, the symptom or disease is not recognized in the culture with which the client identifies. For example, in asking about symptoms of depression, there might be many cultural factors that influence the client's interpretation of the question. In Chinese languages, there is no literal translation for the word *depression*. In Chinese culture it is more acceptable to somaticize emotional pain with expressions of physical discomfort such as chest pain or "heaviness of the heart." If health care providers fail to understand the cultural meaning of the symptom "heaviness of the heart," unnecessary, invasive, and costly tests might be performed to rule out cardiovascular disease. In some instances, clients might be unable to read or write in any language; thus, an assessment of the client's literacy level should precede the use of printed history forms or checklists.

Although there is wide variation in health history formats, most contain the following categories: *biographic data, reason for seeking care, present health or history of present illness, past history, family and social history, and review of systems.* This chapter will not cover a comprehensive overview of all data categories in a health history; it will present only those relative to the provision of culturally congruent and culturally competent nursing care.

Biographic Data and Source of History

In addition to the standard descriptive information about clients (name, address, phone, age, gender, and so forth), it is necessary to record who has furnished the data. Whereas this is usually the client, the source might be a relative or friend. Note whether an interpreter is used and indicate his or her relationship to the client. Be sure to document the *specific language* spoken by the client, e.g., Mandarin Chinese (compared with Cantonese Chinese or other dialects).

Although the biographic information might seem straightforward, several cultural variations in recording age are important to note. In some Asian cultures, an infant is considered to be one year old at birth. Among some South Vietnamese immigrants who migrated to the United States during the Vietnam War, there might be inaccuracies in the reported age. These inaccuracies occurred in response to United States immigration laws in the 1960s and 1970s, which attempted to limit the numbers of Southeast Asians entering the United States.

Among the first areas that you should assess is the client's cultural affiliation. With what cultural group(s) does the client report affiliation? Where was the client born? What is the **ethnohistory** of the client? Knowledge of the client's ethnohistory is important in determining his or her risk factors for genetic and acquired diseases and in understanding the client's cultural heritage. How many years have the client and his or her family lived in this country? If the client is a recent immigrant, ask him or her to describe what the migration experience was like.

Reason for Seeking Care

The *reason for seeking care* refers to a brief statement describing in clients' own words why they are visiting a health care provider. In the past, this statement has been called the *chief complaint,* a term that is now avoided because it focuses on illness rather than wellness and tends to label the person as a complainer. All symptoms are believed to have cultural meanings, and the nurse should realize that they are usually more than manifestations of a biologic reality.

Symptoms are defined as phenomena experienced by individuals that signify a departure from normal function, sensation, or appearance and that might include physical aberrations. By comparison, *signs* are objective abnormalities that the examiner can detect on physical examination or through laboratory testing. As individuals experience symptoms, they interpret them and react in ways that are congruent with their cultural norms. Symptoms cannot be attributed to another person; rather, individuals experience symptoms from their knowledge of bodily function and sociocultural interactions. Symptoms are perceived, recognized, labeled, reacted to, ritualized, and articulated in ways that make sense within the cultural worldview of the person experiencing them (Good & Good, 1980; Wenger, 1993).

Symptoms are defined according to the client's perception of the meaning attributed to the event. This perception must be considered in relation to other sociocultural factors and biologic knowledge. People develop culturally based explanatory models to explain how their illnesses work and what their symptoms mean (Kleinman, Eisenberg, & Good, 1978).

The search for cultural meaning in understanding symptoms involves a translation process that includes both the nurse's worldview and the client's. You need to assess the symptoms within the client's sociocultural and ethnohistorical context. It is important to use the same terms for symptoms that clients use. For example, if the client refers to "swelling" of the leg, refrain from medicalizing that to "edema." Knowledge of the cultural expression of symptoms will influence the decisions you make and will facilitate your ability to provide culturally congruent or culturally competent nursing care (Wenger, 1993).

Present and Past Illnesses

Table 3-1 provides an alphabetic listing of selected diseases and their increased or decreased prevalence among members of certain cultural groups. Accurate assessment and evaluation of the present and past illnesses requires knowledge of the biocultural aspects of acute and chronic diseases. The distribution of selected genetic traits and disorders prevalent among children from selected cultural groups is presented in Chapter 6, Transcultural Perspectives in the Nursing Care of Children.

(Text continues on page 42.)

TABLE 3–1	BIOCULTURAL ASPECTS OF DISEASE

DISEASE	REMARKS
Alcoholism	Indians have double the rate of whites; lower tolerance to alcohol among Chinese and Japanese North Americans
Anemia	High incidence among Vietnamese because of the presence of infestations among immigrants and low iron diets; low hemoglobin and malnutrition found among 18.2% of Native North Americans, 32.7% of blacks, 14.6% of Hispanics, and 10.4% of white children under 5 years of age
Arthritis	Increased incidence among Native North Americans Blackfoot 1.4% Pima 1.8% Chippewa 6.8%
Asthma	Six times greater for Native North American infants <1 year; same as general population for Native North Americans aged 1–44 years
Bronchitis	Six times greater for Native North American infants <1 year; same as general population for Native North Americans aged 1–44 years. Main cause of death for Aboriginal Canadian infants in the postnatal period
Cancer	Nasopharyngeal: high among Chinese North Americans and Native Americans Breast: Black women 1 1/2 times more likely than White Colorectal: Blacks 40% higher than Whites Esophageal: No. 2 cause of death for Black men aged 35–54 years *Incidence:* White men 3.5/100,000 Black men 13.3/100,000 Liver: Highest among all ethnic groups are Filipino Hawaiians Latinos have twice the rate of Whites Stomach: Black men twice as likely as white men; low among Filipinos Cervical: 120% higher in black women than in white women Mexican American and Puerto Rican women 2-3 times higher than Whites Uterine: 53% lower in black women than white women Prostate: Black men have highest incidence of all groups Most prevalent cancer among Native North Americans: biliary, nasopharyngeal, testicular, cervical, renal, and thyroid (females) cancer Lung cancer among Navajo uranium miners 85 times higher than among white miners Most prevalent cancer among Japanese North Americans: esophageal, stomach, liver, and biliary cancer Among Chinese North Americans, there is a higher incidence of nasopharyngeal and liver cancer than among the general population

(continued)

TABLE
3–1

DISEASE	REMARKS
Cholecystitis	*Incidence:*
	Whites 0.3%
	Puerto Ricans 2.1%
	Native Americans 2.2%
	Chinese 2.6%
Colitis	High incidence among Japanese North Americans
Diabetes mellitus	Three times as prevalent among Filipino North Americans as Whites; higher among Hispanics than Blacks or Whites
	Death rate is 3–4 times as high among Native North Americans aged 25–34 years, especially those in the West such as Utes, Pimas, and Papagos
	Complications
	Amputations: Twice as high among Native North Americans vs. general U.S. population
	Renal failure: 20 times as high as general U.S. population, with tribal variation, e.g., Utes have 43 times higher incidence
G-6P-D	Present among 30% of black males
Influenza	Increased death rate among Native Americans aged 45+
Ischemic heart disease	Responsible for 32% of heart-related causes of death among Native Americans; Blacks have higher mortality rates than all other groups
Lactose intolerance	Present among 66% of Hispanic women; increased incidence among Blacks and Chinese
Myocardial infarction	Leading cause of heart disease in Native Americans, accounting for 43% of death resulting from heart disease; low incidence among Japanese Americans
Otitis media	7.9% incidence among school-aged Navajo children versus 0.5% in Whites
	Up to 1/3 of Eskimo children <2 years have chronic otitis media
	Increased incidence among bottle-fed Native Americans and Eskimo infants
Pneumonia	Increased death rate among Native North Americans aged 45+
Psoriasis	Affects 2–5% of Whites but <1% of Blacks; high among Japanese Americans
Renal disease	Lower incidence among Japanese North Americans
Sickle cell anemia	Increased incidence among Blacks
Trachoma	Increased incidence among Native North Americans and Eskimo children (3 to 8 times greater than general population)

(continued)

TABLE 3-1	BIOCULTURAL ASPECTS OF DISEASE *(Continued)*
Tuberculosis	Increased incidence among Native North Americans
	Apache 2.0%
	Sioux 3.2%
	Navajo 4.6%
	Aboriginals living on Canadian reserves are 10 times more likely to have TB than non-Aboriginal Canadians
	Non-Whites 5.2 times more than Whites
Ulcers	Decreased incidence among Japanese North Americans

Based on data reported in T. Overfield (1995). *Biologic Variation in Health and Illness: Race, Age, and Sex Differences.* NY: CRC Press; and Office of Minority Health (Aug. 1995).
Cancer in minority communities. Closing the Gap, Washington, DC: U.S. Govt. Printing Office.
American Cancer Society (2002). Cancer Facts and Figures. http//:www.cancer.org/statistic.
National Center for Health Statistics (2001). http://www.cdc.govt/nchs.
National Vital Statistics Report (2002). Morbidity and Mortality Weekly Report, 49(8), SS-5.
U.S. Department of Health and Human Services (1998). Racial and ethnic disparities in health. http://www.raceandhealth.hhs.gov.
Health Canada (1999). Toward a healthy future: Second report on the health of Canadians. Ottawa, ON: Author. Health Canada (1996). Tuberculosis in First Nations Communities. Ottawa, ON: Author.

Culture-Bound Syndromes

Although all illness might be culturally defined, the term **culture-bound syndromes** refers to disorders restricted to a particular culture or group of cultures because of certain psychosocial characteristics of those cultures. For example, anorexia nervosa is believed to be a Western culture-bound syndrome because the condition is largely confined to Western cultures or to non-Western cultures undergoing the process of westernization, such as Japan. Culture-bound syndromes are thought to be illnesses created by personal, social, and cultural reactions to malfunctioning biologic or psychologic processes and can be understood only within defined contexts of meaning and social relationships (Kleinman, 1980). Table 3-2 summarizes selected culture-bound syndromes found in specific cultural groups.

Current Medications

In the health history you should note the name, dose, route of administration, schedule, frequency, purpose, and length of time that each medicine has been taken. It is also important to note all prescription and over-the-counter medications, including herbs that clients might purchase or grow in home gardens. Because of cultural differences in people's perception of what substances are considered medicines, it is important to ask about specific items by name. For example, you should inquire about vitamins, birth control pills, aspirin, antacids, herbs, teas, inhalants, poultices, vaginal and rectal suppositories, ointments, and any other items taken by the client for therapeutic purposes.

| TABLE 3–2 | SELECTED CULTURE-BOUND SYNDROMES | |

GROUP	DISORDER	REMARKS
Blacks, Haitians	Blackout	Collapse, dizziness, inability to move
	Low blood	Not enough blood or weakness of the blood that is often treated with diet
	High blood	Blood that is too rich in certain things because of the ingestion of too much red meat or rich foods
	Thin blood	Occurs in women, children, and old people; renders the individual more susceptible to illness in general
	Diseases of hex, witchcraft, or conjuring	Sense of being doomed by spell; gastrointestinal symptoms, e.g., vomiting; hallucinations; part of voodoo beliefs
Chinese/ Southeast Asians	*Koro*	Intense anxiety that penis is retracting into body
Greeks	Hysteria	Bizarre complaints and behavior because the uterus leaves the pelvis for another part of the body
Hispanics	*Empacho*	Food forms into a ball and clings to the stomach or intestines, causing pain and cramping
	Fatigue	Asthma-like symptoms
	Mal ojo, "evil eye"	Fitful sleep, crying, diarrhea in children caused by a stranger's attention; sudden onset
	Pasmo	Paralysis-like symptoms of face or limbs; prevented or relieved by massage
	Susto	Anxiety, trembling, phobias from sudden fright
Japanese	*Wagamama*	Apathetic childish behavior with emotional outbursts
Korean	*Hwa-byung*	Multiple somatic and psychologic symptoms; "pushing up" sensation of chest; palpitations, flushing, headache, "epigastric mass," dysphoria, anxiety, irritability, and difficulty concentrating; mostly afflicts married women
Native Americans	Ghost	Terror, hallucinations, sense of danger
North India Indians	Ghost	Death from fever and illness in children; convulsions, delirious speech (or incessant crying in infants); choking, difficulty breathing; based on Hindu religious beliefs and curing practices
Whites	Anorexia nervosa	Excessive preoccupation with thinness; self-imposed starvation
	Bulimia	Gross overeating and then vomiting or fasting

PLANT-DERIVED DRUGS

In particular, it is important to be aware of the widespread use of **plant-derived medications** among various cultures (Table 3-3). Since prehistoric times, people have attempted to identify plants, marine organisms, arthropods, animals, and minerals with healing properties. According the World Health Organization, 80% of people residing in less developed countries use traditional medicine, including medicinal plants, for their major primary health care needs. Of the 119 plant-derived drugs currently used in the United States and Canada, 74% were discovered as a result of chemical studies designed to isolate the active ingredients responsible for the use of the plants in traditional medicine. These drugs are derived from approximately 90 of the 250,000 known species of plants on this planet (Farnsworth, 1993) (Figure 3-1).

Many of the active ingredients in these herbs are unknown and remain largely unregulated by government agencies, except for customs officials who make efforts to control the flow of illegal drugs. Fresh or dried herbs are usually brewed into a tea, with the dosage adjusted according to the chronicity or acuteness of illness, age, and size of the patient. Traditional Chinese medicine usually is used only as long as symptoms persist. Some patients extend the same logic to Western biomedicine. For example, they might stop taking an antibiotic as soon as the symptoms subside instead of completing the course of treatment for the prescribed length of time. Be sure to consider the potential interaction of herbs with Western biomedicines. The root of the shrub *ginseng*, for example, is widely used for the treatment of arthritis, back and leg pains, and sores. Because ginseng is known to potentiate the action of some antihypertensive drugs, you must ask the patient whether he or she is experiencing side effects or toxicity, and monitor blood pressure frequently. It might be necessary to withhold doses of the prescribed antihypertensive medicine if the blood pressure is low or to ask the client to discontinue or reduce the strength of the ginseng. When assessing the patient's use of traditional Chinese medicine, you should be aware that some Chinese North Americans who use herbs topically do not consider them to be drugs. For further information about herbs, the nurse should ask the patient and family, consult with an herbalist, search for reputable sources on the Internet; or check reference books on herbal remedies. Many pharmacists are familiar with the active ingredients of herbal remedies and their uses, side effects, toxicity, and interactions with prescription and over-the-counter drugs, or they can refer the nurse to reliable sources of information.

DOSAGE MODIFICATIONS

As indicated in Table 3-4, there is growing research-based evidence to suggest that modifications in dosages of some drugs should be made for members of some racial and ethnic groups. It might be difficult to develop ethnic-specific norms for drug dosages because of intermarriage, individual differences (e.g., weight and body fat index), and related factors. It is possible, however, to alert nurses and other health care providers to the variations that occur in side effects, adverse reactions, and toxicity so that clients from diverse cultural backgrounds can be monitored for possible untoward symptoms.

(Text continues on page 50.)

TABLE 3-3	HERBAL REMEDIES

Aloe Vera

Aloe Vera

Source	Leaf of *Aloe barbadensis* Mill. (family Liliaceae)
Action	Topical analgesic, anti-inflammatory, antibacterial, and antifungal agent
Traditional Uses	Applied topically for treatment of inflammation, minor burns, sunburn, cuts, bruises, and abrasions.
	Orally, aloe juice was used for gastrointestinal upset, arthritis, diabetes mellitus, and gastric ulcers
Current Uses	Promotes wound healing in soft tissue injuries
	Prevents wound pain by inhibiting the action of the pain-producing agent bradykinin
	May prevent progression of skin damage from electrical burns and frostbite
	Prevention of wound infection because of its antibacterial and antifungal properties
	Used in a wide variety of ointments, creams, lotions, and shampoos
Dosage	Apply topically as needed
Warnings	Rarely, skin rash follows topical application
	May cause burning if applied after removal of acne scars
	To avoid deterioration of active ingredients, use the fresh gel and avoid diluted extracts
	When taken internally as *aloe latex,* it causes intestinal cramping and may lead to ulcers and bowel irritation

Dong-Quai (Chinese Angelica)

Angelica sinensis

Source	Dried root of a member of the parsley family
Action	Smooth muscle relaxant; antispasmodic
Traditional Uses	A highly regarded herb in Chinese medicine, dong-quai means "proper order"; used to suppress menstruation, cleanse the blood, and promote harmony in the body
	In the West, used to regulate menstrual periods, symptoms of menopause, and premenstrual syndrome (PMS)
Current Uses	Relaxes uterine muscle and improves circulation to the uterus
	Improves circulation and lowers blood pressure; reduces inflammation, pains, and spasm; increases number of red blood cells and platelets.
	Protects liver from toxins
Dosage	5–12 g (1 to 3 teaspoons) daily
Warnings	Contraindicated for pregnant and breast-feeding women and persons with abdominal distention or diarrhea
	Large doses may cause contact dermatitis and photodermatitis

(continued)

TABLE 3–3	HERBAL REMEDIES *(Continued)*

Echinacea

Echinacea angustifolia, E. pallida, E. pururea

Source	Member of the daisy family; also known as purple coneflower
Action	Reduces cold symptoms
Traditional Uses	Used by Native Americans in poultices, mouthwashes, and teas for colds, cancer, and other disorders
	Some herbalists consider it a blood purifier and an aid to fighting infections
Current Uses	Enhances the immune system by stimulating the production of white blood cells needed to fight infection or cancer
Dosage	Follow directions on label; needed at onset of symptoms; usually taken for no longer than 2 weeks
Warnings	Contraindicated for pregnant or breast-feeding women, children, and those who are allergic to ragweed
	Not recommended for people with severely compromised immune systems such as those with HIV/AIDS, tuberculosis, or multiple sclerosis
	Look for reputable suppliers, because a high percentage of the root currently marketed is adulterated with less expensive inactive substitutes

Evening Primrose Oil

Oenothera biennis

Source	Seeds of the wildflower evening primrose
Action	Antihypertensive, immunostimulant, weight reduction
Traditional Uses	Used by Native Americans for food; in eastern North America, used to treat obesity and hemorrhoids; new settlers to North America used the plant for gastrointestinal upsets and sore throats
Current Uses	Used as a dietary supplement for essential fatty acids; believed to help asthma, migraine headaches, inflammations, premenstrual syndrome (PMS), diabetes mellitus, and arthritis; also believed to lower blood pressure and lower cholesterol, slow the progression of multiple sclerosis, promote weight loss without dieting, alleviate hangovers, and moisturize dry eyes, brittle hair, and fingernails
Dosage	Follow directions on label; will take at least one month to experience benefits
Warnings	Side effects include occasional reports of headache, nausea, and abdominal discomfort; not recommended for children
	Some capsules may be altered with other types of oil such as soy or safflower

TABLE 3–3	**HERBAL REMEDIES** (Continued)

Ginger

Current Uses	Effective in reducing morning sickness and postoperative nausea for some people; used in China to treat first- and second-degree burns.
Dosage	Boil 1 ounce dried ginger root in 1 cup water for 15 to 20 minutes Follow label directions on ginger supplements
Warning	Large doses may cause central nervous system depression and cardiac arrythmias Side effects include heartburn Contraindicated in the presence of gallbladder disease

Gingko

Gingko biloba

Source	Extract from leaves of the gingko tree, a living fossil, believed to be more than 200 million years old
Action	Antioxidant; improves blood circulation
Traditional Uses	Used in China since the 15th century for cough, asthma, diarrhea, skin lesions, and removal of freckles
Current Uses	Promotes vasodilation and improves circulation of blood May be an effective free radical scavenger or antioxidant Improves short-term memory, attention span, and mood in early stages of Alzheimer's disease by improving oxygen metabolism in the brain
Dosage	Range: 120-160 mg TID. May take 6-8 weeks before results are evident
Warnings	Large doses may cause irritability, restlessness, diarrhea, nausea, and vomiting. Some people (who are also sensitive to poison ivy) are unable to tolerate even low doses Contraindicated for women who are pregnant or breast-feeding. Contraindicated for persons with clotting disorders Not recommended for children

Ginseng (American and Asian)

Panax quinquefolius (American)
Panax gingeng (Asian)

Source	Dried root of several species of the genus *Panax* of the family Aralaceae
Action	Tonic
Traditional Uses	Treatment of anemia, atherosclerosis, edema, ulcers, hypertension, influenza, colds, inflammation, and disorders of the immune system (American) In traditional China, used for treatment of shock, diaphoresis, dyspnea, fever, thirst, irritability, diarrhea, vomiting, abdominal distention, anorexia, and impotence; considered a "heat raising" tonic for the blood and circulatory system (Asian)

(continued)

TABLE 3–3	**HERBAL REMEDIES** *(Continued)*

Current Uses	Used to enhance sexual experience and treat impotence, though there is no current research to support this claim (American)
	In Germany may be labeled as a tonic to treat fatigue, reduced work capacity. In some parts of Asia, used for lack of concentration and for convalescence (Asian)
	Improved sense of well-being (Asian)
Dosage	American: Follow directions on label
	Asian: 100 mg BID
Warnings	American: May cause headaches, insomnia, anxiety, breast tenderness, rashes, asthma attacks, hypertension, cardiac arrhythmias, and postmenopausal uterine hemorrhage
	Should be used with caution for the following conditions: pregnancy, insomnia, hay fever, fibrocystic breasts, asthma, emphysema, hypertension, clotting disorders, and diabetes mellitus
	Asian: Same as American

Gotu-Kola

Centella asiatica

Source	Dried and powdered leaves of a member of the parsley family
Action	Improves memory
Traditional Uses	In ancient India, considered a rejuvenating herb that increases intelligence, longevity, and memory while slowing the aging process
	In China, used as a tea for colds and for lung and urinary tract infections, and topically for snakebite, wounds, and shingles
	Recommended for treatment of mental disorders, hypertension, abscesses, rheumatism, fever, ulcers, skin lesions, and jaundice
Current Uses	Acceleration of wound healing
	Diuretic
	Treatment of phlebitis
Dosage	Follow directions on label; lower dose needed for children and older adults
Warnings	Side effects include headaches and skin rash
	Contraindicated for pregnant or breast-feeding women and children under 2 years.
	Contraindicated when using tranquilizers or sedatives

Saint John's Wort

Hypericum perforatum

Source	Tea made from the leaves and flowering tops of the perennial *Hypericum perforatum,* which is particularly abundant on June 24th, the feast of St. John the Baptist
Action	Antidepressant
Traditional Uses	Used in 1st-century Greece for wound healing and menstrual disorders, and as a diuretic
	In 19th-century North America, used for its astringent, wound healing, diuretic, and mild sedative effects

TABLE 3–3	**HERBAL REMEDIES** *(Continued)*

Current Uses	Treatment of mild to moderate depression; effects are linked to various substances that act as monoamine oxidase (MAO) inhibitors
Dosage	300 mg daily
Warnings	Fair-skinned people may experience urticaria or vesicular skin lesions upon exposure to sunlight
	Reduces effectiveness of some anticancer agents
	Clinical manifestations of depression should be considered seriously
	Encourage client to see a mental health care provider.

Valerian

Valeriana officianalis

Source	Dried rhizome and roots of the tall perennial *Valeriana officinalis*
Action	Mild tranquilizer and sedative
Traditional Uses	Used by the ancient Greeks for the treatment of epilepsy and menstrual disorders, and as a diuretic
	Used by 17th- and 18th-century Europeans as an antispasmodic and sedative
	Listed as an official remedy in the U.S. Pharmacopoeia from 1820 to 1936
Current Uses	Used as a mild tranquilizer and sedative; relieves muscle spasms
	Especially effective for insomniac persons and older adults
Dosage	300–400 mg daily; Take 1 hour before bedtime as a sleeping aid
Warnings	Reported side effects include headache, gastrointestinal upset, and excitability
	Signs of overdose include severe headache, restlessness, nausea, morning grogginess, or blurred vision
	Must not be taken in combination with other tranquilizers or sedatives
	Client should be cautioned against operating a motor vehicle after ingesting

Table developed using data from

Ernst, E., Pittler, M. H., Stevinson, C., & White, A. (2001). *The desktop guide to complementary and alternative medicine: An evidence-based approach.* New York: Mosby.

Fetrow, C. W., & Avila, J. R. (1999). *Professional's handbook of complementary and alternative medicines.* Springhouse, PA: Springhouse.

Fontaine, K. L. (2000). *Healing practices: Alternative therapies for nursing.* Upper Saddle River, NJ: Prentice Hall.

Foster, S. (1996). *Herbs for your health.* Loveland, CO: Interweave Press.

Kuhn, M. A. (1999). *Complementary therapies for health care providers.* Philadelphia: Lippincott Williams & Wilkins.

Kuhn, M. A., & Winston, D. (2000). *Herbal therapy and supplements: A scientific and traditional approach.* Philadelphia: Lippincott Williams & Wilkins.

Monte, T. (1997). *The complete guide to natural healing.* New York: Berkeley Publishing Group.

Tyler, V. E. (1994). *Herbs of choice: The therapeutic use of phytomedicinals.* New York: Pharmaceutical Products Press.

Figure 3–1. Shopkeeper of Indian ancestry sells herbal remedies used in Ayurvedic healing in a neighborhood store that attracts recent immigrants from India. People from diverse backgrounds who embrace Ayruvedic medicine also patronize the store, which sells prepackaged herbal remedies and dried herbs used to brew teas.

MEDICATION ADMINISTRATION

If the medication prescribed, its route of administration, or the substances given with it conflict with clients' adherence to the yin/yang, hot/cold, or other belief system, it is unlikely that they will follow your advice concerning the medication. The nurse should be aware that some clients of Latino, Middle Eastern, and Asian heritage believe that it is important to take medicine with certain beverages or foods to provide the necessary balance for health. If clients give cues that they are uncomfortable with the beverage or food being used in the health care setting, discuss alternatives. For example, in most health care facilities, medications are given with cold water, but they could be given with hot water, tea, coffee, or a similar beverage if the client believes that such a beverage would promote healing. Some Mexican Americans believe that grapefruit juice has healing properties, so you might contact the dietary department to ensure that this juice is available when medications are administered. If the cultural healing beliefs and practices of the client are incorporated into medication administration, there is a higher probability that the client will believe in the healing properties of the drugs and will continue to take them as prescribed after discharge.

Family and Social History

In addition to diagramming a family tree to identify familial relationships and the presence of disease conditions among those related to the client, you should assess the broader socioeconomic factors influencing the client. The health history should include in-depth data pertaining to the client's family and/or close social friends, including identification of *key decision makers.* Although personal financial information is often a very sensitive topic, it is important to determine the overall economic factors that influence a client. For example, regardless of race or ethnicity, people from lower socioeconomic categories have poorer health and shorter lives. Unfortunately, there is a disproportionately high level of poverty among Blacks, Latinos/Latinas, First Nation People of Canada, and North American Indians/Alaska Natives. Economic factors have been identified as causes of less favorable outcomes among clients with cancer. Research suggests that this is caused by a lack of health insurance and/or diminished access to health care services, both of which contribute to a situation in which less affluent clients receive diagnosis and treatment later in the course of the disease. See Appendix B for suggested interview questions aimed at eliciting information about family and social history.

Review of Systems

The purposes of the review of systems are to evaluate the past and present health state of each body system, to provide an opportunity for the client to report symptoms not previously stated, and to evaluate health promotion practices. Knowledge of current research on diseases prevalent in specific ethnic and racial groups might be useful in asking appropriate questions in the review of systems. For example, if the nurse is gathering review of systems information from a middle-aged African-American man, it is useful to know that there is a statistically higher incidence of hypertension, sickle cell anemia, and diabetes in this group than in counterparts from other racial and ethnic groups. This will assist in customizing the review of systems questions and ensuring that symptoms of disease specific to the client's ethnic or racial heritage are included.

• TRANSCULTURAL PERSPECTIVES ON THE PHYSICAL EXAMINATION

The purpose of this discussion is to identify selected **biocultural variations** that nurses sometimes encounter when conducting the physical examination of clients from different cultural backgrounds. Accurate assessment and evaluation of clients require knowledge of normal biocultural variations among healthy members of selected populations. You must also possess assessment skills that will enable you to recognize variations that occur in illness. The following remarks are intended to be illustrative, not exhaustive. As more research on biocultural variations is conducted, undoubtedly there will be additions and perhaps some modifications.

Biocultural Variations in Measurements

Height

Summarized in Table 3-5 are average heights for men and women from selected cultural groups that have been studied. In all groups, *height* increases up to 1.5 inches as socioeconomic status improves. First-generation immigrants might

TABLE 3–4	CULTURAL DIFFERENCES IN RESPONSE TO DRUGS

DRUG CATEGORY	REMARKS
Arab Americans	
Antiarrhythmics	Some may need lower dosage
Antihypertensives	Some may need lower dosage
Neuroleptics	Some may need lower dosage
Opioids	Some may require higher dosage because of diminished ability to metabolize codeine to morphine
Psychotropics	Some may need lower dosage
Asian/Pacific Islanders	
Be aware that drugs are part of the yin/yang belief system embraced by some Asian Americans and that herbal remedies may be used in addition to prescription drugs	
Be sure to consider lower body weight and mass when calculating doses	
Narcotic analgesics	Chinese may be less sensitive to the respiratory depressant and hypotensive effects of morphine but more likely to experience nausea; Chinese have a significantly higher clearance of morphine
Antihypertensives	Respond best to calcium antagonists
Neuroleptics	Require lower dose
Psychotropics	Require lower dose, sometimes as little as one half the normal dose for TCAs and lithium
Fat-soluble drugs	On average, Asian Americans have a lower percentage of body fat, so dosage adjustments must be made for fat-soluble vitamins and other drugs, e.g., Vitamin K used to reverse the anticoagulant effect of Coumadin (warfarin); consider dietary intake of vitamins when calculating doses
Blacks	
Analgesics	Despite decreased sensitivity to pain-relieving therapeutic action of drugs, there are increased gastrointestinal side effects, especially with acetominaphen
Antihypertensives	Respond best to treatment with a single drug (versus combined antihypertensive therapy)
	Research suggests favorable response to diuretics, calcium antagonists, and alpha-blockers
	Less responsive to beta-blockers (e.g., propranolol) and angiotensin-converting enzyme (ACE) inhibitors (e.g., enalapril, imidapril)
	Increased side effects such as mood response (e.g., depression) to thiazides (e.g., hydrochlorothiazide), which may explain reluctance to take drug as prescribed
	There is little justification to use racial profiling to avoid drug classes. Current research is focusing on differences in the causes of hypertension in Blacks to explain differences in drug responses

(continues)

| TABLE 3–4 | CULTURAL DIFFERENCES IN RESPONSE TO DRUGS *(Continued)* |

DRUG CATEGORY	REMARKS
Mydriatics	Less dilation occurs with dark-colored eyes
Psychotropics	Increased extrapyramidal side effects with tricyclic antidepressants (TCAs) such as haloperidol
Steroids	When methylprednisolone is used for immunosuppression in renal transplant patients, there is increased toxicity such as steroid-associated diabetes; although Blacks are four times as likely to develop end-stage renal disease as Whites, they have the poorest long-term graft survival of any ethnic group
Tranquilizers	15–20% are poor metabolizers of Valium (diazepam)
Hispanics	
Psychotropics	May require lower dosage and experience higher incidence of side effects with TCAs
Greeks, Italians, and others of Mediterranean Descent with G-6-PD Deficiency	
Oxidating drugs	The following drugs may precipitate a hemolytic crisis: primaquine, quinidine, thiazolsulfone, furzolidone, nitrofural, naphthalene, toluidine blue, phenylhydrazine, chloramphenicol Aspirin
Jewish North Americans (Ashkenazi)	
Psychotropics	Agranulocytosis develops in 20% when clozapine is used to treat schizophrenia; thus, the granulocyte count should be checked before the drug is administered
Native North Americans	
Muscle relaxants	Alaskan Eskimos may experience prolonged muscle paralysis and an inability to breathe without mechanical ventilation for several hours postoperatively when succinylcholine has been administered in surgery.

Table based partially on data from

Caraco, Y., Langerstrom, P. O., & Wood, A. J. (1996). Ethnic and genetic determinants of omeprazole and effect. *Clinical Pharmacology and Therapeutics, 60*(2), 157–167.

Lawson, W. B. (1996). Clinical issues in the pharmacotherapy of African-Americans. *Psychopharmacology Bulletin, 32*(2), 275–281.

Lin, K., Anderson, D., & Poland, R. (1995). Ethnicity and psychopharmacology: Bridging the gap. *Psychiatric Clinics of North America, 18*(3), 635–647.

Rudorfer, M. (1993). Pharmacokinetics of psychotropic drugs in special populations. *Journal of Psychiatry, 54*(4), supplement, 50–54.

Tornatore, K. M., Biocevich, D. M., Reed, K., Tousley, K., Singh, J. P., & Venuto, R. C. (1995). *Transplantation, 59*(5), 729–736.

Zhou, H. H., Sheller, J. R., Nu, H., Wood, M., & Wood, A. J. J. (1993). Ethnic differences in response to morphine. *Clinical Pharmacology and Therapeutics, 54*(3), 507–513.

TABLE 3–5	**BIOCULTURAL VARIATIONS IN HEIGHT FOR SELECTED GROUPS**

Height (in inches) for all groups

All groups of men	White American	African American	Mexican American	Asian
69.1	69.1	69.2	67.2	65.7

All groups of women				
63.7	63.8	63.8	61.8	60.3

Table developed using data from Overfield, T. (1995). *Biologic variation in health and illness.* New York: CRC Press.

be up to 1.5 inches taller than their counterparts in the country of origin because of (1) better nutrition and (2) decreased interference with growth by infectious diseases. During the past decade, the overall height of men from the U. S. increased by 0.7 inches, whereas women from the U.S. grew an average of 0.5 inches taller (Overfield, 1995).

Body Proportions

Biocultural variations are found in the *body proportions* of individuals, largely because of differences in bone length. In examining sitting/standing height ratios, you will notice that Blacks of both genders have longer legs and shorter trunks than Whites. Because proportionately most of the weight is in the trunk, White men appear more obese than their Black counterparts. The reverse is true of women. Clients of Asian heritage are markedly shorter, weigh less, and have smaller body frames than their white counterparts and/or the overall population (Overfield, 1995).

Weight

Biocultural differences exist in the amount of body fat and the distribution of fat throughout the body. As a general rule, people from the lower socioeconomic class are more obese than those from the middle class, who are more obese than members of the upper class. On average, Black men weigh less than their White counterparts throughout adulthood (166.1 pounds versus 170.6 pounds). The opposite is true of women. Black women are consistently heavier than White women at every age (149.6 pounds versus 137 pounds). Between the ages of 35 to 64 years, Black women weigh on average 20 pounds more than White women. Mexican Americans weigh more in relation to height than non-Hispanic Whites because of differences in truncal fat patterns. Most differences in the amount of body fat are related to socioeconomic factors, which in turn influence nutrition and exposure to communicable diseases. Around the world, people in cold climates tend to have more body fat, whereas those residing in warmer areas have less. Blacks have smaller skinfold thicknesses on their trunks and arms than do their White counterparts. Bottle-fed infants are heavier on average than those who are breast-fed, although their lengths are similar (Overfield, 1995).

Biocultural Variations in Vital Signs

Although the average pulse rate is comparable across cultures, there are racial and gender differences in *blood pressure*. Black men have lower systolic blood pressures than their White counterparts from ages 18 to 34, but between the ages of 35 and 64 it reverses: Blacks have an average systolic blood pressure of 5 mm Hg higher. After age 65 there is no difference between the two races. Black women have a higher average systolic blood pressure than their White counterparts at every age. After age 45, the average blood pressure of Black women might be as much as 16 mm Hg higher than that of White women in the same age group (Overfield, 1995).

Biocultural Variations in General Appearance

In assessing the general appearance, you should survey the person's entire body. You will want to note the general health state and any obvious physical characteristics and readily apparent biologic features unique to the individual. In assessing the client's general appearance, you should consider four areas: physical appearance, body structure, mobility, and behavior. *Physical appearance* includes age, gender, level of consciousness, facial features, and skin color (evenness of color tone, pigmentation, intactness, presence of lesions or other abnormalities). *Body structure* includes stature, nutrition, symmetry, posture, position, and overall body build or contour. *Mobility* includes gait and range of motion. *Behavior* includes facial expression, mood and affect, fluency of speech, ability to communicate ideas, appropriateness of word choice, grooming, and attire or dress (Jarvis, 2000).

In assessing a client's hygiene, it is useful to ask about typical bathing habits and customary use of various hygiene-related products. People in most cultures in the United States and Canada make a great effort to disguise their natural body odors by bathing frequently, using douches, or applying antiperspirants, colognes, and/or perfumes with scents that are deemed to be desirable. Ironically, some colognes and perfumes such as those with musk oil are marketed in the United States and Canada because of their more "natural" odor, which is alleged to give the wearer more sex appeal. Recent immigrants from some arid nations where water is scarce might bathe less frequently than those from countries where water is more abundant.

Biocultural Variations in Skin

An accurate and comprehensive examination of the skin of clients from culturally diverse backgrounds requires that you possess knowledge of biocultural variations and skill in recognizing color changes, some of which might be very subtle. Awareness of normal biocultural differences and the ability to recognize the unique clinical manifestations of disease are developed over time as you gain experience with clients having various skin colors.

The assessment of a client's skin is subjective and is highly dependent on your observational skill, ability to recognize subtle color changes, and repeated exposure to individuals having various gradations of skin color. *Melanin* is responsible for the various colors and tones of skin observed in different people. Melanin protects the skin against harmful ultraviolet rays—a genetic advantage accounting for the lower incidence of skin cancer among darkly pigmented Black and Native North American clients.

Normal skin color ranges widely. Some health care practitioners have made attempts to describe the variations by labeling their observations with some of the following adjectives: *copper, olive, tan,* and various shades of *brown* (*light, medium,* and *dark*). In observing pallor in clients, the term *ashen* is sometimes used. Of most clinical significance, particularly for clients whose health condition might be linked to changes in skin color, is your ability to establish a reliable description of a baseline color and subsequently to recognize when variations occur in the same individual.

Mongolian Spots

Mongolian spots, irregular areas of deep blue pigmentation, are usually located in the sacral and gluteal areas but sometimes occur on the abdomen, thighs, shoulders, or arms. During embryonic development, the melanocytes originate near the embryonic nervous system in the neural crest. They then migrate into the fetal epidermis. Mongolian spots consist of embryonic pigment that has been left behind in the epidermal layer during fetal development. The result looks like a bluish discoloration of the skin.

Mongolian spots are a normal variation in children of African, Asian, or Latin descent. By adulthood, these spots become lighter but usually remain visible. Mongolian spots are present in 90% of Blacks, 80% of Asians and Native North Americans, and 9% of Whites (Overfield, 1995). If you are unfamiliar with Mongolian spots, it is important to exercise caution so as not to confuse them with bruises. Recognition of this normal variation is particularly important when you are dealing with children who might be erroneously identified as victims of child abuse, causing much anguish to the parents or guardians.

Vitiligo

Vitiligo, a condition in which the melanocytes become nonfunctional in some areas of the skin, is characterized by unpigmented skin patches. Vitiligo affects more than 2 million Americans, primarily dark-skinned individuals. Clients with vitiligo also have a statistically higher than normal risk for pernicious anemia, diabetes mellitus, and hyperthyroidism. These factors are believed to reflect an underlying genetic abnormality (Overfield, 1995).

Hyperpigmentation

Other areas of the skin affected by hormones and, in some cases, differing for people from certain ethnic backgrounds are the sexual skin areas, such as the nipples, areola, scrotum, and labia majora. In general, these areas are darker than other parts of the skin in both adults and children, especially among African-American and Asian clients. When assessing these skin surfaces on dark-skinned clients, you must observe carefully for erythema, rashes, and other abnormalities because the darker color might mask their presence.

Cyanosis

Cyanosis is the most difficult clinical sign to observe in darkly pigmented persons. Because peripheral vasoconstriction can prevent cyanosis, you need to be attentive to environmental conditions such as air conditioning, mist tents, and other factors that might lower the room temperature and thus cause vasoconstriction. For the client to manifest clinical evidence of cyanosis, the blood must contain 5 g of reduced hemoglobin in 1.5 g of methemoglobin per 100 mL of blood (Overfield, 1995).

Given that most conditions causing cyanosis also cause decreased oxygenation of the brain, other clinical symptoms, such as changes in the level of consciousness, will be evident. Cyanosis usually is accompanied by increased respiratory rate, use of accessory muscles of respiration, nasal flaring, and other manifestations of respiratory distress. You must exercise caution when assessing persons of Mediterranean descent for cyanosis because their circumoral region is normally dark blue.

Jaundice

In both light- and dark-skinned clients, **jaundice** is best observed in the sclera. When examining culturally diverse individuals, exercise caution to avoid confusing other forms of pigmentation with jaundice. Many darkly pigmented people, e.g., African Americans, Filipinos, and others, have heavy deposits of subconjunctival fat that contains high levels of carotene in sufficient quantities to mimic jaundice. The fatty deposits become more dense as the distance from the cornea increases. The portion of the sclera that is revealed naturally by the palpebral fissure is the best place to accurately assess color. If the palate does not have heavy melanin pigmentation, jaundice can be detected there in the early stages (i.e., when the serum bilirubin level is 2 to 4 mg/100 mL). The absence of a yellowish tint of the palate when the sclerae are yellow indicates carotene pigmentation of the sclerae rather than jaundice. Light- or clay-colored stools and dark golden urine often accompany jaundice in both light- and dark-skinned clients. If you are to distinguish between carotenemia and jaundice, it will be necessary to inspect the posterior portion of the hard palate using bright daylight or good artificial lighting (Overfield, 1995).

Pallor

When assessing for **pallor** in darkly pigmented clients, you might experience difficulty because the underlying red tones are absent. This is significant because these red tones are responsible for giving brown or black skin its luster. The brown-skinned individual will manifest pallor with a more yellowish brown color, and the black-skinned person will appear ashen or gray.

Generalized pallor can be observed in the mucous membranes, lips, and nail beds. The palpebrae, conjunctivae, and nail beds are preferred sites for assessing the pallor of anemia. When inspecting the conjunctiva, you should lower the lid sufficiently so you can see the conjunctiva near the inner and outer canthi. The coloration is often lighter near the inner canthus.

In addition to changes seen on skin assessment, the pallor of impending shock is accompanied by other clinical manifestations, such as increasing pulse rate, oliguria, apprehension, and restlessness. Anemia, particularly chronic iron-deficiency anemia, might be manifested by the characteristic "spoon" nails, which have a concave shape. A lemon-yellow tint of the face and slightly yellow sclerae accompany pernicious anemia, which is also manifested by neurologic deficits and a red, painful tongue. Also, fatigue, exertional dyspnea, rapid pulse, dizziness, and impaired mental function accompany the most severe anemia (Overfield, 1995).

Erythema

You might find that it is difficult to assess **erythema** (redness) in darkly pigmented clients. Erythema is frequently associated with localized inflammation and is characterized by increased skin temperature. The degree of redness is determined by the quantity of blood in the subpapillary plexus, whereas the warmth of the skin is related to the rate of blood flow through the blood vessels. In the assessment of inflammation in dark-skinned clients, it is often necessary to palpate the skin for increased warmth, tautness, or tightly pulled surfaces that might indicate edema, and hardening of deep tissues or blood vessels. You will find that the dorsal surfaces of your fingers will be the most sensitive to temperature sensations. The erythema associated with rashes is not always accompanied by noticeable increases in skin temperature. Macular, papular, and vesicular skin lesions are identified by a combination of palpation and inspection. In addition, it is important that you listen to the client's description of symptoms. For example, persons with macular rashes usually will complain of itching, and evidence of scratching will be apparent. When the skin is only moderately pigmented, a macular rash might become recognizable if the skin is gently stretched. Stretching the skin decreases the normal red tone, thus providing more contrast and making the macules appear brighter. In some skin disorders with a generalized rash, you will observe that the rash is most readily visible on the hard and soft palates (Overfield, 1995).

The increased redness that accompanies carbon monoxide poisoning and the blood disorders collectively known as *polycythemia* can be observed on the lips of dark-skinned clients. Because lipstick masks the actual color of the lips, you should ask the client to remove it prior to inspection.

Petechiae

In dark-skinned clients, **petechiae** are best visualized in the areas of lighter melanization, such as the abdomen, buttocks, and volar surface of the forearm. When the skin is black or very dark brown, petechiae cannot be seen in the skin. Most of the diseases that cause bleeding and the formation of microscopic emboli, such as thrombocytopenia, subacute bacterial endocarditis, and other septicemias, are characterized by petechiae in the mucous membranes and skin. Petechiae are most easily seen in the mouth, particularly the buccal mucosa, and in the conjunctiva of the eye (Overfield, 1995).

Ecchymoses

In assessing **ecchymotic lesions** caused by systemic disorders, you will find them in the same locations as petechiae, although their larger size makes them more apparent on dark-skinned individuals. When you are differentiating petechiae and ecchymoses from erythema in the mucous membrane, pressure on the tissue will momentarily blanch erythema but not petechiae or ecchymoses.

Normal Age-Related Skin Changes

Although aging is accompanied by the growing presence of wrinkles in all cultures, Blacks, Asian Americans, American Indians, and Eskimos wrinkle later in life than their Anglo American counterparts. Light skin shows the effects of sun damage more than dark skin, regardless of race or ethnicity. The area of the skin that is exposed to the sun shows the effects of aging more than protected skin, such as those parts covered by clothing. Regardless of climate, dry skin is inevitable in individuals past 70 years of age. In part, dry skin is caused by transepidermal water loss, which decreases in older adults. African Americans have a significantly higher transepidermal water loss than Whites, which correlates with the water content of the stratum corneum layer of the skin. Because the number of *moles* increases with age, they are thought to be the result of long-term exposure to the sun. People with lighter skin have more moles than those with darkly pigmented skin. Whites have more moles than Asian North Americans or African Americans (Overfield, 1995).

Nurses and other health care providers often over- or underestimate the age when dealing with clients whose cultural heritage is different from their own. Whites tend to underestimate the age of Africans, Asians, and North American Indians, whereas African Americans, Asians, and North American Indians tend to overestimate the age of White clients (Overfield, 1995).

Biocultural Variations in Body Secretions

The *apocrine* and *eccrine sweat glands* are important for fluid balance and for thermoregulation. Approximately 2 to 3 million glands open onto the skin surface through pores and are responsible for the presence of sweat. When they are contaminated by normal skin flora, odor results. Most Asians and Native North Americans have a mild to absent body odor, whereas Whites and African Americans tend to have strong body odor.

Eskimos have made an environmental adaptation whereby they sweat less than Whites on their trunks and extremities but more on their faces. This adaptation allows for temperature regulation without causing perspiration and dampness of their clothes, which would decrease their ability to insulate against severe weather and would pose a serious threat to their survival.

The amount of chloride excreted by sweat glands varies widely, and African Americans have lower salt concentrations in their sweat than do Whites. A study of Ashkenazi Jews (of European descent) and Sephardic Jews (of North African and Middle Eastern descent) revealed that those of European origin had a lower percentage of sweat chlorides (Levin, 1966). This variation might be significant in the care of clients with renal or cardiac conditions or of children with cystic fibrosis (Overfield, 1995).

Biocultural Variation in the Head, Eyes, Ears, and Mouth

Hair

Perhaps one of the most obvious and widely variable cultural differences occurs with assessment of the hair. African Americans' hair varies widely in texture. It is very fragile and ranges from long and straight to short, spiraled, thick, and kinky. The hair and scalp have a natural tendency to be dry and to require daily combing, gentle brushing, and the application of oil. By comparison, clients of Asian backgrounds generally have straight, silky hair.

Obtaining a baseline hair assessment is significant in the diagnosis and treatment of certain disease states. For example, hair texture is known to become dry, brittle, and lusterless with inadequate nutrition. The hair of Black children with severe malnutrition, as in the case of marasmus, frequently changes not only in texture but also in color. The child's hair often becomes straighter and turns a reddish copper color. Certain endocrine disorders are also known to affect the texture of hair.

Although gray hair correlates with age for both men and women, there are cultural differences in the rate of hair graying. Whites gray significantly faster than any other group. The hair of 66% of fair-haired individuals, but only 37% of dark-haired persons, is fully white by age 60 (Overfield, 1995). Among Asian Americans, graying might be delayed significantly, with some in their eighth or ninth decade of life showing little or no graying.

Eyes

Biocultural differences in both the structure and the color of the eyes are readily apparent among clients from various cultural backgrounds. Racial differences are evident in the palpebral fissures. Persons of Asian background are often identified by their characteristic epicanthal eye folds, whereas the presence of narrowed palpebral fissures in non-Asian individuals might be diagnostic of a serious congenital anomaly known as *Down syndrome* or *trisomy 21*.

There is culturally based variability in the color of the iris and in retinal pigmentation: darker irises are correlated with darker retinas. Clients with light retinas generally have better night vision but can experience pain in an environment that is too light. The majority of African Americans and Asians have brown eyes, whereas many individuals of Scandinavian descent have blue eyes (Overfield, 1995).

It is clinically relevant that differences in visual acuity occur among people from different cultures. Blacks have poorer corrected visual acuity than Whites. The visual acuity of Hispanic Americans is between that of Blacks and Whites. American Indians are comparable to Whites in visual acuity, whereas Japanese and Chinese Americans have the poorest corrected visual acuity because of a high incidence of myopia (Overfield, 1995).

Ears

It does not take long to notice that ears come in a variety of sizes and shapes. Earlobes can be freestanding or attached to the face. Ceruminous glands are located in the external ear canal and are functional at birth. Cerumen is genetically determined and comes in two major types: (1) dry cerumen, which is gray and flaky and frequently forms a thin mass in the ear canal, and (2) wet cerumen, which is dark brown and moist. Asians and Native North Americans (including Eskimos) have an 84% frequency of dry cerumen, whereas African Americans have a 99% frequency and Whites have a 97% frequency of wet cerumen (Overfield, 1995). The clinical significance of this occurs when you are examining or irrigating the ears. You should be aware that the presence and composition of cerumen are not related to poor hygiene, and caution should be exercised to avoid mistaking flaky, dry cerumen for the dry lesions of eczema.

Hearing gradually declines with age, especially in the high frequencies. After age 40, men have poorer hearing than women. Blacks have better hearing at high and low frequencies, whereas Whites have better hearing at middle frequencies. Blacks are less susceptible to noise-induced hearing loss (Overfield, 1995).

Mouth

Oral hyperpigmentation also shows variation by race. Usually absent at birth, hyperpigmentation increases with age. By age 50 years, 10% of Whites and 50 to 90% of African Americans will show oral hyperpigmentation, a condition believed to be caused by a lifetime of accumulation of postinflammatory oral changes (Overfield, 1995).

Cleft uvula, a condition in which the uvula is split either completely or partially, occurs in 18% of some Native North American groups and 10% of Asians. The occurrence in Whites and Blacks is rare. *Cleft lip* and *cleft palate* are most common in Asians and Native North Americans and least common in African Americans (Overfield, 1995).

Leukoedema, a grayish white benign lesion occurring on the buccal mucosa, is present in 68 to 90% of Blacks but only 43% of Whites. Care should be taken to avoid mistaking leukoedema for oral thrush or related infections that require treatment with medication (Overfield, 1995).

Teeth

Because teeth are often used as indicators of developmental, hygienic, and nutritional adequacy, you should be aware of biocultural differences. Although it is rare for a White baby to be born with teeth (1 in 3,000), the incidence rises to 1 in 11 among Tlingit Indian infants and to 1 or 2 in 100 among Canadian Eskimo infants. Although congenital teeth are usually not problematic, extraction is necessary for some breast-fed infants (Overfield, 1995).

The size of teeth varies widely, with the teeth of Whites being the smallest, followed by Blacks and then Asians and Native North Americans. The largest teeth are found among Eskimos and Australian Aborigines. Larger teeth cause somFe groups to have prognathic, (protruding) jaws, a condition that is seen more frequently in African and Asian North Americans. The condition is normal and does not reflect a serious orthodontic problem.

Agenesis (absence of teeth) varies by race, with missing third molars occurring in 18 to 35% of Asians, 9 to 25% of Whites, and 1 to 11% of Blacks. Throughout life, Whites have more tooth decay than Blacks, which might be related to a combination of socioeconomic factors and biocultural variation. Complete tooth loss occurs more often in Whites than in African Americans despite the higher incidence of periodontal disease in Blacks. Approximately one third of Whites 45 years or older have lost all their teeth, compared with 25% of Blacks in the same age group (Overfield, 1995).

The differences in tooth decay between African Americans and Whites can be explained by the fact that African Americans have harder and denser tooth enamel, which makes their teeth less susceptible to the organisms that cause caries. The increase in periodontal disease among African Americans is believed to be caused by poor oral hygiene. When obvious signs of periodontal disease are present, such as bleeding and edematous gums, a dental referral should be initiated (Overfield, 1995).

Biocultural Variations in the Mammary Venous Plexus

Regardless of gender, the superficial veins of the chest form a network over the entire chest that flows in either a transverse or a longitudinal pattern. In the transverse pattern, the veins radiate laterally and toward the axillae. In the longitudinal pattern, the veins radiate downward and laterally like a fan. These two patterns occur with different frequencies in the two populations that have been studied. The recessive longitudinal pattern occurs in 6 to 10% of White women and in 30% of Navajos. The only known alteration of either pattern is produced by breast tumor. Although this variation has no clinical significance, it is mentioned so that if nurses note its presence during physical assessment, they will recognize it as a nonsignificant finding (Overfield, 1995).

Biocultural Variation in the Musculoskeletal System

Many normal biocultural variations are found in clients' musculoskeletal systems. The long bones of Blacks are significantly longer, narrower, and denser than those of Whites. Bone density measured by race and sex show that Black males have the densest bones, thus accounting for the relatively low incidence of osteoporosis in this population. Bone density in Chinese, Japanese, and Eskimos is below that of Whites (Overfield, 1995).

Curvature of the body's long bones varies widely among culturally diverse groups. Native North Americans and First Nation People have anteriorly convex femurs, whereas Blacks have markedly straight femurs, and Whites have intermediate femurs. This characteristic is related to both genetics and body weight. The femurs of thin Blacks and Whites have less curvature than average, whereas those of obese Blacks and Whites display increased curvatures. It is possible that the heavier density of the bones of Blacks helps to protect them from increased curvature caused by obesity (Overfield, 1995). Table 3-6 summarizes biocultural variations occurring in the musculoskeletal system that have been identified through observation and study of people from various cultures and subcultures.

Biocultural Variations in Illness

Researchers have abundant evidence that there is a relationship between ethnicity and the incidence of certain diseases across the lifespan, from infancy to old age. The distribution of selected genetic traits and disorders prevalent among infants and children from selected cultural groups is shown in Chapter 6. Table 3-7 provides an alphabetical listing of selected diseases and their increased or decreased prevalence among members of certain cultural groups. A knowledge of normal biocultural variations and those occurring during illness helps nurses to conduct more accurate, comprehensive, and thorough physical examinations of clients from diverse cultures.

• LABORATORY TESTS

You should be aware that biocultural variations occur with some laboratory test results, such as measurement of *hemoglobin, hematocrit, cholesterol, serum transferrin,* and *blood glucose.* You also will want to consider cultural differences in the results of tests conducted during pregnancy. The *multiple-marker screening* test and two tests of *amniotic fluid constituents* are used to screen pregnant women for potential fetal problems. Although the reasons for these differences are unknown, genetic, environmental, dietary, socioeconomic, cultural, and lifestyle factors are being studied to determine the extent to which they contribute to the differences in test results. Table 3-8 identifies biocultural variations and their clinical significance for selected laboratory tests.

• CLINICAL DECISION MAKING AND NURSING ACTIONS

After you have completed a comprehensive cultural assessment, you are ready to analyze your subjective and objective data, set mutual goals with the client, develop a plan of care, make referrals as needed, and implement a plan of care, either alone or with others. Before **clinical decision making** or **nursing actions** can occur, you should identify the client's strengths and limitations, including his or her social support network: family, friends, clergy and other visitors from the

TABLE 3–6	BIOCULTURAL VARIATIONS IN THE MUSCULOSKELETAL SYSTEM

COMPONENT	REMARKS
Bone	
Frontal	Thicker in Black males than in White males
Parietal occiput	Thicker in White males than in Black males
Palate	Tori (protuberances) along the suture line of the hard palate
	Problematic for denture wearers
	Incidence:
	Blacks 20%
	Whites 24%
	Asians Up to 50%
	Native Americans Up to 50%
Mandible	Tori (protuberances) on the lingual surface of the mandible near the canine and premolar teeth
	Problematic for denture wearers
	Most common in Asians and Native Americans; exceeds 50% in some Eskimo groups
Humerus	Torsion or rotation of proximal end with muscle pull
	Whites > Blacks
	Torsion in Blacks is symmetric; torsion in Whites tends to be greater on right side than left side
Radius	Length at the wrist variable
Ulna	Ulna or radius may be longer
	Equal length
	Swedes 61%
	Chinese 16%
	Ulna longer than radius
	Swedes 16%
	Chinese 48%
	Radius longer than ulna
	Swedes 23%
	Chinese 10%
Vertebrae	Twenty-four vertebrae are found in 85 to 93% of all people; racial and sex differences reveal 23 or 25 vertebrae in select groups
	Vertebrae Population
	23 11% of Black females
	25 12% of Eskimo and Native American males
	Related to lower back pain and lordosis
Pelvis	Hip width is 1.6 cm (0.6 in) smaller in Black women than in White women; Asian women have significantly smaller pelvises

(continues)

TABLE 3-6	BIOCULTURAL VARIATIONS IN THE MUSCULOSKELETAL SYSTEM *(Continued)*

Femur	Convex anterior — Native American Straight — Black Intermediate — White
Second tarsal	Second toe longer than the great toe *Incidence:* 　Whites　　　8–34% 　Blacks　　　8–12% 　Vietnamese　31% 　Melanesians　21–57% Clinical significance for joggers and athletes
Height	White males are 1.27 cm (0.5 in) taller than Black males and 7.6 cm (2.9 in) taller than Asian males White females = Black females Asian females are 4.14 cm (1.6 in) shorter than White or Black females
Composition of long bones	Longer, narrower, and denser in Blacks than in Whites; bone density in Whites > Chinese, Japanese, and Eskimos Osteoporosis lowest in Black males; highest in White females
Muscle	
Peroneus tertius	Responsible for dorsiflexion of foot *Muscle absent:* 　Asians, Native Americans, and Whites　　3–10% 　Blacks　　　　　　　　　　　　　　　10–15% 　Berbers (Sahara desert)　　　　　　　24% No clinical significance because the tibialis anterior also dorsiflexes the foot
Palmaris longus	Responsible for wrist flexion *Muscle absent:* 　Whites　　　　　　12–20% 　Native Americans　2–12% 　Blacks　　　　　　5% 　Asians　　　　　　3% No clinical significance because three other muscles are also responsible for flexion

Based on data reported by T. Overfield (1995). *Biologic variation in health and illness: Race, age, and sex differences.* New York: CRC Press.

client's place of worship, ethnic or cultural organizations, or other sources that can be mobilized to assist the client. Next, you will want to determine whether there are client goals or needs for which professional nursing care is required.

(Text continues on page 70.)

TABLE 3–7	DISTRIBUTION OF SELECTED GENETIC TRAITS AND DISORDERS BY POPULATION OR ETHNIC GROUP

ETHNIC OR POPULATION GROUP	GENETIC OR MULTIFACTORIAL DISORDER PRESENT IN RELATIVELY HIGH FREQUENCY
Aland Islanders	Ocular albinism (Forsius-Eriksson type)
Amish	Limb girdle muscular dystrophy (IN—Adams, Allen counties)
	Ellis–van Creveld (PA—Lancaster county)
	Pyruvate kinase deficiency (OH—Mifflin county)
	Hemophilia B (PA—Holmes county)
Armenians	Familial Mediterranean fever
	Familial paroxysmal polyserositis
Blacks (African)	Sickle cell disease
	Hemoglobin C disease
	Hereditary persistence of hemoglobin F
	G6PD deficiency, African type
	Lactase deficiency, adult
	β-thalassemia
Burmese	Hemoglobin E disease
Chinese	α-thalassemia
	G6PD deficiency, Chinese type
	Lactase deficiency, adult
Costa Ricans	Malignant osteopetrosis
Druze	Alkaptonuria
English	Cystic fibrosis
	Hereditary amyloidosis, type III
Eskimos	Congenital adrenal hyperplasia
	Pseudocholinesterase deficiency
	Methemoglobinemia
French Canadians (Quebec)	Tyrosinemia
	Morqulo syndrome
Finns	Congenital nephrosis
	Generalized amyloidosis syndrome, V
	Polycystic liver disease
	Retinoschisis
	Aspartylglycosaminuria
	Diastrophic dwarfism
Gypsies (Czech)	Congenital glaucoma
Hopi Indians	Tyrosinase-positive albinism
Icelanders	Phenylketonuria
Irish	Phenylketonuria
	Neural tube defects
Japanese	Acatalasemia
	Cleft lip/palate
	Oguchi disease

TABLE 3–7	DISTRIBUTION OF SELECTED GENETIC TRAITS AND DISORDERS BY POPULATION OR ETHNIC GROUP *(Continued)*

Jews
   Ashkenazi
        Tay-Sachs disease (infantile)
        Niemann-Pick disease (infantile)
        Gaucher disease (adult type)
        Familial dysautonomia (Riley-Day syndrome)
        Bloom syndrome
        Torsion dystonia
        Factor XI (PTA) deficiency

   Sephardi
        Familial Mediterranean fever
        Ataxia-telangiectasia (Morocco)
        Cystinuria (Libya)
        Glycogen storage disease III (Morocco)

Orientals
        Dubin-Johnson syndrome (Iran)
        Ichthyosis vulgaris (Iraq, India)
        Werdnig-Hoffman disease (Karaite Jews)
        G6PD deficiency, Mediterranean type
        Phenylketonuria (Yemen)
        Metachromatic leukodystrophy (Habbanite Jews, Saudi Arabia)

Lapps   Congenital dislocation of hip
Lebanese   Dyggve-Melchoir-Clausen syndrome
Mediterranean people   G6PD deficiency, Mediterranean type
   (Italians, Greeks)   β-thalassemia
        Familial Mediterranean fever

Navaho Indians   Ear anomalies
Polynesians   Clubfoot
Poles   Phenylketonuria
Portuguese   Joseph disease
Nova Scotia Acadians   Niemann-Pick disease, type D
Scandinavians   Cholestasis-lymphedema (Norwegians)
   (Norwegians,   Sjögren-Larsson syndrome (Swedes)
   Swedes, Danes)   Krabbe disease
        Phenylketonuria

Scots   Phenylketonuria
        Cystic fibrosis
        Hereditary amyloidosis, type III

Thai   Lactase deficiency, adult
        Hemoglobin E disease

Zuni Indians   Tyrosinase-positive albinism

From Cohen, F. L. (1984). *Clinical Genetics in Nursing Practice* (pp. 23–24). Philadelphia: J.B. Lippincott. Reprinted by permission.

| TABLE 3–8 | BIOCULTURAL VARIATIONS AND CLINICAL SIGNIFICANCE FOR SELECTED LABORATORY TESTS |

TEST	REMARKS
Hemoglobin/hematocrit	1 g lower for Blacks than other groups; Blacks < counter parts in other groups
Serum transferrin	Biocultural variation in children aged 1–3 1/2 years Mean for Blacks 22 mg/100 mL > Whites *Note:* May be due to lowered hemoglobin and hematocrit levels found in Blacks *Clinical significance:* Transferrin levels increase in the presence of anemia, thus influencing the diagnosis, treatment, and nursing care of children with anemia.
Serum cholesterol	Biocultural variation across the life span Birth Blacks = whites Childhood Blacks 5 mg/100 mL > Whites Pima Indians 20-30 mg/100 mL > Whites Adulthood Blacks < Whites Pima Indians 50-60 ml/100 mL < Whites *Clinical significance:* Prevention, treatment, and nursing care of clients with cardiovascular disease
High-density lipoproteins (HDL)	Biocultural variation in adults Blacks > Whites Asians ≥ Whites Mexican North Americans < Whites
Ratio of HDL to total cholesterol	Blacks < Whites
Low-density lipoproteins (LDL)	Biocultural variation in adults Blacks < whites *Clinical significance:* Prevention, treatment, and nursing care of clients with cardiovascular disease
Blood glucose	Biocultural variation in adults North American Indians, Hispanics, Japanese > Whites Blacks = Whites (for equivalent socioeconomic groups) *Clinical significance:* Diagnosis, treatment and nursing care of adults with hypoglycemia and diabetes mellitus
Multiple-marker screening	Biocultural variations in blood levels for protein and hormones in pregnant women Alphafetoprotein (AFP), hCG, and estriol levels in Black and Asian women > Whites

TABLE 3–8	BIOCULTURAL VARIATIONS AND CLINICAL SIGNIFICANCE FOR SELECTED LABORATORY TESTS *(Continued)*

TEST	REMARKS
	Clinical significance: High AFP levels signal that the woman is at increased risk for being delivered of an infant with spina bifida and neural tube defects, whereas low levels may signal Down syndrome; Down syndrome also is associated with low levels of estriol and high levels of hCG Black and Asian American women have higher average levels of AFP, hCG, and estriol than White counterparts Using a single median for women of all cultures: • Causes Black and Asian women to be *falsely* identified as being *at risk* for having infants with spina bifida and neural tube defects; by being classified as *high risk,* women are more likely to be subjected to invasive and expensive procedures such as amniocentesis; some may elect to abort the pregnancy based on screening test results. • *Inappropriately lowers* the identified Down syndrome risk for Black and Asian women
Lecithin/sphingomyelin ratio	Biocultural variations in amniotic fluid measures of fetal pulmonary maturity Blacks have higher ratios than Whites from 23 to 42 weeks gestation *Clinical significance:* the ratio is used to calculate the risk of respiratory distress in premature infants: lung maturity in Blacks is reached 1 week earlier than in Whites (34 versus 35 weeks); racial differences should be considered in making decisions about inducing labor or delivering by Cesarean section.

Table based on data from

Allanson, A., Michie, S., & Matreau, T. M. (1997). Presentation of screen negative results on serum screening for Down's Syndrome. *Journal of Medical Screening, 4*(1), 21–22.

Chapman, S. J., Brumfield, C. G., Wenstrom, K. D., & DuBard, M. B. (1997). Pregnancy outcomes following false-positive multiple marker screening test. *American Journal of Perinatology, 14*(8), 475–478.

O'Brien, J. E., Dvorin, E., Drugan, A., Johnson, M. P., Yaron, Y., & Evans, M. I. (1997). Race-ethnicity-specific variation in multiple-marker biochemical screening: Alpha-fetoprotein, hCG, and estriol. *Obstetrics and Gynecology, 89*(3), 355–358.

Overfield, T. (1995). *Biologic variation in health and illness: Race, age, and sex differences.* New York: CRC Press.

Modes to Guide Nursing Judgments, Decisions, and Actions

Leininger (1991) suggests three major modalities to guide nursing judgments, decisions, and actions for the purpose of providing culturally congruent care that is beneficial, satisfying, and meaningful to the people served by nurses. The three modes are *cultural preservation or maintenance, cultural care accommodation or negotiation,* and *cultural care repatterning or restructuring.* Let us briefly examine each of these modes.

Cultural preservation or maintenance refers to "those assistive, supporting, facilitative, or enabling professional actions and decisions that help people of a particular culture to retain and/or preserve relevant care values so that they can maintain their well-being, recover from illness, or face handicaps and/or death" (Leininger, 1991).

Cultural care accommodation or negotiation refers to "those assistive, supporting, facilitative, or enabling creative professional actions and decisions that help people of a designated culture to adapt to, or to negotiate with, others for beneficial or satisfying health outcome with professional care-providers" (Leininger, 1991 p.48). Cultural negotiation is sometimes referred to as *culture brokering.*

Cultural care repatterning or restructuring refers to "those assistive, supporting, facilitative, or enabling professional actions and decisions that help a client(s) reorder, change, or greatly modify their lifeways for new, different, and beneficial health care pattern while respecting the client(s) cultural values and beliefs and still providing a beneficial or healthier lifeway than before the changes were coestablished with the client(s)" (Leininger, 1991, p. 49).

These modes are care-centered and based on use of the client's care knowledge. Negotiation increases understanding between the client and the nurse and promotes culturally congruent nursing care.

Evaluation

Evaluation of the effectiveness of clinical decisions and nursing actions should occur in collaboration with the client and his or her significant others—which may include members of the extended family, traditional healers, those with culturally determined nonsanguine relationships, and friends. A careful evaluation of each component of the transcultural nursing interaction should be undertaken in collaboration with the client. It may be necessary to gather further data, reinterpret existing findings, redefine mutual nurse-client goals, or renegotiate the roles and responsibilities of nurses, clients, and members of their support system.

The previous discussion has focused, to a large extent, on the individual during the period of hospitalization or while being cared for by nurses in the home or community environment. Next, we will look at the issue of evaluation after discharge. In the current managed care environment, there is growing emphasis on patient or client *outcomes* and reported satisfaction with the care provided by nurses and other health care providers. You will need to participate in the establishment of *quality assurance, total quality management,* and/or *continuous quality improvement* initiatives aimed at gathering information from clients/patients about their overall satisfaction with care. You also need to assure that the process and instruments are culturally appropriate. For example, how are the needs of linguistically diverse clients met? Is translation or interpretation available? Are the questions asked in a culturally appropriate manner? It is imperative that nurses be included in all aspects of the evaluation and that they use feedback to improve their nursing care in the future.

SUMMARY

In this chapter we have examined transcultural perspectives on the health history and physical examination, key components of the cultural assessment. In the first section we have provided an overview of the major data categories that nurses should consider if they are to demonstrate cultural competence in conducting the health history. In the second section we have identified biocultural variations in the physical examination in health and illness. In the final section we have examined cultural factors that influence clinical decision making, nursing actions, and evaluation.

REVIEW QUESTIONS

1. In your own words, describe the key components of cultural assessment.
2. Analyze the difference in body proportions, height, and weight among clients from diverse cultural backgrounds, and indicate the reasons for differences among the groups.
3. Compare and contrast your approach to the assessment of light- and dark-skinned clients for cyanosis, jaundice, pallor, erythema, and petechiae.
4. Review the biocultural variations in laboratory tests for hemoglobin, hematocrit, serum cholesterol, serum transferrin, multiple-marker screening, and amniotic fluid constituents.
5. Critically analyze the reasons for the current interest in ethnopharmacology by nurses, physicians, pharmacists, and other health care providers. How does knowledge of ethnopharmacology and cultural differences in response to medications facilitate your ability to provide culturally competent and congruent nursing care?

CRITICAL THINKING ACTIVITIES

1. Critically analyze the instrument, tool, or form used by nurses when conducting an initial patient or resident *admission assessment* at a hospital, extended care facility, or other health care agency in terms of its relevance to the health and nursing needs of persons from diverse cultures. From a transcultural nursing perspective, identify the *strengths* and *limitations* of

the admission assessment instrument. What suggestions would you make to enhance the effectiveness of the instrument in assessing the cultural needs of newly admitted patients or residents? Be sure to consider the *practical* constraints that nurses face in the current managed care environment, such as time limitations, external forces that require us to care for increasingly large numbers of patients, and other constraints, before you suggest modifications.

2. Using the Andrews and Boyle Transcultural Nursing Assessment Guide (Appendix B), answer the questions in each data category as they apply to *yourself*. As you write your responses to the questions, critically reflect on your own health-related cultural values, attitudes, beliefs, and practices.

3. Using the Andrews/Boyle Transcultural Nursing Assessment Guide (Appendix B), interview someone from a cultural background different from your own to assess his or her health-related cultural values, attitudes, beliefs, and practices. After you have completed the interview, compare and contrast those responses with your own responses in Question 2. Identify the ways in which you are *alike*. Critically analyze the *differences* as potential sources of cross-cultural conflict, and explore ways in which they might influence the nurse–client interaction.

4. Conduct a head-to-toe physical examination of a person from a racial background different from your own. Summarize your findings in writing. In a constructively self-critical manner, reflect on what aspects of the exam were (a) easiest and (b) most difficult for you. Try to determine the reason(s) why some aspects were relatively easy or difficult for you. What further information or skill development would assist you in gaining confidence in your ability to conduct physical examinations on people from diverse racial backgrounds?

• References

Andrews, M. M., & Boyle, J. S. (1997). Competence in transcultural nursing care. *American Journal of Nursing, 97*(8), 16AAA–16DDD.

Farnsworth, N. R. (1993). Ethnopharmacology and future drug development: The North American experience. *Journal of Ethnopharmacology, 38,* 145–152.

Good, B. J., & Good, M. J. (1980). The meaning of symptoms: A cultural hermeneutic model for clinical practice. In L. Eisenberg & A. Kleinman (Eds.). *The relevance of social science for medicine.* Boston: D. Reidel.

Jarvis, C. (2000). *Physical examination and health assessment.* Philadelphia: W. B. Saunders.

Kleinman, A. (1980). *Patients and healers in the context of culture.* Berkeley, CA: University of California Press.

Kleinman, A., Eisenberg, L., & Good, B. (1978). Culture, illness and care: Clinical lessons from anthropologic and cross-cultural research. *Annals of Internal Medicine, 88,* 251–258.

Leininger, M. M. (1991). Culture care diversity and universalty; A Theory of Nursing. NY: NLN Press.

Leininger, M. M. (1995). *Transcultural nursing: Concepts, theories, research and practices.* New York: McGraw-Hill.

Leininger, M. M., & McFarland, M. R.(2002). *Transcultural nursing: Concepts, theories, research and practices.* New York: McGraw-Hill.

Levin, S. (1966). Effect of age, ethnic background and disease on sweat chloride. *Israeli Journal of Medical Science, 2*(3), 333–337.

Overfield, T. (1995). *Biologic variation in health and illness.* New York: CRC Press.

Wenger, A. F. (1993). Cultural meaning of symptoms. *Holistic Nursing Practice, 7*(2), 22–35.

The Influence of Cultural and Health Belief Systems on Health Care Practices

Margaret M. Andrews

KEY TERMS

Allopathic medicine
Care meanings
Complementary and alternative medicine
Cultural belief systems
Folk healing system
Folk healers

Health behavior
Health belief system
Holistic health paradigm
Hot/cold theory of disease
Healing system
Illness behavior
Magico-religious paradigm
Metaphor

Paradigm
Professional care system
Scientific paradigm
Self-care
Sick role behavior
Worldview
Yin and yang

OBJECTIVES

1. Describe the major cultural belief systems of people from diverse cultures.
2. Compare and contrast professional and folk healing systems.
3. Identify the major complementary and alternative health care therapies.
4. Describe the influence of culture on symptoms and illness behaviors
5. Critically analyze the efficacy of selected herbal remedies in the treatment of health problems.

In this chapter we shall examine the major cultural belief systems embraced by people from diverse cultures and explore the characteristics of three of the most prevalent worldviews, or paradigms, related to health-illness beliefs: the magico-religious, the scientific/biomedical, and the holistic health paradigms. We shall explore self-treatment, professional care systems, and folk (indigenous, traditional, generic) care systems and their respective healers. After analyzing the influence of culture on symptoms and sick role and illness behaviors, we shall examine selected complementary and alternative therapies used to treat physical and psychologic diseases and illnesses.

• CULTURAL BELIEF SYSTEMS

Cultural meanings and **cultural belief systems** develop from the shared experiences of a group in society and are expressed symbolically. The use of symbols to define, describe, and relate to the world around us is one of the basic characteristics of being human. One of the most common expressions of symbolism is the **metaphor.** In metaphor, one aspect of life is connected to another through a shared symbol. For example, the phrases "what a tangled web we weave" and "all the world's a stage" express metaphorically the relationship between two normally disparate concepts (such as human deception and a spider's web). People often use metaphors as a way of thinking about and explaining life's events.

Every group of people has found it necessary to explain the phenomena of nature. From the explanations developed emerges a common belief system. The explanations usually involve metaphoric imagery of magical, religious, natural/holistic, or biologic form. The range of explanations is limited only by the human imagination.

The set of metaphoric explanations used by a group of people to explain life's events and to offer solutions to life's mysteries can be viewed as the group's **worldview.** A worldview can also be defined as a major paradigm. A **paradigm**, like any general perspective, is a way of viewing the world and the phenomena in it. A paradigm includes the assumptions, premises, and glue that hold together a prevailing interpretation of reality. Paradigms are slow to change and do so only if and when their explanatory power has been exhausted.

The worldview developed reflects the group's total configuration of beliefs and practices and permeates every aspect of life within the culture of that group. Members of a culture share a worldview without necessarily recognizing it. Thinking itself is patterned on this worldview, because the culture imparts a particular set of symbols to be used in thinking. Because these symbols are taken for granted, people do not normally question the cultural bias of their very thoughts. The use in the United States of the term *American* reflects such an unconscious cultural bias. This term is understood by citizens of the United States to refer only to themselves collectively, although in reality it is a generic term referring to anyone in this hemisphere, including Canadians, Mexicans, Colombians, and so on.

Another example of symbolism and worldview can be seen in the way nurses use terms such as *nursing care, health promotion,* and *illness and disease.* Nurses often take for granted that all their clients define and relate to these concepts in the same way they do. This reflects an unconscious belief that the same cultural symbols are shared by all and therefore do not require reinterpretation in any given nurse-client context. Such an assumption accounts for many of the problems nurses face when they try to communicate with others who are not members of the *health profession culture.*

• HEALTH BELIEF SYSTEMS

Generally, theories of health and disease/illness causation are based on the prevailing worldview held by a group. These worldviews include a group's health-related attitudes, beliefs, and practices and frequently are referred to as health belief systems. Three major **health belief systems** or worldviews are embraced by people: magico-religious, scientific, and holistic, each with its own corresponding system of health beliefs. In two of these worldviews, disease is thought of as an entity separate from self, caused by an agent that is external to the body but capable of "getting in" and causing damage. This causative agent has been attributed to a variety of natural and supernatural phenomena.

Magico-Religious Health Paradigm

In the **magico-religious paradigm** the world is an arena in which supernatural forces dominate. The fate of the world and those in it, including humans, depends on the actions of God, or the gods, or other supernatural forces for good or evil. In some cases, the human individual is at the mercy of such forces regardless of behavior. In other cases, the gods punish humans for their transgressions. Many Latino, African American, and Middle Eastern cultures are grounded in the magico-religious paradigm. Magic involves the calling forth and control of supernatural forces for and against others. Some African and Caribbean cultures, e.g., voodoo, have aspects of magic in their belief systems. In Western cultures there are examples of this paradigm, in which metaphysical reality interrelates with human society. For instance, Christian Scientists believe that physical healing can be effected through prayer alone.

Ackerknecht (1971) states that "magic or religion seems to satisfy better than any other device a certain eternal psychic or 'metaphysical' need of mankind, sick and healthy, for integration and harmony." Magic and religion are logical in their own way, but not on the basis of empiric premises; that is, they defy the demands of the physical world and the use of one's senses, particularly observation. In the magico-religious paradigm, disease is viewed as the action and result of supernatural forces that cause the intrusion of a disease-producing foreign body or the entrance of a health-damaging spirit.

Widespread throughout the world are five categories of events that are believed to be responsible for illness in the magico-religious paradigm. These categories, derived from the work of Clements (1932) are sorcery, breach of taboo, intrusion of a disease object, intrusion of a disease-causing spirit, and loss of soul. One of these belief categories, or any combination of them, may be offered to explain the origin of disease. Eskimos, for example, refer to soul loss and breach of taboo (breaking a social norm, such as committing adultery). West Indians and some African and American Blacks believe that the malevolence of sorcerers is the cause of many conditions. *Mal ojo,* or the evil eye, common in Latino and other cultures, can be viewed as the intrusion of a disease-causing spirit.

In the magico-religious paradigm, illness is initiated by a supernatural agent with or without justification, or by another person who practices sorcery or engages the services of sorcerers. The cause-and-effect relationship is not an organic one; rather, the cause of health or illness is mystical. Health is seen as a gift or reward given as a sign of God's blessing and good will. Illness may be seen as a sign of God's special favor, insofar as it gives the affected person the opportunity to become resigned to God's will, or it may be seen as a sign of God's possession or as a punishment. For example, in many Christian religions the faithful gather communally to pray to God to heal the ill or to practice healing rituals such as laying on of hands or anointing the sick with oil.

In addition, in this paradigm, health and illness are viewed as belonging first to the community and then to the individual. Therefore, one person's actions may directly or indirectly influence the health or illness of another person. This sense of community is virtually absent from the other paradigms.

Scientific or Biomedical Health Paradigm

The **scientific paradigm** is the newest and most removed from the interpersonal human arena of life. According to this worldview, life is controlled by a series of physical and biochemical processes that can be studied and manipulated by humans. Several specific forms of symbolic thought processes characterize the scientific paradigm. The first is determinism, which states that a cause-and-effect relationship exists for all natural phenomena. The second, mechanism, relates life to the structure and function of machines; according to mechanism, it is possible to control life processes through mechanical and other engineered interventions. The third form is reductionism, according to which all life can be reduced or divided into smaller parts; study of the unique characteristics of these isolated parts is thought to reveal aspects or properties of the whole. One idea of reductionism is Cartesian dualism: the idea that the mind and the body can be separated into two distinct entities. The final thought process is objective materialism, according to which what is real can be observed and measured. There is a further distinction between subjective and objective realities in this paradigm.

The scientific paradigm disavows the metaphysical. It usually ignores the holistic forces of the universe as well, unless explanations for such forces fit into the symbolic forms discussed above. Members of most Western cultures, including the dominant cultural groups in the United States and Canada, espouse this paradigm. When the scientific paradigm is applied to matters of health, it is often referred to as the biomedical model.

Biomedical beliefs and concepts dominate medical thought in Western societies and must be understood to appreciate the practice of modern health care. In the biomedical model, all aspects of human health can be understood in physical and chemical terms. This fosters the belief that psychologic processes can be reduced to the study of biochemical exchanges. Only the organic is real and worthy of study. Effective treatment consists of physical and chemical interventions, regardless of human relationships.

In this model, disease is viewed metaphorically as the breakdown of the human machine as a result of wear and tear (stress), external trauma (injury, accident), external invasion (pathogens), or internal damages (fluid and chemical imbalances or structural changes). Disease is held to cause illness, to have a more or less specific cause, and to have a predictable time course and set of treatment requirements. This paradigm is similar to the magico-religious belief in external agents, having replaced supernatural forces with infectious agents.

Using the metaphor of the machine, Western medicine uses specialists to take care of the "parts"; "fixing" a part enables the machine to function. The computer is the analogy for the brain; engineering is a task for biomedical practitioners. The discovery of DNA and human genome research have led to the field of genetic engineering, an eloquent biomedical metaphor. The symbols used to discuss health and disease reflect the North American cultural values of aggression and mastery: microorganisms attack the body, war is raged against these invaders, money is donated for the campaign against cancer, and illness is a struggle in which the patient must put up a good defense. The biomedical model defines health as the absence of disease or the signs and symptoms of disease. To be healthy, one must be free of all disease.

Holistic Health Paradigm

The **holistic health paradigm** is similar to the magico-religious worldview. In the holistic paradigm, the forces of nature itself must be kept in natural balance or *harmony*. Human life is only one aspect of nature and a part of the general order of the cosmos. Everything in the universe has a place and a role to perform according to natural laws that maintain order. Disturbing these laws creates imbalance, chaos, and disease. The holistic paradigm has existed for centuries in many parts of the world, particularly in North American Indian cultures and Asian cultures. It is gaining increasing acceptance in the United States and Canada because it complements a growing awareness that the biomedical view fails to account fully for most diseases as they naturally occur.

The holistic paradigm seeks to maintain a sense of balance or harmony between humans and the larger universe. Explanations for health and disease are based not so much on external agents as on imbalance or disharmony among the human, geophysical, and metaphysical forces of the universe. For example, in the biomedical model, the cause of tuberculosis is clearly defined as the invasion of the mycobacterium. In the holistic paradigm, whereby disease is the result of multiple environment-host interactions, tuberculosis is caused by the interrelationship of poverty, malnutrition, overcrowding, and the mycobacterium. The holistic worldview is well illustrated in Silko's 1988 novel *Ceremony,* which is based on the experiences of a young Navajo man confronted with mental illness.

The term *holistic,* coined in 1926 by Jan Christian Smuts, defines an attitude or mode of perception in which the whole person is viewed in the context of the total environment. Its Indo-European root word, *kailo,* means "whole, intact, or uninjured." From this root have come the words *hale, hail, hallow, holy, whole, heal,* and *health.* The essence of health and healing is the quality of wholeness we associate with healthy functioning and well-being.

In this paradigm, health is viewed as a positive process that encompasses more than the absence of signs and symptoms of disease. It is not restricted to biologic or somatic wellness but rather involves broader environmental, sociocultural, and behavioral determinants. In this model, *diseases of civilization,* such as unemployment, racial discrimination, ghettos, and suicide, are just as much illnesses as are biomedical diseases.

Metaphors used in this paradigm, such as *healing power of nature, health foods,* and *Mother Earth,* reflect the connection of humans to the cosmos and nature. Voltaire's statement that an efficient physician is one who successfully bemuses the patient so that nature can effect a cure stems from this belief. The belief system of Florence Nightingale, who emphasized nursing's control of the environment so that patients could heal naturally, was also holistic.

A strong metaphor in the holistic paradigm is exemplified by the Chinese concept of **yin** and **yang**, in which the forces of nature are balanced to produce harmony. The *yin* force in the universe represents the female aspect of nature. It is characterized as the negative pole, encompassing darkness, cold, and emptiness. The *yang,* or male force, is characterized by fullness, light, and warmth. It represents the positive pole. An imbalance of forces creates illness.

Illness is the outward expression of disharmony. This disharmony may result from seasonal changes, emotional imbalances, or any other pattern of events. Illness is not perceived as an intruding agent but as a natural part of life's rhythmic course. Going in and out of balance is seen as a natural process that happens constantly throughout the life cycle. No sharp line is drawn between health and illness; both are seen as natural and as being part of a continuum. They are aspects of the same process, in which the individual organism changes continually in relation to the changing environment.

In the holistic health paradigm, because illness is inevitable, perfect health is not the goal. Rather, achieving the best possible adaptation to the environment by living according to society's rules and caring appropriately for one's body is the ultimate aim. This places a greater emphasis on preventive and maintenance measures than does Western medicine.

Another common metaphor for health and illness in this paradigm is the **hot/cold theory of disease**. This is founded on the ancient Greek concept of the four body humors: yellow bile, black bile, phlegm, and blood. These humors are balanced in the healthy individual. The treatment of disease becomes the process of restoring the body's humoral balance through the addition or subtraction of substances that affect each of these humors. Foods, beverages, herbs, and other drugs are all classified as hot or cold depending on their effect, not their actual physical state. Disease conditions are also classified as either hot or cold. Imbalance or disharmony is thought to result in internal damage and altered physiologic functions. Medicine is directed at correcting the imbalance as well as restoring body functioning. Each cultural group defines what it believes to be hot and cold entities, and little agreement exists across cultures, although the concept of hot and cold is itself widespread, being found in Asian, Latino, Black, Arab, Muslim, and Caribbean societies.

• HEALTH AND ILLNESS BEHAVIORS

The series of behaviors typifying the health-seeking process have been labeled *health and illness behaviors.* These behaviors are expressed in the roles people assume after identifying a symptom. Related to these behaviors are the roles individuals assign to others and the status given to the role players. Kasl and Cobb (1966) first defined the types of behaviors clients assume once they have recognized a symptom. **Health behavior** is any activity taken by a person who believes himself or herself to be healthy for the purpose of preventing disease or detecting disease in an asymptomatic stage. **Illness behavior** is any activity undertaken by a person who feels ill for the purpose of defining the state of his health and of discovering a suitable remedy. **role behavior** is any activity undertaken by a person who considers himself ill for the purpose of getting well.

Three sets of factors influence the course of behaviors and practices carried out to maintain health and prevent disease: (1) one's beliefs about health and illness; (2) personal factors such as age, education, and knowledge or experience with a given disease condition; and (3) cues to action, such as advertisements in the media, the illness of a relative, or the advice of friends.

A useful model of illness behavior has been proposed by Mechanic (1978), who outlines 10 determinants of illness behavior that are important in the help-seeking process (Table 4–1). Knowledge of these factors can help the nurse appreciate the client's behaviors and decisions about seeking and complying with health care. Awareness of these motivational factors can help nurses offer the appropriate assistance to clients as they work through the illness process.

• TYPES OF HEALING SYSTEMS

The term **healing system** refers to the accumulated sciences, arts, and techniques of restoring and preserving health that are used by any cultural group (Smith, 1983). In complex societies in which several cultural traditions flourish, healers tend to compete with one another and/or to view their scopes of practice as separate from one another. In some instances, however, practitioners may make referrals to different healing systems. For example, a gerontologic nurse practitioner may contact a rabbi to assist a Jewish patient with spiritual needs, or a *curandero* may advise a Mexican-American patient to visit a physician or nurse practitioner for an antibiotic when traditional practices fail to heal a wound.

TABLE 4–1	MECHANIC'S DETERMINANTS OF ILLNESS BEHAVIOR

DETERMINANT	DESCRIPTION
Quality of symptom	The more frightening or visible the symptom, the greater is the likelihood that the individual will intervene.
Seriousness of symptom	The perceived threat of the symptom must be serious for action to be taken. Often others will step in if the person's behavior is considered dangerous (e.g., suicidal behavior) but will be unaware of potential problems if the person's behavior seems natural ("he always acts that way").
Disruption of daily activities	Behaviors that are very disruptive in work or other social situations are likely to be labeled as illness much sooner than the same behaviors in a family setting. An individual whose activities are disrupted by a symptom is likely to take that symptom seriously even if on another occasion he would consider the same symptom trivial (e.g., acne just before a date).
Rate and persistence of symptom	The frequency of a symptom is directly related to its importance; a symptom that persists is also likely to be taken seriously.
Tolerance of symptom	The extent to which others, especially family, tolerate the symptom before reacting varies; individuals also have different tolerance thresholds.
Sociocognitive status	A person's information about the symptom, knowledge base, and cultural values all influence that person's perception of illness.
Denial of symptom	Often, the individual or family members need to deny a symptom for personal or social reasons. The amount of fear and anxiety present can interfere with perception of a symptom.
Motivation	Competing needs may motivate a person to delay or enhance symptoms. A person who has no time or money to be sick will often not acknowledge the seriousness of symptoms.
Assigning of meaning	Once perceived, the symptom must be interpreted. Often people explain symptoms within normal parameters ("I'm just tired").
Treatment accessibility	The greater the barriers to treatment—whether psychologic, economic, physical, or social—the greater the likelihood that the symptom will not be interpreted as serious or that the person will seek an alternative form of care.

From Mechanic, D. (1978). *Medical sociology,* 2nd ed. New York: The Free Press, a Division of Macmillan, Inc. Copyright © 1978 by David Mechanic. By permission.

Self-Care

For common minor illnesses, an estimated 70 to 90% of all people initially try **self-care** with over-the-counter medicines, megavitamins, herbs, exercise, and/or foods that they believe have healing powers. Many self-care practices have been handed down from generation to generation, frequently by oral tradition. When self-treatment is ineffective, people are likely to turn to *professional* and/or *folk* (indigenous, generic, traditional) healing systems. Or perhaps it might be more accurate to say that professional health care procedures include those that supplement or substitute for self-care practices. Self-care is the largest component of the North American health care system and accounts for billions of dollars in revenue annually (Lipson & Steiger, 1996).

Professional Care Systems

According to Leininger (1991; 1997), **professional care systems** are formally taught, learned, and transmitted professional care, health, illness, wellness, and related knowledge and practice skills that prevail in professional institutions, usually with multidisciplinary personnel to serve consumers. Professional care is characterized by specialized education and knowledge, responsibility for care, and expectation of remuneration for services rendered. Nurses, physicians, physical therapists, and other licensed health care providers are examples of professionals who constitute professional care systems in North America and other parts of the world.

Folk Healing System

A **folk healing system** is a set of beliefs that has a shared social dimension and reflects what people actually do when they are ill versus what society says they ought to do according to a set of social standards (Wing, 1998). According to Leininger (1991), all cultures of the world have had a lay health care system, which is sometimes referred to as indigenous or generic. Although the terms *complementary, alternative,* or *naturalistic healing* are sometimes used interchangeably with folk healing systems, the key consideration that defines folk systems is their history of tradition. Many folk healing systems have endured over time and rely on oral tradition for the transmission of beliefs and practices from one generation to the next. A folk healing system is a mixture of nonprofessional systems and uses healing practices that are learned informally. The folk healing system is often divided into secular and sacred components.

Most cultures have folk healers (sometimes referred to as traditional, indigenous, or generic healers), most of whom speak the native tongue of the client, sometimes make house calls, and usually charge significantly less than healers practicing in the biomedical/scientific health care system (Leininger, 1997). In addition, many cultures have lay midwives (e.g., *parteras* for Hispanic women), *doulas* (support women for new mothers and babies), or other health care providers available for meeting the needs of clients. Table 4-2 identifies indigenous or folk healers for selected groups.

TABLE 4–2	HEALERS AND THEIR SCOPE OF PRACTICE

CULTURE/FOLK PRACTITIONER	PREPARATION	SCOPE OF PRACTICE
Hispanic		
Family member	Possesses knowledge of folk medicine	Common illnesses of a mild nature that may or may not be recognized by modern medicine
Curandero	May receive training in an apprenticeship; may receive a "gift from God" that enables him or her to cure; knowledgeable in use of herbs, diet, massage, and rituals	Treats almost all of the traditional illnesses; some may not treat illness caused by witchcraft for fear of being accused of possessing evil powers; usually admired by members of the community
Espiritualista or spiritualist	Born with the special gifts of being able to analyze dreams and foretell future events; may serve apprenticeship with an older practitioner	Emphasis on prevention of illness or bewitchment through use of medals, prayers, amulets; may also be sought for cure of existing illness
Yerbero	No formal training Knowledgeable in growing and prescribing herbs	Consulted for preventive and curative use of herbs for both traditional and Western illnesses
Sabador	Knowledgeable in massage and manipulation of bones and muscles	Treats many traditional illnesses, particularly those affecting the musculoskeletal system; may also treat nontraditional illnesses
Black		
"Old lady"	Usually an older woman who has successfully raised her own family; knowledgeable in child care and folk remedies	Consulted about common ailments and for advice on child care; found in rural and urban communities
Spiritualist	Called by God to help others; no formal training; usually associated with a fundamentalist Christian church	Assists with problems that are financial, personal, spiritual, or physical; predominantly found in urban communities

TABLE 4–2	**HEALERS AND THEIR SCOPE OF PRACTICE**	
Voodoo priest or priestess or *Hougan*	May be trained by other priests(esses). In the U.S. the eldest son of a priest becomes a priest; the daughter of a priest(ess) becomes a priestess if she is born with a veil (amniotic sac) over her face	Knowledgeable about properties of herbs; interpretation of signs and omens; able to cure illness caused by voodoo; uses communication techniques to establish a therapeutic milieu like a psychiatrist; treats blacks, Mexican Americans, and Native Americans
Chinese		
Herbalist	Knowledgeable in diagnosis of illness and herbal remedies	Both diagnostic and therapeutic; diagnostic techniques include interviewing, inspection, auscultation, and assessment of pulses
Acupuncturist	3 1/2 to 4 1/2 years (1,500 to 1,800 hours) of courses on acupuncture, Western anatomy & physiology, Chinese herbs; usually requires a period of apprenticeship learning from someone else who is licensed or certified Licensure required in North America	Diagnosis and treatment of yin/yang disorders by inserting needles into *meridians,* pathways through which life energy flows; when heat is applied to the acupuncture needle, the term *moxibustion* is used May combine acupuncture with herbal remedies and/or dietary recommendations Acupuncture is sometimes used as a surgical anesthetic
Amish		
Braucher or baruch-doktor	Apprenticeship	Men or women who use a combination of modalities including physical manipulation, massage, herbs, teas, reflexology, and *brauche,* folk-healing art with origins in 18th and 19th century Europe; especially effective in the treatment of bedwetting, nervousness, and

(continues)

TABLE 4–2	**HEALERS AND THEIR SCOPE OF PRACTICE** *(Continued)*	
		women's health problems; may be generalist or specialist in practice; some set up treatment rooms; some see non-Amish as well as Amish patients
Lay midwives	Apprenticeship	Care for women before, during, and after delivery
Greek		
Magissa "magician"	Apprenticeship	Woman who cures *matiasma* or evil eye May be referred to as doctor
Bonesetters	Apprenticeship	Specialize in treating uncomplicated fractures
Priest (Orthodox)	Ordained clergy Formal theological study	May be called on for advice, blessings, exorcisms, or direct healing
Native Americans		
Shaman	Spiritually chosen Apprenticeship	Uses incantations, prayers, and herbs to cure a wide range of physical, psychologic, and spiritual illnesses
Crystal gazer hand trembler (Navajo)	Spiritually chosen Apprenticeship	Diviner diagnostician who can identify the cause of a problem, either by using crystals or placing hand over the sick person; does not implement treatment

Adapted with permission from Hautman, M.A. (1979). Folk health and illness beliefs. *Nurse Practitioner, 4*(4), 23, 26–27, 31.

If clients use folk healers, these healers should be an integral part of the health care team and should be included in as many aspects of the client's care as possible. For example, you might include the folk healer in obtaining a health history and in determining what treatments already have been used in an effort to bring about healing. In discussing traditional remedies, it is important to be respectful and to listen attentively to healers who effectively combine spiritual and herbal remedies for a wide variety of illnesses, both physical and psychologic in origin. Chapter 14 provides detailed information about the religious beliefs and spiritual healers in major religious groups.

Complementary and Alternative Therapies

Complementary and alternative medicine (CAM) is an umbrella term for hundreds of therapies based on health care systems of people from around the world. Some CAM therapies have ancient origins in Egyptian, Chinese, Greek, and Native North American cultures. Others, such as osteopathy and magnet therapy, have evolved in more recent times (Ernst, Pittler, Stevinson, & White, 2001; Fontaine, 2000; Keegan, 2001; Kuhn, 1999).

Western biomedicine, or **allopathic medicine**, is the reference point, with all other therapies being considered complementary (in addition to) or alternative (instead of) to it. Coined by homeopathic physician Samuel Hahnemann in the nineteenth century, *allopathic medicine* is used most often to refer to conventional medical practice, which emphasizes killing bacteria and suppressing symptoms.

In 1992, the U.S. Congress provided funding for the National Institutes of Health to create the Office of Alternative Medicine to facilitate fair scientific evaluation of therapies that could improve the public's health and well-being. The Office of Alternative Medicine facilitates research on complementary and alternative medicine, provides a research training program, and serves as a clearinghouse for information on research related to the effectiveness of various complementary and alternative practices. The Office of Alternative Medicine defines *alternative medicine* as modalities used instead of conventional medicine, whereas *complementary medicine* refers to the use of modalities together to complement the offerings of conventional medicine.

Integrative medicine is a term introduced by Dr. Andrew Weil to define a hybrid of complementary and conventional medical treatments. It refers to a synergistic combination of therapies that incorporates acupuncture, herbal medicine, manipulation, and related therapies with conventional measures such as antibiotics and surgery.

According to the National Institutes of Health (2002), www.nccam.gov there are seven categories of alternative modalities and therapies:

1. *Mind/body or behavioral interventions* include biofeedback; relaxation; meditation; guided imagery; hypnosis; prayer; art, dance, and music therapy; and yoga.
2. *Alternative systems* of medical practice include traditional Chinese medicine, Ayurveda, homeopathy, naturopathy, environmental medicine, and community-based practices such as shamanism and related practices in various indigenous cultures.
3. *Lifestyle* and *disease prevention* examines the effects of various foods, vitamins, and minerals on acute and chronic diseases and also emphasizes health maintenance and disease prevention.
4. *Biologically based therapies* include natural and biologically based practices, interventions, and products, many of which overlap with dietary supplements. There are four subcategories:
   a. Herbal medicine (see Table 3-3 for selected herbal remedies and the clinical evidence supporting their efficacy)

     b. Special diet therapies (e.g., macrobiotic, vegetarian, Atkins and others);

     c. Orthomolecular medicine, the use of products used as nutritional and food supplements (and not covered in other categories)

     d. Pharmacologic, biologic, and instrumental interventions, including the use of products such as bee pollen and cartilage and procedures such as iridology and neural therapy.

5. *Manipulative and body-based systems* are diagnostic and therapeutic mechanisms based on manipulation or movement of the body, such as osteopathy, massage therapy, hydrotherapy, chiropractic, acupuncture, rolfing, reflexology, and therapeutic touch.

6. *Biofield* involves systems such as therapeutic touch, Reiki, and external qigong that use subtle energy fields in and around the body for medical purposes.

7. *Bioelectromagnetics* explores the relationship between living organisms and electromagnetic fields, including applications for bone repair, wound healing, and stimulation of the immune system.

• CULTURAL VALUES AND CULTURAL CARE MEANINGS

Among the greatest challenges you face is providing care that is congruent with the client's values and **care meanings**. Cultural values and care meanings influence nurse-client interaction, provide useful information about the client's expectations of care, and influence the client's sense of appropriate sick role behaviors, choice of healers, views toward technology, and health-related beliefs and practices. Table 4-3 summarizes the human care expressions and patterns of cultures for selected groups that have been studied by transcultural nurse researchers.

TABLE 4–3	CULTURAL VALUES AND CULTURE CARE MEANINGS AND ACTION MODES FOR SELECTED GROUPS
CULTURAL VALUES	**CULTURE CARE MEANINGS AND ACTION MODES**
Anglo American Culture (Mainly U.S. Middle and Upper Classes)	
1. Individualism—focus on self-reliance	**1.** Stress alleviation by
2. Independence and freedom	-Physical means
3. Competition and achievement	-Emotional means
4. Materialism (things and money)	**2.** Personalized acts
5. Technology dependent	-Doing special things
6. Instant time and actions	-Giving individual attention
7. Youth and beauty	**3.** Self-reliance (individualism) by
8. Equal sex rights	-Reliance on self
9. Leisure time highly valued	-Reliance on self (self-care)

TABLE 4–3	CULTURAL VALUES AND CULTURE CARE MEANINGS AND ACTION MODES FOR SELECTED GROUPS *(Continued)*

CULTURAL VALUES	CULTURE CARE MEANINGS AND ACTION MODES
10. Reliance on scientific facts and numbers	-Becoming as independent as
11. Less respect for authority and the elderly	-Reliance on technology
12. Generosity in time of crisis	4. Health instruction
	-Teach us how "to do" this care for self
	-Give us the "medical" facts

Mexican American Culture*

CULTURAL VALUES	CULTURE CARE MEANINGS AND ACTION MODES
1. Extended family valued	1. Succorance (direct family aid)
2. Interdependence with kin and social activities	2. Involvement with extended family ("other care")
3. Patriarchal (machismo)	3. Filial love/loving
4. Exact time less valued	4. Respect for authority
5. High respect for authority and the elderly	5. Mother as care decision maker
6. Religion valued (many Roman Catholics)	6. Protective (external) male care
7. Native foods for well-being	7. Acceptance of God's will
8. Traditional folk-care healers for folk illnesses	8. Use of folk-care practices
9. Belief in hot/cold theory	9. Healing with foods
	10. Touching

Haitian American Culture**

CULTURAL VALUES	CULTURE CARE MEANINGS AND ACTION MODES
1. Extended family as support system	1. Involve family for support (other care)
2. Religion—God's will must prevail	2. Respect
3. Reliance on folk foods and treatments	3. Trust
4. Belief in hot/cold theory	4. Succorance
5. Male decision makes and direct caregivers	5. Touching (body closeness)
6. Reliance on native language	6. Reassurance
	7. Spiritual healing
	8. Use of folk food, care rituals
	9. Avoid evil eye and witches
	10. Speak the language

African American Culture†

CULTURAL VALUES	CULTURE CARE MEANINGS AND ACTION MODES
1. Extended family networks	1. Concern for my "brothers and sisters"
2. Religion valued (many are Baptists)	2. Being involved
3. Interdependence with "Blacks"	3. Giving presence (physical)
4. Daily survival	4. Family support and "get togethers"
5. Technology valued, e.g., radio, car	5. Touching appropriately
6. Folk (soul) foods	6. Reliance on folk home remedies
7. Folk healing modes	7. Rely on "Jesus to save us" with prayers and songs
8. Music and physical activities	

(continued)

TABLE 4–3	CULTURAL VALUES AND CULTURE CARE MEANINGS AND ACTION MODES FOR SELECTED GROUPS *(Continued)*

CULTURAL VALUES	CULTURE CARE MEANINGS AND ACTION MODES
North-American Indian Culture‡	
1. Harmony between land, people, and environment	1. Establishing harmony between people and environment with reciprocity
2. Reciprocity with Mother Earth	2. Actively listening
3. Spiritual inspiration (spirit guidance)	3. Using periods of silence ("Great Spirit" guidance)
4. Folk healers (shamans) (the circle and four directions)	4. Rhythmic timing (nature, land, and people) in harmony
5. Practice culture rituals and taboos	5. Respect for native folk healers, carers, and curers (use of circle)
6. Rhythmicity of life with nature	6. Maintaining reciprocity (replenish what is taken from Mother Earth)
7. Authority of tribal elders	7. Preserving cultural rituals and taboos
8. Pride in cultural heritage and "nations"	8. Respect for elders and children
9. Respect and value for children	

*These findings were from the author's transcultural nurse studies (1970, 1984) and other transcultural nurse studies in the United States during recent two decades.

**These data were from Haitians living in the United States during the decade 1981–1991.

†These findings were from the author's study of two southern U.S. villages (1980–1981) and from a study of one large northern urban city (1982–1991) along with other studies by transcultural nurses.

‡These findings were collected by the author and other contributors in the United States and Canada over three decades. Cultural variations among all nations exist, so these data are some general commonalities about values, care meanings, and actions.

From M. M. Leininger (1991). *Culture care diversity and universality: A theory of nursing* (pp. 355–357). New York: National League for Nursing Press. Reprinted by permission.

SUMMARY

In this chapter we have examined the major cultural belief systems embraced by people of the world, including the top three: magico-religious, scientific, and holistic health paradigms or worldviews. We examined self-treatment, professional care systems, and folk (indigenous, traditional or generic) care systems and the types of healers who practice in them. After analyzing the influence of culture on symptoms and sick role behavior, we explored complementary and alternative medicine and healing modalities that are frequently used to treat physical and psychologic conditions.

REVIEW QUESTIONS

1. In your own words, describe what is meant by the following terms: (a) cultural belief system, (b) worldview, and (c) paradigm.
2. What are the primary characteristics of the three major health belief systems: magico-religious, scientific, and holistic paradigms?

3. What are the differences between professional and folk care systems?
4. What is allopathic medicine?
5. What are the primary functions of the Office of Alternative Medicine?
6. Identify the seven major categories of complementary and alternative medicine as defined by the Office of Alternative Medicine.

CRITICAL THINKING ACTIVITIES

1. Select a complementary or alternative practice that you would like to know more about, e.g., acupuncture, chiropractic, homeopathy. Search the internet for information about this practice, and go to a library to conduct background research. After you have learned more about the practice, contact a healer who uses the type of practice you're interested in, and ask the following questions:
   a. How did you prepare to be a practitioner of _____?
   b. What do you believe are the major benefits of _____ to clients/patients?
   c. What health-related conditions do you believe respond best to _____?
   d. Are there any risks to clients/patients resulting from the use of _____?
2. According to the World Health Organization, 80% of the people in the world use complementary and alternative medicine for the treatment of common illnesses. Select a common illness such as upper respiratory infection, arthritis, or similar condition and identify the various complementary and alternative approaches to allopathic medicine that clients/patients might use. What is the efficacy of each intervention that you have identified? How effective do you think the complementary and alternative practices are compared with allopathic medicine?
3. The herb echinacea is frequently used for the prevention and treatment of the common cold. If a patient asked your opinion about the use of echinacea, how would you reply? Would you recommend that the patient use this herb for treatment of a cold? Explain why or why not.
4. Visit three of the following web sites for further information about specific types of alternative and complementary medicine.

Acupressure and Massage

Acupressure Institute
   http://www.acupressure.com
American Massage Therapy Association
   http://www.ati-net.com
International Massage Association
   http://www.imagroup.com
Rolf Institute
   http://www.rolf.org

Acupuncture and Chinese Medicine

American Association of Oriental Medicine (provides referrals to acupuncturists in your area)
   http://www.aaom.org

National Acupuncture and Oriental Medicine Alliance
http://www.healthy.netlnaoma or http://acupuncture.com

Aromatherapy

American Alliance of Aromatherapy
http://www.healthy.net/aaoa
National Association for Holistic Aromatherapy
http://www.healthy.net/aromatherapy

Ayurvedic Medicine

Ayurvedic Institute
http://www.ayurveda.com

Biofeedback

Association for Applied Psychophysiology and Biofeedback
http://www.aapb.org

Chiropractic

American Chiropractic Association
http://www.amerchiro.org
International Chiropractors Association
http://www.chiropractic.org

Environmental Medicine

American Academy of Environmental Medicine
http://www.healthy.net/aaem

Guided Imagery

Academy for Guided Imagery
http://www.healthy.net/agi

Herbal Medicine

American Botanical Council
http://www.herbalgram.org
American Herbalist Guild
http://www.healthy.net/herbalist
Herb Research Foundation
http://www.herbs.org

Hypnosis
American Board of Hypnotherapy
http://www.hypnosis.com

Mind/Body Medicine

Center for Mind/Body Medicine
http://www.healthy.net/cmbm
Mind-Body Medical Institute
http://www.med.harvard.edu/programs/mindbody

Music Therapy
American Music Therapy Association
http://www.musictherapy.org

Naturopathic Medicine
http://www.naturopathic.org

Qigong
http://www.healthy.net/qugonginstitute

• References

Ackernecht, E. (1971). Natural diseases and rational treatment in primitive medicine. *Bulletin of the History of Medicine, 19,* 467–497.

Andrews, M. M., Herberg, P., and Rigdon, I. (1983). A comparison of three health-illness paradigms. Unpublished manuscript.

Clements, F. E. (1932). Primitive concepts of disease. *University of California Publications in Archeology and Ethnology, 32(*2), 185–252.

Ernst, E., Pittler, M. H., Stevinson, C., & White, A. (2001). *The desktop guide to complementary and alternative medicine: An evidence-based approach.* New York: Mosby.

Fetrow, C. W., & Avila, J. R. (1999). *Professional's handbook of complementary and alternative medicines.* Springhouse, PA: Springhouse.

Fontaine, K. L. (2000). *Healing practices: Alternative therapies for nursing.* Upper Saddle River, NJ: Prentice Hall.

Foster, S. (1996). *Herbs for your health.* Loveland, CO: Interweave Press.

Kasl, S., & Cobb, S. (1966). Health behavior, illness behavior and sick role behavior. *Archives of Environmental Health, 12,* 246–266.

Keegan, L. (2001). *Healing with complementary and alternative therapies.* Albany, NY: Delmar.

Kleinman, A. (1980). *Patients and healers in the context of culture.* Berkeley, CA: University of California Press.

Kuhn, M. A. (1999). *Complementary therapies for health care providers.* Philadelphia: Lippincott Williams & Wilkins.

Kuhn, M. A., & Winston, D. (2000). *Herbal therapy and supplements: A scientific and traditional approach.* Philadelphia: Lippincott Williams & Wilkins.

Leininger, M. M. (1991). *Culture care diversity and universality: A theory of nursing.* New York: National League for Nursing Press.

Leininger, M. M. (1997). Founder's focus alternative to what? Generic vs. professional caring, treatments and healing modes. *Journal of Transcultural Nursing, 91*(1), 37.

Lipson, J. G., & Steiger, N. J. (1996). *Self-care nursing in a multicultural context.* Thousand Oaks, CA: Sage.

Mechanic, D. (1978). *Medical sociology* (3rd ed.). New York: Free Press.

Monte, T. (1997). The *complete guide to natural healing.* New York: Berkeley Publishing Group.

National Institutes of Health. (2001).

Silko, L. M. (1988). *Ceremonies: A Series of Indian stories.* NY: Penguin Books.

Wing, D. M. (1998). A comparison of traditional folk healing concepts with contemporary healing concepts. *Journal of Community Health Nursing, 15*(3), 143–154.

2

Transcultural Nursing: Across the Lifespan

CHAPTER 5

Transcultural Perspectives in Childbearing

Jana Lauderdale

KEY TERMS

Childbearing
Hot/cold theories
Imbalance
Incarcerated pregnant women
Infant relinquishment
Lesbian couple childbearing

Matrescence
Patrescence
Physical abuse of pregnant
   women
Pollution
Pregnancy

Pregnant homeless women
Prescriptive beliefs
Restrictive beliefs
Taboos

OBJECTIVES

1. Analyze how culturally related issues influence behavior of the childbearing woman and her family during pregnancy.
2. Understand one's own cultural values and norms toward members of vulnerable populations of childbearing women.
3. Understand the childbearing beliefs and practices of diverse cultures.
4. Examine the needs of women making alternative lifestyle choices regarding childbirth and childrearing.
5. Explore how the shared ideologies of vulnerable subcultures of childbearing populations can influence pregnancy outcomes.

This chapter will explore how culture influences the experience of **childbearing**. The experience of the woman as well as of her significant other during pregnancy, birth, and the postpartum period are discussed. Recommendations for practice are outlined in each section for nurses caring for childbearing women and their families. Also included are discussions related to culturally specific circumstances and behaviors that can impose risk to the childbearing woman and her family.

• OVERVIEW OF CULTURAL BELIEF SYSTEMS AND PRACTICES RELATED TO CHILDBEARING

Childbearing is a time of transition and social celebration of central importance in any society, signaling a realignment of existing cultural roles and responsibilities, psychologic and biologic states, and social relationships. For some time, these rites of passage have been described as **matrescence** (mother-becoming) and **patrescence** (father-becoming) (Raphael, 1976). The different ways in which a particular society views this transitional period and manages childbirth are dependent on the culture's consensus about health, medical care, reproduction, and the role and status of women (Dickason, Silverman, & Schult, 1994).

Pregnancy and childbirth practices in contemporary Western society have seen dramatic changes over the past two decades. An increase in the number of women in the work force, advances in reproductive technology, self-care, alternative therapies, the explosion of health information available to consumers on the internet, and the influx of immigrants and refugees are but a few of the trends that require nurses to examine and rethink how we can better care for our clients (Tiedje, 2000). The dominant medical practices related to pregnancy and childbirth in the United States and Canada include the use of various state-of-the-art technologies such as fetal monitoring devices and sometimes cesarean sections. Medical care focuses on the pregnant woman and fetus; the father and other family members or significant others, if they are included at all, are relegated to observer rather than participant status. The dominant cultural practices or rituals in the United States and Canada include formal prenatal care (including childbirth classes), ultrasonography to view the fetus, and hospital delivery. Monitoring fetal status, inducing labor, providing anesthesia for labor and delivery, and placing the woman in the lithotomy position during the birth are all part of routine hospital care in modern North American health care facilities. A highly specialized group of nurses, obstetricians, perinatologists, and pediatricians actively monitors the mother's physiologic status, delivers the infant, and provides newborn care. However, because there is not total cultural agreement about the value of these practices, some health care providers elect to offer their pregnant clients alternative health care services. These alternatives include in-hospital and free-standing birth centers and care by nurse practitioners and nurse midwives, who promote family-centered care and emphasize pregnancy as a normal process requiring minimal technologic intervention.

Additionally, subcultures within the United States and Canada have very different practices, values, and beliefs about childbirth and the roles of women, men, social support networks, and health care practitioners. They include proponents of the "back to nature" movement, who are often vegetarian, use lay midwives for home deliveries, and practice herbal or naturopathic medicine. Other groups that might have distinct cultural practices include Blacks, Native North Americans, Hispanics, Middle Eastern groups, and Asians, among others. Additionally, religious background, regional variations, age, urban or rural background, sexual preference, and other individual characteristics all might contribute to cultural differences in the experience of childbirth.

Great variations exist in the social class, ethnic origin, family structure, and social support networks of women, men, and families in the United States and Canada. Despite these differences, many health care providers assume that the changes in status and rites of passage associated with pregnancy and birth are experienced similarly by all people. In addition, many of the traditional cultural beliefs, values, and practices related to childbirth have been viewed by some professional nurses as "old-fashioned" or "old wives' tales." Although some of these customs are changing rapidly, many women and families are attempting to preserve their own valued patterns of experiencing childbirth. In recent years, nurses and other health professionals have attempted to incorporate the individual's beliefs and cultural practices into health care to reduce some of the cultural conflict surrounding practices in North American obstetrics (Lowdermilk, Perry, & Bobak, 2000).

• FERTILITY CONTROL AND CULTURE

The literature provides limited information regarding cultural beliefs and practices related to the control of fertility. The biologic, or "natural," fertility of a woman varies depending on several factors, which include her monthly probability of conceiving; the probability of intrauterine mortality; the duration of the postpartum period, during which she is unlikely to ovulate or conceive; and the likelihood of sterility (MacCormack, 1982). These biologic variables are further modified by cultural and social variables, including marriage and residence patterns, diet, religion, the availability of abortion, the incidence of venereal disease, and the regulation of birth intervals by cultural or artificial means. The focus of this section is on the cultural and artificial regulation of birth intervals, or spacing.

Commonly used methods of contraception in the United States and Canada include hormonal methods (i.e., "the pill"), intrauterine devices (IUDs), permanent sterilization, and, to a lesser degree, barrier and "natural" methods. Natural methods of family planning are based on the recognition of fertility through signs and symptoms and abstinence during periods of fertility. The religious beliefs of some cultural groups might affect their use of fertility controls such as abortion or artificial regulation of conception; for example, Roman Catholics might follow church edicts against artificial control of conception, and Mormon families might follow their church's teaching regarding the spiritual responsibility to have large families and promote church growth (Stark, 1982). The ability to control fertility successfully also requires an understanding of the menstrual cycle and the times and conditions under which pregnancy is more or less likely to occur—in essence, an understanding of bodily functions. When these functions change, the woman might perceive the changes as abnormal or unhealthy. Because the use of artificial methods of fertility control might alter the body's usual cycles, women who use them might become anxious, consider themselves ill, and discontinue the method. Native American women monitor their monthly bleeding cycles closely and believe in the importance of monthly menstruation for maintaining harmony and physical well-being. Contraceptives such as the IUD are generally better accepted than hormonal methods because of the normal or increased flow associated with the IUD. Because the mechanism of action of an IUD might include the expulsion of a fertilized ovum, some women oppose use of the IUD for religious reasons.

In a study by Yusu, Siedlecky, and Byrnes (1993), 980 Turkish, Lebanese, and Vietnamese immigrant women living in Sydney, Australia, were surveyed regarding family planning. The Lebanese and Turkish women were better informed about the more modern forms of contraception (the pill, condoms, and IUDs) than were Vietnamese women. Currently, the pill and traditional methods (abstinence, prolonged breastfeeding, rhythm, and withdrawal) were the most common forms of birth control, regardless of ethnicity. However, Turkish women continued to rely on abortion as a means of contraception as well. Condom use was low among Lebanese husbands but high among the young Turkish and Vietnamese groups. IUDs were used more often among Turkish women, and sterilization was the contraceptive method of choice for both Lebanese and Turkish women over the age of 40. Only two Vietnamese women reported that their husbands had had vasectomies, probably indicating a similar nonacceptance of vasectomy among immigrants living in North America.

Women living in refugee situations might encounter additional barriers to contraceptive use (see Evidence-Based Practice 5-1). Religious beliefs can also influence birth control choices. For example, the Hindu religion teaches that the right hand is clean and the left is dirty. The right hand is for holding religious books and eating utensils, and the left hand is used for dirty things, such as genitals. This belief complicates the use of contraceptives requiring the use of both hands, such as a diaphragm (Bromwich and Parson, 1990). Buddhism values a celibate life and natural things. Modern contraceptives are not considered natural by this group and are therefore unacceptable. Guatemalan women believe strongly in privacy; therefore, skirts are kept on during intercourse and childbirth. Some Guatemalan women also believe it is improper to touch or expose their genitals, making traditional birth control methods such as abstinence or the rhythm method much more acceptable (Cosminsky, 1982). In some cultures in Africa, the view of birth spacing has traditionally been to impose a taboo on postpartum sexual activity, with some women leaving their home for as long as 2 years to avoid pregnancy (Miller, 1992). The influence of religious beliefs on birth control choices can vary within and between groups. For example, although birth control is strictly forbidden by Islam, it is practiced by most Iranian families living in Canada (Waxler-Morrison, Anderson, & Richardson, 1990).

According to Shain (1982), who reviewed abortion practices and attitudes from a cross-cultural perspective, abortion has been one of the most universally prevalent methods of fertility control throughout recorded history. In a

> ### EVIDENCE-BASED PRACTICE 5-1
> ### *Barriers to Contraceptive Use for Women Living in Khao Phlu Refugee Camp in Thailand*
>
> By use of focus groups, 102 women living in the Khao Phlu refugee camp in Thailand were studied, along with 10 midwives and traditional birth attendants who provided care for the women at the maternal and child health center serving the refugees. Information was gathered regarding the women's knowledge of contraceptives, beliefs, and practices. According to the results, 82% of the women wanted to stop or delay childbearing, but only 12% reported using some sort of contraception. The reasons for lack of contraceptive use included the refugee situation itself (i.e., uncertainty regarding their future), displacement of family or support system, cultural conflicts regarding modern contraceptive use, fear of side effects, lack of information, current illness, and discomfort level for asking about contraception. Additionally, almost 40% of the women had no knowledge of what contraceptive methods were available at the health center that served the camp. Few of the midwives, and none of the women or traditional birth attendants were aware of emergency contraception.
>
> #### Clinical Application
>
> The results suggest that the stress of the refugee situation itself, along with cultural influences and the inaccessibility of contraceptives, had an effect on acceptance and use. Nurses working with refugee women must be aware of the issues to provide culturally competent care in matters regarding contraception practices.
>
> Morrison, V. (2000). Contraceptive need among Cambodian refugees in Khao Phlu camp. *International Family Planning Perspectives, 26*(4), 188–192.

recent study by Otoide, Oronsaye, & Okonofua (2001), Nigerian adolescents participated in focus groups to explore their level of understanding regarding contraception. The researchers were aware that in this particular group there is a low level of contraceptive use but a high reliance on abortion. According to the results, the participants perceived that modern contraceptives would have a prolonged, adverse effect on future fertility, whereas abortion was seen as an immediate solution to unplanned pregnancy. This indicates a need to educate Nigerian adolescents regarding contraceptive action and side effects versus the use of unsafe abortion practices. Few cultural groups give unqualified social approval to abortion. In the United States and Canada, religious affiliation is the variable most closely associated with attitudes toward abortion.

Nurses providing family planning services must take care to be culturally sensitive so that women can be assisted in defining their own attitudes, beliefs, and sense of gynecologic well-being regarding fertility control.

• PREGNANCY AND CULTURE

All cultures recognize **pregnancy** as a special transition period, and many have particular customs and beliefs that dictate activity and behavior during pregnancy. Ford (1964), Mead and Newton (1967), Newton and Newton (1972), and Oakley (1980) have reviewed childbirth from a cross-cultural perspective, surveying the literature on traditional non-Western societies as well as on Western cultural groups. Recent reports of childbirth customs in the United States and Canada have focused on accounts of differing beliefs and practices relative to pregnancy among various ethnic and cultural groups. This section describes some of the biologic and cultural variations that might influence the provision of nursing care during pregnancy.

Biologic Variations

Knowledge of certain biologic variations resulting from genetic and environmental backgrounds is important for nurses who care for childbearing families. For example, pregnant women who have the sickle cell trait and are heterozygous for the sickle cell gene are at increased risk for asymptomatic bacteriuria and urinary tract infections such as pyelonephritis. This places them at greater than normal risk for premature labor as well (Pritchard, MacDonald, & Gant, 1984). It has been established that although heterozygotes are found most commonly among African Americans (8 to 14%), individuals living in the United States and Canada who are of Mediterranean ancestry, as well as of Germanic and Native North American descent, might occasionally carry the trait (Overfield, 1985; Perry, 2000) If both parents are heterozygous, there is a 1 in 4 chance that the infant will be born with sickle cell disease. Presently, of children born with sickle cell disease, 50% live to adulthood (Dickason, Silverman, & Kaplan, 1998). Of those surviving the disease, many experience chronic complications throughout their lives.

Another important biologic variation relative to pregnancy is diabetes mellitus. The incidence of non–insulin-dependent and gestational diabetes is much higher than normal among some Native North American groups—a problem that increases maternal and infant morbidity. Illnesses that are common among European North Americans might manifest themselves differently in Native North American clients. For example, a Native North American woman might have a high blood sugar level but be asymptomatic for diabetes mellitus. It is important to be aware that the mortality rate in pregnant Native North American women with diabetes is higher than in white European American women. Diabetes during pregnancy, particularly with uncontrolled hyperglycemia, is associated with an increased risk of congenital anomalies, stillbirth, macrosomia, birth injury, cesarean section, neonatal hypoglycemia, and other problems. The incidence of gestational diabetes is 10 to 40 times greater among the Pima and Papago Indians of Arizona than in the general population of the United States (Pettit, Knowler, Baird, & Bennet, 1980). Similar patterns exist in Canada. For example, one study found the rate of gestational diabetes among Ojibwa-Cree women in northwestern Ontario to be 8.4%—the highest rate reported so far in a Canadian population (Harris, Caulfield, Sugamori, Whalen, & Henning, 1997). Of the Native North American women who are diagnosed with gestational diabetes in Canada, overt diabetes develops in

70% within 3 years. In the general population, the conversion rate is 25 to 60% over a decade or more (Health Canada, 1999). In Canada and the United States, early detection and blood glucose screening are mandatory among high-risk populations to reduce complications during pregnancy and childbirth.

Other cultural groups whose members might have health conditions that place women or their fetuses at risk are refugees or immigrants from Southeast Asia. Significant numbers of Thais and Cambodians have abnormal hemoglobins (A2 and E), and hemoglobinopathic microcytic anemia coexisting with a dietary or folic acid deficiency anemia is not uncommon. Pregnancies in Southeast Asian women who are recent immigrants to the United States might be complicated by parasites (45–75%), a reactive venereal disease research laboratory (VDRL) test result (signifying treponema syphilis or yaws), tuberculosis (62%), and symptomatic or asymptomatic hepatitis screening results (HbsAg). Obviously, it is important in these cases to rule out active disease or carrier status. Treatment for these conditions might or might not be undertaken during pregnancy because some of the indicated pharmacologic agents might be embryotoxic (Boehme, 1985; Erickson & Hoang, 1980; Nelson & Hewitt, 1983; Pickwell, 1983).

Korea is another area in Southeast Asia where cultural mores might put pregnant women at risk. Evidence-Based Practice 5-2 describes how and why pregnant women in Korea's upper middle class might be at increased risk of HIV transmission to their unborn fetuses.

Cultural Variations

Several cultural variations might influence pregnancy outcomes. Those highlighted in this chapter include alternative lifestyle choices, nontraditional support systems, cultural beliefs related to parental activity during pregnancy, and food taboos and cravings. Nurses must be able to differentiate among beliefs and practices that are harmful, benign, and health promoting. Few cultural customs related to pregnancy are dangerous; although they might cause a woman to limit her activity and her exposure to some aspects of life, they are rarely harmful to herself or her fetus.

Alternative Lifestyle Choices

Despite recent cultural changes that have made it more acceptable for women to have careers and pursue alternative lifestyles, the dominant cultural expectation for North American women remains motherhood within the context of the nuclear family. Changing cultural expectations have influenced many middle-class North American women and couples to delay childbearing until their late 20s and early 30s and to have small families. Some women are making choices regarding childbearing that might not involve a marital relationship.

For another group of mothers who choose not to parent, the choices are not as clear. **Infant relinquishment** is in direct conflict with Western ideal cultural values, which suggest that all parents want a child. Nurses must examine their own cultural values when caring for women in this situation, making

EVIDENCE-BASED PRACTICE 5-2
HIV Knowledge Among Pregnant Korean Women

The findings indicated that Korean women were knowledgeable about HIV infection and AIDS but were less knowledgeable about transmission. A group singled out in the study as being at particular risk of HIV transmission to their unborn fetuses was Korea's upper middle-class pregnant women. Korean women are tolerant of extramarital sex, which is considered a norm within Confucianism. Foreign travel of Korean businessmen, along with their higher socioeconomic status, makes extramarital sex affordable within and outside of Korea. Contact with prostitutes is increased, with subsequent exposure of the wife to sexually transmitted diseases. Koreans' belief that to go outside the family for help when caring for a family member with the HIV virus will bring shame to the family increases the need for health care providers to be culturally sensitive. To prevent rejection and shame, the woman might not reveal her diagnosis, which has obvious implications for prenatal care and subsequent care of the mother and baby.

Clinical Application

Pregnancy is a time when most pregnant women are very aware of the health of their unborn babies. Education focusing on HIV transmission might be especially meaningful to women during this time. Because the family is the mainstay of the support system in this culture, every effort must be made to include selected members in the care of the pregnant woman and her education.

Chang, S. (1996). HIV/AIDS related knowledge, attitudes, and preventive behavior of pregnant Korean women. *Image: Journal of Nursing Scholarship 28*(4), 321–324.

certain to avoid negatively stereotyping mothers who decide to relinquish their babies for adoption. The decision to relinquish is almost always difficult, and the birth mother does not forget the experience. Not all infant relinquishments result merely from the mother "not wanting the baby." For example, Native North Americans living on reservations have been known to relinquish young and older children in the hope that their children will have "a better life off the reservation." Even with such good intentions, the relinquishment is very difficult for all concerned. In a study of the experience of infant relinquishment by Lauderdale and Boyle (1994), the most common reasons given by birth mothers for relinquishment were strictly altruistic: the birth mothers wanted a better life for the baby than they believed they could offer, and they wanted the baby to have both a mother and a father. Box 5-1 lists considerations in the nursing care of relinquishing birthmothers who are making this difficult decision.

Lesbian couple childbearing occurs in another subculture of pregnant women with special needs. This group of women faces psychosocial dilemmas related to their lifestyle and social stigma. The most common fear reported by lesbian mothers is the fear of unsafe and inadequate care from the practitioner once the mother's sexual orientation is revealed (Stine, 1997; Youngkin, Davis,

BOX 5–1	CONSIDERATIONS IN THE CARE OF RELINQUISHING BIRTH MOTHERS

1. During pregnancy, be open to the discussions of single parenting or adoption; be supportive of the woman's decision.
2. Encourage early and appropriate prenatal care.
3. During hospitalization, acknowledge the adoption as a loss; discuss the grief and grieving process with the birth mother.
4. Accept the birth mother as a "real mother," encourage questions, discuss her hospital expectations.
5. The midwife and/or obstetrician and the pediatrician to provide follow-up care to the birth mother.
6. Include the birth mother in postpartum teaching as appropriate.
7. Assist with the creation of memories in the form of picture taking, saving locks of hair, making footprints, or other acts that have meaning to the birth mother.
8. If desired by the birth mother, allow a formal closure ceremony. Examples of closure could be a quiet "good-bye" between mother and infant or a prayer with family and clergy present. This is important because it facilitates the grief and grieving process.
9. After relinquishment, it might be helpful for the birth mother to link with other mothers who have successfully coped with a similar experience. Support groups can be located in association with hospitals, adoption agencies, and other interested community agencies.
10. Encourage postpartum follow-up so that the birth mother's physical and emotional recovery can be monitored.

& Fogel, 1998; Spinks, Andrews, & Boyle, 2000). This situation will require health care providers to examine their own cultural value systems. Keep in mind that lesbian parents are dedicated to bringing a new life safely into the world to love and care for to the best of their ability—the same hopes all parents have for their newborns. There are many similarities in lesbian and heterosexual pregnancies, and the parallels should not be overlooked by health care providers. Issues of sexual activity, psychosocial changes related to attaining the traditionally defined maternal tasks of pregnancy (Rubin, 1984), and birth education all need to be addressed with lesbian couples. Special needs of the lesbian couple requiring assessment include social discrimination, family and social support networks, obstacles in becoming pregnant (i.e., coitus versus artificial insemination), lesbian maternal role development, legal issues of adoption by the partner, and coparenting role management (Tash & Kenney, 1993).

Buchholz's (2000) qualitative study examined the childbirth experiences of lesbian couples. The researcher focused on the positive aspects of the experience and the reasons why they were positive for the mother. Preparation of the nursing staff before the couples' arrival in the delivery area was seen by the couples as helpful. This "preparation" assisted the staff with the execution of the couple's birth plan and helped identify, ahead of time, nurses who would prefer not to work with the couple. The inclusion of the mother's partner by the nurses in the labor and delivery process, in the form of acknowledging of their approaching parenthood and allowing the partner to assist with newborn care after delivery, was seen as positive. Support from the nursing staff was evidenced by comforting gestures, checking with the couple frequently, answering questions, and just "being there" for them (Buchholz, 2000).

Two major concerns of lesbian couples were identified by this study. The first centered on legal issues such as power of attorney, visiting restrictions for the partner, and birth certificate information (father identification). The second dealt with the couple's attention to nurses' behavioral cues and questioning whether "busyness" on the part of the nurses might somehow equate to discomfort with the situation. This study reaffirmed previous findings (Stewart, 1999; Harvey, Carr, & Bernheine, 1989), which indicated that lesbian couples desire an attitude of respect for, and understanding of, their choices.

To meet lesbian parents' special needs and provide sensitive and appropriate care, nurses must come to understand the lifestyle and culture of the lesbian couple and work with them in addressing both their physical and their psychosocial concerns. Equally important, nurses must understand their own cultural values and norms, being careful not to impose them on couples with special needs. Last, hospital policies and procedures might need to be adapted to reflect the changing times, lifestyles, attitudes, and needs of all our clients.

Nontraditional Support Systems

A cultural variation that has important implications is a woman's perception of the need for formalized assistance from health care providers during the antepartum period. Western medicine is generally perceived as having a curative rather than a preventive focus. Indeed, many health care providers view pregnancy as a disaster waiting to happen, a physiologic state that at any moment will become pathologic. Because many cultural groups perceive pregnancy as a normal physiologic process, not seeing pregnant women as ill or in need of the curative services of a doctor, women in these diverse groups often delay seeking, or even neglect to seek, prenatal care.

Pregnant women and their partners are placing increased emphasis on the quality of pregnancy and childbirth, and many childbearing women rely on nontraditional support systems. For couples who are married, white, middle class, and infrequent users of their extended family for advice and support in childbirth-related matters, this kind of support might not be crucial. However, for other cultural groups, including Blacks, Hispanics, Filipinos, Asians, and Native North Americans, the family and social network (especially the grandmother or other maternal relatives) are of primary importance in advising and supporting the pregnant woman (Bryant, 1982; Lantican & Corona, 1992; Rose, 1978). It is essential that the nurse do a thorough cultural assessment to ascertain how much the pregnant woman uses nontraditional support systems and/or Western health care during her pregnancy. Once this assessment is complete and a trusting relationship has been established, the woman's pregnancy can be managed and consideration given to all the components that both she and the nurse believe are important for a successful outcome. Refer to Chapter 2 and the Andrews/ Boyle Assessment Guide in the Appendix A for a review of the components of the cultural assessment.

An example of how women's perceptions for the need of antepartum care might vary is described in Evidence-Based Practice 5-3.

Cultural Beliefs Related to Parental Activity During Pregnancy

Cultural variations also involve beliefs about activities during pregnancy. A *belief* is something held to be actual or true on the basis of a specific rationale or explanatory model. **Prescriptive beliefs**, which are phrased positively, describe expectancies of behavior; the more common restrictive beliefs, which are phrased negatively, limit choices and behaviors. Many people believe that the activities of the mother—and to a lesser extent of the father— influence newborn outcome. Box 5-2 describes some prescriptive and restrictive beliefs and taboos that provide cultural boundaries for parental activity during pregnancy. These beliefs are attempts to increase a sense of control over the outcome of pregnancy.

Positive or prescriptive beliefs might involve wearing special articles of clothing, such as the *muneco* worn by some traditional Hispanic women to ensure a safe delivery and prevent morning sickness. Other beliefs and practices involve ceremonies and recommendations about physical and sexual activity. One event in which a prescriptive belief might cause harm occurs when there is a poor neonatal outcome and the mother blames herself. For example, the mother whose fetus has died as a result of a cord accident, and who believed that hanging laundry caused the cord to encircle the baby's neck or body, might experience severe guilt. The nurse who is sensitive to the mother's anguish might say, "Many people say that if you reach over your head during pregnancy, it will cause the cord to wrap around the baby's neck. Have you heard this belief?" Once the woman responds, the nurse can explore her feelings about the practice. Do others in her family or social support network share her belief? The nurse might share her own views by saying, "I have not read in any medical or nursing books that this practice is related to cord problems, although I know many people share your belief." The discussion can then continue, focusing on the feelings and perceptions of the event as it is experienced by the woman and her family.

Negative or restrictive beliefs are widespread and numerous. They include activity, work, and sexual, emotional, and environmental prescriptions. **Taboos**, or restrictions with serious supernatural consequences, include the Orthodox Jewish avoidance of baby showers and divulgence of the infant's name before the infant's official naming ceremony (Bash, 1980). A Hispanic taboo involves the traditional belief that an early baby shower will invite bad luck, or *mal ojo*, the evil eye (Kay, 1978; Spector, 2000).

EVIDENCE-BASED PRACTICE 5-3
Amish Women and Perinatal Beliefs

Fifteen Amish women from Ohio described their perinatal beliefs and how they used the available health care system during a total of 76 pregnancies. Before the study, local health care providers commonly believed that Amish women underutilized available prenatal and birth care resources. The Amish women used perinatal care based on their beliefs about pregnancy and childbirth and in relation to cost, transportation, and child care. The women reported initiating prenatal care earlier for first pregnancies and progressively later with increasing parity and with the increasing knowledge that pregnancy was indeed a "non-problematic" condition. However, all the women reported seeking immediate medical attention if a serious problem arose, e.g., bleeding. During pregnancy, vitamins and herbal teas were commonly used in preparation for childbirth and usually were recommended by Amish family members or a midwife. Usual daily routines were encouraged to continue throughout pregnancy. A normal pregnancy course for an Amish woman consisted of following recommendations on vitamin and herb use from family and friends, going to a physician for prenatal care, and finally being delivered out of the hospital (either at home or at the Amish birthing center) by a midwife. Hospitals were spoken of positively in terms of "safety" and "getting additional rest." Negative statements about the hospital experience involved "lack of privacy" and "high cost." The findings also indicated that Amish women are not opposed to the technologic aspects of childbirth but that they selected modern technology to meet their individual and cultural needs.

Clinical Application

This finding is consistent with other research, which has shown that selective use of modern technology is a critical means of cultural preservation for the Amish community in modern society (Kraybill, 1989). This study emphasized the need to look beyond conformity and homogeneity when providing health care to the culturally different childbearing woman.

In the preceding examples of nontraditional support during pregnancy, it is evident that women use a variety of sources, including family, friends, and traditional healers. It is the nurse's responsibility to accurately assess each woman's situation, experience, and cultural value system so that culturally competent care can be offered.

Campanella, K., Korbin, J., & Acheson, L. (1993). Pregnancy and childbirth among the Amish. *Social Science Medicine 36*(3), 333–342.

Food Taboos and Cravings

Among many subcultures, women perceive little personal control over the outcome of pregnancy except through the avoidance of foods that are considered taboo. The food taboos in the pregnant Korean woman's diet are thought to have evolved from the danger and uncertainty associated with pregnancy and childbirth (Bauwens, 1978). Traditional Korean food taboos included chicken, duck, rabbit, goat, crab, sparrow, pork, and blemished fruit. These foods were not eaten in an attempt to guard the child from unwanted physical characteristics; for example, eating chicken might cause bumpy skin, or blemished fruit an unpleasant face (Kim & Mo, 1977). A traditional belief in many

| BOX 5–2 | **CULTURAL BELIEFS REGARDING ACTIVITY AND PREGNANCY** |

Prescriptive Beliefs

- Remain active during pregnancy to aid the baby's circulation (Crow Indian)
- Remain happy to bring the baby joy and good fortune (Pueblo and Navajo Indian, Mexican, Japanese)
- Sleep flat on your back to protect the baby (Mexican)
- Keep active during pregnancy to ensure a small baby and an easy delivery (Mexican and Cambodian Canadian)
- Continue sexual intercourse to lubricate the birth canal and prevent a dry labor (Haitian, Mexican)
- Continue daily baths and frequent shampoos during pregnancy to produce a clean baby (Filipino)

Restrictive Beliefs

- Avoid cold air during pregnancy (Mexican, Haitian, Asian)
- Do not reach over your head or the cord will wrap around the baby's neck (African American, Hispanic, White, Asian)
- Avoid weddings and funerals or you will bring bad fortune to the baby (Vietnamese)
- Do not continue sexual intercourse or harm will come to you and baby (Vietnamese, Filipino, Samoan)
- Do not tie knots or braid or allow the baby's father to do so because it will cause difficult labor (Navajo Indian)
- Do not sew (Pueblo Indian, Asian)
- Avoid heavy physical work, eat rich and healthy foods, and get frequent rest (Iranian Canadian)

Taboos

- Avoid lunar eclipses and moonlight or the baby might be born with a deformity (Mexican)
- Do not walk on the streets at noon or 5 o'clock because this might make the spirits angry (Vietnamese)
- Do not join in traditional ceremonies like Yei or Squaw dances, or spirits will harm the baby (Navajo Indian)
- Do not get involved with persons who cast spells or the baby will be eaten in the womb (Haitian)
- Do not say the baby's name before the naming ceremony or harm might come to the baby (Orthodox Jewish)
- Do not have your picture taken because it might cause stillbirth (African American)
- During the postpartum period, avoid visits from widows, women who have lost children, and people in mourning because they will bring bad fortune to the baby (South Asian Canadian)

From Waxler-Morrison, N., Andrews, J., & Richardson, E. (1990). *Cross-cultural caring: A handbook for health professionals in Western Canada.* Vancouver, BC: University of British Columbia Press.

cultures is that a pregnant woman must be given the food that she smells to eat, otherwise the fetus will move inside of her and a miscarriage will be the result (Spector, 2000).

In a Hindu woman's belief system, pregnancy is considered a hot period. Hot foods (i.e., animal products, chilies, spices, and ginger) and gas-producing foods are avoided because they are believed to cause overexcitement, inflammatory reactions, sweating, and fatigue. If eaten too early in pregnancy, hot foods are believed to cause miscarriage and fetal abnormality (Turrell, 1985). Conversely, cold foods (milk products, milk, yogurt, cream, and butter), most vegetables, and foods that taste sour are thought to strengthen and calm the pregnant woman. A study in Saudi Arabia found that pregnant Saudi women craved milk, salt and sour foods, sweets, and dates. They avoided spicy foods and beverages (al-Kanhal & Bani, 1995).

Some pregnant women experience pica: the craving for and ingestion of nonfood substances, such as clay or laundry starch. Some Hispanic women prefer the solid milk of magnesia that can be purchased in Mexico, whereas other women eat the ice or frost that forms inside refrigerator units. The causes of pica are poorly understood, but there are some cultural implications because women from certain ethnic or cultural groups experience this disorder. In the United States, it is common in African-American women raised in the rural South and in women from lower socioeconomic levels. The phenomenon of pica has been described in Kenya, Uganda, and Saudi Arabia. Most often, it is seen in women and appears most frequently during pregnancy. It is occasionally also seen in children (Abrahams, 1997; al-Kanhal & Bani, 1995; Greissler, Mwaniki, Thiong'o, & Friis, 1997).

Cultural Prenatal Care

Morgan's (1996) study of African-American women explored beliefs, practices, and values related to prenatal care. The findings indicated that many of the women in urban areas lacked trust and were apprehensive about their current life circumstances. Establishing a good relationship and providing a safe environment was noted to increase attendance at prenatal clinics. Urban African-American women indicated that they had less support than their contemporaries in the rural South. Nurses should be encouraged to set up peer social and educational groups for women who are similar to those in this study. In addition, the findings indicated that adherence to folk health care beliefs and practices was prevalent among study participants. Nurses must learn more about the practices of their clients and have a nonjudgmental attitude. Acceptance of alternative healers might even be therapeutic and helpful for many clients.

In a study by Berry (1999), Mexican-American women participated in an ethnonursing study focusing on the meanings and experiences attached to generic care (family and extended family pregnancy guidance) and professional care during pregnancy. Significant themes for generic culture care were identified as protection of the mother and fetus by elder Mexican-American women, which was affected by religious and family practices, and the value attached to the family providing care for the mother and being with her. Professional culture care themes included (1) respecting the family roles of caring for the mother in relation to age and gender, (2) expressing concern, knowledge, protection, and explanations and attending to the needs of the mother, (3) using the Spanish language while caring for the mother, and (4) believing that professional prenatal care was valued by the women even though access was in many cases problematic.

Incorporating the value of respect into the culture care of Mexican-American pregnant women can be achieved on many levels and might be demonstrated by the following practices:

1. Supporting the religious or spiritual needs of clients by helping to locate religious advisors and providing time for prayer when indicated
2. Addressing clients by last name and conversing with clients about their families before the initiation of care
3. Acknowledging elder generic guidance during pregnancy and, when appropriate, incorporating these practices into the client's care
4. Respecting the family's beliefs in male authority as protector and final decision maker
5. Encouraging a client to include her spouse in prenatal visits when decisions regarding care must be made, or making the information available for the client to take home for approval, especially when consents are required (Berry, 1999).

Both studies (Morgan, 1996; Berry, 1999) reported similar barriers to prenatal care access, including (1) lack of telephones for communicating with health care providers, (2) lack of transportation to the clinics, (3) legal issues surrounding immigration that affected access, (4) bureaucratic paperwork, and (5) inflexible clinic schedules. Similar barriers to prenatal care access have also been identified in Canada (Waxler-Morrison et al., 1990).

Nurses need to exercise creativity when solving these problems. For instance, they can explore the possibility that city or county governments will provide free transportation to health care sites for women in need of such assistance. They can support the development of telephone health information systems in appropriate languages to explain access to health care, especially for newly immigrated clients. They can rethink and restructure clinic schedules to include weekend and evening appointments as one way of easing the burden of access (Berry, 1999).

Cultural Interpretation of Obstetric Testing

Many women do not understand the emphasis that Western prenatal care places on urinalysis, blood pressure readings, and abdominal measurements. For traditional women, the vaginal examination might be so intrusive and embarrassing that they might avoid prenatal visits or request a female physician or midwife (Bash, 1980; Meleis & Sorrell, 1981; Nelson & Hewitt, 1983; Lipson, Hosseini, Omidian, & Edmonston, 1995). Common discomforts of pregnancy might be managed with folk, herbal, home, or over-the-counter remedies on the advice of a relative (generally the maternal grandmother) or friends (Spector, 2000). Health care providers can attempt to meet the needs of women from traditional cultures by explaining health regimens so that they have meaning within the cultural belief system. However, such explanations are only an initial step. Nursing visits can be made to the home, or group prenatal visits might be made based on self-care models instituted by nurses in local community centers. Additionally, nurses can incorporate significant others into the plan of care. During prenatal visits, nurses can provide information on normal fetal growth and development, and they can discuss how the health and behavior of the mother and those around her can influence fetal outcome.

Cultural Preparation for Childbirth

Preparation for childbirth can be developed through programs that allow for cultural variations, including classes during and after the usual clinic hours in busy urban settings, teen-only classes, single-mother classes, group classes combined with prenatal checkups at home, classes on rural reservations, and presentations that incorporate the older "wise women" of the community. In addition, nurses can organize classes in languages other than English.

• BIRTH AND CULTURE

Beliefs and customs surrounding the experience of labor and delivery are influenced by the fact that the physiologic processes are basically the same in all cultures. Factors such as cultural attitudes toward the achievement of birth, methods of dealing with the pain of labor, recommended positions during delivery, the preferred location for the birth, the role of the father and the family, and expectations of the health care practitioner might vary according to the degree of acculturation to Western childbirth customs, geographic location, religious beliefs, and individual preference.

The concept of achievement versus atonement in birth refers to the way in which a culture defines the birth process as a praised achievement worthy of celebration or a defilement or state of pollution necessitating ritual purification (Newton & Newton, 1972). In general North American culture, birth is often viewed as an achievement—unfortunately not for the mother but rather for the medical staff. The obstetrician "manages" the labor and "delivers" the infant; for this active role, the doctor is often profusely thanked even before the mother is praised or congratulated. Gifts and celebrations are centered on the newborn rather than the mother. The recent consumer movement in childbirth and the upsurge of feminism has caused some redefinition of the cultural focus and has encouraged women and their partners to assume active roles in the management of their own health and birth experiences. Unfortunately, some women who have prepared themselves for a totally "natural" childbirth might feel a sense of personal trauma and failure if they receive analgesia or require delivery by cesarean section (Hott, 1980; Mercer & Stainton, 1984). Nurses must determine how much personal control and involvement are desired by a woman and her family during the birth experience. If expectations and plans made before labor are altered during labor and birth, the nurse should involve the woman and her significant others in all changes and should allow the woman to verbalize her feelings after the birth.

Traditional Home Birth

All cultures have an approach to birth rooted in a tradition in which childbirth occurs at home, within the province of women. For generations, traditions among the poor included the use of "granny" midwives by rural Appalachian whites and southern African Americans and *parteras* by Mexican Americans (Frankel, 1977; Kay, 1978; Barry & Boyle, 1996). A dependence on self-management, a belief in the normality of labor and birth, and a tradition of delivery at home might influence some women to arrive at the hospital only in advanced labor (Frankel, 1977; Nelson & Hewitt, 1983). The need to travel a long distance to the closest hospital might also be a factor contributing to arrival during late labor or to out-of-hospital delivery from many Native North American women living on rural, isolated reservations

Support During Childbirth

Despite the traditional emphasis on female support and guidance during labor, the inclusion of spouses and male partners in North American labor and birth rooms has been seen as positive by women of many cultures. Women from diverse cultures report a desire to have husbands or partners present for the birth. Unfortunately, some North American hospitals still maintain rules that limit the support person to the spouse or that prevent a husband from attending the birth unless he has attended a formal childbirth education program with his wife. Fortunately, this situation has changed a great deal in the past few years, so that husbands or partners now make important contributions in supporting and helping pregnant women during labor (Figure 5-1).

Another source of conflict is the desire of many women to have the mother or some other female relative or friend present during labor and birth. Because many hospitals have rules limiting the number of persons present, the mother might be forced to make a difficult choice among the persons close to her.

Some women and families, particularly those from Orthodox Jewish, Islamic, Chinese, and Asian Indian backgrounds, might follow strict religious and cultural prohibitions against viewing the woman's body by either the husband or any other man, or they might practice separation of the husband and wife once the "bloody show" or cervical dilation has occurred (Bash, 1980; Meleis & Sorrell, 1981; Flint, 1982; Pillsbury, 1982; Callister, Semenic, & Foster, 1999). In cultures in which the husband's presence during labor and delivery is not believed to be appropriate, nurses might mistakenly assume a lack of involvement or interest on his part (Gropper, 1996).

Figure 5–1. These family members provide comfort, emotional support, and coaching throughout the entire labor and delivery. (© Copyright B. Proud)

For particular groups of women, religion or spirituality is central to their belief system and is the guiding factor in the childbirth experience. A recent study by Callister et al. (1999) of Orthodox Jewish and Mormon childbearing women investigated the meaning of culture and religion as they relate to childbirth. Evidence-Based Practice 5-4 highlights the findings and clinical application.

Cultural Expression of Labor Pain

Although the pain threshold is remarkably similar in all persons regardless of gender, social, ethnic, or cultural differences, these differences play a definite role in a woman's perception of labor pain. Because nurses care for women and families from a variety of cultural backgrounds in labor and birth, they must have a knowledge and understanding of how culture mediates pain (Lee & Essoka, 1998; Weber, 1996). In the past it was commonly believed that women from Asian and Native North American cultures were very stoic and did not feel pain in labor (Bachman, 2000). Such views are ethnocentric and should be avoided. Many factors interact to influence labor and the perception of pain. They include cultural attitudes toward the normalcy and conduct of birth, expectations of how a woman should act in labor, the role of significant others, and the physiologic processes involved. For example, when Filipina women were asked how they would act in labor,

EVIDENCE-BASED PRACTICE 5–4
Culture, Religion, and Childbirth.

This descriptive phenomenologic study investigated the spiritual and cultural meanings of childbirth from the perspectives of 30 Canadian Orthodox Jewish and 30 American Mormon childbearing women. Five themes were described and included: (1) the significance of a shared connectedness with others and God, (2) birth was described as a "bittersweet paradox," (3) sense of empowerment, (4) the importance and value placed on childbearing and childrearing, and (5) the spiritual essence of giving birth.

Clinical Application

Listening to women describe significant life events assists nurses as they work with clients to define their health care needs. For these women, spirituality and culture are inextricably woven into the fabric of childbearing practices. Nurses caring for culturally diverse clients must strive to understand the personal meaning and the spiritual essence of birth for each woman and family and respect the expressions of these beliefs by supporting their religious rituals and practices.

Callister, L. C., Semenic, S., & Foster, J. C. (1999). Cultural and spiritual meanings of childbirth. *Journal of Holistic Nursing, 17*(3), 280–295.

many said it was best to lie quietly (Affonso, 1978). By contrast, Middle Eastern women are verbally expressive during labor, sometimes crying and screaming loudly while refusing pain medication (Meleis & Sorrell, 1981; Waxler-Morrison et al., 1990). Samoan women might believe that no verbal expressions of pain are permissible and that only "spoiled" Caucasian women need any analgesia (Clark & Howland, 1978). According to Kay (1978), Hispanic women are traditionally instructed by their *parteras* to endure pain with patience and to close the mouth, for opening the mouth to cry out would cause the uterus to rise.

Callister and Vega (1998) reported that Guatemalan women in labor tend to vocalize their pain. Coping strategies include moaning or breathing rhythmically and massaging the thighs and abdomen. Japanese, Chinese, Vietnamese, Laotian, and other women of Asian descent maintain that screaming or crying out during labor or birth is shameful; birth is believed to be painful but something to be endured (Lee & Essoka, 1998; Weber, 1996; Bachman, 2000). Although many women from diverse cultures are deemed unprepared by some health professionals because they do not use formal breathing and relaxation techniques, women often use culturally appropriate ways of preparing for labor and delivery. These methods might include assisting with childbirth from the time of adolescence, listening to birth and baby stories told by respected elderly women, or following special dietary and activity prescriptions during the antepartal period.

Birth Positions

Numerous anecdotal reports in the literature describe "typical" birth positions for women of diverse cultures, from the seated position in a birth chair favored by Mexican-American women to the squatting position chosen by Laotian Hmong women. The nurse who cares for laboring women must realize, however, that the choice of positions is influenced by many factors other than culture and that the socialization that occurs when a woman arrives in a labor and delivery unit might prevent her from stating her preference.

Economically disadvantaged women from culturally diverse backgrounds have few birth options; most labor and give birth in large public hospitals. Routine patterns of care and decreased individualization are common in these institutions. These and other problems, such as language barriers, make the provision of culturally competent care during the birth process a challenge. However, any special provisions or attempts to understand the client from her perspective will be received with cooperation and gratitude. Recommendations for the intrapartum nursing care of the culturally diverse pregnant woman are presented in Box 5–3.

Cultural Meaning Attached to Infant Gender or Multiple Births

The meaning that parents attach to having a son, a daughter, or multiple births varies from culture to culture. Traditionally, the male gender is highly regarded, which places female infants in a position of "less than favorable." In certain Asian and Islamic cultures, it is felt that a male child is preferable to a female child. Twin births also carry a significance that varies from culture to

BOX 5–3	INTRAPARTUM NURSING CARE FOR CULTURALLY DIVERSE WOMEN

1. If you are unable to speak the woman's language, talk with an English-speaking relative or arrange for an interpreter.
2. If your nursing agency commonly cares for culturally diverse clients, find out whether other nurses have had experiences with similar clients. Share resources and your expertise with staff members.
3. Attempt to gain as much information as possible by completing a cultural assessment.
4. Elicit the mother's expectations about her labor and delivery experience.
5. Does she want a support person with her? If so, have her identify that person.
6. Explore with her any cultural rituals she wants incorporated into her plan of care. If requests are manageable, honor them.
7. Be patient, draw pictures, gesture. Identify key words from family or the interpreter that you will need to be able to express yourself to her; for example, push, blow, pant, stop.

culture. Twins are viewed as a special blessing by the Yoruba tribe and as a curse by the Ibo tribe in the same West African nation of Nigeria. In these situations, the nurse might find the best course of action is simply to point out all the positive attributes of the newborn.

• THE POSTPARTUM PERIOD

Western medicine considers pregnancy and birth the most dangerous and vulnerable time for the childbearing woman. However, other cultures place much more emphasis on the postpartum period. Many cultures have developed practices that balance and cushion this special time of vulnerability for the mother and the infant. Such strategies are thought to serve to mobilize support for the new mother. Interestingly, support that comes from family and friends is usually considered "nontraditional" in approach by Western medicine. These cultural differences, particularly as they relate to restrictive dietary customs, activity levels, and certain taboos and rituals associated with purification and seclusion, might seem unusual to the nurse but have been noted to positively influence the mother's postpartum mental health, thus reducing the incidence of problems such as postpartum depression (Stewart & Jambunathan, 1996). Additional authors (Ross & Mirowsky, 1989; O'Hara, Rehm, & Campbell, 1983) have suggested that lack of social support is one of the highest predictors of both general and postpartum depression. Evidence-Based Practice 5-5 describes postpartum depression among Hmong women.

Routine postpartum nursing care usually includes encouraging a healthy diet, adequate fluid intake, and self-care practices such as good hygiene practices, sitz baths, showering, bathing, ambulation, and exercise. However, these practices, common in North American obstetric care, might seem strange and even dangerous to women of other cultural groups. Nurses must take time not only to teach their clients but to listen to them, making accommodations and being flexible when possible. In many cultures, the concept of postpartum vulnerability is based on one or more beliefs related to imbalance or pollution. **Imbalance** is perceived to be the result of disharmony caused by the processes of pregnancy and birth, and **pollution** is seen to be caused by the "unclean" bleeding associated with birth and the postpartum period (Horn, 1981). Restitution of physical balance and purification might occur through many mechanisms, including dietary restrictions, ritual baths, seclusion, restriction of activity, and other ceremonial events.

Hot/Cold Theory

Central to the belief of perceived imbalance in the mother's physical state is adherence to the **hot/cold theories** of disease causation. Pregnancy is considered a "hot" state. Because a great deal of the heat of pregnancy is thought to be lost during the birth process, postpartum practices focus on restoring the balance between the hot/cold beliefs, or yin and yang. Common components of this theory focus on the avoidance of cold, in the form of either air or food.

EVIDENCE-BASED PRACTICE 5-5
Hmong Women and Postpartum Depression

Postpartum depression in Western culture has been documented. The literature suggests that one cause of postpartum depression is lack of supportive practices surrounding childbirth. This study explored postpartum depression in Hmong women living in the United States. The results indicated these women perceived themselves to be supported during pregnancy and after delivery. The high levels of support received from spouses and family, combined with the practice of a 30-day rest period, might have made them less vulnerable to depression. The only symptoms of depression reported were related to living in a culture and environment different from their own, and having to use a foreign language.

Clinical Application

Be sensitive to the fact that Hmong women have difficulty in learning English because of child care responsibilities and possibly the lack of a formal education. Encourage family involvement in the woman's nursing care plan during and after pregnancy. Provide referrals for opportunities to learn English-speaking skills and employment skills to facilitate the women's adjustment to North American culture.

Stewart, S., & Jumbunathan, J. (1996). Hmong women and postpartum depression. *Health Care for Women International, 17,* 319–330.

One such belief is the Haitian belief that exposure to cold air might cause a uterine cold; the entrance of air into the vagina is thought to be prevented by use of a sanitary pad (Dempsey & Gesse, 1983).

This real fear of the detrimental effects of cold air and water in the postpartum period can cause cultural conflict when the woman and infant are hospitalized. Nurses must assess the woman's beliefs regarding bathing and other self-care practices in a nonjudgmental manner.

Many women will pretend to follow the activities suggested by nurses, to the point of pretending to shower while in reality avoiding the nurses' prescriptions. The common use of perineal ice packs and sitz baths to promote healing can be replaced with the use of heat lamps, heat packs, and anesthetic or astringent topical agents for those who prefer to avoid cold influences. The routine distribution of ice water to all postpartum women is another aspect of care that can be modified to meet women's culturally diverse needs. Offering women a choice of water at room temperature, warm tea or coffee, broth, or another beverage should satisfy most women's needs for warmth, along with the offering of additional bed blankets.

Postpartum Dietary Prescriptions and Activity Levels

Dietary prescriptions are also common in this period. The nurse might note that a woman eats little "hospital" food and relies on family and friends to bring food to her while she is in the hospital. If there are no diet restrictions for health reasons, this practice should be respected. Indeed, the nurse should assess what types of food are being eaten by the woman, documenting them as appropriate.

Regulation of activity in relation to the concept of disharmony or imbalance includes the avoidance of air, cold, and evil spirits. Hispanic women are encouraged to stay indoors and avoid strenuous work. Obviously, if pregnancy and birth cause a "hot" state, the woman should avoid "hot" activities such as ironing. Fruits and vegetables might be avoided because they are considered "cold" foods (Matocha, 1998). Many traditional African-American women view themselves as "sick" during the postpartal lochial flow. They might avoid heavy work, showering, bathing, or washing their hair during this vulnerable time (Carrington, 1978). Cultural prescriptions vary regarding when women can return to full activity after childbirth, but many traditional cultures suggest that a woman can resume normal activities in as little as 2 weeks, and some take up to 4 months.

Postpartum Seclusion

The period of postpartum vulnerability and seclusion in most non–Western cultures varies between 7 and 40 days. Hispanic women, especially primigravidas, might follow a set of dietary and activity rules called *la dieta* (Kay, 1978; Horn, 1981). The Hispanic midwife will stay at the home of the mother for several hours after the delivery and will make a follow-up visit the next day.

A study of traditional Hispanic postpartum practices by Philpotts (1979) described how the midwife disposed of the placenta through burial so that animals would not eat it, because it was believed that if a dog ate the placenta, the mother would be unable to bear subsequent children. Burying the placenta was also believed to prevent the mother from having "afterpains." Placental burial rituals are also part of the traditional Hmong culture, wherein it is believed that proper burial of the placenta is necessary to protect the soul of the deceased from harm after his or her death (Fadiman, 1997).

In some cultures, women are considered to be in a state of impurity or pollution during the postpartum period. Consequently, ritual seclusion and elimination of activity might be practiced to reduce the risk of increasing personal vulnerability to the influence of spirits or of spreading evil and misfortune. In many cultures, this time of seclusion coincides with the period of lochial flow or postpartum bleeding. Common taboos include seclusion and avoidance of contact with others, avoidance of contact with food or objects, and avoidance of sexual relations. Pillsbury (1982) described the Chinese custom of "doing the month," which includes prohibitions against going out into the sunshine, coming into contact with windy drafts, walking about, reading, or crying. A ritual bath might mark the end of the state of pollution; for Navajo women, this might occur on the fourth postpartum day; for Hispanic women, at 2 weeks; and for Orthodox Jewish women, on the seventh day after delivery (Bash, 1980; Kay, 1982).

•CULTURALLY COMPETENT NURSING CARE FOR VULNERABLE CLIENTS DURING PREGNANCY

In this section, culture not only will be viewed from an ethnic or culturally diverse point of view but additionally will examine "cultures within a culture," or subcultures. It will focus on three particular groups or subcultures within the larger culture of pregnant women: the incarcerated pregnant woman, the physically abused pregnant woman, and the homeless pregnant woman. What links these groups of pregnant women as subcultures are shared ideologies or characteristics that influence their behavior and the have profound effects on their pregnancy outcomes. Some of the shared characteristics include stress (physical and emotional), poor lifestyle health practices, delayed prenatal care, lack of support, and exposure to violence. This section will examine the ideologies of each group and offer recommendations about how nurses can offer support to vulnerable pregnant women in these unique circumstances. Other subcultures of the pregnant population that merit consideration in future writings include substance-abusing women, HIV-infected women, migrant laborers, new immigrants or refugees, and pregnant women in rural or remote areas.

Incarcerated Pregnant Women

Incarcerated pregnant women present health care providers with an unusual set of challenges. These women share an unusual and restrictive context that creates a unique subculture. It has been reported that three fourths of incarcerated women are mothers. Most are young, single, undereducated, unskilled, unemployed, and financially disadvantaged, and 10% are pregnant during imprisonment (Osborne, 1995). Normal adaptation to pregnancy is altered by incarceration. According to Hufft (1992), a pregnant woman in prison is vulnerable in four specific areas:

1. Increased stress is caused by inadequate or poor lifestyle health practices, increased risk of suicide, and self-destructive behavior. If a woman becomes pregnant while in a federal prison, it is considered an offense punishable at the very least by isolation, which leads to delays in obtaining prenatal care.
2. Women in prison exist in a restricted environment that fosters aggression and violent behavior, leading to ongoing stress. According to Osborne (1995), prisons have ill-defined provisions for prenatal care and/or plans for labor and delivery. The prison environment dictates the inmates' exercise, diet, mandatory workloads, and clothing, all of which might need alteration during pregnancy.
3. Social support systems are altered during incarceration. The family and social support that usually helps to guide the woman in decision making processes during pregnancy are nonexistent, or at least significantly altered. The social support systems in prison are usually antiauthority, so that if the health care provider is viewed as part of the "establish-

ment," the inmate's own support system might encourage responses that result in noncompliance.

4. There is an alteration in maternal role attainment because learning from the usual sources, such as observing a "good mother role model" and access to appropriate pregnancy literature, is limited.

Rubin (1984) described the maternal role and how the pregnant woman attains it. The attainment of this role focuses on the woman's ability to rehearse the anticipated activities after birth. Incarcerated women know they will not care for their infants after birth, and they understand that they must return to prison after delivery to complete their jail time. The incarcerated woman who has an infant during her prison term has two choices: adoption or placing the infant for guardianship. If she relinquishes her infant for adoption, she is faced with yet another loss that must be addressed. Hufft (1992) suggested that development of the maternal role in incarcerated women must be built on the plans that have been made for the placement of the infant after delivery and must include assessment of the new mother's family situation and her cultural beliefs. Before the birth, the woman must be counseled and assisted to organize her resources. These assessments should ideally be made by either the woman's health care provider or her counselor.

Nurses working in the prison system must be aware of the patterns of behavior that will influence the pregnancy outcomes. They include self-destructive behavior, restrictive environment that increases the exposure to violence, limited prenatal services, and a lack of social support. Nurses are in a position to assist this subculture of pregnant women by developing prenatal programs designed to provide the care and counseling needed to ensure healthy pregnancy outcomes. An additional benefit of such programs would be that learning new coping skills during pregnancy might help with successful coping skills affecting other areas of the woman's life once she is out of prison.

Physically Abused Pregnant Women

Many forms of abuse in the pregnant population warrant attention and discussion. In this section, however, the focus will be on the **physical abuse of pregnant women**.

Information regarding women in abusive situations is scarce, partly because of underreporting. Important information we do know is that abused women are less likely to seek health care because their abuser limits access to resources (King & Ryan, 1989) and that battering occurs more frequently during pregnancy (Taggert & Mattson, 1996). This has implications for the pregnant woman and places her in double jeopardy, not only for herself but for her baby as well, because battering of pregnant women has been associated with adverse pregnancy outcomes (Helton, 1986; Bullock, McFarlane, Bateman, & Miller, 1989; Schei, Samuelsen, & Bakketeig, 1991). A study by Straus and Gelles (1986) reported conservative estimates that 20 to 30% of all women in the United States have experienced physical abuse from their partners at least once. In a recent National Violence Against Women study sponsored by the National Institute of Justice and the Centers for Disease Control and Prevention, it was estimated that 1.9 million women in the United States are assaulted annually (Tjadn & Thoennes, 1998; Rynerson, 2000). During pregnancy, 25 to 45% of women are beaten (Bullock, 1993), and it is estimated that this percentage may be increasing (Rynerson, 2000). Likewise, in Canada, 3 of every 10 women have experienced physical or sexual abuse in a current or previous marital relationship (Statistics Canada, 1993).

Parker, MacFarlane, Soeken, Torres, and Campbell (1993) estimated that 40 to 60% of abused women incur injuries while pregnant. It is reported that violence often begins or escalates during pregnancy and can result in preterm birth or even fetal demise (Schei, et al., 1991; Curry, 1998). It has also been confirmed that abused pregnant women have a two to four times greater risk of being delivered of a low birth weight (LBW) infant (Bullock et al., 1989). One of the associations between abuse and LBW is delay in obtaining prenatal care. Indeed, recent studies suggest that physical and sexual abuse predicts poor health during pregnancy and the postpartum period (Leserman, Stewart & Dell, 1999). Evidence-Based Practice 5-6 discusses delays in obtaining prenatal care as a result of battering.

Campbell and Fishwick (1993) suggested that the most appropriate framework for viewing violence in general, and wife abuse specifically, is the concept of machismo. In Western culture, violence can be viewed as a "clandestine masculine ideal" because male heroes are "Rambo" types and playboys

EVIDENCE-BASED PRACTICE 5–6
Prenatal Care Delays Related to Battering

This study evaluated patterns of abuse during the pregnancies of 132 African American, 208 Hispanic, and 162 White American women from low-income clinics in large metropolitan cities in the West. The researchers found that the incidence of abuse did not vary significantly among ethnic groups and that the abused women from these groups sought prenatal care 6.5 weeks later than did the nonabused group. In this study, 1 in 4 women reported that they had been physically abused since their current pregnancy began, with African-American women experiencing the most severe and most frequent abuse.

Clinical Application

Include questions about abuse in every routine history taken during pregnancy in order to identify abused women. Offer information about abuse and available community resources. Women reporting abuse will need further screening with specific tools. Nurses should be aware of subtle signs of abuse. For example, psychosomatic complaints, injuries inconsistent with the explanation, failure to keep clinic appointments, and overprotective partners might be indications of abuse. Become familiar with community resources for referrals.

Taggart, L., & Mattson, S. (1996). Delay in prenatal care as a result of battering in pregnancy: Crosscultural implications. *Health Care for Women International, 17,* 25–34.

who treat women with disdain. Campbell and Fishwick (1993) suggest that machismo is present to some extent in all men but is more prevalent in lower socioeconomic groups and African Americans. Machismo in African-American men might be related to the systematic degradation and oppression by white racist society. Machismo is also widespread in middle-class white North American society because of the legacy of patriarchy, which is deeply embedded in our culture. Other factors, especially alcohol abuse, often contribute to violence against women.

This section will discuss three ethnically different groups of women and the experience of physical abuse during pregnancy. Attention will be brought to the patterns of behavior that influences their pregnancy outcomes. They includes exposure to physical harm or death, delayed prenatal care because of restricted access by the abuser, restricted support-seeking behavior, and exposure to drugs and alcohol. Recommendations for health care providers will follow each discussion and will emphasize the importance of culturally competent care to these at-risk clients.

Hispanic Pregnant Women

Although there are many different Hispanic groups, they do share some important commonalities, e.g., religion, customs, and language. As with any cultural group, differences do exist among the members. The incidence of wife abuse among pregnant Hispanic women is not clear in the literature. However, Richwald and McClusky (1985) believe that although violence during pregnancy is likely to be the most common form of family violence, it is also the least reported. Campbell and Fishwick (1993) pointed out the irony that prenatal care routinely includes close monitoring for physiologic disorders but does not routinely include screening for physical abuse by the mother's partner.

Access to health care for pregnant Hispanic women is problematic. Barriers to prenatal health care include lack of health care insurance; low levels of education, which encourages the use of traditional healers and remedies and might foster mistrust of physicians and nurses and lead to noncompliance when pregnant women do use modern medicine; lengthy travel time to clinics, followed by long waits; and the lack of Spanish-speaking health care professionals (Torres,1993). Hispanic women tend to be in low-paying jobs whose annual earnings are considerably less than those of non-Hispanic women. They also have less education than White women and large, extended households, often made up of several children and extended family members. The economic status of Hispanics, and therefore their health status, is closely tied to economic levels because economic status often determines access to care (Poma, 1987; Suarez & Ramirez, 1999). These many factors place them at a distinct disadvantage when it comes to accessing prenatal care. Furthermore, these same factors tend to discourage the pregnant Hispanic woman from disclosing a situation of abuse and violence. Her choices are the same as those of other women in abusive situations: she can try to make the relationship work, or she can leave her abuser. If you are poor, have no friends or family members nearby, and have several little children who depend on you, leaving the family provider will be very difficult.

The Hispanic pregnant woman who chooses to leave her abuser must face the reality of language barriers, a poor economic situation, no insurance, and perhaps leaving her traditional family support network. These same factors work to inhibit the seeking of information regarding resources available to abused women. Even when faced with death, some abused women find it very difficult to expose their private situation to someone outside their cultural circle. Furthermore, certain groups of Hispanic women, such as migrants, are at higher risk because they are separated from family support systems, and other barriers such as poverty and language might be exacerbated (Rodriquez, 1993).

Nurses and other health practitioners in prenatal clinics are in an ideal position to facilitate a trusting relationship with an abused woman. Good assessment skills are crucial, because the first sign of abuse might not be an admission of abuse but physical findings of trauma. It is also helpful that the nurse have strong interpersonal skills and a genuine interest in Hispanic culture. In this situation, a Spanish-speaking health care provider might be able to form a trusting relationship more quickly, enabling the woman to share information about domestic violence. Recommendations for assistance of abused pregnant Hispanic women include working with and mobilizing support, using the family and kinship structure; educating the abused woman regarding available resources for abused women; encouraging the woman's inner strength; and assisting in the development of skills necessary to mobilize resources (Torres, 1993).

Black Pregnant Women

Cultural beliefs of Blacks emphasize the larger Black society rather than focusing on individuals, making "all" collectively responsible for one another (McNair, 1992). Therefore, Black women exist in a social context supported by social connectedness versus that of autonomy. It is very difficult to be specific about an assessment of factors related to domestic violence among Black women because of the lack of information. However, Roy (1982) has suggested that poor economic conditions might be the major reason why violence occurs in Black families. Supporting this view, Carlson (1977) reports that the primary basis for domestic violence is environmental stress related to limited social and economic resources. The risk of wife abuse is thought to be greatest when the woman has a higher educational status than her partner or when the man is unemployed or has trouble keeping a job. This is a familiar social situation in Black male-female relationships (Barnes, 1999).

One of the most difficult barriers confronting Black abused women attempting to get help from police or from the legal system is the stereotypical view that suggests that violence among Blacks is normal (Hawkins, 1987). This view can lead to an unequal response to Black victims of violence. In reality, most Blacks do not commit violent crimes, in spite of the tremendous racism, oppression, and discrimination that they experience (Barnes, 1999). Another barrier to reporting of wife abuse is that there might be greater than normal consideration by the wife for her abuser. The women are aware of increased suppression of Black men by society at large and thus might take extra care to protect them (Hare, 1979).

Again, the nurse in the prenatal setting is in an ideal position to gather information and initiate a trusting relationship. As has been pointed out, the abused pregnant woman in this culture might not be willing to incriminate her mate because she already sees him as a "victim of society." The nurse might need to rely heavily on her assessment and history-taking skills, being particularly alert to instances of trauma and to problems with past pregnancies. Education must stress that although the women see their men as "victims," women cannot and must not tolerate abuse. The nurse can identify shelter facilities in the woman's neighborhood and in other areas. If she feels uncomfortable going outside her neighborhood (many do for fear they will not be understood outside their culture) the nurse can encourage her to go to members of her extended family, which might be more acceptable within this culture. What is most important is that she has a plan of what to do, where to go, and who to call for help the next time she is afraid for her own safety. Last, the nurse must realize that in most instances, Black women believe that it is the responsibility of the woman to maintain the family, regardless of other factors. These women have been shown to be more likely to stay in the relationship or to work with professionals to modify the abuser's behavior (White, 1985).

Native North American Pregnant Women

Violence within families has not always been part of Native North American society. Albers and Medicine (1983) noted that before contact with Europeans, Native North American society was based on harmony and respect for nature and all living things, sharing, and cooperation. Contributions from both sexes were valued, and many activities were shared, including the roles of warrior and hunter. Traditionally, cruelty to women and children resulted in public humiliation and loss of honor. Cultural disintegration, poverty, isolation, racism, and alcoholism are just a few of the problems that have fostered violence in Native North American cultures. Nevertheless, despite its prevalence, cruelty to women and children continues to be viewed by Native North Americans as a social disgrace (Green, 1996).

Since the 1970s, Native North American tribes have made an effort to develop programs to meet the needs of their communities. However, abuse among women has not been addressed adequately because of the male-dominated leadership, other needs of the tribes, and the shame associated with abuse (Bohn, 1993). This trend is changing gradually. For example, many Native North American communities in Canada have recently developed programs specifically designed to address family violence and facilitate healing at the individual, family, and community levels (Green, 1996).

Recommendations for health care providers include identification of the abused person by direct questioning in a private setting, but only after a trusting relationship is established. Assessment of the woman's chart or medical record is critical and might provide an opening for discussion of abuse-related questions. A thorough history might indicate signs of abuse through reports of previous problems, injuries, depression, suicide attempts, eating disorders, miscarriages, and complications of pregnancy.

In interviews of Native North American women, a sense of humor is most helpful because they view someone with whom they can laugh as easy to talk to. Open-ended questions are preferable. The nurse should also learn to become comfortable with periods of silence after questions. This does not mean that clients are not listening but rather just the opposite. These women think the question is worthy of thoughtful consideration before answering.

Once abuse has been assessed, the extent of abuse must be ascertained. The nurse or practitioner must then intervene by providing information, discussing alternatives, and supporting the woman in her decision. Options should focus on Native North American resources because they will be culturally sensitive to her needs. If only non-Indian resources are available, the nurse should investigate the experience of Native North American women within these agencies (Bohn, 1993). Variables to be considered in a discussion of options should include the woman's support system, her personal and cultural value system, and her financial status.

Abuse within this culture is traditionally handled within the family first. The abused woman might be reluctant to go outside for help because this might cause both families to ostracize her. It is important to know that a Native North American woman considers it a virtue to stay with her mate no matter what the circumstance, especially if the marriage was performed by a traditional medicine man or woman. Wolk (1982) notes that a woman who chooses to stay with her abuser might do so out of loyalty because he is Native American rather than because he is a man. It is essential to understand that when a woman attempts to leave an abusive relationship, she must know that her health care provider cares about her. Safety for the woman and her unborn baby is the priority. The woman will need phone numbers of shelters, counselors, and legal advisors as well as information about job training and educational opportunities. It is important to focus on her strengths, her sense of humor, and her skills and resources. She must be able to feel hope that both she and her abuser will heal.

An additional factor related to physical abuse for Native North American pregnant women is that of alcohol abuse (Robinson, Armstrong, Moczuk, & Loock, 1992). Living with abuse and becoming dependent on alcohol and other drugs are intertwined problems for many women, especially Native North American women. The use and abuse of alcohol and/or drugs is one way of coping with an abusive relationship, but it also places the woman and her developing fetus at considerable health risk.

Homeless Pregnant Women

Issues related to homelessness are multiple and complex, but for a **pregnant homeless woman**, this time of physiologic and psychologic change without proper medical management is particularly problematic. Evidence-Based Practice 5-7 summarizes a study by Killion (1995) and includes interventions for clinical application.

EVIDENCE-BASED PRACTICE 5–7
Health Care Needs of Pregnant Homeless Women

Using an ethnographic approach, the unique health care needs of pregnant homeless women in southern California over 3 years were studied. Fifteen women from five different shelters participated. The findings included insights into conception while homeless and what effect their homeless state had on the physiologic and psychologic changes of pregnancy.

Clinical Application

1. Many women are ashamed of their homeless state, so it is important that women who "appear" impoverished be assessed carefully, especially regarding housing.
2. Once it is determined that they are living in a shelter or on the street, provide education that is culturally and situationally relevant.
3. "Seize the moment" by providing tools for preventive measures.
4. Encourage the addition or development of "respite rooms" in the office or clinic.
5. Build on existing support systems.

Killion, C. M. (1995). Special health care needs of homeless pregnant women. *Advanced Nursing Science, 18*(2), 44–56.

An additional study with a similar focus investigated perinatal outcomes of homeless women in New York City and showed reasons for poor outcomes, which included poor or no housing, poor access to prenatal care, poor nutrition, and exposure to substance abuse and sexually transmitted diseases (Beal & Redlener, 1995). This study identified two primary groups of homeless pregnant women: runaway youth living on the streets and pregnant women in homeless families, each with different needs. Runaways were found to require the most comprehensive services, health care, housing, education, and some day care, and women in homeless families had complex medical and social needs (Beal & Redlener, 1995). As in the Killion (1995) research, providers often noted that the women were afraid to disclose their homeless status for fear their children would be taken by state authorities. This points to the need for sensitive assessment by the nurse regarding the woman's housing. The researchers observed that one of the initial problems faced by this group is finding a shelter that will accept a pregnant woman, because many will not, for liability reasons. Another issue identified was accessing "homeless-friendly" prenatal services, which the New York State provides. Statistics from the New York Community Family Planning Council indicated that in the homeless pregnant population it serves, women average six to seven prenatal visits with follow-up compliance (New York Community Family Planning Council, 1994).

Housing, although a priority, is not the only need, and providers must be ready to assist clients with information about health care access and social and economic support. Patterns of behavior that providers must take into consideration when caring for this subculture include exposure to violence (living on the street can be most harmful for a pregnant woman), exposure to the elements (extremes in temperature, living in a box, sleeping on the ground), exposure to drugs and alcohol, poor sanitation, lack of nutritional food, and lack of regular meals. Only by being aware of the complexity of homelessness can nurses be prepared to offer empathetic sensitive care to this vulnerable group of pregnant women.

SUMMARY

Culture as it relates to pregnancy and childbirth was discussed from many vantage points. Biologic and cultural variations that can affect childbearing outcomes were identified and analyzed. Women choosing alternative childbearing lifestyles were examined. The importance of nontraditional support systems to pregnant women, along with discussions of cultural beliefs and practices as they relate to pregnancy, birth, and the postpartum period, were presented with suggestions for nursing care.

Vulnerable pregnant subcultures were selected for analysis, including the incarcerated pregnant woman, the physically abused pregnant woman, and the homeless pregnant woman. Nursing care recommendations were offered for each.

Cultural beliefs and practices are continuously evolving, making it necessary for the nurse to acknowledge the various cultures and explore the meaning of childbearing with each family with whom she has contact. It is also important to remember that behavior must be evaluated from within each person's cultural context so that the care provided is not only knowledge based but meaningful.

Cortis (2000), using Leininger's Theory of Culture Care Diversity and Universality, investigated the perceived meaning of care as described by recently hospitalized members of a Pakistani community in Bradford, West Yorkshire, United Kingdom. Although it does not deal with childbearing clients, the study merits inclusion for consideration from the "culture and care" aspect. The findings indicate that the participants did not believe their expectations for "care" by nurses were realized while they were in the hospital. The study suggests one possible reason: that a therapeutic nurse-client relationship did not develop. The Pakistani participants gave evidence of a lack of cultural care by nurses. The researcher noted that a nurse, if not careful, might find that "innate racism" might keep him or her from acknowledging and addressing a client's cultural needs. In keeping with these findings, Cortis discussed the importance of effective cultural assessment, the use of assessment guides as a framework, and the importance of developing the nurse-client relationship as a way to come to understand not only clients' normative needs but their cultural needs as well (Cortis, 2000).

These types of studies should serve to heighten our awareness of not only the need for sound nursing knowledge but the significance of genuine concern, interest, and respect for our clients' differing backgrounds. Only when these aspects are fully realized can we develop and provide culturally appropriate care for childbearing women and their families.

REVIEW QUESTIONS

1. List the biologic variations discussed and the implications for nursing care of the childbearing woman and her family.
2. Identify nursing interventions for women who relinquish infants during the postpartum period. Identify the typical cultural values in North American society about women who relinquish their infants.
3. Describe the special needs of lesbian couples during the childbearing process. What are common pejorative values about lesbian mothers?
4. Compare traditional Western medical support for pregnant women with nontraditional support, and describe why both might be critical for successful pregnancy outcomes in culturally diverse women.
5. Describe the differences between prescriptive and restrictive beliefs about a mother's behavior during pregnancy.
6. Describe two barriers that face Black women as they attempt to get help in abusive situations.
7. Describe the culturally competent care that must be available to pregnant women who experience domestic violence. Why is this care important?
8. Identify what you believe to be important considerations in adapting a cultural assessment for use with a homeless pregnant woman.

CRITICAL THINKING ACTIVITIES

1. Critically analyze the culturally competent nursing interventions for a Hispanic woman after fetal demise from a cord accident.
2. Develop a prenatal assessment tool that takes account of the cultural context of incarcerated pregnant women. How would you implement the use of such a tool? What argument would you use?
3. Analyze the responses the culturally competent postpartum nurse should initiate when a Black woman refuses to get out of bed and shower?
4. Discuss and critically analyze how you would respond to your labor patient's request to allow her lesbian partner to participate in the birth of "their" child. What activities would you include in the plan of care? Why?
5. Describe and analyze how the nurse might offer culturally appropriate support to the husband of a Middle Eastern laboring woman who has followed his cultural traditions and leaves the labor room once the bloody show occurs.

• References

Abrahams, P. W. (1997). Geophagy (soil consumption) and iron supplementation in Uganda. *Tropical Medicine and International Health, 2*(7), 624–630.

Affonso, D. D. (1978). The Filipino American. In A. L. Clark (Ed.). *Culture, childbearing, and health professionals.* Philadelphia: F. A. Davis.

Albers, P., & Medicine, B. (1983). *The hidden half: Studies of plains Indian women.* Lanham, MD: University Press of America.

al-Kanhal, M. A., & Bani, I. A. (1995). Food habits during pregnancy among Saudi women. *International Journal for Vitamin and Nutrition Research, 65*(3), 206–210.

Bachman, J. A. (2000). Management of discomfort. In D. L. Lowdermilk, S. E. Perry, & I. M. Bobak (Eds.). *Maternity and women's health care* (7th ed., pp.463–487). St. Louis, MO: Mosby.

Barnes, S. Y. (1999). Theories of spouse abuse: Relevance to African Americans. *Issues in Mental Health Nursing, 20,* 357–371.

Barry, D., & Boyle, J. S. (1996). An ethnohistory of a granny midwife. *Journal of Transcultural Nursing, 8*(1), 13–18.

Bash, D. M. (1980). Jewish religious practices related to childbearing. *Journal of Nurse-Midwifery, 25*(5), 39–42.

Bauwens, E. E. (1978). *The anthropology of health.* St. Louis, MO: Mosby.

Beal, A. C., Redlener, I. (1995). Enhancing perinatal outcome in homeless women: The challenge of providing comprehensive health care. *Seminars in Perinatology, 19*(4), 307–313.

Berenstein, J. L., & Kidd, Y. A. (1982). Childbearing in Japan. In M. A. Kay (Ed.). *Anthropology of human birth.* Philadelphia: F. A. Davis.

Berry, A.B. (1999). Mexican American women's expressions of the meaning of culturally congruent prenatal care. *Journal of Transcultural Nursing, 10*(3), 203–212.

Boehme, T. (1985). Hepatitis B: The nurse-midwife's role in management and prevention. *Journal of Nurse-Midwifery, 30*(2), 79–87.

Bohn, D. K. (1993). Nursing care of Native American battered women. *AWHONN's Clinical Issues in Perinatal and Women's Health Nursing, 4*(3), 424–436.

Bromwich, P., and Parsons, T. (1990). *Contraception: The facts.* 2nd ed. Oxford: Oxford University Press.

Bryant, C. A. (1982). The impact of kin, friend, and neighbor networks on infant feeding practices. *Social Science & Medicine, 16,* 1757–1765.

Buchholz, S. (2000). Experiences of lesbian couples during childbirth. *Nursing Outlook, 48*(6), 307–311.

Bullock, L., McFarlane, J., Bateman, L., & Miller, V. (1989). Characteristics of battered women in a primary care setting. *Nurse Practitioner, 14*(6), 47–55.

Bullock, L. (1993). Nursing interventions for abused women on obstetrical units. *AWHONN's Clinical Issues in Perinatal Women's Health Nursing, 4*(3), 371–377.

Bushy, A. (1998a). Health issues of women in rural environments: An overview. *Journal of American Medical Women's Association, 53*(2), 53.

Callister, L. C., Semenic, S., & Foster, J. C. (1999). Cultural and spiritual meanings of childbirth: Orthodox Jewish and Mormon women. *Journal of Holistic Nursing, 17*(3), 280–295.

Callister, L. C., & Vega, R. (1998). Giving birth: Guatemalan women's voices. *Journal of Obstetric, Gynecologic, and Neonatal Nursing, 27,* 289–295.

Campanella, K., Korbin, J., & Acheson, L. (1993). Pregnancy and childbirth among the Amish. *Social Science Medicine, 36*(3), 333–342.

Campbell, J., & Fishwick, N. (1993). Abuse of female partners. In J. Campbell & J. Humphreys (Eds.). *Nursing care of survivors of family violence* (2nd ed., pp. 68–104). St. Louis, MO: Mosby.

Carlson, B. (1977). Battered women and their assailants. *Social Work, 22,* 455–471.

Carrington, B. W. (1978). The Afro-American. In A. L. Clark (Ed.). *Culture, childbearing, and health professionals.* Philadelphia: F. A. Davis.

Clark, A. L., & Howland, R. I. (1978). The American Samoan. In A. L. Clark (Ed.). *Culture, childbearing, and health professionals.* Philadelphia: F. A. Davis.

Cosminsky, S. (1982). Childbirth and change: A Guatemalan study. In C.P. MacCormack (Ed.). *Etiology of fertility and birth.* New York: Academic Press.

Cortis, J. D. (2000). Caring as experienced by minority ethnic patients. *International Nursing Review, 47,* 53–62.

Curry, M. (1998). The interrelationships between abuse, substance use, and psychosocial stress during pregnancy. *Journal of Obstetric, Gynecologic, and Neonatal Nursing, 27*(6), 692–699.

Dempsey, P. A., & Gesse, T. (1983). The childbearing Haitian refugee: Cultural applications to clinical nursing. *Public Health Reports, 98*(3), 261–267.

Dempster, J. (1996). Continuing education forum. Fetal alcohol syndrome: The nurse practitioner perspective. *Journal of the American Academy of Nurse Practitioners, 8*(7), 343–352.

Dickason, E. J., Silverman, B. L., & Schult, M. O. (1994). *Maternal infant nursing care* (2nd ed.). St. Louis, MO: Mosby.

Dickason, E. J., Silverman, B. L., & Kaplan, J. A. (1998). *Maternal infant nursing care* (3rd ed.). St. Louis, MO: Mosby.

Erickson, R. V., & Hoang, G. N. (1980). Health problems among Indochinese refugees. *American Journal of Public Health, 70*(9), 1003–1005.

Fadiman, A. (1997). *The spirit catches you and you fall down: A Hmong child, her American doctors, and the collision of two cultures.* New York: Noonday Press.

Flint, M. (1982). Lockmi: An Indian midwife. In M. A. Kay (Ed.). *Anthropology of human birth.* Philadelphia: F. A. Davis.

Ford, C. S. (1964). *A comparative study of human reproduction.* New Haven, CT: Human Relations Area Files Press.

Frankel, B. (1977). *Childbirth in the ghetto: Folk beliefs of Negro women in a North Philadelphia hospital ward.* San Francisco: R & E Research Associates.

Geissler, P. W., Mwaniki, D. L., Thiong'o, F., & Friis, H. (1997). Geophagy among school children in western Kenya. *Tropical Medicine and International Health, 2*(7), 624–630.

Green, K. (1996). *Family violence in aboriginal communities: An aboriginal perspective.* Ottawa, ON: National Clearing House on Family Violence.

Gropper, R. C. (1996). *Culture and the clinical encounter.* Yarmouth, ME: Intercultural Press.

Hare, N. (1979). The relative psycho-socio-economic suppression of the black male. In W. D. Smith, K. H. Burlew, M. H. Moseley, & W. M. Whitnew (Eds.). *Reflections on black psychology* (pp. 359–381). Washington, DC: University Press.

Harris, S. B., Caulfield, L. E., Sugamori, M. E., Whalen, E. A., & Henning, B. (1997). The epidemiology of diabetes in pregnant Native Canadians. *Diabetes Care, 20*(9), 1422–1425.

Harvey, S. M., Carr, C., & Bernheine, S. (1989). Lesbian mother's health care experiences. *Journal of Nurse Midwifery, 34*(3), 115–119.

Hawkins, D. F. (1987). Devalued lives and racial stereotypes: Ideological barriers to the prevention of family violence among blacks. In R. H. Hampton (Ed.). *Violence in the black family: Correlates and consequences* (pp. 190–205). Lexington, MA: Lexington Books.

Health Canada (1999). *Diabetes in Canada: National statistics and opportunities for improved surveillance, prevention, and control.* Available at: *http://www.hc-sc.gc.ca/hpb/lcdc/publicat/diabet99/pdf/diab99_e.pdf.* Accessed January 18, 2002.

Helton, A. (1986). *Protocol of care for the battered woman.* White Plains, NY: March of Dimes Birth Defects Foundation.

Horn, B. M. (1981). Cultural concepts and postpartal care. *Nursing and Health Care, 2*(9), 516–517.

Hott, J. R. (1980). Best laid plans. *Nursing Research, 29,* 20–27.

Hufft, A. G. (1992). Psychosocial adaptation to pregnancy in prison. *Journal of Psychosocial Nursing, 30*(4), 19–23.

Johnston, M. (1980). Cultural variations in professional and parenting patterns. *Journal of Obstetric, Gynecologic, and Neonatal Nursing, 9*(1), 9–13.

Kay, M. A. (1978). The Mexican American. In A. L. Clark (Ed.). *Culture, childbearing, and health professionals.* Philadelphia: F. A. Davis.

Kay, M. A. (1982). Writing an ethnography of birth. In M. A. Kay (Ed.). *Anthropology of human birth.* Philadelphia: F. A. Davis.

Killion, C.M. (1995). Special health care needs of homeless pregnant women. *Advances in Nursing Science, 18*(2), 44–56.

Kim, K., & Mo, S. (1977). A study of food taboos on the Jeju island: Focused on pregnancy. *Korean Journal of Nutrition, 10,* 49–57.

King, M. C., & Ryan, J. (1989). Abused women: Dispelling myths and encouraging intervention. *Nurse Practitioner, 14,* 47–58.

Kraybill, D. B. (1989). *The riddle of Amish culture.* Baltimore: The John Hopkins University Press.

Lantican, L. S., & Corona, D. F. (1992). Comparison of the social support networks of Filipino and Mexican-American primigravidas. *Health Care for Women International, 13,* 329–338.

Lauderdale, J., & Boyle, J. (1994). Infant relinquishment through adoption. *Image Journal of Nursing Scholarship, 26*(3), 213–217.

Lee, M. & Essoka, G. (1998). Continuing education. Patient's perception of pain: Comparison between Korean-American and Euro-American obstetric patients. *Journal of Cultural Diversity, 5*(1), 29–40.

Leserman, J., Stewart, J., & Dell, D. (1999). Sexual and physical abuse predicts poor health in pregnancy and postpartum. *Psychosomatic Medicine, 61,* 92.

Lipson, J. G., Hosseini, M. A., Omidian, P. A., & Edmonston, F. (1995). Health Issues among Afghan in California. *Health Care for Women International,* 16(4), 279–286.

Logan, B. B., & Dawkins, C. E. (1986). *Family centered nursing in the community.* Menlo Park, CA: Addison-Wesley.

Lowdermilk, D. L., Perry, S. E., & Bobak, I. M (Eds.). (2000). *Maternity and women's health care* (7th ed.). St. Louis, MO: Mosby.

MacCormack, C. P. (1982). Biological, cultural, and social adaptation in human fertility and birth: A synthesis. In C. P. MacCormack (Ed.). *Ethnography of fertility and birth.* New York: Academic Press.

Matocha, L. K. (1998). Chinese-Americans. In L. D. Purnell & B. J. Paulanka (Eds.). *Transcultural nursing: A culturally competent approach* (pp. 163–188). Philadelphia: F. A. Davis.

McClain, C. (1982). Toward a comparative framework for the study of childbirth: A review of the literature. In M. A. Kay (Ed.). *Anthropology of human birth.* Philadelphia: F. A. Davis.

McNair, L. D. (1992). African American women in therapy: An Afrocentric and feminist synthesis. *Women and Therapy, 12,* 5–19.

Mead, M., & Newton, N. (1967). Cultural patterning of perinatal behavior. In S. A. Richardson & A. F. Guttmacher (Eds.). *Childbearing: Its social and psychological aspects.* Baltimore: Williams & Wilkins.

Meleis, A. I., & Sorrell, L. (1981). Bridging cultures: Arab American women and their birth experiences. *Maternal Child Nursing, 6,* 171–176.

Mercer, R. T., & Stainton, M. C. (1984). Perceptions of the birth experience: A cross-cultural comparison. *Health Care for Women International, 5,* 29–47.

Miller, M. A. (1992). Contraception outside North America: Options and popular choices. *NAACOG's Clinical Issues in Perinatal and Women's Health Nursing, 3*(2), 253–265.

Morgan, M. (1996). Prenatal care of African American women in selected USA urban and rural cultural contexts. *Journal of Transcultural Nursing, 7*(2), 3–9.

Morrison, V. (2000). Contraceptive need among Cambodian refugees in Khao Phlu camp. *International Family Planning Perspectives, 26*(4), 188–92.

Nelson, C. C., & Hewitt, M. A. (1983). An Indochinese refugee population in a nurse-midwifery service. *Journal of Nurse-Midwifery, 28*(5), 9–14.

New York Community Family Planning Council. (1994). A network of community-based health centers [press release].

Newton, N., & Newton, M. (1972). Childbirth in crosscultural perspective. In J. G. Howells (Ed.). *Modern perspectives in psycho-obstetrics.* New York: Brunner/Mazel.

Oakley, A. (1980). *Women confined: Towards a sociology of childbirth.* New York: Schocken Books.

O'Hara, M., Rehm, L., & Campbell, S. (1983). Postpartum depression: A role for social network and life stress variables. *Journal of Nervous Disorders, 171,* 336–341.

Okamoto, N. I. (1978). The Japanese American. In A. L. Clark (Ed.). *Culture, childbearing, and health professionals.* Philadelphia: F. A. Davis.

Osborne, O. (1995). Jailed mothers: Further explorations in public sector nursing. *Journal of Psychosocial Nursing, 33*(8), 23–28.

Otoide, V. O., Oronsaye, F. & Okonofua, F. E. (2001). Why Nigerian adolescents seek abortion rather that contraception: Evidence from focus-group discussions. *International Family Planning Perspectives, 27*(2), 77–81.

Overfield, T. (1985). *Biologic variation in health and illness.* Menlo Park, CA: Addison-Wesley.

Parker, B., McFarlane, J., Soeken, K., Torres, S. and Campbell, J. (1993). Physical and emotional abuse in pregnancy: a comparison of adult and teen women. *Nursing Research 42,* 173–177.

Perry, S. E. (2000). Medical-surgical problems in pregnancy. In D. L. Lowdermilk, S. E. Perry, & I. M. Bobak (Eds.). *Maternity and women's health care* (7th ed., pp. 887–911). St. Louis, MO: Mosby.

Pettit, D. J., Knowler, W. C., Baird, H. R., & Bennet, P. H. (1980). Gestational diabetes: Infant and maternal complication of pregnancy in relation to third-trimester glucose tolerance in Pima Indians. *Diabetes Care, 3*(3), 458–464.

Philpott, L. L. (1979). *A descriptive study of birth practices and midwifery in the lower Rio Grande valley of Texas.* Dissertation Abstracts International Vol. 40-11B. p. 5217.

Pickwell, S. (1983). Health screening for Indochinese refugees. *Nurse Practitioner, 8*(4), 20–21, 25.

Pillsbury, B. (1982). "Doing the month": Confinement and convalescence of Chinese women after childbirth. In M. A. Kay (Ed.). *Anthropology of human birth.* Philadelphia: F. A. Davis.

Poma, P. A. (1987). Pregnancy in Hispanic women. *Journal of the National Medical Association 79,* 929–935.

Pritchard, I. A., MacDonald, P. C., & Gant, N. F. (1984). *William's obstetrics* (17th ed.). Norwalk, CT: Appleton-Century-Crofts.

Raphael, D. (1976). Matrescence, becoming a mother, a new/old rite de passage. In F. X. Grollig & H. B. Haley (Eds.). *Medical anthropology.* Paris: Mouton Publishers.

Richwald, G. A., & McClusky, T. E. (1985). Family violence during pregnancy. In D. B. Jeliffe & E. F. T. Jeliffe (Eds.). *Advances in international maternal and child health* (pp. 87–96). New York: Oxford University Press.

Robinson, G., Armstrong, R., Moczuk, B., & Loock, C. (1992). Knowledge of fetal alcohol syndrome among native Indians. *Canadian Journal of Public Health, 83*(5), 337–338.

Rodriguez, J. (1998). Culture Tips. Cuban Americans. Cross-cultural-connection. 4(1):5 July-Sept.

Rose, P. A. (1978). The Chinese American. In A. L. Clark (Ed.). *Culture, childbearing, and health professionals.* Philadelphia: F. A. Davis.

Ross, C. E., & Mirowsky, J. (1989). Explaining the social patterns of depression: Control and problem solving—or support and talking? *Journal of Health and Social Behavior, 30,* 206–219.

Roy, M. (1982). Four thousand partners in violence: A trend analysis. In M. Roy (Ed.). *The abusive partner* (pp. 17–35). New York: Van Nostrand.

Rubin, R. (1984). *Maternal identity and the maternal experience.* New York: Springer.

Rynerson, B. C. (2000. Violence against women. In D. L. Lowdermilk, S. E. Perry, & I. M. Bobak (Eds.). *Maternity and women's health Care* (7th ed., pp. 225–246). St. Louis, MO: Mosby.

Schei, B., Samuelsen, S., & Bakketeig, L. (1991). Does spousal physical abuse affect the outcome of pregnancy? *Scandinavian Journal of Social Medicine, 19,* 26–31.

Shain, N. S. (1982). Abortion practices in cross cultural perspective. *American Journal of Obstetrics and Gynecology.* 142(3), 245–251.

Smitherman, C. (1994). The lasting impact of fetal alcohol syndrome and fetal alcohol: Effect on children and adolescents. *Journal of Pediatric Health Care, 8*(3), 121–126.

Spector, R. (2000). *Cultural diversity in health and illness* (5th ed.). Upper Saddle River, NJ: Prentice Hall Health.

Spinks, V. S., Andrews, J., & Boyle, J. S. (2000). Providing health care for lesbian clients. *Journal of Transcultural Nursing, 11,* 137–143.

Stanton, M. E. (1979). The "myth" of natural childbirth. *Journal of Nurse-Midwifery 24*(2), 25–28.

Stark, S. (1982). Mormon childbearing. In M.A. Kay (Ed.). *Anthropology of human birth.* Philadelphia: F. A. Davis.

Statistics Canada (1993). The violence against women survey. Available at: *http://stcwww.statcan.ca/english/sdds/3896.htm.* Accessed January 18, 2002.

Stewart, S., & Jambunathan, J. (1996). Hmong women and postpartum depression. *Health Care for Women International 17,* 319–330.

Stine, K. (1997). Health care for lesbians: Issues and influences. *ADVANCE for Nurse Practitioners, 5*(11), 60–62.

Straus, M. A., & Gelles, R. J. (1986). Societal change and change in family violence from 1975 to 1985 as revealed by two national surveys. *Journal of Marriage and the Family 48,* 465–479.

Stevens, P. E., & Hall, J. M. (1988). Stigma, health beliefs, and experiences with health care in lesbian women. *Image: Journal of Nursing Scholarship 20*(2), 69–73.

Stevens, P. E., & Hall, J. M. (1991). Stigma, health beliefs and experiences with health care in lesbian women. In K. Saucier (Ed.). *Perspectives in family and community health* (pp. 378–385). St. Louis, MO: Mosby.

Stewart, M. (1999). Women's health: Lesbian parents talk about their birth experiences. *British Journal of Nurse Midwifery 7*(2), 96–101.

Stringfellow, L. (1978). The Vietnamese. In A. L. Clark (Ed.). *Culture, childbearing and health professionals.* Philadelphia: F. A. Davis.

Suarez, L., & Ramirez, A. G. (1999). Hispanic/Latino health and disease. In R. M. Huff & M. V. Kline (Eds.). *Promoting health in multicultural populations* (pp.115–136). Thousand Oaks, CA: Sage.

Taggart, L., & Mattson, S. (1996). Delay in prenatal care as a result of battering in pregnancy: Crosscultural implications. *Health Care for Women International 17,* 25–34.

Tash, D., & Kenney, J. (1993). The lesbian childbearing couple: A case report. *Birth 20*(1), 36–40.

Thompson, J., & Thompson, M. (1983). *Genetics in medicine* (3rd ed.). Philadelphia: W. B. Saunders.

Tiedje, L. B. (2000). Returning to our roots: 25 years of maternal/child nursing in the community. *Maternal/Child Nursing, 25*(6), 315–317.

Tjadin, P. & Thoennes, N. (1998). *Prevalence, incidence and consequences of violence against women: Findings from the national violence against women survey.* U.S. Department of Justice Research in Brief, November. Washington, D.C.: U.S. Department of Justice.

Torres, S. (1993). Nursing care of low-income battered Hispanic pregnant women. *AWHONN's Clinical Issues in Perinatal and Women's Health Nursing, 4*(3), 416–425.

Turrell, S. (1985). Asians' expectations: Customs surrounding pregnancy and childbirth. *Nursing Times 81*(18), 44–49.

Waxler-Morrison, N., Anderson, J. & Richardson, E. (1990). *Cross-cultural caring: A handbook for health professionals in Western Canada.* Vancouver, BC: University of British Columbia Press.

Weber, S. (1996). Cultural aspects of pain in childbearing women. *Journal of Obstetrics, Gynecology, and Neonatal Nursing, 25*(1), 67–72.

White, E. (1985). *Chain, chain, change.* Seattle: The Leaf Press.

Wolk, L. E. (1982). *Minnesota's American Indian battered women: The cycle of oppression.* St. Paul: Battered Women's Project, St. Paul American Indian Center.

Youngkin, E. Q., Davis, M. S., & Fogel, C. I. (1998). Health needs of lesbians. In E. Q. Youngkin & M. S. Davis (Eds.). *Women's health: A primary care clinical guide* (2nd ed., pp. 125–135). Stamford, CT: Appleton & Lange.

Yusu, F., Siedlecky, S., and Byrnes, M. (1993). Family planning practices among Lebanese, Turkish and Vietnamese women in Sydney. *Australian New Zealand Journal of Obstetrics and Gynecology, 33*(1), 8–16.

CHAPTER **6**

Transcultural Perspectives in the Nursing Care of Children

Margaret M. Andrews

KEY TERMS

Adolescence
Bicultural
Black English
Caida de la mollera (sunken fontanel)
Child abuse
Chronic illness
Cosleeping
Cradleboard
Cross-cultural communication
Cultural identity
Culture-bound syndromes
Culture-specific childrearing

Culture-universal childrearing
Curandero (male), *curandera* (female)
Developmental milestones
Disabilities
Elimination
Empacho
Extended family
Ghost illness
Ghost possession
Growth patterns
Infant attachment
Intermarriage

Mal ojo (evil eye)
Menstruation
Mixed heritage
Nuclear family
Pandanus mat
Parent-child relationship
Premasticate
Prematurity
Pujos (grunting)
Single-parent family
Socialization
Socialization goals
Susto

OBJECTIVES

1. Examine cultural beliefs and practices related to infants, children, and adolescents.
2. Explore cultural similarities and differences in normal growth and development.
3. Examine biocultural influences on selected acute and chronic conditions affecting infants, children, and adolescents.
4. Apply the transcultural concepts that promote culturally competent care for infants, children, and adolescents.

Society depends on its children for its future and provides its offspring with care, nurturance, and socialization. Cultural survival depends on the transmission of values and customs from one generation to the next: a process that relies on children for its success. In this chapter, the cultural influences on

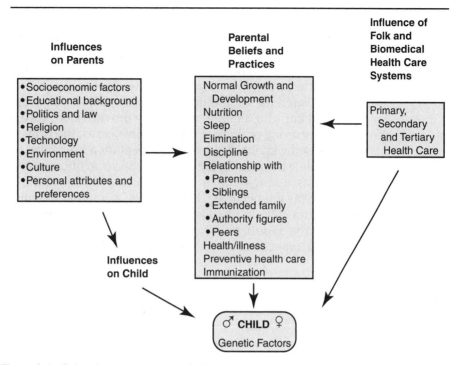

Figure 6–1. Cultural perspectives on childrearing.

child growth, development, health, and illness will be examined. Figure 6-1 provides a schematic representation of the cultural factors that influence parents' childrearing beliefs and practices. Figure 6-2 provides a visual representation of the interrelationship among culture, communication, and parental

Figure 6–2. Culture, communication, and parental decisions about childrearing practices.

decisions and actions related to childrearing. The *clinical relevance* of this information for nurses caring for infants, children, and adolescents from diverse cultures will be examined throughout the chapter.

Because the majority of children are cared for by their natural or adoptive parents, the term *parent* is frequently used in the chapter. However, some children are cared for by grandparents, aunts, uncles, cousins, or those who are unrelated but who function as primary providers of care and/or parent surrogates for varying periods of time. In some cases, the primary provider of care looks after the infant, child, or adolescent for a brief time, perhaps for an hour or two, while the parents are unable to do so. In other cases, this person might function as a long-term or permanent parent substitute even though legal adoption has not occurred. For example, a grandparent might assume responsibility for a child in the event of parental death, illness, disability, or imprisonment. You should be aware that the same factors influencing the parents' cultural perspectives on childrearing also influence others who might care for the child.

• CHARACTERISTICS OF THE CHILD POPULATION

Racial and Ethnic Composition

According to the U.S. Census Bureau (2000), there are 79.9 million children in the United States; 65% are White, 15% Black, 4% Asian/Pacific Islander, and 1% Native American/Alaska Native. The number of Hispanic children has increased faster than that of any other group, growing from 9% of the child population in 1980 to 16% in 2000. By 2020, it is projected that more than 1 in 5 children in the United States will be of Hispanic origin. The percentage of Asian/Pacific Islander children doubled from 2 to 4% of all children between 1980 and 2000. Their percentage is projected to increase to 6% by 2020. Increases in the percentages of Hispanic and Asian/Pacific Islander children are the result of both fertility and immigration. The percentages of Black and Native American/Alaska Native children have been fairly stable between 1980 and 2000—a trend that is projected to continue during the next 20 years. The percentage of children who are White has decreased from 74% in 1980 to 65% in 2000. It is estimated that by 2020, 40% of school-aged children in the United States will be from federal minority groups.

According to the U.S. Bureau of the Census, Population Division, Education and Social Stratification Division (1990), more than 2 million children in the United States are foreign-born, and millions more are the children of recent immigrants. Many of these children constitute the 6.3 million school-aged children (14% of the population of the United States aged 5 to 17) who speak a language other than English at home. Approximately two thirds of these children come from Spanish-speaking homes, and a large percentage of the remainder speak a variety of Asian languages. Some children of immigrants live in *linguistically isolated* households: those in which no member aged 14 or older speaks English "very well." Nationwide, 4% of children aged 5 to 17 live in such households (U.S. Census Bureau, 2000).

Although immigrants and their children are found throughout the United States and Canada, they tend to cluster in certain geographic areas. According to the U.S. Bureau of the Census (2000), California, Texas, and New York are homes for almost two thirds of all foreign-born children. New Mexico, Arizona, New Jersey, and Florida also have relatively high numbers of children whose parents recently migrated to the United States. In Canada, Toronto, Vancouver, and Montreal are home for the majority of children of recent immigrants.

Children's Health Status

Indicators of child health status include birthweight, infant mortality, and immunization rates. In general, children from diverse cultural backgrounds have less favorable indicators of health status than their White counterparts. Health status is influenced by many factors, including access to health services. There are numerous barriers to high-quality health care services for minority children such as poverty, geography, lack of cultural competence by health care providers, racism, and other forms of prejudice. Families from diverse cultures might experience difficulties in their interactions with nurses and other health care providers, and these difficulties might have an adverse impact on the delivery of health care. Because ethnic minorities are under-represented among health care professionals, parents and children often have different cultural backgrounds from their health care providers.

Children are very dependent on their families, and when parents or other adult family members are unfamiliar with the social and health care systems, children are at risk of being underserved. In the current environment, this risk might be compounded when parents, siblings, and/or the children themselves are in the United States or Canada illegally. For many undocumented immigrants, frequent contact with public institutions might place them or their continued residence in the United States or Canada in jeopardy.

Socialization of Children from Racial and Ethnic Minorities

In socializing their children, parents from racial and ethnic minorities have distinctive beliefs and behaviors that are determined by their cultural and socioeconomic situation. **Socialization** is often aimed at preparing children for the society they will encounter—a society in which children find out that the color of their skin or their parental background determines how others relate to them. How parents socialize their children is influenced by the circumstances in which the parents themselves developed throughout life, their experience with prejudice and discrimination, their educational opportunities, and historical and political events involving members of their racial or ethnic heritage.

By following culturally influenced values and beliefs, parents try to foster competencies for successful functioning during childhood and in later years.

Parents frequently have developed *adaptive strategies* based on their beliefs about what it means to be a member of a racial or ethnic minority group. Adaptive strategies arise from a need to survive and maintain continuity from one generation to the next. These strategies are the observable social behaviors that become linked with cultural patterns. Families formulate **socialization goals** to teach their children the strategies necessary for survival in a multicultural society. These goals are derived essentially from cultural knowledge of the tasks their children will have to face as adults, including ways of dealing with being a member of a racial or ethnic minority in a class-conscious and race-conscious society. Research reveals that some children of African-American, Hispanic, Asian, and Native-American heritage are socialized to be **bicultural**, i.e., to acquire the skills needed to function in both the minority culture and the majority culture (Cross, 1987; Zayas & Solari, 1994). By comparison, White parents who are second- or third-generation immigrants tend to embrace a monocultural framework when socializing their children for life in contemporary society. Further study of children of so-called **mixed heritage** needs to be conducted to determine how socialization occurs.

The competencies needed to function in the real world come from socialization goals and are instilled through close interaction between children and older family members, whereby more experienced members of the culture guide children to acquire the skills needed to function in the culture. One result of this mentorship and skills development is that the child's **cultural identity** is enhanced. The presence of nurturing, supportive, and disciplined mentors is essential in transmitting the values, beliefs, and behaviors of a culture.

One example of an adaptive strategy and socialization goal occurs when families emphasize solidarity and the individual's sense of obligation to the family. This strategy helps protect the family's continuity and preserve its culture—or multiple cultures in the case of intermarriage. It should be noted that the extended family members might serve as the primary mentors for transmitting important values of the culture when parents are unavailable or unable to do so, for example, when financial constraints require parents to rely on extended family members for child care while they work outside the home. The socialization goal then is to have children accept the family as the central focus of their lives. A childrearing practice that incorporates these goals is the insistence on children's conformity to parental and extended-family authority, which often extends to conformity to the authority of other adults as well. In addition to giving esteem to elder members of the culture, this reinforces the importance of family relatedness and helps in identity development.

• NORMAL GROWTH AND DEVELOPMENT

Although the growth and development of infants and children is similar in all cultures, important racial, ethnic, and sex differences can be identified. From the moment of conception, the developmental processes of the human life cycle take place in the context of culture. Throughout life, culture exerts an all-pervasive influence on the developing infant, child, and adolescent. For example, there is cross-cultural similarity in the sequence and timing of **developmental milestones** in infant development: smiling, separation anxiety, and language acquisition. Developmental researchers who have worked in other cultures have become convinced that human functioning cannot be separated from the cultural and more immediate context in which children develop.

Not all developmental theories formulated on the basis of observations with Western children have cross-cultural generalizability. Investigations of the universality of the stages of development proposed by Piaget, the family role relations emphasized by Freud, and patterns of mother-infant interaction that are taken to indicate security of attachment have resulted in modifications as a result of cross-cultural data.

Demographic Data

In assessing the growth and development of a child, it is important to determine the child's correct age. Stated age might vary according to culture. For example, the Vietnamese consider that infants are 1 year old at birth and that they become another year old at the next *Tet,* or New Year. Furthermore, some Vietnamese who migrated around the time of the Vietnam War learned that it was necessary to give inaccurate information about their children's ages to meet legal requirements for entrance into the United States. Thus, an apparently simple question about a child's age is a potential source of miscommunication. Moreover, an apparently straightforward question about a child's age is more complex than you might expect, and it might adversely affect the nurse-parent relationship, particularly if the parent misperceives the reason underlying the question.

Growth Patterns

Certain **growth patterns** can be identified across cultural boundaries. For example, regardless of culture, there is a pattern of general-to-specific abilities, from the center of the body to the extremities (proximal to distal development) and from the head to the toes (cephalocaudal development). Adult head size is reached by the age of 5 years, whereas the remainder of the body continues to grow through adolescence. Physiologic maturation of organ systems such as the renal, circulatory, and respiratory systems occurs early, whereas maturation of the central nervous system continues beyond childhood.

Other growth patterns seem to be specific to cultural groups. For example, in some cultures, the standard Western developmental pattern of sitting—creeping—crawling—standing—walking—squatting is not followed. The Balinese infant goes from sitting to squatting to standing. Hopi children begin walking about a month and a half later than Anglo-American children, which is paradoxical, given the advanced motor development that generally characterizes members of traditional societies. Tooth eruption occurs earlier in Asian and African-American infants than in their White counterparts (Overfield, 1995).

Height and Weight

In the United States, African Americans and Whites differ in mean birthweight, with African Americans being 181 to 240 grams lighter. This explains in part why **prematurity**, defined as birthweight less than 2,500 grams (5 pounds, 8 ounces), is twice as common in African Americans as it is in Whites. Chinese, Filipinos, Hawaiians, Japanese, and Puerto Ricans also have lower mean birthweights than Whites in the United States. Significant intertribal variation occurs in the birthweights of Native Americans. For example, the average birthweight among Hopi infant girls is 3,097 grams, whereas Cheyenne infant girls weigh, on average, 3,459 grams. Native North Americans from British Columbia and Northwestern Ontario have higher mean birthweights than non-Native Canadians. Overall, Native North Americans have a larger number of infants weighing 4,000 grams or more at birth—a fact that is believed to be associated with the high incidence of diabetes in Native North Americans (Overfield, 1995).

Although it is difficult to separate nongenetic from genetic influences, some populations are shorter or taller than others during various periods of growth and in adulthood. African-American infants are approximately three-fourths of an inch shorter at birth than Whites. In general, African-American and White children are tallest, followed by Native Americans; Asian children are shortest. Children of higher socioeconomic status are taller in all cultures. Data on African-American and White children aged between 1 and 6 years show that at age 6, African-Americans are taller than Whites. Around age 9 or 10, White boys begin to catch up in height. White girls catch up with their African-American counterparts around 14 or 15 years of age. Around puberty, African-American children begin to slow down in growth, and White children catch up, so that the two races achieve similar heights in adulthood. Their sitting/standing height ratios, however, differ. Mexican-American children have sitting/standing height ratios similar to those of White children, indicating similar stature and leg proportions. African-American children have longer legs in proportion to height than other groups (Overfield, 1995).

The growth spurt of adolescence involves the skeletal and muscular systems, leading to significant changes in size and strength in both sexes but particularly in boys. According to Overfield (1995), North American Caucasian youths aged 12 to 18 years are 22 to 33 pounds heavier and 6 inches taller than Filipino youths the same age. African-American teenagers are somewhat taller and heavier than White teens up to age 15 years. Japanese adolescents born in the United States or Canada are larger and taller than Japanese who are born and raised in Japan, owing to differences in diet, climate, and social milieu. Adolescence also involves changes in the physiologic functioning of body systems, including the reproductive system.

Infant Attachment

When **infant attachment** is examined, cross-cultural differences become apparent from research on the topic. For example, researchers have discovered that German mothers expect very early autonomy in the child and have few physical interventions as the child plays alone. Among Japanese, there are infrequent mother-child separations, and the mother has close physical interaction with the child during play. Japanese mothers tend to stay near their infants a great deal, to do many things for them, and to have close physical contact with them. Similarly, Hispanic mothers of Puerto Rican and Dominican ancestry display close mother-child relationships and more verbal and physical expression of parental affection than do European-American parents. Anglo-American mothers tend to have few physical interventions when the child is playing, and they encourage exploration and independence: behaviors that reflect the cultural values of the mothers. Anglo-American mothers tend to give greater emphasis to qualities associated with the mainstream American ideal of individualism such as autonomy, self-control, and activity, whereas Puerto Rican mothers describe children in terms congruent with Puerto Rican cultural emphasis on relatedness, such as affection, dignity, respectfulness, responsiveness to mother and others, and proximity-seeking (Zayas & Solari, 1994). Studies suggest that differences in infant attachment are linked to cultural variations in parenting behavior and life experiences. The parents' socialization, values, beliefs, goals, and behaviors are determined in large measure by what their culture defines as good parenting and preferred child behaviors for each gender (Figure 6-3).

Crying

Cultural differences exist in mothers' developmental goals for their infants and in the way they perceive, react, and behave in response to their infants' cues, behaviors, and demands. A knowledge of cultural differences in parental responses to crying is relevant for nurses who base their assessment of the severity of an infant's distress according to the parent's interpretation of the crying. You might overestimate or underestimate the seriousness of a problem because of cultural differences in the parent's perception of the infant's distress. You also might misinterpret the degree of parental concern toward an infant if your cultural beliefs and practices differ from those of the parent or other provider of care.

• CULTURE-UNIVERSAL AND CULTURE-SPECIFIC CHILDREARING

In the following section, some **culture-universal** and **culture-specific childrearing** values, attitudes, beliefs, and practices will be examined. In reviewing the literature on cultural perspectives on children and adolescents, you will note similarities and differences in the way parents and other primary providers of care relate during various developmental stages. A discussion of

Figure 6–3. This Chinese-American family is in the process of developing a strong parent-child bond. (© Copyright Caroline Brown, RNC, MS, DEd)

culture-universal practices in childrearing will be followed by some remarks about culture-specific practices.

Culture-Universal Childrearing Practices

In all cultures, infants and children are valued, treasured, loved, and nurtured because they represent the promise that the human race will continue in future generations. From the moment of birth, differentiation between the sexes is recognized. The early differentiation of sex roles is manifest in terms of sex-specific tasks, play, and dress (Figure 6-4). Throughout infancy, childhood, and adolescence, girls and boys undergo a process of socialization aimed at preparing them to assume adult roles in the larger society into which they have been born or to which have migrated. Parents and other primary providers of care use various forms of discipline to encourage certain types of behavior and discourage other behaviors in children and adolescents. As children grow and develop, their interaction with others—siblings, extended family members, teachers, religious leaders, peers, and so forth—increases. Children learn communication, language, and other skills needed to interact with people within a cultural context. All parents want to be treated respectfully by their children and want their children to show respect toward selected others in society, the manifestations of which are expressed verbally and nonverbally. When children behave in a manner that is culturally appropriate, they become a source of pride to their parents and bring honor to their family and cultural heritage.

Figure 6–4. Male and female role differences are taught to children early in life and form the basis for adult roles within a culture. Playing with a construction set is an enjoyable and meaningful way to learn adult roles. (© Copyright B. Proud)

Culture-Specific Childrearing Practices

Although there are many universals, most research has focused on culture-specific childrearing values, attitudes, beliefs and practices. In other words, there has been a greater interest in cultural differences than in similarities.

A few caveats will be presented before childrearing practices specific to certain groups are discussed. First, childrearing practices are interrelated with the social, educational, religious, and cultural backgrounds of the parents or other providers of care. Second, it is important to distinguish between cultural practices and those that reflect the *economic* well-being of the parents and extended family. For example, stereotypes of African Americans suggest that premarital teenage pregnancy is more common and acceptable than among counterparts in other cultures. When socioeconomic factors are considered, however, the myth is shattered. Although African-American adolescents from the lower socioeconomic class have higher rates of teen pregnancy, this is not the case for middle- and upper-class African Americans.

You need to be sensitive to a wide variety of childrearing practices when caring for children from different cultural backgrounds . The following discussion will focus on *clinically significant* childrearing behaviors among families from diverse cultures. Although it might be interesting to know, for example, that children are viewed as a gift from God among various ethnic and religious groups, your primary concern is with knowledge that has clinical relevance, such as nutrition, sleep, elimination, parent-child relationships, discipline, and related concepts. Of course, in addition to being aware of these generalized cultural practices, you should observe parent-child interactions and discuss childrearing practices with the parents.

Nutrition: Feeding and Eating Behaviors

In many cultures, breastfeeding is traditionally practiced for varying lengths of time after the birth of an infant: 1 year, 2 years, until the birth of the next child, and so forth. With the growing availability and convenience of bottled formula, manufacturers of these products have launched effective marketing campaigns during recent decades, which has resulted in a decrease in the number of women who breastfeed. The findings of a study on Puerto Rican cultural beliefs and infant feeding practices are summarized in Evidence-Based Practice 6-1.

You need to be aware that cultural feeding practices might result in threats to the infant's dental health. Studies involving Navajo, Black, Mexican North

EVIDENCE-BASED PRACTICE 6–1
Puerto Rican Cultural Beliefs and Infant Feeding Practices

The purpose of this study was to examine the cultural beliefs and practices of Puerto Rican families that influence feeding practices of infants and young children as well as their nutritional status. Recognition of the influences of extended family was also critical to understanding the cultural factors that affect infant feeding practices. The goal of the study was to identify strategies that enable nurses to provide culturally congruent care for Puerto Rican infants and young children. Leininger's Theory of Culture Care Diversity and Universality guided the research. Using an ethnonursing methodology, the investigator interviewed 10 key informants and 5 general informants.

Clinical Implications

Culture care preservation includes reinforcing the family caring values of nurturance and succorance, respecting and understanding the use of religious and protective care symbols, touching the infant or child and saying, "God bless you," maintaining eye contact, and promoting continuity of care.

Culture care accommodation modalities include using the Spanish language, reinforcing intergenerational caregiving, promoting *respeto* (respect) and *confianza* (confidence, trust) by accommodation or deference to family and community values, encouraging the introduction of healthy traditional foods such as rice, beans, and eggs at the appropriate time, and developing a bilingual assessment guide to improve anticipatory guidance.

Culture care restructuring modalities include involving grandmothers and other kin in a collaborative participatory approach to feeding, providing anticipatory guidance about overfeeding formula and introducing solid foods, developing Spanish-language pamphlets linking feeding practices, advertising infant feeding classes on Spanish-speaking radio and TV stations, and developing a nutritional outreach program for Puerto Rican mothers interested in nutrition and health.

Higgins, B. (2000). Puerto Rican cultural beliefs: Influence on infant feeding practices in Western New York. *Journal of Transcultural Nursing, 11*(1), 19–30.

American, and other groups demonstrate that caregivers frequently prop a bottle filled with milk, juice, or soda pop when the infant goes to sleep; this practice is known to cause dental caries. You should teach new mothers about the dangers of propping bottles and encourage them to return to breastfeeding unless there are contraindications to breastfeeding.

In some cultures, mothers might **premasticate**, or chew, the food for infants and young children in the belief that this will facilitate digestion. The practice has been most frequently reported among Black and Hispanic mothers of lower socioeconomic status. From a nutritional perspective, this practice might remove some of the vitamins and minerals from the food before it reaches the infant and make it more acidic. You should warn the mother to refrain from premasticating the food if she has an upper respiratory infection, sore throat, or other condition that could be transmitted to the baby.

Health status is dependent in part on nutritional intake, thus integrally linking the child's nutritional status and health. Although the United States is the world's greatest food-producing nation, nutritional status has not been a priority for many people in this country. An estimated 1 million children in the United States have malnutrition that is serious enough to interfere with brain development. Many Southeast Asian refugees, for example, were in a prolonged state of malnutrition before emigrating, and undocumented aliens, migrants, poor African Americans in rural and inner-city areas, residents of Appalachia, and others living at the poverty level might be unable to provide their children with an adequate food intake. Likewise, Canadian children living in poverty and those accepted as refugees are more likely to have serious problems associated with malnutrition.

Malnutrition is not found exclusively among children from the lower socioeconomic class. Many middle- and upper-class children, including some obese children, are also malnourished. Obesity frequently begins during infancy, when mothers succumb to pressures to overfeed. For example, among many who identify themselves as Filipino, Vietnamese, and Mexican, to name a few cultures, fat babies generally are considered healthy babies. In most African tribes, fat babies are considered healthy, and mild to moderate obesity is considered a sign of affluence and health later in life.

The popularity of fast-food restaurants and "junk" foods has resulted in a high-calorie, high-fat, high-cholesterol, and high-carbohydrate diet for many children. Parents are frequently involved in numerous activities outside the house and have little time for traditional tasks such as cooking meals. The prevailing attitude among many couples with children is that cooking and housekeeping chores are a choice rather than a necessity. Parents from both affluent and less affluent populations often hold this view toward domestic chores. Because fast foods have intrinsic nutritional value, their benefit needs to be evaluated on the basis of age-specific requirements. For example, the total caloric needs of children of specific ages should be calculated and then compared with total caloric intakes during a typical day (Figure 6-5).

Figure 6–5. Culture determines the type of foods eaten and the manner in which they are consumed. Parents and children can choose foods that are culturally appealing and nutritionally beneficial. (© Copyright Jeff Greenberg/Science Source/Photo Researchers)

The extent to which families retain their cultural practices at mealtime varies widely (Evidence-Based Practice 6-1.) Because a hospitalized child's recovery might be enhanced by familiar foods, you need to assess the influence of culture on eating habits. For hospitalized children, you should foster an environment at mealtime that closely simulates the home. Family members can be encouraged to visit during mealtime or to eat with the child if this is appropriate. For example, most Vietnamese parents believe that children should be fed separately from adults and that they should acquire "good table manners" by the age of 5 years. Depending on dietary restrictions necessitated by the child's medical condition, parents should be encouraged to prepare familiar foods at home and bring them to the hospital. The child should be encouraged to eat in the manner that is customary at home. For example, the Asian-American child who eats with chopsticks at home should be encouraged to do so in the hospital.

Sleep

Although the amount of sleep required at various ages is similar across cultures, differences in sleep patterns and bedtime rituals exist. The sleep practices in a family household reflect some of the deepest moral ideals of a cultural community. Nurses working with families of young children in both community and inpatient settings frequently encounter cultural differences in family sleeping behaviors.

Community health, psychiatric, and pediatric nurses who work with young children and their families often assess the family's sleep and rest patterns. On the issue of cofamily sleeping, nurses traditionally have taken a rigid approach that excludes common cultural practices. Although some degree of

cosleeping—the practice of parents and children sleeping together for all or part of the night—is common in families with young children, there are marked cultural differences in the proportion who regularly cosleep all night (more than 2 to 3 times per week). In a survey of parents of 3- and 4-year olds of African-American, Hispanic, Vietnamese, Russian, Middle Eastern, and Eastern European descent, Canuso (1996) found that the majority bring their children into bed with them at some time. Some parents allow the child into their bed only occasionally, after a nightmare or if the child is upset, whereas others routinely have children crawl in bed with them. A few parents indicated that they sleep with their children all the time.

According to Lozoff, et al. (1996) regular all night cosleeping is most common among African American families (50%), intermediate among Hispanic families (21%), and lowest among White families (<10%). Children might also sleep in the same bed with siblings or members of the extended family. Although the socioeconomic status of the family is known to be a factor, with more cosleeping occurring in families of lower socioeconomic status, some middle- and upper-class families also practice cosleeping. Most White middle-class North Americans believe that infants and children should sleep alone. According to Shweder, Jensen, and Goldstein (1990), the values that underlie the custom of having children sleep alone—autonomy, privacy, independence, and the primacy of the couple's relationship over the parent-child relationship—are not necessarily shared by parents from diverse cultures who place a higher value on protection of the vulnerable child. As indicated in Evidence-Based Practice 6-2, children who cosleep are more likely to wake at night or to have trouble falling asleep alone at bedtime.

To promote rest in the inpatient setting, you need to identify the child's usual pattern by asking the parents about the normal bedtime routine at home. The child might have a favorite toy or story. Depending on the family's religious persuasion, parents might encourage the child to say a prayer at bedtime. You should encourage the child's familiar routine to be continued in the hospital as much as possible.

The type of bed familiar to the child also might vary considerably. In a traditional American Samoan home, infants sleep on a **pandanus mat** covered with a blanket, and sometimes a pillow is used. A **cradleboard** is used by several Native North American tribes. Constructed by a family member, a cradleboard is made of cedar, pine, or piñon wood and might be decorated in various ways, depending on the affluence of the family and on tribal customs (Figure 6-6). After completion, the cradleboard is blessed in a traditional manner. The cradleboard helps the infant feel secure and can be moved around with ease while the family engages in work, travel, or other activities. Although cradleboards have been blamed for exacerbating hip dysplasias in Native infants, diapering counterbalances this by causing a slight abduction of the hips.

In the United States and Canada, the common developmental milestone of sleeping for 8 uninterrupted hours by age 4 to 5 months is regarded as a sign of neurologic maturity. In many other cultures, however, the infant sleeps with the mother and is allowed to breastfeed on demand with minimal disturbance of adult sleep. In such an arrangement, there is less parental motivation to

EVIDENCE-BASED PRACTICE 6-2
Cultural Perspectives on Cosleeping and Early Childhood Sleep Problems

This study examined ethnic differences in the relationship between cosleeping and sleep problems among children, taking socioeconomic status (SES) into consideration. The sample consisted of 186 urban families (90 Black and 96 White) with a healthy child between the ages of 6 and 48 months who had been seen for well-child care at pediatric health care facilities in a large urban midwestern city. The children were divided into categories based on race and SES, and parents were interviewed about cosleeping and perceived sleep problems. For the purpose of this study, cosleeping was defined as parents and children sleeping in body contact with each other for all or part of the night.

The findings reveal that cosleeping was associated with increased night waking and/or bedtime protests among lower SES White children and higher SES Black children. Among families who coslept, White parents were more likely than Black parents to consider their child's sleep behavior to be a problem, that is, stressful, conflictual, or upsetting as well as regularly occurring. The researchers suggest that one explanation for this is that differing childrearing attitudes and expectations influenced how parents interpreted their children's sleep behavior.

Clinical Application

At the time of each well-child ambulatory visit, home care visit, and pediatric hospital admission, the nurse usually asks how the infant or child has been sleeping. Because difficulties surrounding sleep may indicate the presence of an illness or be the source of concern to parents or other primary providers of care, the nurse must be knowledgeable about cultural beliefs and practices about sleep. Anticipatory guidance aimed at prevention of a problem surrounding the child's sleep is better than rectifying a problem once it has been created. Nurses should examine the cultural context in which cosleeping occurs, assess parental reactions to children's sleep behaviors, and tailor the advice they give about cosleeping and sleep problems. The researchers suggest the following: Ask parents of infants how they feel about cosleeping with a toddler or preschooler or staying with their child at bedtime when he or she is older. If the parents do not like these ideas, suggest that they avoid cosleeping or plan to stop doing so well before the end of the first year of life, when attachment and separation issues become more intense.

Lozoff, B., Askew, G. L., & Wolf, A. W. (1996). Cosleeping and early childhood sleep problems: Effects of ethnicity and socioeconomic status. *Developmental and Behavioral Pediatrics, 17*(1), 9–15.

enforce "sleeping through the night," and infants continue to wake up every 4 hours during the night to feed, which is approximately the frequency of feeding during the day. Thus, it appears that this developmental milestone, in addition to its biologic basis, is a function of the context in which it develops.

Elimination

Elimination refers to ridding the body of wastes—a function that is accomplished by the combined work of the gastrointestinal, genitourinary, respira-

Figure 6–6. In most cultures, parents and other care providers use devices that enable the child to sleep while being transported from place to place with relative ease. The use of cradleboards, created many centuries before the infant seat to promote infant mobility and safety, is still prevalent among many Native American tribes.

tory, and integumentary systems. Of primary concern to parents is bowel and bladder control, which is the focus of considerable attention by parents of toddlers and preschoolers. Toilet training is a major developmental milestone, perhaps more for the parents than for the child, and is taught through a variety of cultural patterns.

Most children achieve dryness by 2½ to 3 years of age. Bowel training is more easily accomplished than bladder training. Daytime, or diurnal, wetting is less frequent than nighttime, or nocturnal, wetting. Some cultures start toilet training a child before the end of the first year and consider the child a "failure" if dryness is not achieved by 18 months. In other cultures, children are not expected to be dry until 5 years of age. Boys have a more difficult time achieving bladder control than girls.

Constipation in a child is a persistent concern among parents who expect a ritualistic daily pattern. In some cultures, infants are given herbs aimed at purging them when they are a few days, weeks, or months old to remove evil spirits from the body. You should advise the parents against using purgatives in infants because fluid and electrolyte imbalance occurs and dehydration can ensue rapidly.

The role of the nurse is to acknowledge that toilet training can be taught through a variety of cultural patterns but that physical and psychosocial health are promoted by accepting, flexible approaches. A previously toilet-trained child might become incontinent as a result of the stress of hospitalization but will regain control quickly when returned to his or her familiar home environment. You should reassure parents that regression in hospitalized children is normal and expected.

Menstruation

Ethnicity is the strongest determinant of the duration of menstrual bleeding and of the likelihood that heavy bleeding will occur. In a study of 248 12- to 14-year-old girls of African-American and European descent. Harlow and Cambell (1996) reported that the average duration of bleeding was 5.1 days for African-American girls and 5.6 days for European-American girls. European-American girls were less likely to have an episode of heavy bleeding than were African-American girls. These findings reveal that cultural differences exist in **menstruation** among girls from different groups. The roles of diet, exercise, and stress must also be examined because these factors are known to influence menstruation in women of all ages. Further investigation of potential differences in characteristics of bleeding among various cultural groups might help us understand the reasons for differences in risk of menstrual and uterine abnormalities.

Attitudes toward menstruation are often culturally based, and the adolescent girl might be taught many folk beliefs at the time of puberty. Among Mexican Americans, menstruation is often considered an unpleasant but natural condition requiring circumspect behavior. For example, in traditional Mexican-American families, menstruating girls and women are not permitted to walk barefooted, wash their hair, or take showers or baths. In encouraging hygienic practices, you should respect cultural directives by encouraging sponge bathing, frequent changing of sanitary pads or tampons, and other interventions that promote cleanliness without violating cultural mandates.

Some Mexican Americans believe that sour or iced foods cause menstrual blood to coagulate, and some Puerto Rican teenagers have been taught that drinking lemon or pineapple juice will increase menstrual cramping. You should be aware of these beliefs and should respect personal preferences concerning beverages. The teenager has probably been taught the folk practices by her mother or by another woman in her family, who might be watchful during the girl's menstrual periods. If menstruation coincides with hospitalization, you need to respect the teenager's preferences and might need to reassure the mother or significant other that cultural practices will be respected.

Some Mexican Americans believe that delayed menses are caused by the stoppage of blood flow—a condition treated by the administration of certain herbs. Among other cultural groups, menstrual cramping might be treated with a wide variety of home remedies. You should ask the adolescent girl whether she takes anything special during menstruation or in the absence of menstrual flow. It might be necessary to verify the amount and type of home remedy and to determine its interactive effect with prescription medicines.

Adolescent girls of Islamic religious persuasion, whose heritage might be Palestinian, Lebanese, Jordanian, or Saudi Arabian or from other Near or Middle Eastern nations or some African nations, have cultural/religious prohibitions and duties during and after menstruation. In Islamic law, blood is considered unclean. The blood of menstruation, as well as blood lost during childbirth, is believed to render the female impure or potentially polluting.

Because one must be in a pure state to pray, menstruating girls and women are forbidden to perform certain acts of worship such as touching the

Qur'an (Koran), entering a mosque, praying, and participating in the feast of Ramadan. During the menstrual period, sexual intercourse is forbidden for both men and women. When the menstrual flow stops, the girl or woman performs a special washing to purify herself.

In Islam, sexual pollution applies equally to men and women. For men, sexual intercourse and the discharge of semen is an act that renders a man impure. A *junub* is a man or woman who has become "impure" because of sexual intercourse and must then perform a ritual washing before being able to perform the prayer (Luna, 1989).

Parent-Child Relationships and Discipline

In some cultures, both parents assume responsibility for the care of children, whereas in other cultures, the relationship with the mother is primary and the father remains somewhat distant. With the approach of adolescence, the gender-related aspects of the **parent-child relationship** might be modified to conform with cultural expectations.

Some cultures encourage children to participate in family decision making and to discuss or even argue points with their parents. Some African American families, for example, encourage children to express opinions verbally and to take an active role in all family activities. Many Asian parents value respectful, deferential behavior toward adults, who are considered experienced and wise. Many Asian children are discouraged from making decisions independently. The witty, fast reply that is viewed in some European cultures as a sign of intelligence and cleverness might be punished in some non-Western circles as a sign of rudeness and disrespect.

Physical punishment of Native North American children is rare. Instead of using loud scoldings and reprimands, Native North American parents generally discipline with a quiet voice, telling the child what is expected. During breastfeeding and toilet training, Native North American children are typically permitted to set their own pace. Parents tend to be permissive and nondemanding.

With the approach of adolescence, parental relationships and discipline generally change. Teens are usually given increasing amounts of freedom and are encouraged to try out adult roles, but in a supervised way that enables parents to retain considerable control. In many cultures, adolescent boys are permitted more freedom than girls of the same age.

Child Abuse vs. Folk Healing

Child abuse and neglect have been documented throughout human history and are known across cultures. In the early 1960s, child maltreatment in the United States and Canada became prominent as pediatricians documented radiologic evidence and other symptoms of abuse and neglect in well-publicized reports. International attention to child maltreatment emerged in the late 1970s, and the International Society for the Prevention of Child Abuse and Neglect (ISPPCAN) has held international congresses and regional meetings to explore physical abuse and neglect, sexual molestation, child prostitution, nutritional deprivation, emotional maltreatment, and institutional abuse from a cross-national perspective (Doek, 1991; Korbin, 1991).

Cross-cultural variability in childrearing beliefs and practices has created a dilemma that makes the establishment of a universal standard for optimal child care, as well as definitions of child abuse and neglect, extremely difficult.

Korbin (1991) has identified three levels in formulating culturally appropriate definitions of child maltreatment: (1) cultural differences in childrearing practices and beliefs, (2) idiosyncratic departure from one's cultural continuum of acceptable behavior, and (3) societal harm to children.

The *first level* encompasses practices that are viewed as acceptable in the culture in which they occur but are considered abusive or neglectful by outsiders. For example, in Turkey and many Middle Eastern cultures, despite warm temperatures, infants are covered with multiple layers of clothing and might be observed to sweat profusely because parents believe that young children become chilled very easily and die of exposure to the cold. Many African nations continue to practice rites of initiation for boys and girls, usually at the time of puberty. In some cases, ritual circumcision—of both boys and girls—is performed without anesthesia, and the ability to endure the associated pain is considered to be a manifestation of the maturity expected of an adult. In the United States and Canada, the African-American family's focus on physical forms of discipline might present controversial and ethical issues for the nurse.

The *second level,* idiosyncratic abuse or neglect, signals a departure from the continuum of culturally acceptable behavior. Some societies (Turkish, Mexican, and others), for example, permit fondling of the genitals of infants and young children to soothe them or encourage sleep. However, such fondling of older children or for the sexual gratification of adults would fall outside of the acceptable cultural continuum (Korbin, 1991).

At the *third level,* societal conditions such as poverty, inadequate housing, poor maternal and child health care, and lack of nutritional resources either contribute powerfully to child maltreatment or are considered maltreatment in and of themselves. African-American children are three times as likely as White children to die of child abuse, but considerable disagreement exists about whether race differences exist in the prevalence of child abuse independently of socioeconomic factors such as income and employment status. You need to become knowledgeable about folk beliefs, childrearing practices, and cultural variability in defining child maltreatment. Four Southeast Asian folk healing practices that produce physical marks on the child's body are summarized in Table 6-1.

Gender Differences

In all known human societies, adult men differ from adult women in both primary and secondary sex characteristics. On average, men have a higher oxygen-carrying capacity in the blood, a higher muscle to fat ratio, more body

(Text continues on page 153.)

TABLE 6-1	SOUTHEAST ASIAN FOLK HEALING PRACTICES

Coining (Cao gio)

Appearance	Superficial ecchymotic, nonpainful areas with petechiae, usually appearing between the rib bones on the front and back of the body and resembling strap marks. Coining may also be done along the trachea or on either side of the trachea, vertically along the linner aspect of both upper arms, or along both sides of the spine.
Conditions treated	Pain, colds, heat exhaustion, vomiting, headache.
Procedure	A special menthol oil or ointment is applied to the painful or symptomatic area. Then the edge of a coin is rubbed over the area with firm downward strokes. The procedure is mildly uncomfortable.
Belief	The "coining" exudes the "bad wind." Appearance of a deep reddish-purple skin color is confirmation that the person indeed had "bad wind" in the body and that coining was the appropriate treatment. If only redness appears, the client must consult a healer or doctor for another treatment.
Age of patient	Infants a few months old through seniors.
Practiced by	Mien, Vietnamese, Cambodian (rare), Lao (rare), ethnic Chinese.
Who applies the treatment	Any adult.

Burning (Poua)

Appearance	Asymmetric, superficial, painful burns 1/4 inch in diameter, appearing either as a single burn in the center of the forehead or as two nearly symmetrical vertical rows down the front or back of the body, often including the neck.
Conditions treated	Any kind of pain—including pain from a cough or diarrhea—as well as serious conditions such as failure to thrive.
Procedure	A tall, weedlike grass is peeled and allowed to dry. The end is dipped in heated, melted pork lard, and the tip is then ignited and applied to the skin in the area requiring treatment (e.g., joints are burned for failure to thrive). The treatment is painful and always the *treatment of last resort*.
Belief	The burning exudes the noxious element causing the pain or illness.
Age of patient	Infants a few months old through seniors.
Practiced by	Mien, Cambodian (rare).
Who applies the treatment	In Mien culture, the treatment is performed only by a skilled healer. In Cambodian culture, any experienced adult may do it.

Cupping (Ventouse)

Appearance	Circular, nonraised, ecchymotic, painful burn marks 2 inches in diameter, usually appearing in symmetric, vertical rows

(continued)

TABLE 6-1	SOUTHEAST ASIAN FOLK HEALING PRACTICES *(Continued)*
	of two to four cups on the left and right sides of the chest, abdomen, and back, or singly as one cup on the forehead. Cupping is rarely practiced in the United States.
Conditions treated	Pain, bodyache, headache.
Procedure	Though borrowed from the French, the specific procedure in southeast Asia varies among ethnic groups. The principle is to create a vacuum inside a special cup by igniting alcohol-soaked cotton inside the cup. When the flame extinguishes; the cup is immediately applied to the skin of the painful site. Suction is created, and the skin is pulled up inside the mouth of the cup. The cup remains in place 15 to 20 minutes or until the suction can be easily released. The procedure is painful.
Belief	The suction exudes the noxious element. The greater the "bruise," the greater the seriousness of the illness.
Age of patient	Adults, occasionally teens.
Practiced by	H'mong, Mien, Lao (rare), Cambodian (rare), Vietnamese, ethnic Chinese.
Who applies the treatment	Any adult, except in Vietnamese culture, in which only a skilled nurse or healer may do it.
Pinching (Bat gio)	
Appearance	Intensely ecchymotic, isolated, nonsymmetric areas. May be present anywhere on the body, including on the forehead between the eyes, vertically along the trachea, in a "neck-lace" pattern around the base of the neck, on both sides of the upper chest, on the upper arms (left and right), along the spine, or on either side of the spine.
Conditions treated	Localized pain and a variety of minor and more serious conditions, including lack of appetite, heat exhaustion, dizziness, fainting, blurred vision, any minor illness, cough, fever. Pinching is a *very common* practice.
Procedure	Index and middle finger of one hand are flexed and firmly applied to the skin in a quick, pinching motion. Tiger balm, a penetrating, mentholated ointment, may be massaged into the area before pinching. The H'mong may pinch first, then prick the area with a sharp needle to draw blood and thus "draw out" the noxious elements.
Belief	Pinching exudes the bad wind or noxious element.
Age of patient	Children over 10 years old in most cultures; adults only in H'mong culture.
Practiced by	H'mong, Mien, Laotian, Vietnamese, and Cambodian.
Who applies the treatment	Any adult.

From Schreiner, D., Multnomah County Health Services Division. (1981). S.E. Asian folk healing practices/child abuse? Indochinese Health Care Conference, Eugene, Oregon. September 18, 1981, pp. 2–5. Reprinted by permission.

hair, a larger skeleton, and greater height. Behaviorally, there are also differences between the two sexes, especially in the division of labor.

For children, gender differences can be identified cross-culturally in six classes of behavior: nurturance, responsibility, obedience, self-reliance, achievement, and independence (Barry, Bacon, & Child, 1967). Differences between boys and girls appear early in life and form the basis for adult roles within a culture. Newborn boys are larger and more vigorously active and have more muscle development, a higher basal metabolic rate, and a higher pain threshold than newborn girls. Newborn girls react more positively to comforting than do newborn boys. By 14 weeks of age, girls might be conditioned through the use of auditory reinforcers, and boys might be conditioned through the use of visual reinforcers, but not vice versa. By the age of 4 months, girls focus longer than boys on facelike masks, indicating that girls are more interested in faces or facelike configurations (Overfield, 1995).

Variability in sex-role behavior is common. Most people in a society adopt most of the behavior defined as appropriate to their biologic sex, but there are many exceptions. Sex roles are themselves highly variable—by age and by social class, among other ways. The stringency of expectations also varies, so that girls and women in the United States and Canada can violate sex-role norms with fewer explicit sanctions than can boys and men. Across cultures, even the number of sex roles is subject to variations.

Affective Development

In an effort to understand how people from various cultures construe their private and social worlds, social scientists have identified various ways to describe the modes that people find comfortable and socially acceptable. For example, there are some cultures in which a predominantly *cognitive* mode prevails, whereas others are characterized by an *emotional* one. For many Anglo North Americans, the attributes of cognitive behavior such as an emphasis on logic, rationality, and control are dominant, whereas members of many North American subcultural groups emphasize feeling states, and emotional encounters are of more importance. These different constructions of the world are not accidental cultural developments but rather reflect different philosophic legacies. Also, these constructions occur on a continuum and are not intended to be dichotomous categories.

Among White middle- and upper-class Anglo North Americans, for example, children are socialized from a very early age to learn to control their feelings and emotions, especially in public places. By contrast, they are trained to become independent, self-determining, achievement-oriented, and *work-centered* and *activity-centered*. In a work- and activity-centered society, relationships are formed on the basis of shared commonalities. One is expected to "work" at a relationship—in a marriage, in a family situation, with colleagues at work, and with friends at a social level.

In a *relationship-oriented* society, feelings and emotions are not repressed, and their expression is generally encouraged. Crying, dependence on others, and high levels of emotionality are socially acceptable. No agenda of shared commonalities is necessary for the cultivation of a relationship. Examples of subcultures that are relationship-oriented include Italian, Hispanic, and East Indian.

•HEALTH AND HEALTH PROMOTION

The concept of *health* varies widely across cultures. Regardless of culture, most parents desire health for their children and engage in activities that they believe to be health promoting. Because health-related beliefs and practices are such an integral part of culture, parents might persist with culturally based beliefs and practices even when scientific evidence refutes them, or they might modify them to be more congruent with contemporary knowledge of health and illness.

•ILLNESS

The family is the primary health care provider for infants, children, and adolescents. It is the family that determines when a child is ill and decides to seek help in managing an illness. The family determines the acceptability of illness and sick-role behaviors for children and adolescents. Societal trends in illness orientation and economic stress both influence the cultural beliefs that are passed from generation to generation. Health, illness, and treatment (cure/healing) are part of every child's cultural heritage (Figure 6-7). Every society has an organized response to defined health problems. Certain people are designated as being responsible for deciding who is sick, what kind of sickness the person has, and what kind of treatment is required to restore the person to health.

Figure 6–7. Among the healing rituals associated with fractures in children is having expressions of support and concern written on the cast by family and friends.

EVIDENCE-BASED PRACTICE 6–3
Racial and Ethnic Differences in the Use of Prescription Medications for Children

This study examined differences in probability and number of prescribed medications for children from African-American, Hispanic, and White backgrounds, and whether the differences remain if socioeconomic factors, indicators of need, and number of health care visits are taken into account. Using data from a national survey, multivariate regression analysis was used to examine the probability of receiving a prescription medication for two samples of children, aged 1 to 5 (n = 1347) and aged 6 to 17 (n = 2155).

The findings reveal that when compared with White children, African-American and Hispanic children are less likely to receive a prescribed medication and have, on average, fewer medications. These differences persist after adjustment for socioeconomic factors, health conditions, and number of health care visits.

In discussing the findings, the researcher analyzed reasons for the differences in prescribing medications for the groups studied, which included five major considerations: (1) better health care access for poor minority children through Medicaid may result in increasing the number of visits and decreasing the number of prescriptions per visit; (2) families without private insurance may increase their use of over-the-counter drugs instead of purchasing prescription medicines; (3) the parents of White, non-Hispanic children are more likely to report repeated ear infections, tonsillitis, pneumonia, and urinary tract infections compared with African-American or Hispanic parents, but it is unknown whether these differences are due to socioeconomic, demographic, or biologic characteristics; (4) differences may be due to lack of compliance by African-American or Hispanic families compared with Whites, which may reflect cultural biases that prohibit prescribed medicines, language differences, and other communication issues; and (5) limitations in the data collection fail to enable the researcher to address all of the unanswered questions without further data collection.

Clinical Application

Pediatric and family nurse practitioners can examine their prescriptive practices for differences when prescribing medicines for children from diverse cultures. If differences are identified, analyze the reasons for them by considering the answer to the following questions: Are differences by race and ethnicity due to factors such as income, insurance, or poor health? If the primary provider of care does not follow the advice given with the prescription, why not?

All nurses, whether they have prescriptive privileges or not, can examine the instructions they provide to the primary provider of care concerning medications. For example, it might be useful to ask, How do I ensure that the instructions have been understood correctly? What resources are available for primary providers of care who do not speak or read English? Is there a pharmacy available to the family that will provide written and verbal instructions in languages other than English? Do I request the primary provider of care to repeat the instructions? Is it clear by what route the medication is to be administered? Is the person who received the instructions the same one who will be responsible for administering the medication at home? Be aware that extended family members or nonrelatives may assist with child care, including medication administration.

Hahn, B. A. (1995). Children's health: Racial and ethnic differences in the use of prescription medications. *Pediatrics 95*(4), 727–732.

Research has consistently demonstrated that African-American and Hispanic children are less likely to have seen a physician than are Whites. They also have a lower average number of ambulatory visits than their White counterparts. Even when children are hospitalized, minorities receive fewer services than do Whites. Summarized in Evidence-Based Practice 6-3 are the findings from a nationwide study of racial and ethnic differences in the use of prescription medications for African American, Hispanic, and White children. Unfortunately, the findings reveal that children from federally defined minority groups receive fewer prescription medications than Whites, contributing to a disturbing trend in which minority children are deprived of medications that would facilitate their healing, foster recovery from disease, and ameliorate symptoms.

Health Belief Systems and Culture-Bound Syndromes

Among many cultural groups, traditional health beliefs coexist with Western medical beliefs (Figure 6-8). Members of a cultural group choose the components of traditional or folk beliefs that seem appropriate to them. A Mexican-American family, for example, might take a child to a physician and either a **curandero** (male) or **curandera** (female)—a traditional healer. After visiting the physician and the *curandero* or *curandera,* the mother might consult with her own mother and then give her sick child the antibiotics prescribed by the physician and the herbal tea prescribed by the traditional healer. If the problem is viral in origin, the child will recover because of innate immunologic defenses, independently of either treatment. Thus, both the herbal tea of the *curandero* or *curandera* and the penicillin prescribed by the physician might

Figure 6–8. This premature Mexican-American infant is cared for at a modern hospital facility. After the child returns home, the family might integrate folk-healing practices with physician-prescribed interventions. (© Copyright Caroline Brown, RNC, MS, DEd.)

be viewed as folk remedies; neither intervention is responsible for the child's recovery.

Belief systems about specific symptoms are culturally unique. These are referred to as **culture-bound syndromes**. In Hispanic culture, **susto** is caused by a frightening experience and is recognized by nervousness, loss of appetite, and loss of sleep. Mexican-American babies must be protected from various illnesses. **Pujos** (grunting) is an illness manifested by grunting sounds and protrusion of the umbilicus. It is believed to be caused by contact with a woman who is menstruating or by the infant's own mother if she menstruated sooner than 60 days after delivery.

The evil eye, **mal ojo**, is an affliction feared throughout much of the world. The condition is said to be caused by an individual who voluntarily or involuntarily injures a child by looking at or admiring him or her. The individual has a desire to hold the child, but the wish is frustrated, either by the parent of the infant or by the reserve of the individual. Several hours later, the child might cry and experience fever, vomiting, diarrhea, and loss of appetite. The child's eyes might roll back in the head, and he or she will become listless.

Because the most serious threat to the infant with *mal ojo* is dehydration, the nurse encountering this problem in the community health setting needs to assess the severity of the dehydration and initiate a plan for fluid and electrolyte replacement. You should emphasize the potential seriousness of dehydration to the parents and teach them the warning signs that will alert them to impending danger in the future. A simple explanation of the causes and treatment of dehydration is warranted. If the parents adhere strongly to traditional beliefs, you should respect their desire for the *curandera* to participate in the care. Parents or grandparents might wish to place an amulet, talisman, or religious object such as a crucifix or rosary on the child or near the bed.

Caida de la mollera, or fallen fontanel, has a variety of causes for the Mexican American, such as failure of the midwife to press preventively on the palate after delivery. Falling on the head, abrupt removal of the nipple from the infant's mouth, and failure to place a cap on the infant's head have also been identified as causes of *caida de la mollera*. The signs of this condition include crying, fever, vomiting, and diarrhea. Given that health care providers frequently note the correspondence of these symptoms with those of dehydration, many parents see *deshidratacion* (dehydration) or *carencia de agua* (lack of water) as synonymous with *caida de la mollera*. Although regional differences exist, treatment usually is directed at raising the fontanel.

Empacho, a digestive condition recognized by Mexicans, is caused by the adherence of undigested food to some part of the gastrointestinal tract. This condition causes an internal fever, which cannot be observed but which betrays its presence by excessive thirst and abdominal swelling caused by drinking water to quench the thirst. Children, who are prone to swallowing chewing gum, are most likely to have *empacho,* but it can affect persons of any age.

Among some Hindus from northern India, there is a strong belief in **ghost illness** and **ghost possession**—culture-bound syndromes or folk illnesses based on the belief that a ghost enters its victim and tries to seize its soul. If the ghost is successful, it causes death. Illness and the supernatural world are linked by the concepts of fever and the ghost, a supernatural being discussed in the *Mahabharata* and the *Puranas,* the Hindu sacred scriptures.

One sign of ghost illness is a voice speaking through a delirious victim; this may occur in children and adults. Other signs are convulsions and body movements, indicating pain and discomfort, and choking or difficulty breathing. In the case of an infant, incessant crying is a sign (Freed & Freed, 1991). The psychologic state of the parents is often involved in the diagnosis, and some believe that ghosts might be cultural scapegoats for the illness and death of children. When an infant or small child becomes ill and dies, a mother or father might be relieved of psychic tension from feelings of personal guilt by transferring the blame for the death to a ghost.

Biocultural Influences on Childhood Disorders

Children are born with a genetic constitution inherited from their parents, who in turn have inherited their own genetic compositions. The child's genetic makeup affects his or her likelihood of both contracting and inheriting specific conditions.

In both children and adults, genetic composition has been demonstrated to affect the individual's susceptibility to specific diseases and disorders. It is often difficult to separate genetic influences from socioeconomic factors such as poverty, lack of proper nutrition, poor hygiene, and such environmental conditions as lack of ventilation, inadequate sanitary facilities, lack of heating during cold weather, and clothing that is insufficient to provide protection during winter months. Other factors responsible for differing susceptibilities to specific conditions are variations in natural and acquired immunity, intermarriage, geographic and climatic conditions, ethnic background, race, and religious practices. Some studies have attempted to explain differences in susceptibility solely on the basis of cultural heritage, but they have not succeeded in doing so. This section examines some common conditions in which genetic constitution seems to be a factor; it is based on research reported by Overfield (1981, 1985).

Immunity

Perhaps one of the most frequently cited examples of the connection between immunity and race is that of malaria and the sickle cell trait in Africans. Black Africans possessing the sickle cell trait are known to have increased immunity to malaria, a serious endemic disease of the tropics. Thus, Blacks with the sickle cell trait survived malarial attacks and reproduced offspring who also possessed the sickle cell trait. As dictated by mendelian probability, eventually the sickle cell anemia disease developed.

Intermarriage

Intermarriage among certain cultural groups has led to a wide variety of childhood disorders. For example, there is an increased incidence of ventricular septal defects among the Amish and of mental retardation in several other groups. In the extreme, intermarriage among groups having few members can lead to total extinction; the number of Samaritans in Israel, for example, has dwindled to a handful of surviving, aging members.

Geography and Climate

Geographic and climatic factors can be illustrated by the classic example of a common communicable disease of childhood, rubeola (measles). Owing either to mutation of the rubeola virus or to increased individual resistance to the virus, measles became a virtually universal benign childhood disease in many parts of the world during the 19th century. Although the majority of children experienced few ill effects from measles, certain populations, such as children in the Hawaiian Islands, were severely or even mortally affected when explorers and missionaries brought the virus to their lands.

Ethnicity

Although the role of socioeconomic factors in tuberculosis—such as overcrowding and poor nutrition—cannot be disregarded, ethnicity also appears to be a factor in this disease. Groups with a relatively high incidence of tuberculosis are Native North Americans living in the Southwest U.S. and in northern and prairie regions of Canada, Vietnamese refugees, and Mexican Americans. Ethnicity is also linked to several noncommunicable conditions. For example, Tay-Sachs disease, a neurologic condition affecting Ashkenazic (but not Sephardic) Jews of northeastern European descent, and phenylketonuria (PKU), a metabolic disorder primarily affecting Scandinavians, are congenital abnormalities known to be most prevalent among specific ethnic groups (Overfield, 1981, 1985).

Race

Race has been linked to the incidence of a variety of disorders of childhood. For example, the endocrine disorder cystic fibrosis primarily affects White children, whereas sickle cell anemia has its primary influence among Blacks and those of Mediterranean descent. Black children are known to be at risk for inherited blood disorders, such as thalassemia, G6PD deficiency, and hemoglobin C disease. An estimated 70 to 90% of Black children have an enzyme deficiency that results in difficulty with the digestion and metabolism of milk.

Hereditary Predisposition to Disease

The predisposition to certain diseases also has been linked to cultural influences. For example, the incidences of pneumonia and diabetes are especially high among Blacks, and those of dysentery, alcoholism, and suicide are high among Native North American children and adolescents. Mexican-American children are known to succumb to pneumonia more frequently than Anglo North American children of similar socioeconomic status.

Chronic Illness and Disability in Children

Chronic illnesses and **disabilities** have become the dominant health care problem in North America and are the leading causes of morbidity and mortality.

Beliefs Regarding the Cause of Chronic Illnesses and Disabilities

Illness is viewed by many cultures as a form of punishment. The child and/or family with a chronic illness or disability might be perceived to be cursed by a supreme being(s), to have sinned, or to have violated a taboo. In some cultural groups, the affected child is seen as tangible evidence of divine displeasure, and its arrival is accompanied throughout the community by prolonged private and public discussions about what wrongs the family might have committed.

Inherited disorders and illnesses are frequently envisioned as being caused by a family curse that is passed along from one generation to the next through blood. Within such families, the nurse's desire to determine who is the carrier for a particular gene might be interpreted as an attempt to discover who is at fault and might be met with family resistance.

Folk beliefs mingled with eugenics, particularly throughout western and southern Europe, have resulted in the idea that many chronic conditions, particularly mental retardation, are the products of intermarriage among close relatives. The belief that a chronically ill or disabled child might be the product of an incestuous relation can further complicate attempts to encourage parents to seek assistance.

In societies in which belief in reincarnation is strong, such as Indian Southeast Asian groups, a disability is frequently seen as direct evidence of a transgression in a previous life, on the part of either the parents or the child. Those who are disabled are frequently avoided or discounted because of their past lives and are encouraged to lead particularly virtuous lives this time around. They are answerable to both the past and the future, and often too little time and energy can be devoted to improving life in the present.

Among those who believe that chronic illness and disability are caused by an imbalance of hot/cold or yin/yang, the burden of responsibility lies with the affected individual. For many individuals from Latino or Southeast Asian cultures, the cause and potential cure lie within the individual. He or she must try to reestablish equilibrium through regaining balance. Unfortunately for those with permanent disabilities who cannot be fully healed within this conceptual system, society might perceive them as living in a continually impure or diseased state.

Traditional beliefs are tenacious and tend to remain even after genetic inheritance or physiologic patterns of chronic disease progression are explained to the family. Often new information is quickly integrated into the traditional system of folk beliefs, as is evidenced by the addition of currently prescribed medications to the hot/cold classification system embraced by many Hispanic families. An explanation of the genetic transmission of disease might be given to a family, but this does not guarantee that the older belief in a curse or "bad blood" will disappear.

When disability is seen as a divine punishment or an inherited evil, or as the result of a personal state of impurity, the very presence of a child or adult with a disability might be something about which the family is deeply ashamed or with which they are unable to cope. In addition to public disgrace, among some families, especially immigrant groups from eastern Europe and Southeast Asia, parents might fear that disabled children will be taken away and institutionalized against their will.

Finally, it must be emphasized that some cultural explanations of the cause of chronic disease or disability are quite positive. For example, some Mexican-American parents of chronically ill children believed that a certain number of ill and disabled children would always be born into the world. Many Mexican-American parents who embrace Roman Catholicism believe that they have been singled out by God for the role because of the past kindnesses to a relative or neighbor who was disabled. They often stated that they welcome the birth of the disabled infant as God's will.

Expectations for Survival

Regardless of cultural heritage, parents of disabled and chronically ill children are concerned with the prognosis for conditions affecting their loved ones. Although sophisticated technology in North America can now ensure the physical survival of many children with congenital anomalies, the parents might be influenced by cultural attitudes and practices. Such attitudes might compromise attempts to encourage parents to plan realistically for their child's future. Either neglecting or overprotecting an ill or disabled child can have adverse implications for healthy psychologic development.

Cultural expectations are not easily categorized or compartmentalized into groups in which long-term survival is expected and groups where it is not. How one is believed to be restored to health can also be an important issue and has implications for long-term planning. For example, in some African American households, particularly those that are strongly affiliated with Christian churches, hope for even the most critically ill child is frequently encouraged, with families praying for miracles in the face of somber medical prognostications.

Studies of Asian-American children with disabilities indicate that parents tend to be more pessimistic about their child's outcome than peers from other cultural groups whose children have equivalent disabling conditions (Elfert, Anderson, & Lai, 1991; Kelley, 1996). Although infants are treated very indulgently, there are strict demands on school-aged Chinese children to behave and help with household chores; thus, they serve a useful purpose in the family unit. Siblings of disabled and chronically ill children are frequently admonished that it is their obligation to look after the affected child's education and future. Similarly, adult members of society are expected to look after their aging parents. The birth of a disabled child might cause Chinese parents to worry about their own future well-being.

For many Chinese North American parents, once the immediate crisis of survival has passed, the child's illness is interpreted in terms of how it will affect the child's future. Parents might be dissatisfied with treatment that they see as only treating the symptoms but not getting at the root of the problem, e.g., asthma or epilepsy. Chinese North American parents might not encourage the use of a prosthesis, such as an artificial arm or a hearing aid, because they believe it does not really change anything for the child. If the prosthesis is unable to make the child well, why bother with it? Parents might gradually discontinue visits to health care providers when they perceive that "nothing is happening" (i.e., the child is not being restored to "normal"). You should be cautioned against labeling this behavior as noncompliant or neglectful; rather, the cultural context of the parent's behavior needs to be examined carefully.

• SPECIAL CONSIDERATIONS FOR ADOLESCENTS

Culture and Adolescent Development

Adolescence is a developmental passage to adulthood marked by major physical, emotional, and social changes. In many ways, adolescents from different cultural backgrounds grow and develop in similar ways and experience common physical, emotional, and social changes. It is believed that all adolescents show concerns over changes occurring during puberty such as identity, self-image, increased autonomy, relationships with peers of the opposite sex, and career aspirations. Cultural forces, however, influence the manner in which adolescents respond to these developmental changes.

Havighurst (1974) suggests eight subtasks that adolescents must complete before entering adulthood: (1) develop new and more relationships with peers, (2) accept a sex role, (3) accept one's physical appearance, (4) become emotionally independent from parents, (5) prepare for marriage and family life, (6) prepare for economic independence, (7) acquire an ideology and value system, and (8) achieve and accept socially responsible behavior. Each task is believed to be important in accomplishing the central task of adolescence: achieving an identity.

Havighurst indicates that the tasks are both historically and culturally relative and acknowledges that variations exist in the type and timing of the tasks faced by adolescents raised in different cultural or subcultural settings. In a cultural-ecologic model, Ogbu (1981) theorizes that development occurs along multiple pathways and suggests that successful development is defined by the culture's "implicit theory of success." This theory is important because it defines for members of the culture the range of available cultural tasks or social positions, their relative value or importance, the competencies essential for attainment or performance, the strategies for attaining the positions or obtaining the tasks, and the expected penalties and rewards for failure and successes.

To achieve culturally defined success, individuals must demonstrate competency at the series of tasks that confront them across the life course. Because the demands and opportunities differ in various cultures or subcultures, however, the competencies required for mastery of cultural tasks also might differ.

From a cultural and developmental task perspective, competent development occurs with successful completion of the tasks that confront the individual at different points in the life course and concomitant development of the social and cognitive skills required by the task and permitted by the culture. Adolescents from a wide range of cultural backgrounds are believed to face different tasks at different points in their lives.

As children grow older they are likely to encounter more people from other cultures and therefore to become increasingly influenced by factors external to their family. By making comparisons between themselves and members of other cultures, adolescents develop a better awareness of their own culture and might begin to select values, behaviors, or attitudes from cultural groups outside the family (Figure 6-9). The increased sensitivity to cultural differences experienced by adolescents is largely the result of three factors: (1) increased mobility and independence, which permits greater exposure to the world outside the home; (2) growing cognitive ability, which permits greater awareness and understanding of cultural issues; and (3) widening social networks in which diversity manifests itself (Evidence-Based Practice 6-4).

Adolescents who identify with traditionally underrepresented or so-called minority groups are frequently faced with choices about maintaining separateness or going through the process of assimilation or acculturation to the

Figure 6–9. Adolescents have a need to interact with peers to learn more about themselves and others. (Photo by Melissa Olsen)

EVIDENCE-BASED PRACTICE 6-4
Ethnic Identity, Self-Esteem, and Assimilation Among Offspring of Immigrants

In a study of ethnic identity formation among 5,000 8th- and 9th-grade offspring of first-generation immigrants from Asia, Latin America, and the Caribbean, Rumbaut (1994) found that instead of a single uniform assimilation path, these adolescents followed multiple or segmented paths to identity formation and resolution. The findings reveal that 27% identified by national origin, 40% chose a hyphenated-American identity, 11% identified as unhyphenated Americans, and 21% selected racial or ethnic identity labels. The researcher reported that two thirds of the adolescents ethnically identified with their own or their parents' immigrant origins, and the remaining one third identified with an American heritage.

The findings indicated that gender is significant in ethnic self-identification. Girls were much more likely to choose additive or hyphenated identities and to choose a Hispanic panethnic label. Boys were more likely to choose an unhyphenated national identity (whether American or national origin) and, among those of Mexican descent, to identify as Chicano. Gender also was a main determinant of psychologic well-being outcomes; girls were much more likely than boys to report lower self-esteem, higher depression, and a greater level of parent-child conflict.

The researcher found that perceptions of discrimination affect the way the adolescents define their ethnic identities. Those who have experienced being discriminated against and those who believe discrimination will persist regardless of educational level are less likely to identify as American and undercut the prospect that they will assimilate or finish high school. They are also likely to exhibit higher levels of depressive symptoms and greater parent-child conflict.

Youths in inner city schools, where most students belong to racial or ethnic minorities, are more likely to define themselves in terms of those identities, particularly Black and Chicano, and less likely to identify ancestrally by national origin. The opposite effect is seen for those attending upper-middle class private schools. Virtually no Asian-origin youth chose the panethnic labels Asian or Asian American. A Black or Black American racial identity was chosen by only 10% of those from Afro-Caribbean backgrounds. A Hispanic identity was picked by more than 20% of those from Spanish-speaking countries.

Clinical Application

In caring for the adolescent offspring of recent immigrants, the nurse should be aware that developing a U.S. or Canadian self-identity takes different forms, has different meanings, and is reached by different paths. The process, however, is one in which all adolescents of immigrants are engaged, in addition to the other developmental tasks appropriate for their age. The process is complex, conflictual, and stressful for parents and teens alike. Based on study findings, the nurse should refrain from using panethnic labels (e.g., Black, Hispanic, Asian, or Asian American) when referring to the teen's ethnic identity unless he or she does so. The nurse should be aware that these teens are at higher risk for interpersonal conflict in relationships with parents, teachers, and peers; depression; and suicide. The nurse should provide emotional support for teen offspring of first-generation immigrants struggling with identity issues, observe for clinical manifestations associated with mental disorders, and, when appropriate, refer them to a school guidance counselor, psychiatric nurse, or other mental health professional.

Rumbaut, R. G. (1994). The crucible within: Ethnic identity, self-esteem, and segmented assimilation among children of immigrants. *International Migration Review, 28*(4), 748–793.

majority group. In assimilation, adolescents take on the values, beliefs, and behaviors of the majority culture and abandon their original ethnic traditions. In acculturation, they accept both their own culture and other cultures, adapting elements of each. Acculturated teenagers demonstrate flexibility in adapting their behavior to multiple cultures and are sometimes referred to as having bicultural or multicultural competence.

Special Health Care Needs of Adolescents

There are approximately 22 million adolescents in the United States and Canada. Teenagers are in a process of evolving from childhood to adulthood, and they belong not only to the cultural groups that have formed the basis for their values, attitudes, and beliefs but also to the subculture of adolescents. This subculture links the adolescent with other adolescents through a system of socially transmitted behaviors and belongings, such as clothing, music, and status symbols, including motorcycles, automobiles, videocassettes, compact discs, and stereos. The adolescent subculture has its own set of values, beliefs, and practices that might or might not be in harmony with those of the cultural group that previously guided the teenagers' behaviors.

The society of adolescents is a subculture that is vaguely structured and lacks formal written laws or codes, in which conformity with the peer group is emphasized. One of the most outstanding characteristics of the adolescent subculture is preoccupation with clothing, hairstyles, and grooming. Clothing mirrors the personal feelings of the adolescent and ensures identity with the peer group (Klaczynski, 1990).

In the hospital setting, gowns might stifle the individual's sense of identity, so the adolescent should be permitted to wear familiar clothing whenever the style does not interfere with safety, comfort, or hygiene. There is no harm in allowing a small amount of makeup, jewelry, or other items of apparel that might be important to the adolescent.

Whether or not you personally approve of the adolescent's taste in apparel, you should ask the following questions:

- Is the preferred clothing or accessory consistent with the teenager's cleanliness and hygiene? You have the right and responsibility to prohibit the wearing of soiled clothing or to request that clothing be laundered before it is worn.
- Does the clothing or accessory item permit adequate blood circulation? If clothing is tight or constricting, it might interfere with healing or safety.
- To gain the cooperation of the adolescent, you should explain the rationale underlying any concerns about clothing. The adolescent's need to conform to peer norms is important. Rejection by members of the peer reference group might be seen as a fate worse than the illness for which the adolescent is hospitalized.

You might notice that some female refugees or recent immigrants prefer to dress in traditional clothing. Some boys also might elect to wear traditional clothing, but Western-style attire is likely to be more acceptable for men and boys than for women and girls. It is important for the nurse to determine what the adolescent finds most comfortable to wear during hospitalization.

Because of the relationship between some diseases and socioeconomic status, many low-income adolescents from African-American, Puerto Rican, Mexican-American, and Native American/Canadian subgroups have a higher than normal incidence of infectious diseases, orthopedic and visual impairments, mental illness, and untreated dental caries. This group of teenagers from low-income, culturally diverse backgrounds is more vulnerable than normal to illness and is more likely to live in an area in which health care is inadequate or absent. Consequently, low-income teenagers have a wide range of diagnosed and undiagnosed diseases. As these adolescents change from dependent children into independent adults, these disorders might interfere with their development of a positive body image, sexual and personal identity, and value system; with their preparation for citizenship; and with their independence from their parents.

Although some adolescent behaviors are believed to be culturally universal—such as the physiologic changes associated with puberty, rebellion, and testing of independence and autonomy—the expression of these changes might vary with the individual and might be related to the individual's cultural heritage. In other words, the cultural expression of the conflicts resulting from the changes of adolescence varies. For example, playing loud music might be an acceptable expression of asserting autonomy for an African-American youth but not for a Southeast Asian teen.

Communicating with Adolescents

Without minimizing the importance of nonverbal communication, this section focuses primarily on verbal communication. For adolescents from many cultural groups, English is a second language. In the case of adolescent members of refugee families, English might not be spoken, written, or understood at all. For example, because of a 1984 agreement between the governments of Vietnam and the United States, many Vietnamese children of American service personnel have emigrated to this country and are now in foster homes throughout the 50 states. Although most Vietnamese teenagers are fluent in English, it is sometimes necessary to use an interpreter, especially during severe illness. It has long been recognized that all people regress under the stress of illness, and this regression can manifest itself as a return of the adolescent to his or her primary language.

The nurse should be aware of gender- and age-related customs before selecting an interpreter. For example, an adolescent girl might be uncomfortable with an older male interpreter, and an older boy or man might find a young interpreter of either sex unacceptable. You must be careful to identify correctly the national origin of the client before seeking an interpreter. Vietnamese, Cambodians, and Laotians, for example, are all Southeast Asians, but there are vast differences in their languages as well as in their health-related attitudes, values, and beliefs.

Even when English is the client's primary language, you should not take for granted that communication is occurring. People from culturally diverse groups might have their own unique vocabulary that can be misinterpreted by the nurse. For example, the African-American adolescent might use the expression "tripping out" to mean intentionally acting silly or foolish. If you erroneously think this refers to substance abuse, the results of the miscommunication could be problematic for both parties. **Black English** is highly functional in some circles of the African-American community and is widely spoken and understood.

You should avoid adopting expressions used by teenagers unless you are certain of the meaning of these expressions. A nurse who attempts to use teenage jargon but instead misuses it will appear foolish. You might find that teenagers voluntarily abandon jargon when you interact with them. The use of certain vocabulary gives the user a sense of insider status and a feeling of pride and self-worth through group identification. Thus, it is frequently more important for you to translate ethnic expressions, slang, Black English, or other special language than to use it. It is your responsibility to assess the level of comprehension when providing care for teenagers and to communicate effectively.

Teenagers from non–English-speaking families often have mastered the art of being bicultural or multicultural. At home they speak, dress, and behave in a manner that will gain them acceptance by their ethnic group, whereas in school or the work world they speak English, dress in keeping with the fashions of the dominant culture, and behave in a manner similar to that of the group from which they seek acceptance.

You should realize that adolescents from different groups might express themselves in different ways. For example, Filipino teenagers often avoid direct expression. Japanese adolescents might find the open expression of feelings and confrontational behavior to be in direct conflict with cultural values. Some Chinese adolescents are discouraged from showing emotions, especially anger, because this is in conflict with a very deeply rooted belief that harmonious relationships with others are more important than individual feelings.

You must be aware of nonverbal communication when caring for adolescents, especially the significance of touch. Even though many adolescent boys exchange hugs with other boys as they celebrate athletic victories, some might perceive this and other types of physical contact as a threat to their masculinity. In touching adolescents, handshakes and gentle taps on the shoulder are usually acceptable. Public expression of any emotion might be prohibited for some Japanese, Chinese, and Filipino North Americans. When caring for teenagers from cultural groups in which expression of emotions is encouraged, you might misperceive the intensity of degree of feeling that is being expressed.

For most cultural groups, nudity is unacceptable. The need to undress for a physical examination should be explained, and modesty should be protected. The Hispanic or Latina patient might refuse to be examined by a male physician or nurse. Every effort must be made to have the adolescent and the nurse be of the same gender. If the physician or nurse performing a physical assessment or procedure is of the opposite sex, there should be a health care provider of the same sex present throughout.

• CULTURALLY COMPETENT NURSING CARE FOR CHILDREN AND ADOLESCENTS

A few principles of care for specific cultural groups have been provided to illustrate the practical ways in which culturally competent nursing care should be provided. The examples are intended to be illustrative, not exhaustive.

Nursing Assessment of the Family

Cultural Background

Culture, like language, is acquired early in life, and cultural understanding is typically established by age 5. Every interaction, sound, touch, odor, and experience has a cultural component that is absorbed by the child even when it is not taught directly. Lessons learned at such early ages become an integral part of thinking and behavior. Table manners, the proper behavior when interacting with adults, sick role behaviors, and the rules of acceptable emotional response are anchored in culture. Many beliefs and behaviors learned at an early age persist into adulthood.

Over time, culture has influenced family functioning in many ways, including marriage forms, choice of mates, postmarital residence, family kinship system, rules governing inheritance, household and family structure, family obligations, family-community dynamics, and alternative family formations. These traditions have given families a sense of stability and support from which members draw comfort, guidance, and a means of coping with the problems of life, including physical and mental illness, handicaps, disability, dying, and death.

Each family modifies the culture of the larger group in ways that are uniquely its own. Some beliefs, practices, and customs are maintained, whereas others are altered or abandoned. Although it is helpful for you to have a basic knowledge of children's cultural backgrounds, it is also necessary to view each family on an individual basis. Assumptions or biased expectations cannot be allowed to replace accurate assessment. It is essential for you to remember that not all members of a cultural group behave in a stereotypical fashion. For example, although many Chinese North American children behave in the manner congruent with the stereotype—showing respect for authority, polite social behavior, and a moderate to soft voice—some are disrespectful, impolite, and boisterous. Individual differences, changing norms over time, the degree of acculturation, the length of time the family has lived in a country, and other factors account for variations from the stereotype.

Family Belief Systems

The behavior of children and adolescents is influenced by childrearing practices, parental beliefs about involvement with children, and the type and frequency of disciplinary measures. Although both parents exert an influence on the child's orientation to health, research indicates that a wide cultural variability exists, with the mother being the most influential parent in most cultural groups. Thus, identifying the attitudes, values, and beliefs about health and illness held by the parents and other providers of child care is an important part of the cultural assessment of the family (Figure 6-10).

According to Richman, Miller, and LeVine (1992), mothers' attitudes toward health and illnesses are related to their educational level. Mothers with little formal education tend to be more fatalistic about illness and less concerned with detecting clinical manifestations of disease in their children than are well-educated mothers. The former are also less likely to follow up on precautionary measures suggested by health care providers. A mother who believes that people have no control over whether they become sick is unlikely to have an approach to health in which there is anticipatory guidance or accident prevention and might not comply with recommended immunization schedules. Nursing interventions with a mother who believes that there is much a person can do to keep from becoming ill will be different with regard to the nature of health education and counseling you provide.

With a knowledge of the belief system(s) of the family, you have data from which to choose approaches and priorities. For a mother who is not oriented to prevention of illness or maintenance of health, focusing energies on teaching might not be very productive; it might be more useful to spend time designing family follow-up care or establishing an interpersonal relationship that invites the parent to follow recommended immunization schedules, well-child care, and other aspects of health promotion. You also should be prepared to understand why the mother who is less educated and embraces a fatalistic philosophy might fail to show up for scheduled well-child appointments but will arrive for an appointment when she believes her child is sick. You might attempt to improve the attendance at well-child care appointments by offering to send reminders (by mail, phone, computer); encouraging moth-

Figure 6–10. The nurse involves the family in the assessment of the child to identify cultural attitudes, values, and beliefs about health and illness.

ers to bring grandparents, cousins, friends, or others in a manner that mobilizes the culturally appropriate social support system; and ensuring that the waiting period is reasonable and pleasant (e.g., providing magazines and toys that are culturally appropriate).

Extended Family

Early in the nurse-parent relationship, it is necessary to identify members of the **extended family** who play a significant role in the care of the child (Figure 6-11). Among families worldwide, the **nuclear family** is a rarity. In only 6% of the world's societies are families as isolated and nuclear as in the United States and Canada. The extended family is far more universally the norm. Kin residence sharing, for example, has long been acknowledged as characteristic of many African-American, Mexican-American, Amish, and other groups.

In societies where the extended family is the norm, parents—particularly those who married at a young age—might be considered too inexperienced to make major decisions on behalf of their child. In these groups, key decisions are frequently made in consultation with more mature relatives such as grandparents, uncles, aunts, cousins, or other kin. Sometimes non-kin are considered to be part of the extended family. In many religions, the members of one's church, synagogue, temple, or mosque are viewed as extended family members who might be relied on for various types of support, including child care. Not coincidentally, members of some congregations refer to one another as brothers and sisters. The Amish family pattern is referred to as *freindschaft*, or three-generational family structure. Amish parents know that they can rely on the support of their entire church community. For example, a young Amish

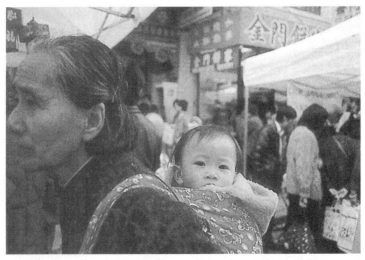

Figure 6–11. In some cultures, extended family members, such as grandparents, take an active part in caring for children. (© Copyright Kathy Sloane.)

couple might turn to that community for assistance with decision making, finances, and emotional and spiritual support when a child is ill.

You should ask the parents if anyone else will be participating in the decision making that affects their child. Once that information is known, you should include the person(s) identified by the parents in the child's plan of care.

Cultural groups might differ not only in the central role played by families but also in the way they are structured hierarchically. In many parts of the world, distinct lines are drawn between members of society based on family connections, education, and wealth, and all members of the society are keenly aware of where they fit within this hierarchy. For example, in nations such as India, the caste system has been an integral component of the social order for many centuries. Members of the royal families in many European, Middle Eastern, and African nations enjoy positions of status not afforded to their subjects. Royals, aristocrats, and members of the upper class from various nations sometimes seek treatment from specialists in the United States or Canada for cardiac, renal, and other serious or life-threatening diseases. It should be noted that nurses and other health care providers are also assigned a hierarchical position.

The influence of the extended family or of the social support network on the child's development becomes particularly important when the number of **single-parent families** in some culturally diverse groups is considered. According to the U.S. Census Bureau (2000), 32% of all children in the United States live with only one parent; 23% of them reside with their mothers; 4% with their fathers; and 4% with neither parent. White non-Hispanic children are much more likely than Black children and somewhat more likely than Hispanic children to live with two parents. Seventy-seven percent of White non-Hispanic children live with two parents. Children born to single mothers are likely to have greater health risks because the social, emotional, and financial resources available to the family are more limited.

The nuclear family is the unit on which most health care programs are designed. Consider the implicit message about the family when you note the number of chairs for visitors typically placed in hospital rooms, physician or nurse practitioner offices, and other health care settings. Although a handful of rural hospitals make special accommodations for the extended and church family of Amish patients to hitch their horses and buggies adjacent to the facility, seldom are the needs of the extended family network accommodated by the majority of health care facilities.

Nursing Interventions

Hair Care

Despite its importance, hair care is sometimes omitted for Black children because White, Hispanic, Asian, and Native American nurses might be unfamiliar with proper care. The hair of Black children varies widely in texture and is usually fragile. Hair might be long and straight, or short, thick, and kinky. The hair and scalp have a natural tendency to be dry and to require daily combing, gentle brushing, and application to the scalp of a light oil, such as Vaseline or mineral oil. For girls and women (and some adolescent boys), the hair might be rolled on curlers, braided, or left loose according to personal preference. Bobby pins or combs might be used to keep the hair in place. If an individual has corn-rowed braids, the scalp might be massaged, oiled, and shampooed without unbraiding the hair.

Some Blacks prefer straightened hair, which might be obtained chemically or thermally. Hair that has been straightened with a pressing comb will return to its naturally kinky state when exposed to moisture or humidity or when hair growth occurs. Box 6-1 provides a regimen for shampooing the hair of Black children and adolescents.

Children of Asian descent tend to have straight hair that does not require the same amount of care as the hair of most African Americans or Whites. Principles related to personal hygiene apply to children of all racial and ethnic backgrounds, but the specific manner in which care is given might vary widely. When in doubt, you should ask the child's parent or extended family member how hair care is carried out at home. Children might feel more secure if a parent or close family member actually provides the care. If you determine that the child would benefit from care by a familiar caregiver from home, the rationale for requesting family intervention should be explained. Comments that the nursing staff is too busy or uninterested in providing hair care should be avoided; rather, the benefit to the child's security and sense of well-being should be emphasized.

Facial Hair Care

Textural variations are found in the facial hair of culturally diverse boys and men during adolescence and adulthood. Many Asian teenage boys have light facial hair and require infrequent shaving, whereas African-American boys and men tend to have a heavy growth of facial hair requiring regular attention.

Some Black teenage boys have tightly curled facial hair, which when shaved curls back on itself and penetrates the skin. This results in a local

BOX 6–1	SHAMPOOING THE HAIR OF BLACK CHILDREN AND ADOLESCENTS

1. Select a mild shampoo. Dandruff is best controlled by shampoos containing zinc pyrithione.
2. Wet hair and apply shampoo directly to scalp. Lather and rinse with warm water.
3. If additional luster and body are desired, add protein conditioner. Allow conditioner to remain in contact with skin for at least 1 full minute, or as directed.
4. Rinse with warm water.
5. Remove excess water with towel, using squeezing motion.
6. Apply small amount of light oil to scalp, using fingertips. Vaseline or mineral oil may be used unless client has a preference for a commercial formula.*

*Note: Chemical relaxers should be applied only by licensed beauticians.

foreign-body reaction on the face that can lead to the formation of papules, pustules, and multiple small keloids. Some African-American boys and men might prefer to grow beards rather than shave, particularly when they are ill.

Before shaving a client, you should determine the client's usual method of facial grooming and should attempt to shave or apply depilatories (agents that remove hair) in a similar manner. When using depilatories, you should protect the skin from irritation by keeping the chemical from contacting the client's nose, mouth, eyes, and ears. Straight and safety razors are contraindicated when depilatories are used because they can cause local irritation to the skin.

Skin Care

When bathing a client, you should remember that the washcloth removes some parts of the outermost skin layer. Such sloughed skin, which will be evident on the washcloth and in the bath water, will vary in color depending on the ethnic group of the person being bathed. The sloughed skin of an African-American child, for example, will be a brownish black color. This does not mean that the child was dirty; the normal sloughing of skin is simply more evident in African Americans than in other lightly pigmented groups. The more melanin that is present, the darker will be the skin color. Because dryness is more evident on darkly pigmented skin, Vaseline, baby oil, lanolin cream, and lotions can be applied after the bath to give the skin a shiny, healthy appearance.

Evaluation of the Nursing Care Plan

To evaluate the effectiveness of the nursing care plan in providing culturally competent care, first you should ask a few probing questions to determine whether the plan was successful in achieving the desired *outcomes,* including the mutual goals established with the child's parents. Second, if the goals were not met, you should ask a few probing questions to determine the reasons for failure. Were the child's parents included in the planning and implementation of the nursing care? Were extended family members included in the plan? Did the true decision maker in the family participate in the care plan? For example, it might be that the grandmother, grandfather, uncle, aunt, or other extended family member—not the biologic mother or father—is the family decision maker. Third, if the goals were met, the reasons for their success should be evaluated and communicated to other nurses for future reference. Other members of the health care team should be involved in the evaluation, including traditional healers or folk practitioners.

• APPLICATION OF CULTURAL CONCEPTS TO NURSING CARE

Case study 6-1 is presented to demonstrate the application of transcultural nursing concepts, theories, and research findings to clinical nursing practice.

CASE STUDY	6–1

Maria Gonzalez, an enthusiastic new graduate, argues heatedly with her nursing supervisor, certain that her persuasive, rational approach will win her case, if not the pure "rightness" of her cause. Located approximately 50 miles from a sophisticated urban university medical center is a rural Amish community. With frequent intermarriages have come some serious, but surgically correctable, cardiac defects among the offspring of the Amish. Members of the Amish community have become a familiar nursing "problem" for the staff of this large children's hospital. Arriving in "unreasonably large groups," several adults, adolescent girls, and younger children often come to visit Jeremiah, a 6-month-old with a ventricular septal defect. The problem of overnight accommodation for the extended family, which includes members of the biologic family as well as of the extended Amish community, has become a topic of lively debate among the nursing staff. Sensitive to the cultural practices and beliefs of the Amish child and his family, the new graduate begins her argument on behalf of the family's right to adhere to Amish cultural practices.

The supervisor listens impatiently as Maria argues her case for cultural sensitivity and quickly interrupts Maria with her decision. "These people are such a nuisance. They don't even know how to flush the toilets when they visit the hospital. This isn't a hotel. They can just go back to their horses and buggies, outhouses, and old-fashioned ways. The answer is *NO!* The natural, biologic mother or father may spend the night. Everyone else is to go home. And that's final."

The use of the Amish in this case is illustrative of many cultural groups characterized by an extended family network and by cultural beliefs and practices that differ from those of the health care providers of the dominant health care delivery system. The case example warrants attention for the many issues it raises. The cultural concepts relevant to nursing practice in this situation are illustrated in Box 6-2. As shown, the nursing problem is complex and multifaceted. The interconnectedness of the various components of the child's situation with the larger system is often minimized or disregarded. The values and beliefs of both the nurses within the health care delivery system and the Amish extended social network must be considered. For the purpose of analysis, some fundamental conflicts in values and beliefs have been identified. Similarities and differences also have been indicated in the nursing plan of care.

After conducting a cultural assessment, identified mutual goals, and compared underlying attitudes, values, and beliefs among the Amish parents and the health care providers, you are ready to engage in activities that will promote health or identify nursing care problems (sometimes referred to as nursing diagnoses). Having done this, you examine potential nursing interventions from a transcultural perspective. When nursing care decisions or actions are made, Leininger's (1991, Leininger and McFarland, 2002) cultural care preservation/maintenance, cultural care accommodation/negotiation, and cultural care repatterning/restructuring will be useful in the provision of culture-congruent care. Finally, the nurse, in collaboration with the parents and signifi-

BOX 6–2	**NURSING PLAN OF CARE: HOSPITALIZATION OF AN AMISH CHILD**

Goal: Child's recovery and ultimate discharge from the hospital (return to parents) in an optimal state of health.

This is a mutual goal of the Amish child's parents and of the health care providers within the health care system.

In order to plan care for this child, the nurse needs to examine the underlying attitudes, values, and beliefs of the two groups that are in conflict. Points on which there is agreement must be identified as well.

Amish	**Health Care Providers**
Family	
Large families, agricultural lifestyle, extended sociocultural-religious network of Amish community members who can be counted on to assist the natural parents.	Small family units, urban lifestyle, nuclear family.
Cooperation and support among extended family, especially in stressful "crisis" times such as hospitalization of a child.	Individual responsibility by nuclear family, mother and father primarily responsible.
Amish community members show interest and concern by visiting.	Visiting by grandparents and siblings accepted only under specified conditions (i.e., at times and places convenient for the nurses).
Concept of family includes non–blood relatives.	Concept of family includes only biologically related persons.
Parental obligations	
Children are a part of a larger cultural group, adult members of the larger community have various relationships and obligations to the children and parents even though they are not biologically related.	Mother and father are responsible for children; *one* adult may stay with patient overnight, preferably natural mother or father. Hospital facilities do not allow for a larger number of visitors, who clutter rooms, violate fire safety rules, and hinder work. A request for information from every visitor is time-consuming and perceived as an interruption to the nurse's work.
Economic considerations	
Communal sharing of resources; hospital bill is paid from a common fund; entire bill is paid in cash upon discharge.	Rely on health insurance; Using large pools of money derived from insurance premiums for claim payment. Sense of anonymity and impersonal. Government regulation of health care

(continued)

BOX 6–2	**NURSING PLAN OF CARE: HOSPITALIZATION OF AN AMISH CHILD** *(Continued)*

Amish	**Health Care Providers**
Traditional and religious values	
Religious values permeate all aspects of daily living; time set aside daily for prayer and reading of scripture.	Religion is important, in some families often in proportion to the degree of illness; usually worship is limited to a single day of the week, such as Saturday or Sunday.
Illness afflicts both the just and the less righteous and is to be endured with patience and faith.	Illness is part of a cause-effect relationship; science and technology will one day conquer illness.
Protestant work ethic (in an agricultural, rural sense).	Protestant work ethic (in an urban sense).
Dress is according to 19th-century traditions; specific colors and styles indicate marital status.	Fashions occur in trends; wide range of "acceptable" dress.
Married men wear beards; single men are clean-shaven.	Whether a man shaves is a matter of personal preference.
Simple, rural lifestyle; family-oriented living. For religious reasons, avoid "modern" conveniences such as electricity; use candle/kerosene lights, outdoor sanitary facilities.	Use electricity/nuclear energy; indoor plumbing is the norm; view flush toilets as "ordinary."

cant others who might be members of the extended family, should evaluate the effectiveness of the nursing care from a transcultural nursing perspective.

The key to successful nursing care is conducting a comprehensive cultural assessment during which appropriate and relevant cultural information is gathered. In addition, you need to compare these data with what you know about the health care system within your institution or agency. How does change occur? What parts of the system need to be manipulated to bring about the desired change? Who are the key persons to involve in effecting change? In the case involving the Amish child, the nurse is clearly pushing for a policy change, for which she has no support from her immediate nursing supervisor. Is a compromise possible? How legitimate are the arguments against having the extended family room in with the child? Are there legal implications? What ramifications does the proposed change have for the welfare of other patients? Can fire safety regulations be met without necessitating expensive changes in the hospital building? What are the adverse effects on the child if the extended family cannot spend the night? Are the natural parents able to understand the rules of the hospital and to adapt to the situation?

There are no definitive solutions or answers to these questions. This case study is intended to demonstrate the complexity of the problem and to emphasize the necessity for thoughtful analysis of various facets of the problem. The ability to apply knowledge from the liberal arts—psychology, anthropology, religion and theology, history, economics, sociology, and others—to the nursing care of children from culturally diverse backgrounds is invaluable.

If nurses want to provide excellent transcultural nursing care, cultural assessment is the foundation on which it is based. With practice and repeated experiences with assessing children and adolescents from various cultural backgrounds, you will gain the knowledge and skill needed to conduct comprehensive, meaningful cultural assessments. In reflecting on the practical aspects of conducting cultural assessments, some nurses comment on the busy and rapid pace of a typical pediatric unit and argue that there is insufficient time to conduct cultural assessments of their patients. The few minutes needed to take a cursory admission history might be the only time a professional nurse spends in assessing the aspects of the child and family that have cultural significance. Cultural assessment should be an integral part of the admission routine for all children and adolescents, not an additional data category that is perceived to be optional. Other members of the health team frequently overlook cultural information that the nurse fails to obtain during the cultural assessment as well. The missing cultural data might result in an unnecessarily prolonged period of recovery or in care that is culturally inappropriate.

SUMMARY

Culture exerts an all-pervasive influence on infants, children, and adolescents and determines the nursing care appropriate for the individual child, parents, and extended family members. Knowledge of the cultural background of the child and family is necessary for the provision of excellent transcultural nursing care. Your **cross-cultural communication** must convey genuine interest and allow for expression of expectations, concerns, and questions.

Culture influences the child's physical and psychosocial growth and development. Basic physiologic needs such as nutrition, sleep, and elimination have aspects that are culturally determined. Parent-child relationships vary significantly among families of different cultures, and individual differences among those with the same background add to the complexity. Cultural beliefs and values related to health and illness influence health-seeking behaviors by parents and determine the nature of caring and curing expected.

There is a dearth of specific information about adolescents from different cultures. Therefore, health professionals need to learn about, study, and document findings about teenagers. Regardless of the cultural background of an adolescent, the transition has to be made from childhood to adulthood. This can be complicated when the adolescent's values, beliefs, and practices conflict with traditional cultural values or with those of the dominant culture of the United States or Canada in which the teenager lives. The blending of an old culture with a new culture by an adolescent presents problems for the family as well as for the individual.

REVIEW QUESTIONS

1. Analyze the cultural factors that influence parents' childrearing beliefs and practices. From a transcultural perspective, explore the ways in which parental beliefs influence children's growth and development.
2. Critically examine the framework for socialization of children in the racial and ethnic minorities presented in this chapter. Identify the strengths and limitations of the framework. What challenges do adolescents who are the offspring of mixed marriages face in the process of cultural identification?
3. Compare and contrast the childrearing practices of at least three cultural groups. Explore the role of extended family members in raising children for each of the three groups. How does the nurse identify key decision makers in the child's family? Critically examine the ways in which extended family members can assist parents during a child's illness.
4. Critically examine the culturally perceived causes of chronic illness and disability in children from diverse cultures. How are the parents' philo-sophic and religious beliefs interconnected with their explanations for the causes of chronic illness and disability?
5. Compare and contrast the following Hispanic culture-bound syndromes affecting children:
   a. *pujos* (grunting)
   b. *mal ojo* (evil eye)
   c. *caida de la mollera* (fallen fontanel)
   d. the digestive disorder known as *empacho*
6. Critically explore the cultural influences on teen pregnancy. Compare and contrast cultural beliefs about contraceptives for adolescents from different cultures.
7. Analyze the major three causes of death during adolescence and young adulthood: unintentional injuries, homicide, and suicide. Critically examine the risk factors for teens from diverse cultural backgrounds that contribute to their early deaths.

CRITICAL THINKING ACTIVITIES

1. Arrange for an observational experience in a classroom at a school known to have children from various cultures. Compare and contrast the behav-iors observed. Does the student-teacher interaction vary according to cul-tural background? What culturally based attitudes, values, and beliefs are reflected in the children's behaviors? If possible, ask the students how they believe they should relate to teachers, nurses, and other adults. Ask the teacher(s) to discuss cultural similarities and differences in the classroom.

2. When caring for a child from a cultural background different from your own, spend time talking with the child's parents or primary provider of care about child-rearing beliefs and practices (e.g., discipline, toilet training, diet, and related topics). Who is the primary provider of care? Compare and contrast the parental responses with your own beliefs and practices.

3. When assigned to the pediatric unit, observe the number and relationship of visitors for children from various cultures. Who visits the child? If non-related visitors come, what is their relationship to the child? How do various visitors interact with the child? With the parent(s)?

4. When caring for a child from a cultural background different from your own, ask the parent(s) or primary provider(s) of care to tell you what they believe causes the child to be healthy and unhealthy. To what cause(s) do they attribute the current illness/hospitalization? What interventions do they believe will help the child to recover? Are there any healers outside of the professional health care system (e.g., folk, indigenous, or traditional healers) whom they believe could help the child return to health?

5. If your hospital has a playroom, observe the types of toys and books available. For which group(s) are the majority of these items intended? Do books and toys represent various cultures? What is the role of nurses in determining culturally appropriate books and toys? Are there any items you believe should be added to (or removed from) the playroom to better meet the cultural needs of hospitalized children?

• References

Barry, H., Bacon, M. K., & Child, I. L. (1967). Definitions, ratings, and bibliographic sources of child-training practices of 110 cultures. In C. S. Ford (Ed.). *Cross-cultural approaches (pp. 293–331).* New Haven: HRAF Press.

Canuso, R. (1996). Co-family sleeping: Strange bedfellows or culturally acceptable behavior? *Journal of Cultural Diversity, 3*(4), 109–111.

Cross, W. E. (1987). A two-factor theory of black identity: Implications for the study of identity development in minority children. In J. S. Phinney and J. M. Rotherman (Eds.). *Children's ethnic socialization: Pluralism and development (pp. 117–133).* Newbury Park, CA: Sage.

Doek, J. E. (1991). Management of child abuse and neglect at the international level: Trends and perspectives. *Child Abuse and Neglect, 15*(Suppl. 1), 51–56.

Elfert, H., Anderson, J. M., & Lai, M. (1991). Parents' perceptions of children with chronic illness: A study of immigrant Chinese families. *Journal of Pediatric Nursing, 6*(2), 114–120.

Erikson, E. H. (1969). *Identity, youth and crisis.* New York: Norton.

Freed, R. S., & Freed, S. A. (1991). Ghost illness of children in North India. *Medical Anthropology, 12,* 401–417.

Havighurst, R.J. (1974). *Developmental Tasks and Education.* NY: David McKay.

Henry, F., Tator, C., Mattis, W., & Roes, T. (2000). *The color of democracy: Racism in Canadian Society* (2nd ed). Toronto: Harcourt Brace & Company.

Kelley, B. R. (1996). Cultural considerations in Cambodian childrearing. *Journal of Pediatric Health Care, 10*(1), 2–9.

Klaczynski, P. A. (1990). Cultural-developmental tasks and adolescent development: Theoretical and methodological considerations. *Adolescence, 25*(100), 811–823.

Korbin, J. E. (1991). Cross-cultural perspectives and research directions for the 21st century. *Child Abuse and Neglect, 15* (Suppl. 1), 67–77.

Leininger, M. M. (1991). Culture Care Diversity & Universality: A Theory of Nsg. PY: NLN Press

Leininger, M. M. & McFarland, M. R. (2002). Transcultural Nursing: Concepts, Theories, Research and Practices NY: McGraw-Hill.

Lozoff, B., Askew, G. L., and Wolf, A. W. (1996). Cosleeping and early childhood sleep problems: Effects of ethnicity and socioeconomic status. *Developmental and Behavioral Pediatrics, 17*(1), 9–15.

Luna, L. J. (1989). *Care and cultural context of Lebanese*

Muslims in an urban U.S. community: An ethnographic and ethnonursing study conceptualized within Leininger's theory. Unpublished doctoral dissertation, Wayne State University, Detroit, MI.

McShane, D. (1988). An analysis of mental health research with American Indian youth. *Journal of Adolescence, 11,* 87–116.

Mead, M. (1928). *Coming of age in Samoa.* New York: William Morrow.

Ogbu, J. (1981). Origins of human competence: A cultural-ecological perspective. *Child Development, 52,* 413–429.

Overfield, T. (1981). Biological variation: Concepts from physical anthropology. In G. Henderson and M. Primeaux (Eds.). *Transcultural health care.* Menlo Park, CA: Addison-Wesley.

Overfield, T. (1985). *Biologic variation in health and illness: Race, age and sex differences.* Menlo Park, CA: Addison-Wesley.

Overfield, T. (1995). *Biologic variation in health and illness: Race, age and sex differences.* 2nd edition. New York: CRC.

Richman, A. L., Miller, P. M., & LeVine, R. A. (1992). Cultural and educational variations in maternal responsiveness. *Developmental Psychology, 28,* 614–621.

Statistics Canada (2001). *Canada Year Book:* 2001. Ottawa, ON: Author.

Statistics Canada (1996). *Visible Minority population by age, 1996 Census.* Available at: http://www.statscan.ca/english/pgbb/People/Poulation/demo41.htm. Accessed June 18, 2002.

U.S. Census Bureau (2000). *Population estimates and projections: 2000 Census.* Washington, DC: U.S. Government Printing Office.

Zayas, L. H., and Solari, F. (1994). Early childhood socialization in Hispanic families: Context, culture, and practice implications. *Professional Psychology: Research and Practice, 25*(3), 2100–2206.

CHAPTER 7

Transcultural Perspectives in the Nursing Care of Adults

Joyceen S. Boyle

KEY TERMS

Adulthood
Caregiving
Civic responsibility
Developmental crises
Developmental tasks
Empty middle
Empty nest syndromes
Generativity
"High blood"
HIV/AIDS

Humanist models of personality
  development
Middle adult
Middle-class value system
Midlife crisis
"Nerves" ("bad nerves")
Physiologic development
Psychosocial development
Sandwich generation

Situational crises
Situational stressors
Social age
Social responsibility
Social roles
Stable adulthood
Stroke belt
"The virus"
Young adult

OBJECTIVES

1. Understand how culture influences adult development.
2. Explore how health-related situational crises might influence adult development.
3. Analyze the influences of culture on caregiving in the Black culture.
4. Analyze the influences of culture on women's development in the Black family.
5. Evaluate cultural responses in adulthood that assist individuals and families to manage during health-related situational crises.
6. Assess the ways in which gender, religious views, and culture influence adult development.

This chapter discusses transcultural perspectives of health and nursing care associated with developmental events in the adult years. The first section presents an overview of cultural influences on adulthood, with an emphasis on the stages of psychosocial development and cultural variations. The second section gives an example of problems faced by a middle-aged Black woman who is experiencing a situational crisis, as well as personal health problems. Developmental transitions occur when HIV illness develops in her young son, and he returns home to live with her. The influences of culture on individual and family responses to health problems and developmental transitions are described.

• OVERVIEW OF CULTURAL INFLUENCES ON ADULTHOOD

Until recently, little interest, attention, or research has been directed toward developmental processes and health concerns in adulthood. Yet, the middle years are a time of physical and psychosocial change. These changes are usually gradual and reflect the processes of normal aging. **Physiologic development** is evident in the hormonal changes that take place in midlife in both men and women, whereas **psychosocial development** may be more subtle. These changes, both physiologic and psychosocial, are influenced by cultural values and norms.

Physiologic Development During Adulthood

Women undergo menopause, a gradual decrease in ovarian function, with subsequent depletion of progesterone and estrogen. While these physiologic changes occur, self-image and self-concept change also. The influence of culture is relevant because women learn to respond to menopause within the context of their families and culture. The perception of menopause and aspects of the experience of menopausal symptoms vary across cultures (Beyene, 1986). It has sometimes been assumed that non-Western women do not experience menopausal problems because their status increases as they age; however, this assumption has been challenged. Although there are not many studies on the perimenopausal transition, there do appear to be cultural differences in the reporting of symptoms associated with menopause and in the use of health care services, as well as prescribed treatments for menopausal symptoms. This reinforces an earlier statement that women (as well as others) learn to respond to menopause within the context of their families and culture.

Men also have physical changes from the decreased levels of hormones. Loss of muscle mass and strength and a possible loss of sexual potency occur slowly. However, developmental differences among both men and women have not been examined cross-culturally, and most existing theoretic and conceptual models of adult health do not provide insight into cultural variations. Recognition of the cultural belief that aging, however gradual, is a normal process and not a cause for medical intervention may be more culturally appropriate for persons of diverse cultural groups.

Psychosocial Development During Adulthood

Development in adulthood was termed the **empty middle** by Bronfenbrenner (1977)—an indication of Western culture's lack of interest in the adult years. Traditionally, these years have been viewed as one long plateau that separates childhood from old age. It was assumed that decisions affecting marriage and career were made in the late teens and that drastic changes seldom occurred afterward. Some developmental theorists saw adulthood as a period to adapt and come to terms with aging and one's own mortality. For example, Baruch and Brooks-Gunn (1984, p. 1) observed that adulthood was often depicted as little more than a "staging area on the way to old age."

However, over the past several decades, the concept of a **stable adulthood** in North American society has undergone dramatic changes, and we now conceptualize adulthood in vastly different ways. Sociocultural factors have precipitated tremendous changes, producing crises and other unpredictable events in adult lives. Divorce, career change, increased mobility, the sexual revolution, and the women's movement have had a profound impact on the adult years. The middle-aged adult may be caught in the **sandwich generation**—still concerned with older children (and sometimes grandchildren) but increasingly concerned with the care of aging parents. Middle age can be a time of reassessment, turmoil, and change. Society acknowledges this with common terms such as **midlife crisis** or **empty nest syndrome** along with other terms that imply stress, dissatisfaction, and unrest. However, adulthood is not always a tumultuous, crisis-oriented state; many middle-aged persons welcome the space, time, and independence that middle age often brings.

Chronologic Standards for Appropriate Adult Behavior

Neugarten (1968) observed that each culture has quite specific chronologic standards for appropriate adult behavior and that these cultural standards prescribe the ideal ages at which to leave the protection of one's parents, choose a vocation, marry, have children, and so on. Neugarten (1968) argued that the events themselves do not necessarily precipitate crises or change. What is more important is the timing of these events. As a result of each culture's sense of social time, individuals tend to measure their accomplishments and adjust their behavior according to a kind of social clock. Awareness of the social timetable is frequently reinforced by the judgments and urging of friends and family, who say, "It's time for you to..." or "You are getting too old to . . ." or "Act your age." Problems often arise when social timetables change for unpredictable reasons. An example is the recent trend of adult children, frequently divorced or unemployed or both, returning to live with their parents, often bringing along their own children. Grandparents caring for grandchildren are now a common phenomenon in our society. Being widowed in young adulthood or fired close to retirement are other examples that are more likely to cause stress and conflict because they occur outside of our notions of social order.

Culture exerts important influences on human development in that it provides a means for recognizing stages in the continuum of individual development throughout the life span. It is culture that defines **social age**, or what is judged appropriate behavior for each stage of development during the phases of the life cycle. In nearly all societies, adult role expectations are placed on young people when they reach a certain age. Several cultures have defined rites of passage that mark the line between youth and adulthood.

Menarche is a milestone in women's development and a psychologically significant event, providing a rather dramatic demarcation between girlhood and womanhood. In North American culture, menstruation is not openly discussed, and menarche is treated more like a hygiene crisis (Golub, 1983; Block, Coutts, & Berg, 1993) than a rite of passage. Most girls think of it as too embarrassing to discuss with anyone but their mothers and closest friends.

In modern North American society, there are no definitive boundaries that mark adulthood for either young girls or young boys, although legal sanctions confer some rights and responsibilities at the ages of 18 and 21 years. Examples are the age requirements for obtaining a driver's license, for voting, and for purchasing alcohol and tobacco. There is no single criterion for the determination of when young adulthood begins, given that different individuals experience and cope with growth and development differently and at different chronologic ages. Even though there are broad norms, social time varies even by subculture in the United States and Canada.

Adulthood as such is usually divided into young adulthood (late teens, 20s, and 30s) and middle adulthood (40s and 50s), but the age lines can be fuzzy. Generally, a **young adult** in his or her late teens and early 20s struggles with issues related to intimacy and relationships outside the family of origin. Role changes occur while the young adult is pursuing an education and establishing a career. A **middle adult** concentrates on making a contribution to society through work and/or family (Behler, Tippett, & Mandle, 1994). However, as previously mentioned, adulthood is not necessarily a stable or predictable plateau. Experiences at work have a direct bearing on the middle-aged adult's development through exposure to job-related stress, levels of physical and intellectual activity, and social relations formed with coworkers. At home, family life can be chaotic, with role changes and other transitions occurring with dizzying frequency. Often adults are faced with the realization that they are getting older and have left many things still undone. This realization can lead to **developmental crises**, **situational stressors**, and **situational crises**. How well individuals cope with and manage the challenges of adulthood are influenced by their cultural values, traditions, and background.

Developmental Tasks

Throughout life, each individual is confronted with **developmental tasks**: responses to life situations encountered by all persons experiencing physiologic, psychologic, spiritual, and sociologic changes. Although the developmental tasks of childhood are widely known and have long been studied, the critical experiences of adulthood are less familiar to most nurses.

Several theorists have studied and defined the developmental tasks of adulthood. For example, **humanist models of personality development** propose that middle adulthood brings with it the opportunity for continued growth. Many personality theorists, such as Freud, Erikson, and Fromm, cite maturity as the major criterion of adulthood. Jung recognized young adulthood as a time of coping with the demands of emotional involvements in family, work, and community (Hill & Humphrey, 1982). According to Erikson (1963), the developmental task of middle adulthood is the attainment of generativity versus stagnation. **Generativity** is accomplished through parenting, working in one's career, participating in community activities, or working cooperatively with peers, spouse, family members, and others to reach mutually determined goals. Hill and Humphrey (1982) suggested that the mature adult has a well-developed philosophy of life that serves as a basis for leadership, stability, and objectivity. Individuals in adulthood assume numerous **social roles**, such as spouse, parent, child of aging parent, worker, friend, organization member, and citizen. Each of these social roles involves expected behaviors established by the values and norms of society. Through the process of socialization, the individual is expected to learn the behaviors appropriate to the new role (see Evidence-Based Practice 7–1).

In many ways, Erikson's and other theorists' views of what occurs in adulthood are the biases of middle-class "Anglo" values and experiences. This constellation of characteristics has been attributed to predominantly White, Anglo-Saxon, Protestant (WASP) views and behaviors. For many cultural groups in Western society, the mastery of mainstream developmental tasks is not easily managed, and in some cases, it may even be undesirable. For some groups, developmental tasks may be accomplished through culturally defined patterns that are different from or outside the norm of what is expected in the dominant culture. Furthermore, some authors now suggest that developmental stages and the associated developmental tasks of adulthood have been derived primarily from studies of men, and thus women may experience adult development somewhat differently (Gilligan, 1982a, 1982b; Belenky, Clinchy, Goldberger, & Tarule, 1986). Women's traditional location of responsibility was in the home, nurturing children and husband as well as parents. This view is changing, prompted by societal changes and informed by scholars who are addressing women's psychosocial development in new ways. Some of these differences are described in the next section.

Although the applicability of many of developmental theories to diverse cultural groups within the United States and Canada can certainly be called into question, it is important to consider the work of Havighurst (1974). Havighurst's theories have been similarly criticized; however, his work does reflect traditional thinking about adulthood and the norms that are associated with that particular stage of life. Havighurst (1974) identified seven developmental tasks or stages of middle adulthood.

TASK 1: REACHING AND MAINTAINING SATISFACTORY PERFORMANCE IN ONE'S CAREER

Havighurst (1974) defines the first task as reaching and maintaining satisfactory performance in one's career. Success in a career seems based on behaviors and attitudes that arise in a traditional White **middle-class value system** that emphasizes the male working role. A successful career is enhanced for a middle-aged man if his wife has assumed primary responsibility for manage-

EVIDENCE-BASED PRACTICE 7–1
"So That Our Souls Don't Get Damaged": The Impact of Racism on Maternal Thinking and Practice Related to the Protection of Daughters

This study suggests that racism influences the conceptualization of motherhood and the practice of mothers in Black culture. Understanding Black culture requires a thoughtful appreciation of the experiences of the diaspora and the institution of slavery in the Americas. This research reaffirms that living in a racist society has a profound impact on maternal thinking and the practice of mothering in Black women as they actively engage in ways of protecting their daughters. Mothers were intensely involved in advocating for their children and teaching them survival skills. Protection of children was viewed as a common responsibility. Mothering practices, such as nurturing intellectual growth and preparing children to be productive members of society, were integral to the success of promoting the mental health and well-being of young Black women.

CLINICAL APPLICATION

- Recognize that mothering practices of Black mothers remain largely invisible and unappreciated within dominant society.
- Know that respite from ongoing challenges and safe spaces to vent frustrations, as well as opportunities to celebrate the wonderfulness of being a Black woman, are important to the success of promoting mental health in this population.
- Realize that self-help groups composed of Black women can be especially helpful; mental health providers should become familiar with a range of self-help groups that may be beneficial to their clients or populations of interest.
- Recognize that studying development in diverse cultures is important to clinical practice; to be effective, mental health providers must have an understanding of the contexts in which Black clients live.
- Acknowledge that many conceptual frameworks used in mental health care were developed using predominantly White middle-class values and often reflect gender biases as well.
- Provide a safe environment to work through issues stemming from real or perceived racism within the context of the therapeutic relationship.

Banks-Wallace, J., & Parks, L. (2001). "So that our souls don't get damaged": The impact of racism on maternal thinking and practice related to the protection of daughters. *Issues in Mental Health Nursing, 22,* 77–98.

ment of the household and supervision of their children. For men and women without spouses (or an equivalent person to manage domestic tasks and child rearing), success in a career may seem less important or may be more difficult because of division of time and energy. It could also be argued that economic goals may be more quickly attained if both husband and wife are employed outside the home. However, managing a household with children in a two-career family brings about its own challenges and stressors.

In studies of Afghan refugees, it has been found that although family life is the core of Afghan culture, role conflict and stress occur within the family as gender roles begin to change during contact with American culture (Lipson, Hosseini, Kabir, Omidian, & Edmonston; Lipson & Omidian, 1996). For example, sometimes the male head of household is unable to find employment; if he was a professional in Afghanistan, he may be reluctant to accept the menial jobs that are traditionally filled by immigrants or refugees when they first come to this country. Frequently, low-status jobs are more available to immigrant women. The traditional Afghan woman's role is closely tied to the home and family. When the Afghan woman seeks employment (e.g., as a hotel maid), this threatens her husband's traditional patriarchal role and alters the power structure between them as well as changing her role as wife and mother. Husbands who do not adjust to new cultural roles and expectations often drink heavily and become abusive. Afghan women are expected to prepare traditional food, which takes hours to prepare, and Afghan housekeeping standards are high. It is the woman's responsibility to take care of the children and do all the housekeeping, even if the man is unemployed and stays at home (Lipson & Miller, 1994). The lack of adequate social supports, such as affordable day care and adequate compensation for work, and the additional physical and emotional stress result in an unacknowledged toll on refugee women and their families, including their husbands. Similar experiences have been reported in other immigrant groups (see Box 7-1).

At present, to expect members of certain groups such as poor ethnic minorities, newly arrived immigrants or refugees, or the homeless or the

BOX 7–1	SOME CHARACTERISTICS OF IMMIGRANT AND REFUGEE FAMILIES

1. Traditional family values are evident; for example, roles of men and women are differentiated. Women's role is in the home, with the family. Men are heads of household and family providers.
2. Families tend to be extended; if members do not actually live in the same household, there is frequent visiting and contact.
3. Many immigrants come to Canada and the United States because they already have family members here.
4. Most immigrants and refugees are poor and struggle to earn an adequate income. Often men in refugee communities have been professionals in their home country but are unable to be employed in the same capacity in their new host country.
5. Refugees may be fleeing war and political persecution. Many may experience symptoms of posttraumatic stress syndrome.
6. Traditional health and illness beliefs may influence behavior. Immigrant and refugee families may combine traditional health practices with modern Western health care. The use of traditional practices is fairly common in some groups.
7. Language is a significant barrier for the first few years immigrants and refugees live in the United States and Canada. Children tend to learn English more quickly and to become acculturated faster than their parents.

unemployed to achieve satisfaction from jobs that interest them or from status derived from succeeding in a career is unrealistic and indicates a lack of sensitivity to the problems faced by these groups. In addition, plant closings, downscaling in workplaces, decreased production, and unemployment have posed problems for many workers, including health care professionals. Thus, although the work role is valued in North American society, the attainment of a successful career may not be realistic for some minority groups, immigrants, or even certain individuals within the majority culture, some of whom are returning to school in the hope of preparing for a second career.

TASK 2: ACHIEVING SOCIAL AND CIVIC RESPONSIBILITY

Havighurst (1974) defines the second major task of adulthood as achieving **social responsibility** and **civic responsibility**. Social and civic responsibilities are in part culturally defined. Whereas members of the dominant North American culture may value achieving an elected office in the local PTA or Rotary Club, other cultures may emphasize different goals. For example, in some groups, religious obligations may be given priority over civic responsibilities. Becoming an elder or a lay pastor may be highly valued by some Blacks. Among religious groups such as the Latter-Day Saints (Mormons) or the Amish, being appointed a lay bishop may be more valued than career success. Usually, traditional religious groups have not encouraged the emergence of women in leadership roles within the church structure or the wider society.

When women seek roles outside the traditional family, the result is often censure or criticism because broadly defined developmental tasks that include recognition and acknowledgment outside the family group may conflict with the traditionally defined role of women. Some religious and ethnic or cultural groups believe that a woman's place is in the home, and women who attempt to succeed in a career or in activities outside the home or group are frowned on by other members of the group. Civic responsibilities that relate to children or domestic matters may be viewed as appropriate for women to assume, whereas others may be viewed as more within the province of men. Middle Eastern and Southeast Asian cultures emphasize responsibilities and contributions to the extended family or clan rather than to the wider society. Lipson and Miller (1994) report that Afghan women in the United States continue to socialize almost exclusively with other women, usually extended family members. They do not talk with male strangers, no matter how unusual the circumstances. Family ties are of great importance to many traditional cultural groups residing in the United States and Canada as well as to immigrant groups who have arrived within the last few years.

Members of diverse cultures have encountered barriers such as racism or prejudice in North American society. For example, Black women, both historically and presently, have had to deal with limitations in their social environment. Faced with the need to accommodate these experiences into their own identities over time, they have developed capacities to compensate for the environment, and they have become productive citizens against many odds. However, as these women age they are faced with challenges to their identity, often intensified by poverty and ill health. Black women are at high risk for strokes, hypertension, and other cardiovascular diseases (Casper, et al., 1999).

Many individuals and groups living in Canada also experience the negative consequences of racism and prejudice. One Canadian study estimated that about 60,000 hate crimes were committed in nine major urban centers in 1994; 61% of these crimes were directed against racial minorities, and 23% were directed toward religious minorities (Canadian Heritage, 1998). Prejudice, discrimination, hate crimes, and violence cannot help but have a negative impact on the health of those at the receiving end. However, little research is available in Canada that explores the effects of such discrimination and violence on the health of immigrants and minorities (Health Canada, 1999).

TASK 3: ACCEPTING AND ADJUSTING TO THE PHYSIOLOGIC CHANGES OF MIDDLE AGE

The third developmental task of adulthood (Havighurst, 1974) is to accept and adjust to the physiologic changes of middle age. Age-related physical changes begin in middle adulthood and ultimately necessitate adjustments in activities of daily living, lifestyle, and attitude. Over all, North American culture values youth and beauty. The rapid acceptance of hair coloring, contact lenses versus eyeglasses, and cosmetic surgery and the interest in procedures such as suction lipectomies say much about the way some members of North American culture resist or attempt to delay the physiologic changes associated with late adulthood. By contrast, the effects of aging may be more easily accepted by members of cultural groups such as Native North Americans or Asian North Americans, whose traditional values include respect for and deference to the elderly.

TASK 4: HELPING TEENAGE CHILDREN BECOME RESPONSIBLE ADULTS

The fourth developmental task of middle-aged adults (Havighurst, 1974) is to help teenaged children become responsible adults. The age at which young persons marry and become independent varies by custom or cultural norm as well as by socioeconomic status. Generally speaking, adults of lower socioeconomic status leave school, begin work, marry, and become parents and grandparents at earlier ages than middle-class or upper-class adults. It is relatively common in North American society for an 18-year-old, for example, to marry and move away from home or to leave home to pursue higher education or find employment. Indeed, many American and Canadian families encourage early independence, or "leaving home," although this trend decreases when the economy declines. Other cultural groups, such as those from the Middle East and Latin America, place more emphasis on the extended family. Even after marriage, a son and his new wife may choose to live very close to both families and to visit relatives several times each day. Families from some cultural groups such as Hispanics, or traditional religious groups such as the Hutterites or the Amish, may be reluctant to allow their young daughters to leave home until they marry.

Many couples who have delayed childbearing, perhaps because of the woman's career or for other reasons, or couples who have chosen to have children in a second marriage are having children in later childbearing years. These parents confront many unique issues. They may have less in common with parents of their children's playmates or even their own peers whose children are grown. Energy, agility, and emotional flexibility may be lacking as parents nearing 50 years of age attempt to keep up with their young children. Young children born to older parents may not know their grandparents, who have played an important role in extended family relationships in the past.

TASK 5: CHANGING THE ROLES AND RELATIONSHIPS OF INDIVIDUALS WITH THEIR PARENTS

The fifth developmental task of adulthood (Havighurst, 1974) involves a change in the roles and relationships of individuals with their parents. This stage in life has been described as the sandwich generation. Caring for and launching their own children and caring for their own aging parents place some middle-age adults between the demands of caregiving from parents and those from children. Primarily, caregivers have been women, and the excessive stress resulting from the demands of caregiving places them at increased risk to health problems. In cultures that value and maintain extended family networks, the responsibilities of caring for both children and older parents can be shared (Figure 7-1).

Figure 7–1. American families, such as the extended family of Teresa and Neil Cooper of Carlsbad, California, are multiethnic in each generation, yet maintaining close family ties is a priority. This emphasis on family has continued through three generations. The children look forward to seeing each other. Their parents and grandparents believe that this is the beginning of the fourth generation of close family ties.

Adjusting to aging parents and responsibilities toward them, as well as finding appropriate solutions to problems created by aging parents, are challenges faced by many adult North Americans as they approach middle age. Placing an aged mother or father in a nursing home may be a decision made with reluctance and only when all other alternatives have been exhausted. Such actions may be totally unacceptable to some members of other cultural groups, in which family and community structures would facilitate the complex care required by an aged ill person and would exert a great deal of social pressure on an adult son (or especially a daughter) who failed in this obligation.

TASKS 6 AND 7: EMPHASIZING THE ROLE OF WIFE OR HUSBAND, STRONG FRIENDSHIPS, AND LEISURE ACTIVITIES

The sixth and seventh developmental tasks defined by Havighurst (1974) place emphasis on the role of wife or husband and the establishment of strong friendships along with increasing enjoyment of leisure activities. The relationship of wife and husband is often enhanced in middle adulthood, although divorce at this time, while declining in Canada (Statistics Canada, 1999), is becoming more frequent in the United States. In both Canada and the United States, the frequent need for both spouses to work may conflict with traditional roles and cause feelings of guilt and shame on the part of the husband. Some women continue to assume all responsibility for domestic chores while working outside the home, and they experience considerable stress and fatigue as a result of multiple role demands. If either or both spouses are working in low-paying jobs and still struggling to make ends meet, the enjoyment of leisure activities may be sharply curtailed.

In addition, an emphasis on an emotionally close interpersonal relationship between a husband and wife may be a culturally defined value. Studies have suggested that in some groups, such as Hispanic cultures, women develop more intense relationships or affective bonds with their children or relatives than with their husbands. Latin men, in turn, may form close bonds with siblings or friends—ties that meet the needs for companionship, emotional support, and caring that might otherwise be expected from their wives (O'Kelly, 1980; Boyle, 1996). Touch between men and between women is acceptable. Gender roles and how men and women go about establishing personal ties with either sex are heavily influenced by culture. New paradigms that examine women's development suggest that female identity is formed not by individuation but within relationship contexts (Lewis & Bernstein, 1996). In North American society, women are more likely to have intimate, self-disclosing friendships with other women than men have with other men. A man's male friends are likely to be working, drinking, or playing "buddies." In southern Europe and the Middle East, men are allowed to express their friendship with each other with words and embraces. Such expressions of affection between men are uncommon in North American culture and might be attributed to homosexuality.

Thus, affiliation and friendship needs in adulthood and the satisfaction of these needs are facilitated or hindered by cultural expectations. How individuals are approached and greeted as well as the kind and type of relationship established may be closely tied to cultural expectations and norms. Health care professionals should inquire about the appropriate manner to use in approaching clients and their family members. Table 7-1 provides some suggestions and guidelines to use in approaching clients and using their names in interpersonal relationships. Social support, family ties, and friendship needs can be met through the extended family and kinship system or through other culturally prescribed groups such as churches, singles bars, work, and civic associations. An individual's health may be affected by such ties: persons who have a reliable set of close friends and an extensive network of acquaintances are usually healthier—both emotionally and physically—than those without friends. Lifestyle, a powerful influence on health status, involves the practice of health habits and a guiding philosophy of life to promote a positive outlook. Individual and family lifestyles vary according to resources and cultural values and traditions. Changing North American lifestyles are creating realignment of the division of labor, roles, and values of the family. In turn, adult growth and development in middle age are undergoing profound changes.

• HEALTH-RELATED SITUATIONAL CRISES

The preceding section described cultural influences, developmental tasks, and selected cultural variations in adulthood. This section contains a case study of a middle-aged Black woman who experienced health problems compounded by social and cultural factors as well as by situational or developmental crises. In addition to the developmental or maturational changes discussed in the preceding section, situational crises resulting from a serious illness may impinge on individuals in middle age. For example, the leading causes of death in middle adulthood are heart diseases, lung cancer, cerebrovascular disease, breast cancer, colorectal cancer, and obstructive lung disease (U.S. Department of Health and Human Services, 2000). These conditions affect individuals, but they also occur within a family system and affect children, spouses, aging parents, or other close relatives. Since middle-aged adults may be responsible for aging parents or ill adult children as well as for grandchildren, the illness of any one individual must be evaluated very carefully for the myriad ways in which it affects all members of the family.

Health care professionals need a better understanding of how families influence the health-related behavior of their members, because definitions of health and illness and reactions to them form during childhood within the family context. Yet, there are many gaps in our knowledge. Health promotion, disease prevention, and the treatment of illness are influenced by cultural beliefs and values. When the illness has social and/or cultural connotations, the issues become more complex. Medical treatment and nursing care must take into account the cultural history, values, beliefs, and practices that influence

TABLE 7–1	**GUIDELINES FOR NAMES**
Arab	Both male and female children are given a first name. The father's first name is used as the middle name; the last name is the family name. Usually, a person is called formally by the first name as Mr. Mohammed or Dr. Anwar.
Chinese	The family name is stated or written first and then the given name, just opposite of European and North American tradition. Only very close friends use the given name. Politeness and formality are stressed; always use the whole name or family name. Use only the family name to address men, e.g., if the family name is Chin and the man's given name is Wei-jing, address the man as Chin. Many Asians take an English name that they use in their North American host country. Use the title Mr. or Mrs. preceding the English name, because the use of only the first name is considered rude. Some Asians switch the order of their names to be like Western names, and this can be very confusing to outsiders.
	Women in China do not use their husband's name after marriage. If the woman has lived in Hong Kong, Taiwan, or a Western country for a long time, her name may be the same as her husband's name.
Latin American	The use of surnames may differ by country. Many Latin Americans use two surnames, representing the mother's and father's sides of the family. "Maria Cordoba Lopez" indicates her that father's name is Cordoba and her mother's surname is Lopez. When Maria marries, she will retain her father's name and add the last name of her husband. Thus, Maria becomes Maria Cordoba de Reclnos. Many Latin Americans drop their mother's surnames after they immigrate to the United States. In approaching clients of traditional Latin cultures, it is appropriate to use the Spanish terms *Señor* or *Señora,* followed by the primary surname (the husband's), if the nurse is comfortable with those terms.
Native North American	Native North American names differ by tribal affiliation. Many tend to follow the dominant cultural norms. In the Navajo culture, a health care provider may call an older Navajo client "grandfather" or "grandmother" as a sign of respect. In the past, some tribes have tended to convert traditional names into English surnames. Thus, there are names like Joe Calf Looking and Phyllis Greywolf.

The above-mentioned examples are very general. If in doubt, always ask, because it can be embarrassing for the nurse and the client if the nurse uses a name in an inappropriate manner. Members of cultures that adhere to traditional values might be confused by our current practice of using Ms. as a designation for women. Generally speaking, it is *always best and most appropriate* to be formal and to use the surname with the appropriate title of Mr. or Mrs. preceding the name.

Adapted from Purnell, L. D., & Paulanka, B. J. (1998). *Transcultural health care: A culturally competent approach.* Philadelphia: F. A. Davis.

the client's and family's ability to cope with the illness as well as assessing whether the interventions are congruent with their culture.

Caregiving and Black Women

Black women, like all women, receive and provide health care in the context of the families in which they perform multiple caregiving roles: as wives, mothers, daughters, widows, single childless women, and so on. Women's assumption of the caregiving role is in line with traditional expectations of women's domestic role, and the majority of caregivers are women (Ward & Brown, 1994). It is not surprising that the caregiving roles of women often predispose them to interrupted employment and limited access to health care insurance, pension plans, and retirement plans. Leigh (1995) observed that these general problems and characteristics of caregivers are compounded for Black women by the special circumstances of their lives and the lives of the men about whom they care. In the case of Black caregivers, "prejudice, discrimination, and poverty all interact to generate the daily diet of stresses that bear on their health" (Leigh, 1995, pp. 112–113).

Caregiving implies the provision of long-term help to an impaired family member or close friend (Wright, Clipp, & George, 1993). Caregiving usually is labor intensive, time-consuming, and stressful, although the exact effects on the physical and emotional health of caregivers are still being documented. The most commonly studied caregiving situation has been that of an elderly individual, usually a woman, caring for a spouse with Alzheimer's disease. When caregiving activities for other family members are necessary in middle adulthood, the roles and challenges obviously are different, although this factor has not been extensively documented. In addition, culture and ethnicity influence beliefs, attitudes, and perceptions of what is normal and what is sickness. Culture and ethnicity also influence how often individuals engage in self care versus seeking formal health services, how many medications they take, how often they rest and exercise, and what type of foods they consume (Wykle & Haug, 1993). Yet, we know very little about caregiving in diverse cultural groups. Wright (1997) observed that "caregiver research is based predominantly on White subjects, and ethnic differences are rarely analyzed. Further, very few studies focus specifically on minority caregivers" (Wright, 1997, p. 277).

Studies of Black caregivers have found that they tend to use religious beliefs to help them cope with the stress of caregiving. Boyle, Ferrell, Hodnicki, and Muller (1997) found that Black caregivers' belief in a personal God and their intense, daily relationship with Him provided them with support during the illness of a family member and helped them cope with death and loss. Poindexter, Linsk, and Warner (1999) and Picot (1995) also found that a major source of support for Black caregivers was their personal relationships with "Jesus," "God," or "the Lord." Church attendance may not be the key to understanding spirituality or religiosity in Black culture; several studies (Picot, Debanne, Namazi, & Wykle, 1997; Poindexter, Linsk, & Warner, 1999) suggest that spirituality is both personal and empowering and is related to the deepest motivations in life (Roof, 1993). Spirituality is expressed in the context of the daily life of Black caregivers, not in formal attendance at religious events.

Although several studies show the positive results of caregiving, researchers warn that Black caregivers pay a high emotional and physical price for their care. Caring for a family member who has HIV disease can be an intensively personal event; it brings the caregiver closer to the loved one but involves sadness and grief (Poindexter & Linsk, 1999). Some studies on depression in caregivers show that Blacks are less depressed than Whites (Haley, et al., 1995) and Hispanic caregivers (Cox & Monk, 1990). There is also some indication that Black caregivers may solve problems of caregiving differently and that these differences may result from social and cultural factors. For example, Black mothers who care for adult children with HIV disease may not always exhibit a proactive, problem-solving approach to the disease (Boyle, Bunting, Hodnicki, & Ferrell, 2001). This is not because Black caregivers are not interested in their adult children's health or cannot understand the complexity of medical regimens. Such behavior may be related more to the racial discrimination and racism that have remained significant factors in the health care of Blacks over time. In addition, there may be cultural influences that shape human behavior in such a way that problems arising from illness and caregiving are solved by different approaches.

The Context of HIV/AIDS and the Black Community

Quam (1994) argued that the epidemic of **HIV/AIDS** must be viewed in the larger context of developments in the political economy of the United States. This context includes a close examination of the distribution of wealth and changes in control over production that have eroded the living standards of most American citizens and have undermined the ability of the federal and state governments to meet the health needs of the American people. Other groups, both governmental and private, also have insisted that the AIDS epidemic cannot be understood apart from the context of racism, homophobia, poverty, and unemployment (National Commission on Acquired Immune Deficiency Syndrome, 1991). Although there is often a fine line between what is cultural, what is political, and what is economic, it is important for health care professionals to become advocates for new policies that provide services needed for the health and well-being of everyone, especially those whose lives have been blighted by social and economic deprivation. From a public health standpoint, education has been stymied by an unwillingness to talk frankly about sexual and drug use behaviors, and this has been a substantial barrier in effective HIV preventive programs. In essence, the AIDS epidemic has forced society to examine and attempt to alter cultural behaviors and values that were largely ignored in the past.

Over the past two decades in the United States, the practice of high-risk HIV behaviors has changed from selected populations of White homosexual men with no history of drug use to heterosexuals having multiple sex partners and using drugs (Siegal, Carlson, & Falck, 1993). The HIV disease disproportionately affects selected groups, especially Blacks and Hispanics, and risk patterns are different for men and women (Centers for Disease Control, 1993). Of equal concern, large epicenters are giving way to rural areas with regard to HIV infection rates (Kalichman, 1995), and minority women seem at particular risk. A phenomenon that is becoming more common is to see HIV-affected caregivers, either mothers or grandmothers, who are caring for family members who are also HIV positive. Some caregivers are caring for one or more family members who need care and attention in addition to the persons with HIV, and such caregivers are often caught between multiple sets of responsibilities. It is generally agreed by most researchers and public health officials that preventive efforts and other interventions should match the social, cultural, linguistic, psychologic, developmental, and behavioral characteristics of the risk group of interest (Sumartojo, Carey, Doll, & Gayle, 1997). However, implementing such interventions has proved extremely difficult.

Culturally Competent Nursing Care of a Black Woman in Situational Crisis

Much of the caregiving literature has focused on predominantly European North American caregivers who provide care to elderly spouses or parents. In the past decade or so, the nature of caregiving has changed with the impact of the AIDS epidemic because AIDS affects a much younger population. At first, caregivers to persons with AIDS often were men; however, mothers and other family members have become more involved as the incidence of HIV disease has changed from White homosexual men to the heterosexual population. Many Blacks living in the rural South first learned about HIV/AIDS from television programs, and many thought of AIDS as a disease that was common in large cities; few thought it was something that could happen in small southern towns or to a member of their own family. Like many other Americans, most Blacks thought AIDS was a disease of White homosexual men, so it was something of a shock when rural Black families learned that one of their own family members had HIV disease. Many Blacks, especially younger adults or teenagers, now commonly refer to HIV/AIDS as **"the virus."** Case 7-1 provides an example of a middle-aged Black woman who provides care to her retarded sister and to her 26-year-old son with AIDS. Culturally appropriate ways in which the nurse might implement nursing care are subsequently suggested. The use of traditional family and religious systems is encouraged because these ties are of particular significance in rural Black culture.

Health Promotion Strategies and Nursing Interventions

Black women are at high risk for cardiovascular diseases, particularly hypertension and stroke. Mrs. Pollard lives in that area of the south known as the **stroke belt** because morbidity and mortality from cardiovascular diseases are so prevalent in this region (Graham-Garcia, Raines, Andrews & Mensah, 2001).

CASE STUDY	7–1

Mrs. Ernestine Pollard, a 52-year-old Black woman, lives in a small town in rural South Carolina. Mrs. Pollard cares for an older sister, who is now 65 years old. Mrs. Pollard explains that her sister "can't talk, and her mind's not good."

Her sister has always lived with her and her husband. Mr. Pollard died a few years ago. Recently the sister's health has been deteriorating because of a series of "little strokes." Then, just a few months ago, Mrs. Pollard's 26-year-old son, Steve, returned home to live with her. Steve was living and working in Florida, where he became very ill. He was taken by friends to the emergency room and then admitted to the hospital. During this hospitalization, the results of a test for HIV disease were positive. After discharge from the hospital, he decided to return home to live with his mother. Mrs. Pollard welcomed this move because she worried about Steve living so far away from her.

Mrs. Pollard explains that sometimes with the stress of caregiving and worrying about Steve, her "pressure goes sky high." She has had "high blood" for several years. Her physician prescribed medication for her blood pressure, and she tries to take it on a regular basis, but sometimes she forgets. Lately, as Steve has become more ill, Mrs. Pollard is not sleeping well, and she is very worried about Steve's condition. She told her doctor that she has "bad nerves" and explained that she was unable to sleep at night. The physician prescribed sleeping pills for her, but Mrs. Pollard is unwilling to take them because she fears that she will not hear Steve during the night if he needs her. In addition to her worry about Steve, she is concerned about her sister's health. Mrs. Pollard has two daughters who are older than Steve, and they try to help their mother with her caregiving activities.

The nursing management priorities for Mrs. Pollard will be support of her caregiving role and health promotion strategies to control her blood pressure and help reduce the stress she is currently experiencing. In terms of blood pressure management, a nurse might advise Mrs. Pollard to lose weight and incorporate changes in eating habits and regular exercise into her lifestyle. However, these health goals maybe compromised by social and cultural factors as well as the caregiving situation. Nurses can become more culturally sensitive to cultural norms and values of clients like Mrs. Pollard by listening carefully, being empathetic, recognizing the client's self-interest and needs of her family members, being flexible, having a sense of timing, using the client's and family's resources, and giving relevant information at the appropriate time.

Although Mrs. Pollard does have a private physician and tries to seek care when appropriate, she considers Steve's needs before her own. Steve is the only member of the Pollard family who is receiving regular health care. He attends an infectious disease clinic at a health science center about 50 miles away from where his mother lives. His medications are provided through Ryan White legislation, a state and federal cooperative agreement to provide care for persons with AIDS. As his illness progresses, a home health care nurse visits several times each week. Even though the nurse's focus is on Steve's illness, he or she will want to support and help Mrs. Pollard care for her son, because she is directly responsible for most of his care and is with him much of the time. Of considerable importance, Mrs. Pollard knows his health history and probably understands him better than anyone else.

Like many other adults, Mrs. Pollard has fairly definite preferences about food and the way it is prepared and served. She believes that the proper kinds of food will promote and enhance good health. The Pollard family frequently eats foods that are high in fat; for example, they enjoy servings of fatback or "fat meat" for breakfast several times each week. They prefer their vegetables cooked with bacon for flavoring. Mrs. Pollard is primarily concerned about Steve's appetite and his ability to eat regular meals. One morning, Steve told his mother that he thought he would like a steak. Mrs. Pollard hurried to the grocery store to buy a steak and cook it for him, and he obviously enjoyed eating it. Symbolism is attached to food in every culture, and Mrs. Pollard believes that Steve will gain some of his strength back by eating healthful foods like meat. In her concern for Steve, she neglects her own diet or eats whatever is convenient, often "fast foods" or those high in carbohydrates and sodium. Mrs. Pollard needs to be gently reminded by the nurse that it is important for her to pay some attention to her own nutrition also.

Clark (1996) suggested that "food can function as a focus of emotional association [and as] a channel for interpersonal relationships, or as a means of communicating love, disapproval, or discrimination" (p. 303). Being able to prepare food that her son will eat and enjoy is a source of satisfaction for Mrs. Pollard and a reinforcement of her successful caregiving. Her focus is now on Steve and his worsening health problems. At the same time, she must maintain her own health to continue to provide care for Steve. A priority is that she take her medication to control her blood pressure. Taking her medication regularly, resting as often as she can, and avoiding foods that are high in fat and/or sodium or eating them only in small or moderate amounts may be realistic goals for Mrs. Pollard during Steve's illness.

Nurses providing care to clients like Mrs. Pollard will need to consider other cultural factors that ultimately influence the nursing goals. Rural Blacks often have cultural ways to view health and illness. **"High blood"** is an illness condition that is associated with Blacks in the rural south. Many health care professionals make the wrong assumption that "high blood" is the same as high blood pressure, and although there are similarities, the cultural explanation of "high blood" is different from the biomedical explanation of high blood pressure. "High blood" is conceptualized in terms of blood volume, blood thickness, or even elevations of the blood in the body (e.g., "blood rushes to your head").

"High blood" is believed to be caused primarily by factors that "run blood up," such as salt, fat, meats, and sweets. This condition results in an increased "pressure" or high blood pressure. Sometimes "high blood" leads to a feeling of faintness that may cause the afflicted person "to fall out" or faint. Other causal factors that result in "high blood" are emotional upsets or prolonged stress. Sometimes it is thought to be caused by a falling out with God, or by eternal forces such as enemies putting a "hex" on someone. Many older Black clients believe that eating slightly acidic foods, such as greens with vinegar or dill pickles, will lower "high blood." Thus, although there are similarities between "high blood" and high blood pressure, the explanations and treatments are not always the same in the cultural prescriptions as in the biomedical model. Mrs. Pollard tries to be conscientious about taking her blood pressure medication, but she does sometimes forget when caring for Steve and her sister. The nurse should acknowledge Mrs. Pollard's concern and her active involvement in her own health promotion and encourage her to take her blood pressure medication as prescribed.

"Nerves" or even **"bad nerves,"** while not unique to the rural south, are commonly described by many southerners. "Bad nerves" are often equated with anxiety and worry but may refer to something as serious as a "mental breakdown" or severe emotional disorder. Mrs. Pollard uses the term to refer to her worry, concern, and anxiety about Steve's deteriorating health status and her anticipation of loss. Sometimes she has "crying spells" that she describes as "just crying and crying, and not being able to stop." She gets up several times at night to answer Steve's call or to check on him and make certain that he is all right. Lack of sleep and continued worry and anxiety accelerate her psychologic distress. Again, recognition from the nurse that she is providing excellent care to her son is reassuring for her. She should be encouraged to rest and should be assured that crying and feeling sad are normal reactions to her son's illness and impending death.

Because of a lack of economic resources, Black midlife women are likely to be subjected to many stressful life events such as job and marital instability, lack of male companions as heads of households, erratic income, and frequent changes and relocations (Lewis & Bernstein, 1996). Even before Steve's illness, Mrs. Pollard experienced many life stresses that were related to the lack of economic resources. In the beginning of Steve's course of illness with HIV disease, Mrs. Pollard continued working in the housekeeping department of a local technical college. However, as Steve's illness progressed and he became increasingly unable to care for himself, Mrs. Pollard quit her job to stay home and take care of him. She faces numerous situational crises: Steve's illness and impending death, the poor health and aging of her older sister, and economic hardship because Mrs. Pollard is the family provider.

Stress and anxiety are normal reactions in the lives of middle-aged adults like Mrs. Pollard. However, limited resources, lack of access to high-quality health care, and discrimination during a severe illness of a family member compound the stress and complicate a situational crisis. Mrs. Pollard's physician prescribed sleeping medication for her, assuming that would take care of her inability to sleep. Unfortunately, this reaction is fairly common: physicians sometimes tend to prescribe medications for the symptoms reported by clients rather than probing more deeply into the situation. The nurse can reinforce Mrs. Pollard's decision not to take this medication and explore with her how to set aside time during the day when she might be able to take a nap. In addition, Mrs. Pollard's anxiety and inability to sleep well are directly related to the stress of caregiving. This can be dealt with in a more culturally acceptable manner than the routine prescription of sleeping medication. Some ways to support and help Mrs. Pollard deal with stress and anxiety may be family support, participation in religious activities, and coping through traditional spirituality.

Close family and spiritual ties within the Black family and community support the caregiving role. Extended and nuclear family members willingly care for sick persons and assume these roles without hesitation. Mrs. Pollard's two daughters try to help their mother and Steve as much as possible. They visit daily and bring their children with them. Steve enjoys being with his nieces and nephews, and he enjoys reading to the younger ones. The teenagers can help him with small tasks such as folding his clothes when they have helped with the laundry. Even Mrs. Pollard's sister tries to help out as best she can by sweeping the floor and wiping the dishes. After a family discussion that involved Steve, Mrs. Pollard, and his two older sisters, it was decided to disclose Steve's HIV diagnosis to his older teenaged nieces and nephews. Steve felt very strongly that he could help his nieces and nephews acknowledge the value of prevention of HIV/AIDS. By preventing others from contracting HIV/AIDS, Steve can find that his life and potential death will assume meaning and purpose.

Many individuals with HIV disease and their close family members are reluctant to disclose the diagnosis to others outside the family, because the stigma of disclosure in a small community can affect all members of the family. Mrs. Pollard's minister is aware of Steve's condition, as are a few members of Mrs. Pollard's "church family." The primary stressor of women during the midlife years is the loss of relationships and friendship networks, often because of competing demands on time (Lewis & Bernstein, 1996). It is extremely important for Mrs. Pollard's health and coping abilities that she continue to participate in church activities and to maintain those friendships and networks.

Spiritual beliefs form a foundation for Mrs. Pollard's daily life. Like other Blacks who live in the same rural community, Mrs. Pollard attends a small Protestant church whose membership is exclusively Black. Many, but not all, Blacks strongly believe in the use of prayer for all situations they may encounter. They use prayer as a means of dealing with everyday problems and concerns. Mrs. Pollard relies a great deal on prayer, and her religious beliefs and practices provide her with support and strength in her caregiving role.

Mrs. Pollard has a lifetime experience with her church; she attended church services as a child and has continued this pattern in her adult years. The role of the church in the Black community has always been important; the church was the center of activities for Blacks for decades (Poindexter, Linsk, & Warner, 1999). Mrs. Pollard's religious beliefs are integrated into her daily life as a caregiver, and her belief in God enhances her ability to care for Steve. She, like many other Blacks, has a personal relationship with God and is able to share her worries and concerns through prayer. Her traditional spirituality and church support provide a foundation for an active approach to coping with problems (see Evidence-Based Practice 7–2).

Psychosocial Development and Nursing Interventions

An important priority of nursing care for Steve and his family is to help them understand and adjust to the impact of HIV disease. The diagnosis of HIV/AIDS precipitated a situational crisis for the Pollard family. Such a situation can best be resolved by the provision of culturally relevant health-promotion and risk-reduction strategies. The health teaching and nursing interventions provided to

EVIDENCE-BASED PRACTICE 7–2
Sources of Support in a Sample of HIV-Affected Older Minority Caregivers

"HIV-affected" is the commonly used term in the field of HIV services and research to designate persons who have personally experienced the impact of HIV disease, because of their own infection or their concern about a loved one. Older persons are now more responsible for the well-being of ill or orphaned family members at a time when they may be at risk for their own health or social losses. We know very little about the social support patterns of older adults, especially among minority populations, who serve as caregivers to family members who have HIV/AIDS. There were two sources of support in this study. The first was support from the family and friends of the caregiver and the HIV-affected person. This kind of support was limited because seeking support from outside required disclosure of the HIV diagnosis, and caregivers and the HIV-affected person were wary of disclosure because of the stigma of HIV/AIDS. The greatest source of support received by the sample members in this study was religious or spiritual. Caregivers did not necessarily attend church services but reported that they communicated with "God," "Jesus," or "the Lord." This study highlights the social isolation of this population resulting from fears of stigma related to HIV illness.

CLINICAL APPLICATION

- Recognize that caregivers may experience a high degree of social isolation and network constriction because of the stigma of HIV/AIDS.
- Understand the deleterious effects that social isolation and decreased support can have on the physical and mental health of caregivers.
- Identify hidden and vulnerable caregivers, and provide aggressive outreach to them.
- Provide meaningful support and assistance to caregivers by listening to their moving stories.
- Encourage and participate in the development of church-based and community-based educational efforts and support services for HIV-affected individuals.
- Develop an awareness of the role of nursing in affecting policy in community, state, and national programs.

Poindexter, C. C., & Linsk, N. L. (1998, September/October). Sources of support in a sample of HIV-affected older minority caregivers. *Families in Society: The Journal of Contemporary Human Services*, 491–503.

the Pollard family should focus on wellness and health promotion. The nurse can continue this emphasis by helping Mrs. Pollard successfully manage the situational crises as well as the developmental tasks common to adulthood.

Mrs. Pollard may face problems in completing the developmental tasks discussed earlier. Havighurst (1974) suggests that an important developmental task for middle-aged adults is career success. Mrs. Pollard has worked outside the home most of her adult life; yet, rural Black culture does not place the kind of emphasis on work and career that the wider American society does. Mrs. Pollard's ties of affection to Steve and her maternal role are reinforced by Black cultural values. Family ties and the lifelong attachments, as well as the extension of the maternal role to an adult child, are valued in the Black culture (Boyle, Hodnicki, & Ferrell, 1999). These values are emphasized over women's careers outside the home. In a historical study of Black women in America, Hine and Thompson (1998) suggested that Black women have always been the financial providers in Black families and that women's work roles have been culturally viewed as an inherent part of Black motherhood, not as individual careers.

Many Black women of Mrs. Pollard's generation obtain meaning in their lives by caring for family members. Their feelings, behavior, and attitudes go beyond a simple sentiment of affection or of family ties. In explaining why she cares for her older retarded sister, Mrs. Pollard says, "We were little girls together. I always knew that I was going to take care of her." In many societies, women disproportionally provide caregiving services and social policies, and programs are organized around the assumption of women's availability and willingness to provide care (Ward & Brown, 1994). At the same time, it is important to understand that Mrs. Pollard values the traditional caregiving role and that she needs support and assistance in providing the care she believes her family members need (see Evidence-Based Practice 7–3).

Family caregivers should be recognized for their unique knowledge of the care receiver's preferences, values, needs, and life history (Rutman, 1996). It is important for the nurse to assess and acknowledge that Mrs. Pollard is valued, recognized, and respected for her competence and expertise as a caregiver. The nurse could begin by including Mrs. Pollard, Steve, and his sisters in developing mutual goals for his care. Mrs. Pollard should be encouraged in her role of providing help and care to family members and in promoting the health of her son and others. It is also important that her attention be directed toward her own needs on occasion, as she tends to focus on meeting the needs of Steve and her sister before her own. Of particular concern is the timing of Steve's serious illness. A terminal condition in a young, previously healthy adult child will cause unique trauma and conflict because of society's expectations that older parents will die before their adult children do.

The second task of adulthood defined by Havighurst (1974) involves relationships with others and the community. Social and civic responsibilities among rural, older Blacks in the South are met almost entirely at the level of the extended family and the Black church. These ties and associations are very strong, are often complex, and are not readily understood by outsiders.

EVIDENCE-BASED PRACTICE 7-3
Women as Family Caregivers: Why Do They Care?

Forty Francophone Québécois female family caregivers of frail elderly or mentally ill adult relatives were interviewed about the motives that led to their decision to provide this care. Fourteen motives emerged and were clustered into three major categories: (1) motives associated with the caregiver (e.g., feelings of closeness with family, gender role conditioning, feelings of duty and obligation); (2) motives related to family, institutional, and community resources (e.g., availability or of family resources that could offer an alternative caregiving situation); and (3) motives related to the care receiver (e.g., imposition of the decision by the dependent person). These findings contribute to our general understanding of why women are vastly overrepresented as caregivers, by revealing how the sexual division of labor operates and is maintained at both individual and societal levels.

CLINICAL APPLICATION

- Encourage caregivers to discuss their feelings about and reasons for providing care to a dependent adult relative (e.g., love, family ties, obligation, guilt, religious convictions, family tradition).
- As needed, explore the availability of family, community, or institutional resources that could provide caregivers with respite or caregiving alternatives.
- Explore the nature of the relationship between the caregiver and the care receiver. For example, is the care receiver imposing himself or herself upon the caregiver, or is the relationship reciprocal and mutually rewarding?
- Challenge governmental programs and policies that assume women's availability and willingness to provide unpaid care to the growing number of frail elderly in North American society.

Guberman, N., Maheu, P. & Maillé, C. (1992). Women as family caregivers: Why do they care? *The Geronotologist, 32*(5), 607–617.

Black pastors are key players in the lives of their congregation and in their communities. Mrs. Pollard should be encouraged to attend church services and to seek the help and support available to her through this important cultural resource. Mrs. Pollard sings in the church choir and tries to attend choir practice every Wednesday evening. One of her daughters comes by to stay with Steve while Mrs. Pollard is away for the evening. The Black church has been a traditional source of support, and congregations are frequently made up of middle-aged or older adults. Because Blacks are at high risk for high blood pressure, stroke, and other cardiovascular diseases, the church would be an excellent site for health education. Perhaps the nurse could help set up a blood pressure clinic for church members. Several women who are active in the church are also nurses, and they could be included in the planning and implementation of the clinic.

The third developmental task of adulthood proposed by Havighurst (1974) is acceptance and adjustment to the physiologic changes of middle age.

Because hypertension is common in Blacks, it is sometimes seen as normal in the middle or late ages. The health-promotion strategies and nursing interventions described earlier will help Mrs. Pollard adjust to other health-related changes.

The fourth developmental task for adults (Havighurst, 1974) is helping teenagers become responsible adults. In Mrs. Pollard's situation, two of her daughters and her son Steve have attained adulthood. However, this developmental task is complicated by Steve's illness and his returning home for care during a terminal illness. Although he has lived independently for several years, he is now dependent on his mother for support and care. As discussed earlier in this chapter, the social timetable for what is considered socially and culturally important can influence how families and individuals respond to life events. The nurse can help Mrs. Pollard evaluate Steve's independence and respond in a sensitive and appropriate ways. The personal tasks of caregiving—bathing, hygiene, toileting, etc.—may pose special concerns as Mrs. Pollard assumes more responsibility for these tasks. Different stressors, however, may have different effects on caregivers because personality factors and experience influence each person's perception of and reaction to a stressful situation. Coping strategies such as prayer, and resources such as family and church support, may help mediate Mrs. Pollard's reaction to stressful situations.

Other developmental tasks pertinent to this case study (Havighurst, 1974) involve relationships with spouse and friends. Mrs. Pollard's life revolves around her family and church. The nurse must understand the importance of cultural ties with kin and others. The support provided by these ties is crucial when an illness develops and is necessary to successful health promotion and maintenance in care-giving activities. Although social support is very important in situations like Mrs. Pollard's, some researchers have found that that many Black caregivers of persons with HIV illness have not disclosed the presence of HIV in the family to anyone outside the immediate family, including church members and ministers (Poindexter, Linsk, & Warner, 1999). When asked where they obtained help and support, these caregivers answered, "Jesus," "God," or "the Lord." It is not uncommon for older Blacks to cope without the amount of social support that would usually be expected in such a crisis, relying instead on internal spiritual resources (Poindexter, Linsk, & Warner, 1999, p. 231). Mrs. Pollard's daughters are crucial to support and assistance during this stressful time. Their contributions should be acknowledged and encouraged by the nurse. In addition, they should be involved in planning Steve's home care and the support of their mother.

The last task suggested by Havighurst (1974) involves increased enjoyment of leisure activities. Mrs. Pollard can be encouraged to continue with leisure activities that are congruent with cultural practices. It is important for her to attend church services and activities because her social life is derived from her participation in the activities of her church. Arranging for one of Steve's sisters to stay with him while Mrs. Pollard attends church services and choir practice would be appropriate. It is possible that it will be the church family who will be instrumental in providing emotional support and help when Steve's condition worsens. After his death, the church will offer spiritual support as well as the opportunity for Mrs. Pollard to find meaning and to cope with her loss and grief.

SUMMARY

All individuals are confronted with developmental tasks: those culturally defined ways of responding to life situations. The challenge to create new paradigms of adult development reflecting a more holistic picture of adult life seems evident in the example just described. It may well be that existing models of adult development are androcentric, meaning that they are based on the life experiences and situations of men. Using these models to understand and interpret women's lives may obscure women's life structures and developmental pathways. Bryant (1989) suggested that we need to examine more closely "both men and women, who are out of sync with their time, the forerunners of new criteria for normal adult development—the women who could not be patently subservient to men, the men who could not be independent of emotions, the oldsters in physical and sexual vigor...." (pp. 3–4).

REVIEW QUESTIONS

1. List and describe the developmental tasks proposed by Havighurst (1974) and outlined in this chapter.
2. How are these developmental tasks of adulthood influenced by culture? For example, explain how a woman from a traditional culture such as those in the Middle East might experience adulthood differently.
3. Discuss how gender might influence adult development in White "mainstream" North American culture.
4. Describe how social factors such as mobility, increased education, and changes in the economy have influenced adult development in mainstream North American culture.
5. How might caregiving for a family member influence development in middle-aged adults? Would this differ for cultural groups such as Chinese Americans or Mexican Americans? How?
6. Describe how culture influences the role of the caregiver in some Black cultures.

CRITICAL THINKING ACTIVITIES

1. Interview a middle-aged colleague, a client, or a person from another cultural group. Ask about family adult roles and how they are depicted. How are these role descriptions typical of traditional roles that are described in

the literature? If not, how are they different? What are some of the reasons why they have changed?

2. Interview a middle-aged client from another cultural group. Ask about the client's experiences within the health care system. What were the differences the client noted in health beliefs and practices? Ask the client about his or her health needs during middle age.

3. Using the cultural assessment guidelines provided in Appendix A conduct a cultural assessment of a middle-aged client of another cultural group. Critically analyze how the client's culture affects the client's role within the family and the timing of developmental tasks. How might the assessment data differ if the client were older? Younger?

4. Review the literature on Mexican American culture. Describe the traditional Mexican American family. What are the cultural characteristics of Mexican Americans to consider in assessing the developmental tasks of adulthood in this group?

5. Christina Calderon Salazar is a refugee from El Salvador who now lives in California and has residency status in the United States. Several weeks ago, she underwent a mastectomy. Señora Calderon has recently experienced menopause. She lives with her husband in a small suburb of Los Angeles, fairly near her two grown sons and their families. Critically analyze the cultural factors that are important to consider in providing nursing care to Señora Calderon. For example, how does Latin American culture view breast surgery? Menopause? How might you assist her in meeting her developmental tasks? What will be some problems that Señora Salazar might encounter in the United States health care system?

• References

Banks-Wallace, J., & Parks, L. (2001). "So that our souls don't get damaged": The impact of racism on maternal thinking and practice related to the protection of daughters. *Issues in Mental Health Nursing, 22,* 77–98.

BarucBaruch, G., & Brooks-Gunn, J. (1984). *Women in midlife.* New York: Plenum.

Behler, D., Tippett, T., & Mandle, C. L. (1994). Middle adult. In C. L. Edelman & C. L. Mandle (Eds.), *Health promotion through the lifespan* (3rd ed., pp. 607–631). St. Louis, MO: C. V. Mosby.

Belenky, M. F., Clinchy, B. M., Goldberger, N. R., & Tarule, J. M. (1986). *Women's ways of knowing.* New York: Basic Books.

Beyene, Y. (1986). Cultural significance and physiological manifestations of menopause: A biocultural analyis. *Culture, Medicine & Psychiatry, 10,* 47–51.

Boyle, J. S. (1996). Central Americans. In J. G. Lipson, S. L. Dibble, & P. A. Minarik (Eds.), *Culture & nursing care: A pocket guide* (pp. 64–73). San Francisco: School of Nursing, University of California Nursing Press.

Boyle, J. S., Ferrell, J. A., Hodnicki, D. R., & Muller, R. B. (1997). Going home: African-American caregiving for adult children with human immunodeficiency virus disease. *Holistic Nursing Practice, 11*(2), 27–35.

Boyle, J. S., Ferrell, J. A., Hodnicki, D. R., & Muller, R. B. (1998). Connections of care: African American mothers and adult children with HIV disease. Manuscript submitted for publication.

Boyle, J.S., Hodnicki, D. R., & Ferrell, J. A. (1999). Patterns of resistance: African American mothers and adult children with HIV illness. *Scholarly Inquiry for Nursing Practice 13,* 111–133.

Canadian Heritage (1998, December). Hate and bias activity in Canada. *The evidence series: Facts about multiculturalism, 4,* 4.

Casper, M. L., Barnett, E., Halveson, J. A., Elmes, G. A., Braham, V. E., Majeed, Z. A, Bloom, A. S., & Stanley, S. (1999). *Women and health disease: An atlas of racial and ethnic disparities in mortality.* Morgantown: West Virginia University, Office for Social Environment and Health Research.

Centers for Disease Control (CDC) (1993, October). *HIV/AIDS surveillance report.* Atlanta: U. S.

Department of Health and Human Services, Public Health Service.

Clark, M. J. (1996). Cultural influences on community health. In M. J. Clark (Ed.), *Nursing in the community* (pp. 273–333). East Norwalk, CT: Appleton & Lange.

Cox, C., & Monk, A. (1990). Minority caregivers of dementia victims: A comparison of black and Hispanic families. *Journal of Applied Gerontology, 9*(3), 340–354.

Danielson, C. B., Hamel-Bissell, S., & Winstead-Fry, P. (1993). *Families, health and illness: Perspectives on coping and intervention.* St. Louis, MO: C. V. Mosby.

Erikson, E. (1963). *Childhood and society* (2nd ed). New York: Norton.

Erikson, E. H. (1980). *Identity and the life cycle.* New York: Norton.

Gilligan, C. (1982a). Adult development and women's development: Arrangement for a marriage. In J. Z. Giele (Ed.), *Women in the middle years* (pp. 89–114). New York: John Wiley & Sons.

Gilligan, C. (1982b). *In a different voice: Psychological theory and women's development.* Cambridge, MA: Harvard University Press.

Golub, S. (1983). *Menarche: The transition from girl to woman.* Lexington, MA: Lexington Book.

Graham-Garcia, J., Raines, T., Andrews, J., & Mensah, G. (2001). Race, ethnicity, and geography: Disparities in heart disease in women of color. *Journal of Transcultural Nursing 12*, 56–67.

Guberman, N., Maheu, P., & Maillé, C. (1992). Women as family caregivers: Why do they care? *The Gerontologist, 32*(5), 607–617.

Haley, W. E., West, C. A. C., Wadley, V. G., Ford, G. R., White, E. A., Barrett, J. J., Harrell, L. F., & Roth, D. L. (1995). Psychological, social, and health impact of caregiving: A comparison of black and white dementia family caregivers and noncaregivers. *Psychology and Aging, 10*, 540–552.

Havighurst, R. J. (1974). *Developmental tasks and education.* New York: David McKay.

Health Canada (1999). Canadian research on immigration and health. Available at: http://www.hc-sc.gc.ca/iacb-dgiac/nhrdp/metropolis/cirh_pdf_index_e.htm. Accessed November 23, 2001.

Hill, P. M., & Humphrey, P. (1982). *Human growth and development throughout life: A nursing perspective.* New York: John Wiley & Sons.

Hine, D. C. & Thompson, K. (1998). *A shining thread of hope: The history of black women in America.* New York: Broadway Books.

Kalichman, S. C. (1995). *Understanding AIDS: A guide for mental health professionals.* Washington, DC: American Psychological Association.

Kirkpatrick, S., & Cobb, A. (1990). Health beliefs related to diarrhea in Haitian children: Building transcultural

nursing knowledge. *Journal of Transcultural Nursing, 1*(2), 2–12.

Leigh, W. A. (1995). The health of African American women. In D. L. Adams (Ed.), *Health issues for women of color* (pp. 112–132). Thousand Oaks, CA: Sage.

Lewis, J. A., & Bernstein, J. (1996). *Women's health: A relational perspective across the life cycle.* Sudbury, MA: Jones and Bartlett Publishers.

Lipson, J. G. & Miller, S. (1994). Changing roles of Afghan refugee women in the United States. *Health Care for Women International, 15,* 171–180.

Lipson, J. G., Hosseini, M. A., Kabir, S., Omidian, P. A., & Edmonston, F. (1995). Health issues among Afghan women in California. *Health Care for Women International 16*(4), 279–286.

Lipson, J. G., & Omidian, P. (1997). Afghan refugee issues in the U. S. social environment. *Western Journal of Nursing Research 19*(1), 110–126.

National Commission on Acquired Immune Deficiency Syndrome. (1991). *America living with AIDS: Report of the National Commission.* Washington, DC: U.S. Government Printing Office.

Neugarten, B. (1968). *Middle age and aging: A reader in social psychology.* Chicago: University of Chicago Press.

O'Kelly, C. G. (1980). *Women and men in society.* New York: Van Nostrand.

Picot, S. J. (1995). Rewards, costs, and coping of African American caregivers. *Nursing Research, 44,* 147–152.

Picot, S. J., Debanne, S. M., Namazi, K. H., & Wykle, M. L. (1997). Religiosity and perceived rewards of Black and White caregivers. *The Gerontologist, 37,* 89–101.

Poindexter, C. C., Linsk, N. L. (1998, September/October). Sources of support in a sample of HIV-affected older minority caregivers. *Families in Society: The Journal of Contemporary Human Services,* 491–503.

Poindexter, C. C., & Linsk, N. L. (1999). "I'm just glad that I'm here": Stories of seven African-American HIV-affected grandmothers. *Journal of Gerontological Social Work, 32,* 63–81.

Poindexter, C. C., Linsk, N. L., & Warner, R. S. (1999). "He listens...and never gossips:" Spiritual coping without church support among older, predominantly African-American caregivers of persons with HIV. *Review of Religious Research, 40,* 231–243.

Purnell, L. D., & Paulanka, B. J. (1998). *Transcultural health care: A culturally competent approach.* Philadelphia: F. A. Davis.

Quam, M. D. (1994). AIDS policy and the United States political economy. In D. A. Feldman (Ed.). *Global AIDS policy.* Westport, CT: Bergin & Garvey.

Roof, W. C. (1993). *A generation of seekers: The spiritual journeys of the baby boom generation.* San Francisco: Harper.

Rutman, D. (1996). Caregiving as women's work: Women's experiences of powerfulness and powerlessness as care-givers. *Qualitative Health Research, 6,* 90–111.

Siegal, H. A., Carlson, R. G., & Falck, R. S. (1993). HIV infection/serostatus outside epicenters. Human immunodeficiency virus (HIV-1) infection: A comparison among injection drug users in high and low seroprevalence areas. In B. S. Brown & G. M. Beschner (Eds.), *Handbook on risk of AIDS: Injection drug users and sexual partners* (pp. 38–71). Westport, CT; Greenwood Press.

Statistics Canada (1999, May). Divorces. *The Daily,* May 18. Available at: http://www.statcan.ca/Daily/English/990518/d990518b.htm. Accessed January 23, 2002.

Sumartojo, F., Carey, J. W., Doll, L. S., & Gayle, H. (1997). Targeted and general population interventions for HIV prevention: Towards a comprehensive approach. *AIDS, 11,* 1201–1209.

U. S. Department of Health and Human Services. (2000). Healthy people 2010: National health promotion and disease prevention objectives. Available at: http: www. health.gov/healthypeople/document. Accessed June, 2002.

Ward, D. & Brown, M. A. (1994). Labor and cost in AIDS family caregiving. *Western Journal of Nursing Research, 16*(1), 10–25.

Wiese, J. (1976). Maternal nutrition and traditional food behavior in Haiti. *Human Organization, 35*(2), 193–200.

Wright, L. K. (1997). Health behavior of caregivers. In D. S. Gochman (Ed.), *Handbook of health behavior research III: Demography, development, and diversity* (pp. 267–283). New York: Plenum Press.

Wright, L. K., Clipp, E. C., & George, L. K. (1993). Health consequences of caregiver stress. *Medicine, Exercise, Nutrition, and Health, 2,* 181–195.

Wykle, M., & Haug, M. R. (1993, Fall). Multicultural and social class aspects of self-care. *Generations,* 25–28.

CHAPTER 8

Transcultural Nursing Care of Older Adults

Margaret A. McKenna

KEY TERMS

Case manager
Community-based settings
Formal support

Illness behavior
Informal social support networks
Traditional medicine

OBJECTIVES

1. Demonstrate knowledge of socioeconomic factors and community resources that influence the experiences of older adult clients in the health care system.
2. Apply concepts of cultural variation, life experiences, and acculturation to plan and implement nursing care for the older adult client in community and institutional settings.
3. Integrate concepts of informal and formal support systems, patterns of caregiving, and available resources to plan appropriate nursing care of the older adult.
4. Develop nursing interventions for older adult clients in a variety of caregiving contexts that will be perceived as culturally acceptable.

Nurses and other health care professionals are becoming increasingly aware that improved health and longevity among older clients is contributing to our aging society. Care of the older adult client is an important focus in the education and clinical training of nurses in response to the expected demands that a sector of the older population will place on the health care system. Nurses have traditionally cared for the older adult client in acute care hospitals and long-term care facilities, but they are now expanding their roles in the care of older adults, as individuals and in groups, in community-based settings. As used in this chapter, the term **community-based settings** refers to community health or social agencies that are based in the community rather than in a hospital setting.

These expanded roles for nurses in community settings are available because many older adults retain significant capabilities and continue to reside in their communities. Nurses will provide care to clients in various environments: the care of many older clients will occur in multiple settings, including independent residences, active adult retirement communities, board and care facilities, and long-term care facilities. Older adults are a heterogeneous group and will have a range of strengths as well as various needs that require different levels of care, assistance, and support. Nurses will likely fill roles as long-term care case managers, direct care providers, discharge planners, and nursing consultants.

Culture shapes the way individuals view aging and explains the variability between groups of older clients in their adjustments to aging and in their health- and illness-related behavior and practices. Although culture is not the sole determinant of behavior, an awareness of it is critical for understanding the interactions of older clients, both in their families and in their wider social context. When attention is given to a client's cultural background, nurses will implement care that is more individualized to the strengths and needs of each client, and care will be most appropriate to each individual's circumstances.

To appropriately plan and implement care, nurses should assess the evolving socioeconomic, cultural, and family contexts in which the older adult exists. By examining the variations in an older adult client's interactions in their family, community, and societal contexts, nurses can determine the relative impact of these variables on the individual client. Nurses should understand that the older client participates in the culturally influenced patterns of care within a family. The available resources in a community, along with the institutions, long-term care funding, and interventions available at the societal level, will affect both the older clients' options for care and the individual's movement on a continuum of care. The three factors that nurses will find relevant in planning appropriate and acceptable care for older adults are (1) the encompassing social and economic factors that influence the older client's plans for long-term care and help-seeking behavior; (2) community level factors that include cultural values, practices, patterns of caregiving, and the informal and formal sources of help that are available to older clients; and (3) how the interaction of factors at the society and local community level affects older adults and their families, who respond to illness and make decisions during a continuum of care and services.

Nurses must assess, within the broader societal context, the cultural variations that should be considered when they plan and implement the care of older adults. Older clients' cultural traditions and values will influence their preferences for residence, lifestyles, and expectations of who will be their caregivers. The cultural traditions and related practices among older adults are, of course, varied, and their retention is influenced by social, economic, and acculturation factors. When assessing the needs of older adults, nurses must consider individuals in a broad societal context, in the context of their cultural upbringing, and in the context of their families, which have varying strengths, resources, and capacities for the care of aging family members. Doing so has implications for how nurses can assess and plan nursing care for individuals in both community and institutional care settings.

• THE OLDER ADULT IN SOCIETY

The broadest context to consider in the development of culturally appropriate care for older clients is the societal level. The help-seeking behavior of the older adult population has been influenced by social and economic factors that include government interventions intended to improve the experiences and care of older adults in the health care system. For example, Medicare, a federal program to finance health care services, was intended to provide health care access for persons over the age of 65 years. See Box 8-1 for highlights of factors that interact and shape the context for older adult clients who seek care or use health care services. Important factors to consider at the societal level include the demographics of the aging population, the variables that increase the proportion of older adults in the human services system, and social theories of aging that explain how adults in Western society perceive growing older.

Demographics

The number of people under 65 years of age in the United States tripled during the 20th century—a significant increase that calls attention to the needs of children, youth, and middle-aged adults. At the same time, however, the

BOX 8–1	**FACTORS THAT INFLUENCE OLDER ADULTS' RESPONSES IN SEEKING HEALTH CARE**

At the Societal Level

• Social and economic factors and changes affect the experiences of older adults in the health care system.
• Interventions to control Medicare expenditures force shorter hospital stays.
• Gaps in health care services put greater burdens on older patients for home and community-based care.

Cultural Variation Within a Societal Context

• Different cultural traditions have values that influence patterns in caring for older adult family members as they require more assistance.
• Younger family members become acculturated and change traditional behaviors that may differ from older adults' expectations.

At the Individual Level

• Female family members who were considered primary caregivers for older family members are entering the work force.
• Families' economic situations, proximity to the older adult, and sources of formal support in the community will determine options for residence and care needs of the older adult.

number of adults age 65 years or over increased by a factor of 11 (U.S. Department of Commerce, 1995). Similar trends are found in Canada, where the number of Canadians age 65 and over has increased by almost 60 percent since 1981 (Statistics Canada, 2000a). Improved living conditions, increased life expectancies, and decreasing fertility rates all contribute to an increase in the proportion of older adults in the population of the United States and Canada as well as of other developed countries. In Japan, the nation with the longest life expectancy at birth, more than 25% of the population will be age 65 or older by the year 2025 (Angel & Angel, 1997; Murashima, Zerwekh, Yamada, & Tagami, 1998). In the Northern European nations of Iceland, Finland, Norway, Sweden, and Denmark, 20.5% of the population is projected to be over the age of 65 years in 2025 (Giarchi, 1996).

Whereas in 1900 only 1 out of every 25 Americans was over 65 years old, in 1994 1 out of 8 were over 65 years old, and in 2030 1 out of 5 are projected to be so (U.S. Department of Commerce, 1995). The number of Americans and Canadians age 65 years or over will double between now and 2050. The group 85 years and older was the fastest-growing sector of the last U.S. and Canadian censuses (Department of Health and Human Services, 1997; Rodin & Iris, 1998; Statistics Canada, 2000b), and projections are that the number of centenarians in the U.S. will increase to 47,000 by 2040 (Elsner, Quinn, Fanning, Gueldner, & Poon, 1999). Ethnic populations of color, which include Hispanic, American Indian, Eskimo, Aleut, Asian, Pacific Islander, and Arab American populations, are expected to represent 25% of the elderly by 2030. In Canada, however, only 6% of seniors belong to visible minority groups. Nevertheless, this number is expected to rise, due to changing immigration patterns (Health Canada, 1998).

Disability

Disability is not an inevitable result of growing older, and evidence shows that today's population aged 65 years and older in the United States is less disabled than earlier cohorts (Department of Health and Human Services, 1997). The majority of older adults in North American settings do not have disabling conditions, and this is true in other countries as well. In the United Kingdom, approximately 80% of the population 75 years and older are not disabled, and in Belgium and France, 70% of the older adult population are similarly able (Giarchi, 1996).

For approximately 20% to 25% of the older adult population, however, the care and management of chronic conditions becomes more problematic and costly with advancing age. Health care systems in the United States, Canada, and other developed countries must face the expanded demands of some older clients who require care for multiple chronic conditions. By 2050, the number of older adults in the U.S. who have dementia, for example, may increase to 14 million, and 45% or more of those over 85 years may be affected (Beresford, 1997). Similarly, in Canada, dementia and depression are the two most common mental health problems encountered by seniors (Health Canada, 2002). Older adults who are Black, Hispanic, and North American

Indian have a higher prevalence of cardiovascular disease and diabetes than do White (non-Hispanic) populations (Federal Interagency Forum, 2000; Heart and Stroke Foundation of Canada 1999, October). Diabetes, the seventh leading cause of death in the United States and Canada, is especially problematic in older North American Indians and Alaskan Natives, who die of diabetes at a rate nearly three times higher than that in populations of White older adults. Older Pacific Islanders have a higher prevalence of diabetes and obesity than do White populations. And the American Heart Association 1998 Statistical Update reported that Filipino, Japanese, and Southeast Asian populations in the United States had a higher prevalence of hypertension than did White populations. In Canada, more research is needed to better determine and track such rates of cardiovascular disease among various ethnic groups and visible minorities (Heart and Stroke Foundation of Canada, 1999, October). No simple correlation exists between the need for care and increased age because health status and the need for care are affected by many other factors, including social class and ethnicity. Elderly Blacks have often experienced functional declines at earlier ages than White Americans. Older Black women have a much higher proportion of disabling conditions than do older Black men and older White adults. Older Black women in the southern United States are also at higher risk for functional impairments than are Black women living in other regions (Martin & Panicucci 1996).

The demands that the older population will place on the health care field are complex. A subgroup of the older adult population will experience significant physical decline or functional disability that requires extended use of hospital, community, or home-based personal health services.

To serve the growing proportion of older clients, nurses should be aware that social and economic factors, cultural variation, and available support will interact and affect the **illness behavior** (i.e., behavior taken in response to symptoms of a disease or illness) and related help-seeking responses of older clients. As nurses prepare to care for older clients they must assess the heterogeneity of the population, because ethnicity, cultural traditions, social and economic situations, living arrangements, employment status, and migration history are as varied for older adults are they are for younger adults. These background factors contribute to older adults' varied responses to illnesses that require care and management in the health care system.

Economic Factors

The cost of long-term care for older adults in the United States and Canada has contributed to growing health care expenditures for adults aged 65 years and older as more patients have required management of chronic illness and not just of acute care episodes. Because the numbers of older adults who will require long-term community-based or institutional care is likely to rise, the financial burdens on national, state, provincial, and local systems is likely to rise as well. These elderly North Americans may have set aside resources for retirement, but they may not be sufficient for their longer life spans. As the number of elderly has increased they have continued to have the highest poverty rate of adult Americans. In Canada, the poverty rates among seniors have declined. However, a large proportion of Canadian seniors, especially females, continues to live below the poverty line (Lee, 2000).

Forty percent of the elderly of color, including Hispanic Americans and Blacks, have no private savings for their retirement and will depend on state and federal reimbursement programs for their health and social service needs. More than 20% of older Hispanic persons have incomes below the poverty level, compared with less than 10% for non-Hispanic White elderly. Poverty among one sector of the Mexican American elderly may be attributed to a history of low wage jobs, periods of unemployment, and lower educational levels. The proportion of Hispanic elderly with no formal education is eight times higher than the rate for non-Hispanic White elderly (U.S. Department of Commerce, 1995; Federal Interagency Forum, 2000).

Many ethnic elderly persons of color have accumulated fewer financial assets: they have a lower household income, fewer dividends, and less income from private pensions than do elderly Whites (Angel & Angel, 1997). One in five elderly persons of color rely on Supplemental Security Income for their primary source of income after age 65, whereas only 1 in 20 elderly White clients do (Angel & Angel, 1997). Similar economic disadvantages are disproportionately experienced by elderly members of visible minority groups living in Canada. Many older adults and their families in particular ethnic groups face limited tangible assets and lower equity in their homes, and this may limit care options because they cannot afford costly long-term care or community-based care. In some Native North American families, each adult child, in a serial fashion, assumes the burden of responsibility and cost of care for aging parents, using up their limited personal financial resources.

Because of the needs of older Americans, many states or communities are developing or implementing managed care systems to integrate health care and long-term care (Collins, Butler, Gueldner, & Palmer, 1997). Although several state demonstration projects in which older clients benefited from chore services and skilled nursing care at home were successful, proving their cost-effectiveness has remained a challenge. One model now being replicated is the Program of All-Inclusive Care for the Elderly (PACE), which is built around attendance at an adult day health care center where interdisciplinary health care team members provide restorative, social, medical, and supportive care (Murashima, et al. 1998). Nurses working on teams with social workers, aides, and therapists develop care plans to help frail older individuals live independently for as long as possible (Graber & Kilpatrick, 2001). According to one evaluation, PACE participants are experiencing fewer hospital days and less nursing home use than the general Medicare population (Kunz & Shannon, 1996). Another model for long-term care is the Social Health Maintenance Organization (SHMO), which uses Medicare and Medicaid funding to cover such comprehensive services as homemakers, adult day care, transportation, personal care, and short-term institutional care (National LTC Resource Center, 1996; Zablocki, 2001). Evaluations of these managed care strategies are just becoming available. One study suggests that frail elderly persons who meet eligibility criteria and are carefully assessed may receive community-based services at a lower cost than that required by comparable nursing home care (Weissert, Lesnick, Musliner, & Foley, 1997). Evidence that community-based and home-based care options can be cost-effective will likely lead to broader implementation of similar services that will enable more elderly persons to reside longer in their preferred community residences. Comparable initiatives to support independent living among seniors are underway in Canada. For example, the province of Alberta has introduced a Community Supports Model designed to support independent living by providing technical and personal services in the home (e.g., in-home nursing care, housekeeping, respite care, personal care, wheelchairs, etc.) (Health Canada, 1995, February).

The majority of older adults prefer to "age in place"—that is, stay in their homes and in their neighborhoods as long as possible. By considering the needs of older adults and designing health and social services programs to accommodate these needs, communities can be successful in keeping older adults among them. Demonstration projects to provide community-based services to older adults have proved several approaches to be successful: (1) Care of the elderly at home requires comprehensive services from a multidisciplinary team of providers along a continuum of care. (2) Providing services at home in place of institutionalization may be less costly but requires a broad spectrum of services that often use formal and informal networks of caregivers. (3) Nurses who provide primary care have a vital role in assessing the older adult's physical, mental, and social well-being within the contexts of family, culture, and community.

A nurse may be a **case manager** for older adult clients in active retirement communities or other settings. As a case manager, a nurse has responsibility to help clients and families meet specific health care needs by using health care resources appropriately. One example from the caseload of a nurse who provides preventive health care and assessments in a low-income housing complex for older adults illustrates individuals' different experiences have in their use of health care services and Medicare. An 82-year-old woman who worked as a housekeeper did not seek health care until she had a stroke related to untreated hypertension. She had made limited contributions to Social Security because of her episodic work, and her savings were depleted by her illness. She received Medicare-funded services and continues to receive home health care through Medicaid, which is state-funded health care coverage for individuals with low income. This is representative of the situations faced by many older adults of lower socioeconomic status who are affected by societal interventions that provide health care coverage for older clients, including Medicare.

As a home health nurse, you may assess that older patients on your caseload would benefit from nursing assessments and medication monitoring, but discover that the patient's insurance and Medicare will not cover such services. Medicare pays only a small portion of home health care services, and the patient must be medically eligible to qualify. Older adults who have other insurance may have some additional home health services covered. Similarly in Canada, the cost and accessibility of home care services to seniors is variable and largely dependant upon senior's income and/or personal health insurance coverage. For example, in New Brunswick, seniors with lower incomes and limited health insurance coverage will have a proportion of the costs of home care paid by the province.

The care received by older adults is influenced by their environment. For example, clients in poor rural areas may not have the variety of services that are available to clients in affluent urban environments. An older adult's needs for care, requests for assistance, and sources of caregivers are all culturally influenced. In the United States and Canada, nurses and health care professionals see many variations in the community caregiving support resources, both formal and informal, that are provided for older adults.

• SOCIAL THEORIES OF AGING

In addition to demographic and economic factors, psychosocial factors shape the experiences of older adults. The older client's requests for services and the reactions of others to older adults are shaped in part by the prevailing social theories of aging. Important traditional Western theories of aging include the following:

- The disengagement theory, which focused on the withdrawal of older adults who were forced into retirement or who incurred disabilities.
- The activity theory, which focused on the selective substitution of activities by retired individuals.
- The continuity theory, which focused on the adaptation or continuation of patterns and behaviors from younger adulthood.

These Western theories provided frameworks for assessing clients' responses to growing older and making decisions about living arrangements, and they anticipated care needs that were useful in working with older adults brought up with Western values. In North American society, the values of independence, self-reliance, and productivity contributed to attitudes held by many, including older adults, that they were not as valuable as they once were when they were working, productive individuals. Unfortunately, some older adults experienced lowered self-esteem once they retired, believing that they were no longer contributing members of society. Traditionally, in mainstream North American culture, many older individuals felt that they were forced to retire for various reasons; as a result, they often withdrew from social interaction with others and became isolated and disengaged. In 1997, however, international collaboration between researchers who study aging resulted in the "active aging" paradigm. Active aging reflects the reality that industrialized nations have older populations who may remain engaged in economically and socially productive activities (Department of Health and Human Services, 1997). Older adults are perceived not as imposing a financial burden but as being involved in socially important activities such as volunteering, providing household and childcare help, aiding the disabled elderly, and supporting social service organizations. Industrialized societies are using this paradigm to promote social and economic integration of older people that recognizes individual choices and circumstances (Department of Health and Human Services, 1997). The traditional theoretic frameworks and new paradigm are highlighted in Box 8-2.

Evidence of active aging may be seen in both organizations and individuals. The Gray Panthers advocate for creative, productive lifestyles in older adults that are aimed at counteracting the losses of roles and status experienced by many older clients. A recent study of 213 women who were monitored for more than 30 years found that women with more roles had higher self-esteem and improved health as they grew older, which lends support to the activity theory and the active aging paradigm (Moen, Dempster-McClain, & Williams 1995).

• THE OLDER ADULT IN A CULTURAL COMMUNITY

The stressful life experiences of some older adults may make them reluctant to seek services or to trust care provided by health care professionals who are very different from themselves. Life experiences that shape their responses in seeking health care include living through the Depression; being inundated by advances in technology such as television, computers, and high-tech medical equipment; migrating to find employment; and fighting in an international conflict. European North Americans in their 80s may have fled Poland or Czechoslovakia as young adults before World War II. Many Southeast Asians fled Cambodia because of conflict and political unrest there. Political refugees

BOX 8–2	THEORIES OF REACTIONS TO AGING

Disengagement Theory

- A pattern of withdrawal is usually considered desirable by the older person
- Time is allocated for reflection and leisure activities

Activity Theory

- Substitute activities for the tasks, such as employment, that are regulated and have been withdrawn from the worker
- Maintain activity levels and resist changes that would mean withdrawal

Continuity Theory

- Continue lifelong activities that contribute to self-perceptions
- Find meaning in adapting behaviors from younger adulthood

Active Aging Paradigm Themes

- Improvements in active life expectancy
- Employment opportunities in an aging society
- Strengthened pension systems
- Role of caregiving and volunteerism
- Planning for age-related health and long-term care needs

who lived through civil wars and political revolution may have depleted their coping mechanisms and may experience adjustment problems that warrant physical or mental care, but they may also distrust the health care system.

Nurses providing care to clients whose background differs from their own are often sensitive to assessing the client's culture. But individuals who have immigrated from the same country or region will differ in their needs and in the ways their cultural background influences their health- and illness-related actions. These differences may be based on factors such as the following:

- their regional or religious identity
- the situation in their homeland that prompted them to emigrate
- the length of time they have spent in the United States or Canada
- whether they came to be close to immediate family or extended family members
- whether they have a network of friends and social support from their homeland
- whether they have a link with ethnic social and health-related institutions.

The Hispanic American population in the United States illustrates the wide variety of experiences in a single ethnic group. Persons of Mexican descent, the largest group, constitute 54% of the total Hispanic American population, followed by Cubans with 14%, Puerto Ricans with 9%, and other Spanish-speaking persons with 24%. The patterns of immigration and repatriation vary among these Hispanic groups and lead to substantial differences in the proportion of elderly Hispanic Americans in them. Cuban Americans, for example, have a high proportion of elderly (13.3%) because many well-educated and professionally established Cubans immigrated to the United States in the 1960s and have stayed and retired here. They may also have longer life expectancies because of their better socioeconomic conditions. Families leaving Mexico, however, have been younger. Older Mexican Americans do not have as long a life expectancy as their Cuban American peers. More attention should be given to understanding the diversity in Asian North American elderly as well. Asian North Americans and Pacific Islanders are a heterogeneous collection of more than 40 distinct ethnic groups. Filipinos are the most numerous of the older immigrant groups, which also include the Chinese and Japanese. Newer immigrants include Koreans and Thais. Among the refugees, Vietnamese are more numerous than Cambodians and Laotians.

Traditional Medicine

Culture also influences how individuals view aging and how persons manage interpersonal crises and the alterations in health that often accompany aging. Culture influences the older person's expectations of what constitutes illness and whether he or she will continue using traditional sources of health care in place of, or in addition to, biomedical sources of care. Some older clients prefer to use **traditional medicine** from their native countries or practices that they recall from their childhood traditions. The use of traditional sources of health care concurrently with, or in place of, the biomedical health care system is not limited to members of recently migrated cultural groups but is common to nearly all individuals in these groups. The lingering chronic conditions that often accompany age increase the likelihood that older adults will use traditional sources to treat their symptoms. The older adult may resort to an over-the-counter medication or popular remedies before, during, or after the use of prescribed sources of care. Nurses can show an interest in clients and can ask them about any actions they take to treat their conditions, to assess their concurrent use of traditional practices, folk medicine, or popular medicine.

Older adult clients may also use traditional medicine that they recall from their cultural upbringing to prevent illness. Preventive measures may include magical or religious elements, such as burning a candle, offering cornmeal to the spirits, wearing an amulet, or reciting a prayer. The nurse may reinforce those preventive actions that the older client views as promoting health with other actions that prevent illness and maintain health. To assess cultural beliefs and practices, the nurse can demonstrate a nonjudgmental attitude and ask questions such as the following:

- Have you eaten any foods that made your problem better?
- Have you used some herbs to make you feel better?
- Have you bought or used pills or medicine to help your problem?
- Did you talk to someone else and follow his or her advice about your problem?
- What do you expect your treatment to be?
- What would you like us to do to make you comfortable?

Case Study 8-1 illustrates that assessing the client's use of alternative sources of treatment is useful in developing a care plan that the client will accept. Older clients who choose to use alternative sources of care and decide not to

---

CASE STUDY	8–1

Mr. S.L. was a 78-year-old retired machinist who had degenerative joint disease that caused recurring pain in his elbows and knees. He referred to his condition as "arthritis" and attributed his pain to the wear and tear of his long career working around machinery, hauling parts, handling equipment, and standing for long intervals. He was raised in West Virginia and recalled that his mother used rubbing liniment and kerosene to relieve aching joints. He lived outside a major Northwest city when he was interviewed by a nurse researcher about his use of alternative sources of treatment for his joint pain. He said that in addition to over-the-counter pain medication, he regularly rubbed kerosene and sheep liniment on his affected joints. He explained that his joints were not well lubricated and that they felt like gears that were clashing. An oil-based rubbing compound penetrated the joints and relieved his discomfort.

Clinical Application
The nurse assessed that the use of the rubbing compound did not interfere with the prescribed medications. The patient's belief that rubbing compound improved his condition and decreased his pain allowed him to participate in a prescribed exercise program. The nurse would continue to assess the treatment to determine whether the use of an alternative source of treatment interfered with the prescribed care plan.

follow prescribed treatment plans may do so based on their beliefs about the causes of their illness and their expectations for treatment. Because older clients may blend biomedical beliefs about the cause of illness with traditional and popular beliefs, it follows that clients may adhere to some traditional practices and to some biomedical treatments. For example, a study of rural Black older clients found that the study participants held beliefs about high blood pressure that were fairly congruent with biomedical concepts. Even though the clients acknowledged their traditional practices surrounding "high blood," they still preferred prescribed medications. This study is described in Evidence-Based Practice 8–1 and indicates how important it is that nurses assess each client's beliefs and practices individually, because of intragroup variations.

EVIDENCE-BASED PRACTICE 8–1
Health Beliefs of Black Rural Elders

A sample of Black elders living in a rural area in Florida maintained selected traditional beliefs along with biomedical explanations about the causes of high blood pressure. Most study participants believed that high intake of certain foods and a genetic predisposition could cause hypertension. They also believed that they would always have high blood pressure, and, although they knew of the "old way remedies to reduce high blood," the participants tended to prefer to use prescribed medications. This finding, though limited in its generalizability, is useful because it describes the beliefs and practices of one group of Blacks and therefore highlights the heterogeneity of this population. The research findings remind nurses to (1) assess rather than assume knowledge of older clients' beliefs about the cause of an illness and treatment expectation, (2) avoid stereotypical views from previous research that clients are homogeneous and adhere to traditional ways, and (3) recognize that culture is dynamic, so older clients' views of illness will change as they blend some biomedical explanations with traditional concepts.

CLINICAL APPLICATION

- The views and advice offered by nurses were highly regarded and were well received by study participants. This reminds nurses to take appropriate responsibility to work with the older clients toward mutually agreed-upon goals for care.
- Nurses who are culturally competent will recognize that prescribed diets such as low-sodium diets may not be region specific, or they may not include foods common in rural older clients' diets, so nurses should help clients with adjustments.
- Nurses should assess how older clients prepare their foods; "greens," for example, may be prepared with pork and therefore be high in sodium.
- Nurses are in a good position to reinforce older clients' beliefs (that may be based in religion) that they should live life in moderation and modify their dietary intake, because these behaviors will support a prescribed regimen that is intended to improve the clients' well-being.

Schoenberg, N. E. (1997). A convergence of health beliefs: An "ethnography of adherence" of African-American rural elders with hypertension. *Human Organization, 56*(2), 174–181.

Culture will also determine the older adult's expectations for family caregiving. Culture is not the only determinant of behavior, but it significantly influences the interactions of older clients in their society, their access to and use of the health care system, and their relationships with family members and friends in a support network.

The National Family Caregivers Association (NFCA) conducted a survey and compiled the following profile of family and informal caregivers in the U.S. (National Alliance for Caregiving, 1997):

- 81% are women
- 54% care for a spouse
- 21% care for a parent
- 55% help with activities of daily living (ADLs)
- 60% have been providing care for 5 years or more.

Approximately half of the informal caregivers of chronically disabled seniors are spouses who are themselves aged 65 or older (Department of Health and Human Services, 1997). Likewise, in Canada, women are more likely than men to provide informal personal care, 46% of which is provided to a parent and 16% to a spouse. Canadians most likely to provide some unpaid senior care are between 45 and 54 years of age (23%) (Health Canada, 1999).

The hardships that older clients have endured may increase their desire for autonomy and time to reflect on their decisions in later years. This desire may in turn diminish an older client's readiness to accept health restorative care from the nurse and push the client toward self-reliance. A study found that older Appalachian adults tended to regard health care very cautiously. (Lewis, Messner, & McDowell, 1985). Their harsh lives led the clients to be fatalistic about many losses in life and to weigh any options about health care in relation to their fatalistic views and their roles and interactions in their families.

Several recent studies have described the implications of cultural backgrounds for appropriate health care of the older adult. Although the situations of cultural groups are unique, some similarities across these groups are relevant in planning nursing care. Older clients from different backgrounds may share, for example, in experiences of migration, changing social and family structures, structural forces such as discrimination, and historical events that included political conflict. These studies indicate that older clients retain their traditional beliefs while modifying aspects of their behavior to adapt to new surroundings. Older adult clients may vary from total acceptance of their traditional practices to some blending of traditional and biomedical care to total acceptance of biomedical care. That older clients preserve their traditional values indicates that a connection to their origins gives meaning to their lives. These studies are highlighted in Table 8–1.

Nurses can provide culturally appropriate care after assessing whether the older client retains traditional values or blends traditional values and practices with biomedical beliefs and practices. Many older clients, now in their 80s, may have grown up with limited preventive care and may associate health care only with emergency conditions, so nurses should assess the older client's previous experiences in the health care system.

TABLE 8–1	HIGHLIGHTS OF SELECTED TRANSCULTURAL STUDIES OF OLDER ADULT CLIENTS, 1996–2001	
STUDY (AUTHOR, DATE) AND GROUP STUDIED	**CULTURAL VALUES RELEVANT IN CARE OF OLDER ADULT CLIENT**	**IMPLICATIONS FOR NURSING CARE**
Murashima, Zerwekh, Yamada, & Tagami (1998): Frail elderly Japanese living at home receiving visiting nurse services	Family caregivers are becoming less available, and the extended family is separating into smaller family units. The numbers of households with an older adult who requires assistance are rising.	Teams of skilled nurse managers and support workers providing care in early morning and late night hours supported family care givers who could be sustained in providing help with daily activities during the day and evening hours.
Subgranon & Lund (2000): Caregivers in Thailand caring in their homes for elderly relatives who had strokes	Buddhist caregivers believed their actions repaid their past deeds and earned them merit. Muslim caregivers believed their deeds would help them experience good things and get into heaven.	Nurses can encourage caregivers to share their personal knowledge and experiences and can also help develop programs to assist caregivers.
Martin & Panicucci (1996): 40 Black women, over 65 years old, members of a Southern, urban Baptist church	Sample had a high adherence to 20 recommended health behaviors, including abstinence from alcohol and smoking, that may have been related to participants' religious doctrines.	Assess each client's interest in preventive behavior and make preventive practices relevant for client's lifestyle. Identify whether cost is a factor in preventive care. Tailor approaches to individuals; do not take a global approach.

(Continued)

The Effects of Immigration

Some older adults have been lifelong residents of the U.S. or Canada and have resided in the same city or state/province for all of their adult lives. Others have migrated to different regions of these countries or have made significant transitions and relocations in their late adult years to be close to younger family members. Older clients may have the common experience of relocating or migrating, but their lengths of residence in one area may vary. Other older adults are recent immigrants and refugees. Whereas immigrants in previous

TABLE 8–1	*(Continued)*	
STUDY (AUTHOR, DATE) AND GROUP STUDIED	**CULTURAL VALUES RELEVANT IN CARE OF OLDER ADULT CLIENT**	**IMPLICATIONS FOR NURSING CARE**
Bonura, Fender, Roesler, & Pacquaio (2001): Professional hospice caregivers and family caregivers in a large Jewish community in New Jersey	A common worldview is that suffering is a part of life. There are differences in the concept of afterlife among Orthodox, Conservative, and Reform Jews.	Nurses may find that Jewish patients and their family members are more comfortable in a grief support group of their peers. Nurses should assess, understand, and work with differences among Jewish groups.
Kim, Juon, Hill, Post, & Kim (2001): 205 Korean American elderly, 60-69 years old, who lived in Maryland and were identified from social organizations	The stresses related to acculturation most likely adversely affect blood pressure. Many Korean American elderly use herbal medications to reduce blood pressure.	Nurses should try to reduce language barriers by requesting interpreters but should also assess for adverse effects from regimens that clients may be reluctant to discuss
Schiavenato (1997): Hispanic elders, cultural heritage distinguished among Mexican, Spanish, Central American, South American, Cuban, Spanish	Traditional gender roles, values, respect, courtesy are features of Hispanic culture that positively affect an individual's health status. The term "Hispanic" masks the cultural identities and traditions of diverse groups.	Assess for increased severity of the illness that may be related to delay in seeking treatment. Communication barriers may lead to distrust. Assess use of traditional medicine that may be incorporated in plan of care.

centuries came primarily from northern and western European countries, increasing numbers of older adults migrate from nations all over the world to relocate with other family members in the United States and Canada. Nurses and health care professionals may find that recent immigrants have a stronger family orientation and an expectation of caregiving by adult children to their parents.

Older adults who have immigrated may have lost social position or status, or left behind careers, and may be clinging to their family roles because of the stress of acculturation. The psychologic stress related to cultural change is more intense for older refugees. Older adults who reside with immediate family members may adjust to such a change in living arrangements with less difficulty than do older adults who share a living space with many extended family members and non-kin.

Mai Bliatout's experience illustrates the impact of migration. She fled Laos in the late 1970s and settled in the Pacific Northwest with her husband and three daughters, then gave birth to a fourth daughter in the United States. Although some Laotians are Buddhists or animists, Mai and her family are Roman Catholic, because her family had been friends with missionaries. Mai lived with her oldest daughter, her son-in-law, and her two granddaughters in an urban neighborhood where there were other Laotian, Vietnamese, and Korean families. Her other three daughters lived within two hours of Mai and visited her at least once a week. Mai traveled with one of her daughters to a church in another part of the city to hear mass in her native language rather than in English. She lived where she could shop in a market and buy Vietnamese noodles similar to those she used to have at home. She had contact with immigrants whose experience was similar to hers. Although she had lived in the United States for 30 years, Mai preferred to speak her native language while at home with her husband. Mai and her husband are representative of approximately 85% of older Southeast Asian refugees who have traditional expectations of living with and receiving support from their children. Case Study 8-2 illustrates an older immigrant parent who found a new role and source of status in her family.

Under current immigration policies, some recent immigrants have a financial responsibility to their older family members. Older adults usually do not have the option to work or to receive public assistance, so their families must provide for them. In Hispanic and other traditional cultures, older family members often provide child care to younger children and actively assist in family decisions. As part of a nursing assessment, the nurse should note whether older adults are primary care providers for grandchildren or other family members and whether an illness episode in the older adult disrupts the family.

Many immigrants who have migrated after the age of 50 years experience depression associated in part with their increased dependence. One study of Mexican American elderly persons found that the rate of depression among those who immigrated to the United States after they were 50 years old was nearly 35%. Immigrants between the ages of 40 and 49 had the lowest rates of depression, 23%, and the rate of depression among Mexican Americans born in the United States was 22.8% (Markides, 1992).

For many Mexican American older adults, some socioeconomic factors suggest that they are at risk for higher morbidity and mortality rates than Whites. Their rates of heart disease and cancer, however, are actually somewhat lower than those of non-Hispanic Whites. This suggests that traditional Mexican American culture may have protective aspects, such as the integration of older adults into the extended family, and providing care for them at home frequently contributes to a slightly better than expected health status (Scribner, 1996; Schiavenato, 1997). These protective aspects of Mexican American culture may diminish over time in families as they become more acculturated. With increases in the length of residence and extent of acculturation in families with older adult members, the families may face the economic necessity of adults working outside of the house. This will decrease their availability for family care of the older adult, and the family may have to rely on community and institutional sources of care.

CASE STUDY	8–2

Mrs. D.R. is a 79-year-old native of the Philippines. She moved to an urban area in California to be near her four children, who live in the same state. She had lived in the same town in the Philippines for her entire adult life and had stayed there to care for her husband and her sister, who both required care for chronic conditions. She is representative of Filipinos who migrate at a later age to join family members in North America. Although she was a much needed and highly esteemed member of her household in the Philippines, she, like many other immigrants, experienced role reversal when she lost the once dominant position within the family and became financially dependent on adult children during relocation. Mrs. D.R. was also like other older Filipino adults who had a more active social network before relocation. She, like many older Filipinos, spoke a dialect and did not speak Tagalog, the language spoken by many younger residents of the Philippines. After her relocation to the United States, her communication and interaction became restricted to her extended family because she did not feel confident using her limited English and did not find other speakers of her dialect. Mrs. D.R. found increasing comfort through prayer and attendance at the Roman Catholic Church to buffer the disequilibrium she felt as a result of her migration.

An older Filipino adult's status changes if he or she assumes child care or other duties within an adult child's home. Doing so maintains the older member's respect within the family, and this reciprocal relationship may lead to the perception of filial obligation between the generations of family members. After Mrs. D.R. assumed the care of her two daughters' children, her self-esteem, personal dignity, and pride in her family increased. The nurse who treated Mrs. D.R. in the emergency department after she fractured her wrist in a fall assessed that Mrs. D.R.'s injury would place a strain on the family because they would temporarily be without their child care provider. The nurse was able to involve her family members in the discharge plan for Mrs. D.R. so her recovery could be assured, she would not lose respect, and she would not feel responsible to assume her usual duties until she felt better.

Clinical Application

The nurse caring for Mrs. D.R. assessed the following areas, which are relevant concerns for any older adult client:

- Dynamics of the family system
- Interaction of the older client within the family
- Environment to which the older client will return
- Adherence of the client and the family to traditional values
- Isolation of the older client associated with speaking native language

All of the above-mentioned factors may vary among older Filipino migrants, and nurses must assess the extent to which individuals retain their traditional practices and the related underlying values.

Older adults who share membership in a cultural group or the experience of immigrating from the same country are not necessarily similar. Their life experiences, occupations, education, and acculturation all affect their needs and expectations for care in their advancing years. Thus, there are tremendous differences among individuals within a cultural group as well as between cultural groups.

Three cultural values are held by many Asian North American cultural groups: respect for the aging, intergenerational duty, and the primacy of family bonds. In these groups, the majority of individuals most likely expect, and find, that care for older adult family members is assumed by younger family members. In traditional Japanese culture, for example, the expectation is that daughters and daughters-in-law will care for older family members as their health declines.

Although some Asian North American families continue to uphold traditional values, signs of conflicting traditional values and popular culture values are increasing. Increased education and career opportunities for women, as well as the economic necessity of their entering the labor force, may influence female family members to work outside the home and not be full-time caregivers. Nurses may need to assess disparities between what the older client expects for care and what the younger family members can realistically provide.

Family Support

It is important to involve the family in the care of the older adult, although the extent of the involvement and the decisions made about care may vary according to the culture of the family. Family members are participants in **informal social support networks** (places where the older adult prefers to live and where his or her health and social needs are best met). The preferences of the older person and his or her family members should be assessed by the nurse, who should also consider the capacities of the older adult for self-care, and the willingness and capabilities of the families to offer support and assistance with care. The type and duration of support that can be provided by family members must be considered in relation to sources of **formal support** that could be used to sustain the family care. Formal support is usually considered to be help, support, and assistance from outside the family, from formal health care agencies such as home health care, assisted living facilities, and nutritional centers. This includes the skilled assessment, care, and evaluation of care that are provided by nurses and other health care professionals in different settings.

What constitutes formal support and the contexts for formal support and health care for the older adult have been evolving steadily over the past two decades. The traditional paradigm of care for older adults being given in skilled nursing facilities has given way to a continuum of services for older adults that includes self-care, supported self-care, assisted care, and skilled care. The roles taken by family members in each of these levels of care vary according to cultural, socioeconomic, and demographic characteristics, which are discussed later in this chapter. Family members are learning more about the care of older family members from books that have been written by and for adults caring for aging parents. Some adults are sandwiched between the responsibilities of caring for their own children and caring for their aging parents. All families have culturally influenced patterns of responsibility to meet the care needs of older family members. Nurses and health care professionals must be aware of the social and economic factors that alter families' retention of traditional values that affect caring for older family members. The economic necessity for two adults to work in many households has contributed to a decline in the availability of adult female children as caregivers to parents and grandparents, which was formerly taken for granted.

The effect of family structure on the type of support offered by family members to older clients is one example of the influence of culture on care. Some families, including Yankee Americans, German North Americans, and families of English extraction, have a linear structure. Adult children are expected to assume care responsibilities for aging parents, and grandchildren are expected to assume caregiving for aging parents and grandparents when needed. Other families, including Irish, Polish, and Black families, have a collateral structure. In a collateral family structure, the perceived bonds are more diffuse and include parents, aunts, uncles, grandparents, and family friends. Families with a collateral structure expect to receive and to provide informal support among all collateral contacts. The expectation for care in many Irish families, for example, is that relatives must assist one another when needed. Two assumptions describe this mutual support within kinship relations: (1) a person must act like a relative in order to be thought of as one, and (2) relatives are obliged to enter into generalized reciprocity (Giarchi, 1996). Research among Black families has indicated that church members may also provide assistance that supports family members' care. Non-kin—that is, individuals who are friends but are not related—may be very significant helpers in the informal network for older Blacks.

The participation of women in the workplace and the decline in the numbers of adult children in many families have also contributed to families' not being available to provide personal care to older adult family members. Adult children and other family members may be available only to provide episodic assistance, emotional support through short visits, or some financial assistance to purchase in-home services. Older adults and their families are not a homogeneous group: cultural diversity and lifestyle choices influence and determine many different options for care of the older adult. Nurses working in acute care, community, and long-term care settings will be asked to support family members who are involved in and contributing to the care of older family members in different ways: through tangible support, emotional support, and financial assistance and as personal caregivers and relief caregivers.

Some older adults experience forms of disabilities in their functional status. Culture can influence the extent to which functional disabilities will be perceived as disabling or merely annoying, and will influence the extent to which individuals seek help for their disabilities.

Demographic and Socioeconomic Variation

Socioeconomic status, in addition to cultural variations, will influence the amount and level of assistance that family members provide to older adult family members. Two types of factors affect how family members provide support to their older members: (1) demographic factors such as family size, migration patterns, rural/urban residence, and (2) socioeconomic factors including income level and educational level. Both sets of factors may determine the availability of family members to offer assistance and may influence the type of support that is offered. Nurses must assess the relative influence of these factors on the older adult's social support network and realize that demographic factors and socioeconomic factors may be blended with culturally influenced patterns of behavior.

Some sectors of the Native North American elderly population have lived in urban areas and assimilated more than their rural peers who live on reservations. Elder Native North Americans tend to socialize less outside their extended families and expect that the needs of clan members and extended family members will come before those of the individual. Native North American values support the care of older family members in the home, but the pool of available caregivers is diminishing because of declining fertility and employment mobility.

Generally, more older adults in rural areas tend to live with their family members than do urban older adults. Older adults in rural areas are also more likely to see their adult children every day than are urban older adults (Angel & Angel, 1997).

The elderly in our society's working class families are more likely to have family assistance with ADLs and household chores. Families in higher socioeconomic levels are more inclined to purchase goods or gifts for older family members (Angel & Angel, 1997; Giarchi, 1996).

An older Mexican or Chinese adult living in a traditional or immigrant family is more likely to live with and receive help from an adult child than is an older person of European descent. This suggests that economic necessity or the presence of larger families may lead to the observed pattern of residence and assistance for some families. Nurses and other health care professionals must be sure to identify the variations within groups and not just between groups. They should not assume that all Hispanic families are family-oriented or that this is a characteristic only of Hispanic families. Other groups also have strong family ties and value older family members, and some Hispanic families do not demonstrate this characteristic to any greater extent than do other families in our society.

Social Support

Older individuals with adequate support systems may maintain their health and remain in a community-based setting such as the home or some type of assisted living facility for a longer time before institutional care becomes necessary. Mexican American institutionalized elderly persons were more physically and functionally impaired than their Caucasian peers (Sutherland & Murphy, 1995). This fact lends support to theories that informal networks that provide help with ADLs, transportation, nutrition, respite care, and social support defer the necessity of nursing home placement. Older Mexican Americans also interacted more frequently with younger family members than their Anglo counterparts, owing in part to closer geographic proximity. Social support assumes special relevance for older clients because many of them sustain social deprivation because of several factors:

- Separation from immediate family members as a result of geographic mobility
- Age-related segregation resulting from increase of nuclear families in neighborhoods
- Loss of spouse by death or illness
- Loss of leisure pursuits or entertainment resulting from illness or loss of income

Having social, emotional, and physical sources of support is especially important for many older adults remaining as independent as possible. Understanding the patterns of support that older adults might need, and assessing the cultural variations in these patterns of support, is good preparation for nurses who may be working in acute care, extended-care, or community settings. The types of social support include the following:

- Affective support: expressions of respect and love
- Affirmational support: receiving endorsement of one's behavior and perceptions
- Tangible support: receiving aid or physical assistance, such as accompanying a person to an appointment

Nurses should identify the importance placed by the older client on these types of social support. In one study, older clients in two community settings indicated that the need for affective support was highest, followed by tangible support (Sutherland & Murphy, 1995). Nurses should also assess the older client's sources of affective, affirmational, and tangible support. One nursing study of older adult participants in a community center group and in a geriatric day treatment center group identified the members of their respective groups as important sources of social support (Sutherland & Murphy, 1995). The community center group also identified family, friends, and clergy as additional sources of support (Sutherland & Murphy, 1995).

Nurses and other health care professionals can gain insight into understanding the older adult's social support network from cross-cultural work in nursing and anthropology. Anthropologists who study the structure and functions of support networks have described the intricacies and multiple relations that individuals have within a support network. Nursing researchers have discovered that the kinds, amounts, and sources of social support vary in health and illness situations, and that they are situation specific (Sutherland & Murphy, 1995). Table 8-2 describes several different types of support networks and shows what older adults in different community settings do and do not have in common. Understanding these differences can help nurses assess the strengths of older clients as well as anticipate the type of support that they might need.

TABLE 8–2	SOCIAL NETWORKS COMMON TO OLDER CLIENTS IN COMMUNITY SETTINGS	
NETWORK	**PARTICIPANTS IN NETWORK**	**CHARACTERISTICS OF NETWORK**
Integrated support network with local support	Family members living nearby, friends, neighbors	Family members do not live in proximity, friends may be available, neighbors more accessible. Family members accessible by phone for affective support, friends may not be in good health to help, younger neighbors who are available help as they can for tangible support.
Community-based support network	Family members do not live in proximity, friends may be available, neighbors more accessible	Family members accessible by phone for affective support, friends may not be in good health to help, younger neighbors who are available help as they can for tangible support.
Family-dependent network	Adult children, other relatives, minimal or no contact with friends, contact with neighbors for emergencies or occasional relief support	Adult children and other relatives provide most sources of support. Network may depend on a primary caregiver with planned relief. Would benefit from some formal source of support: homemaker, aide.
Restricted support network	Spouse or adult children of the older client are primary caregivers; friends do not maintain contact or are not available because of their own illness or distance	Older client may be out of touch with peers. Older client may live in the adult child's home. Usually frailer older adult. Network may fall apart if the one primary caregiver becomes ill or loses touch with peers. Older unable to provide support. Usually needs formal source of support to be maintained.

Intragroup Variation

Nurses and health care professionals should move beyond generalizations and appreciate the cultural differences among older adults in cultural groups. Hispanic older adults, for example, differ in their patterns of daily contacts, church attendance, and socialization with friends (Angel & Angel, 1997). Older Cubans are more likely than Mexicans and older Puerto Ricans to meet often with friends. Older Mexicans are more likely than either Cubans or Puerto Ricans to attend church and to have daily contact with their children (Angel & Angel, 1997). Older Asian North Americans and Pacific Islanders also vary significantly. Older Korean North Americans may have immigrated with their highly educated adult children, but a high proportion of them wish to live independently from the adult children. Korean North American elderly may socialize with their peers through Korean churches, but they are more likely to be lonely and isolated than Chinese, Japanese, and Filipino elderly.

Supporting their ties to their native lands may help enhance the self-esteem of elders from some ethnic groups. Nurses working in the community may look for opportunities to do this. An older adult can be invited to talk to a group of children at an ethnic community center, such as the Ukrainian Community Center, El Centro, or the Polish Association. Older adults can also tell the history of their immigration to adolescents who may be tracing their cultural heritage for an oral history project. Senior adults may also be connected to school-age children to walk them to and from school or to tutor them after school.

Nurses working with elderly clients from various ethnic groups may want to look for resources in the local community to do outreach to these community members and involve them in their care. One example of such a program is the Spanish Speaking Council RAICES, in Brooklyn, New York. It was founded to respond to the unmet needs of Hispanic, Black, and other low-income families through outreach and targeted services focused especially on the needs of older adults (Spanish Speaking Elderly Council RAICES, 1998). Similar organizations exist in Canada, such as Pride of Race, Unity and Dignity Through Education Incorporated (P.R.U.D.E. Inc.) located in Saint John, New Brunswick, which offers programs and services for the visible minority, including special programs for seniors.

• THE OLDER ADULT AS AN INDIVIDUAL

The social and cultural variables discussed in the previous sections affect older clients as individuals, especially in their efforts to meet the developmental tasks of aging. The developmental tasks that older adults achieve include both the satisfaction of basic needs, such as safety, security and dignity, and the fulfillment of integrity and self-actualization. For the majority of older adults, these needs are intertwined with their lifestyle and residence. The options that older adults have for community or institutional care, therefore, are important to consider because they provide safety, security, and an opportunity to possess dignity and autonomy. The older adult usually exerts some control over planning where he or she will live and exercises self-determination and self-esteem. In conjunction with his or her community or institutional residence, the individual may find an outlet for individual or group activity, volunteer efforts, artistic activity, or socialization that increase self-esteem, give meaning to life, and contribute to positive fulfillment of the developmental tasks of aging.

Nurses are especially well prepared to work with older clients when they understand that aging is a positive developmental experience for individuals who are in a stage of reflecting on life experiences and finding meaning in their lives. Older adults may have many transitions, both those that are chosen and those that are inevitable with growing older. These transitions include retirement, grandchildren, changed living arrangements, family mobility, declining health, and the deaths of family members, including spouse, siblings, or children. Older adults may assume new roles, and nurses can do much to help them adjust to change and reframe their challenges as opportunities for positive growth (Cutillo-Schmitter, 1996). Nurses often view the strengths and residual abilities that older clients possess rather than dwelling on their losses and, by doing so, promote optimal functioning when the older adult may be experiencing unavoidable dependency.

Cultural factors such as cultural group history, and life experiences such as immigration, will interact and determine the success of the older client's efforts to achieve security, autonomy, and integrity. Achieving integrity requires the older client to bring closure to his or her life and accept eventual death. A nurse may assess this need in a client's family and be a sensitive listener as the client works through the steps of achieving integrity. Older clients need time for a purposeful life review. The older adult may relinquish tasks such as paying bills to an adult child, so he or she may be free to reflect on life successes and failures.

The hardships that older clients have endured may increase their desire for autonomy and time to reflect on their decisions in later years. This desire may in turn diminish the readiness of the older client to accept health restorative care from the nurse and may push the client toward self-reliance. In some cultural groups (e.g., those in Appalachian culture), some older clients tend to regard health care services with some suspicion. Their economic and social situation has led them to be fatalistic about many losses and disappointments in life; thus, they tend to weigh any options about health care carefully and with some pessimism. They make decisions only after extended consultation with family members.

All older clients require culturally appropriate communication and intervention that is specific to their background. Additionally, the older population requires three types of care: (1) intensive personal health service, depending on the presence of acute and chronic conditions; (2) health maintenance and restorative care, depending on the presence of chronic conditions; and (3) coordinated nursing, social services, and ancillary services that may be provided on an episodic basis for older clients in the community.

Choosing the Care Environment

Depending on the level of disability experienced by an older person, he or she may be faced with a choice between continuing to live at home with assistance and living with family members, in an assisted living residence, or in a skilled nursing facility. Older clients express different attitudes, ranging from resignation to acceptance, when they must change residences. The nurse should assess whether the older client's attitudes about community or facility residence have been influenced by social and peer groups, and can be sensitive to the older client's reactions.

Researchers who have studied the elderly in North America have found that for nearly two decades the most consistent factor in determining the placement of an older person in a skilled nursing facility is the lack of an adequate informal network. Families vary in their capacities to provide care for the older relative who declines in functional abilities. The nurse should assess the following: Does the family modify the environment and assist in home care so that the older adult remains at home? Do children and grandchildren share tasks, provide meals, and run errands so the grandparents can live alone? Do family members have a plan to have relatives share responsibility to provide support and supervision for an older family member? Does the older family member have caregivers and alternates who can provide care as needed if the older adult wishes to remain at home? Some differences have been noted in the patterns of living arrangements according to ethnic background. Even when single older Blacks lose functional abilities, they are less likely than Whites with similar losses to enter skilled nursing facilities.

This finding indicates that some older Blacks may be able to reside in the community with family assistance and social support, both informal and formal, longer than White clients. One study of Puerto Ricans in skilled nursing facilities in New York City found that they had higher levels of disability than did a comparison group of other facility residents (Yu, Kim, Liu, & Wong, 1993). That finding suggested that Puerto Rican family members may have been more inclined to care for family members with declining health status and for a longer time than members of other families. Nurses must also be aware that the values of independence and self-reliance may be very strong for some older clients and that they may refuse any assistance from family members. Some elderly persons may be reluctant to let their family members make decisions for them because they believe the decision about where they live should be up to them. By contrast, some grown children may respect their elderly loved one's independence and be reluctant to make decisions about assisted living or a nursing home placement. The nurse should evaluate the client's and the family members' values and norms that relate to how such decisions are made.

Nursing facility admissions in the U.S. show that the percentage of Whites over the age of 65 years who reside in a nursing facility on a typical day is 6%, whereas the percentage of Hispanics who do is only 3%, and that of Asian Americans is 3% (U.S. Department of Commerce, 1995). White elderly clients aged 85 years old and older constitute 23% of the nursing home residents in the United States. Hispanic and Asian/Pacific Islander older adult clients who are 85 years or older constitute 10% of the nursing home population aged 85 years or older.

In some ethnic and cultural groups, cultural traditions may influence the perceived responsibility of adult children to care for their parents at home. Historically, a higher proportion of older adults from diverse cultures have been cared for in home environments than have White older adults. The availability, acceptability, and affordability of a skilled nursing facility close to the ethnic populations also affects the overall residence patterns by members of cultural and ethnic groups.

Older foreign-born Chinese American residents who were asked about the desired residence for older adults with diminishing capacities for self-care indicated that a nursing home was a good choice for the older person to recover from an illness, but they did not believe a nursing home was appropriate for someone who was incapacitated. They believed that a nursing home environment would only increase the loss of control experienced by an incapacitated person. Therefore, they expected that adult children would care for them. Nearly one third of elderly Korean respondents, however, indicated that a nursing home was the best living arrangement for a chronically ill or disabled person. Although 41% of the elderly Korean respondents still preferred to remain in their own homes, they also expressed reluctance to be a burden to their adult children if they became incapacitated (Yu, Kim, Liu, & Wong, 1993).

Older adults who have spoken their native language for most or all of their lifetimes and who have surrounded themselves with friends who also shared their customs may find it enormously difficult to enter a skilled nursing facility that appears quite foreign in its practices. Much of the action and behavior of professionals in health care facilities is the result of acculturation to the biomedical culture. Nurses and other health care professionals are not always aware, however, that such behavior as an insistence on schedules, order, and cleanliness may not be valued equally by older adults from different cultural groups. Elders from various ethnic groups may feel especially uncomfortable if they do not understand why they are awakened at a certain time, required to be dressed, or asked to participate in group socialization activities. Such an elder may find the skilled nursing facility to be hostile and unfriendly.

Some older adults who have immigrated to North America from other nations may have negative perceptions of skilled nursing facilities based on experiences in their native countries. Nurses can do much to ease the entry of these elders into skilled nursing facilities when they assess each resident's cultural background, food preferences, choices for daily care and personal schedule, and interaction with family members. An individual's life experiences and personality will shape his or her reaction to being in a skilled care facility. A nurse may ask questions on topics that are meaningful to older clients, for example, what is most important for them to maintain in their daily routines, and what they would like to do to remain as independent as possible. Older clients in long-term care facilities for care of debilitating physical conditions have expressed the desire to maintain their quality of life by controlling their personal care and making decisions about their personal affairs whenever possible.

The skilled nursing facility is only one option for extended care of the older adult and, according to experts in the field, is usually used only when an individual has exhausted the opportunities for care in the community. This individual usually enters a facility only after home care and levels of assisted living have been implemented. Long-term care nursing consultants and nurses working in ambulatory care settings are often asked to assess older clients to help determine the best care option for aging individuals with declining functional abilities. Nurses often consider the following criteria when recommending the appropriate level of care or residential placement for an older client:

- mental orientation
- physical mobility restrictions (use of assistive devices and ability to walk unaided)
- degree of assistance needed to complete ADLs
- frequency of incontinence
- level of risk for accident or injury if living independently

Long-term care facilities that offer culture-specific care are optimal options for older clients. For example, several long-term care facilities provide culture-specific care for Native North American elders. They incorporate traditional spiritual care with biomedical care. The distinguishing aspects of the facilities are listed in Box 8-3.

Assessing the Older Adult's Needs

Nurses can assess the social and cultural factors influencing the care older adults will need, the resources to meet those needs, and the locations for residence and care that are most acceptable to the client. Nurses must assess the physiologic status of older adults and how safe a residential setting would be for them. The nurse must also consider medication management for the older client, and the physiologic changes in aging that must be considered for every client. A nurse should also reduce potential misunderstandings resulting from language differences in a care plan for any older client. The nurse should assess an older client's understanding of medication directions, because the client's eyesight may be failing, and directions such as "take with meals" may be open to multiple interpretations. Other factors to assess include cultural values that affect the older adult's expectations for care by family members.

Nurses and health care professionals who are aware of the older adult client's preference for in-home care or residence in a skilled nursing facility should realize that the client's economic resources may affect preferred care options. Purchasing a part-time personal health care service or attendant care that is needed for safe living at home may not be an option for the poor elderly person, so he or she will manage in living situations that are less than desirable or potentially unsafe. Nurses working with individual clients and those who are assigned a caseload of older adults in community settings, such as apartment complexes and assisted living centers, will assess the client's

| BOX 8–3 | **RESERVATION LONG-TERM CARE FACILITIES PROVIDING CULTURE-SPECIFIC CARE TO NATIVE AMERICANS** |

Blackfeet Nursing Home, Blackfeet Indian Reservation, Browning, Montana

First and only nursing home in the state operated by the tribe; 95% of residents are Native American and are eligible for Indian Health Services.

Morning Star Manor, Wind River Reservation, Fort Washaskie, Wyoming

Owned and managed by the Shoshone tribe.

Nokimis-Mishomis Place, Sault Ste. Marie, Michigan

Administered by the Sault tribe. The facility combines biomedical care and traditional Ojibway practices. Planned programs include traditional arts and crafts, elders' gatherings, and Native American spiritual events.

Chinle Nursing Home, Navajo Nation, Chinle, Arizona

First Indian owned and operated health care facility on an Indian reservation; 100% of the residents and 91% of the staff are Navajo. Services are planned to meet the spiritual, social, and cultural needs of residents.

Gila River Indian Care Center, Gila River Indian Community, Laveen, Arizona

Facility serves the Maricopa, Pima, and Navajo tribes; 95% of the staff are American Indian. Activities include traditional arts and crafts, music, and spiritual activities.

Colville Tribal Convalescent Center, Colville Reservation, Nespelem, Washington

Long-term health care services for 52 residents; includes emotional, social, and spiritual services to meet residents' needs.

needs, available sources of support from the family, and formal sources of support that are affordable to the client in a total plan of care for each client. Local programs through the Division of Aging or Aging Services or a comparable agency may leverage available state/provincial or federal funds in innovative programs to reduce rental costs and enable elderly clients to remain in the community.

Local or church-affiliated agencies that recruit and train volunteer visitors and caregivers for the elderly may be used in conjunction with agency programs for the aging to enable a fragile older adult to function at home. These organized sources of support, such as a weekly visitor or a person to do chores for the elderly client, may supplement the care and support provided by family members. Nearly all older adults indicate their preferences for remaining in the community and in their homes over receiving institutional care. The desire to be independent is a cultural value that is highly regarded by many older adults, who proudly proclaim how they have supported and cared for themselves for years. For the majority of older North American adults, the long-held value to be independent is so strong that the person would rather live alone even in poor health than be a burden to his or her family.

Options for Community Residence

Older individuals who are independent or self-sufficient in the above-mentioned areas are most likely candidates for continuing care retirement communities. These are common residential locations that offer the older adult a comfortable apartment, a range of levels of assistance with ADLs, meals, social activities, and supervised exercise programs. Some residential communities have attached facilities for skilled nursing care. Many of these communities have accommodations to move clients to higher and lower levels of care on the basis of their needs, which may change over time. Factors that warrant transfer from one level of care to another include acute exacerbations of chronic illness, new illness episodes, surgical care, and declines in functional abilities associated with falls or accidents.

These continuing care retirement communities offer older adults the security of being able to summon health care assistance if needed and the opportunity to interact with peers. Remaining in a community setting increases their likelihood of taking advantage of community resources, such as cultural events, shopping trips, and entertainment provided by younger adults or school children. Some older adults, however, feel stigmatized by residence in such a facility and prefer to live in an independent location in the community. Other older adults may prefer the stimulation of intergenerational contact available outside an age-related residence and prefer living on their own with other means of informal and formal support.

The challenge faced by most older individuals is the high cost of paying for levels of care in residential communities or in skilled nursing facilities. Many older clients and their families assume that Medicare will pay for such care. Medicare, however, is limited to reimbursement for stays in acute care nursing facilities after hospital discharge; it does not cover custodial or maintenance care of the older client. In Canada, some provinces include some home care cost coverage under their extended care programs. However, such coverage is inconsistent from province to province, as there is no national home care program. In both countries, older individuals and their families may exhaust their personal resources to cover extended care needs and custodial care. Ambulatory care nurses are finding many new opportunities caring for older adult clients in short-term posthospital care and assessing clients who need extended care.

Formal Support for Community-Based Care

In the past decade, communities have increasingly developed day programs that provide nursing assessment, physical or occupational therapy, group

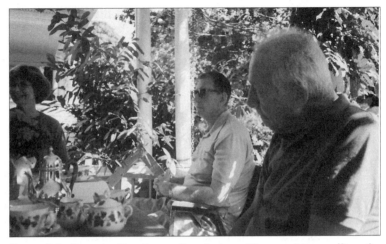

Figure 8–1. Opportunities to recall and share life experiences affirm the older client's identity and self-esteem. (Elderwise, Seattle, Washington.)

socialization, and nutrition for older adults. These programs supplement the affective support and tangible assistance that families give, and they provide settings that affirm the older clients' dignity (Figures 8-1 and 8-2). The range of services, including volunteers and professional staff, provided at each site varies with the support of the local community. Some sites provide group socialization and a nutritional lunch. Older adults may be transported to the sites by public or private means. Older adults attending this type of nutrition program are usually oriented and independently ambulatory. Another effective way of providing services to elders, used by Asian North American elders in urban areas who are caregivers for their grandchildren, is to offer services for both generations at the same site. The grandparent may bring the grandchild for well child examinations and also have access to a health care provider for himself or herself.

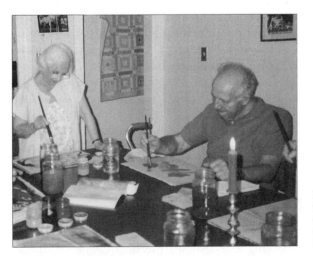

Figure 8–2. Creative expression through painting stimulates discussion among participants in an older adult enrichment program. (Elderwise, Seattle, Washington.)

Other communities may offer more comprehensive programs, such as the On Lok adult day care program pioneered in San Francisco's Chinatown. Here, a unique multidisciplinary team provides comprehensive services to very frail elderly persons who otherwise would be candidates for nursing home placement. The participants are transported from their homes to the centers and may receive occupational and physical therapy as part of coordinated services in a treatment plan that is monitored and evaluated for the participants' progress. Other programs have adapted aspects of the On Lok service delivery model in different locations, because it has been successful in operating under a Medicaid waiver and receives a higher per capita Medicaid payment for serving high-risk clients. The Cherokee Nation of Oklahoma's Program of All-Inclusive Care for the Elderly (PACE) is a culturally specific approach to providing services for the frail elderly in rural Oklahoma communities that have a high Cherokee population.

Options for the older client who wishes to continue to reside in the community and participate in an adult day program are expanding. One example is Elderwise, a senior enrichment program in Seattle, Washington, that offers older adults the opportunities to share experiences and be heard by supportive listeners in a nurturing environment. Activities at Elderwise include art, exercise, lunch, and discussion topics. Discussion of current events, history, and psychologic issues stimulate the older participants to reflect and learn with each other. As older adults review events in their personal histories they are validated as the authorities on their lives, needs, and abilities.

Nurses may want to assess the availability of enrichment programs in local settings and encourage attendance at such programs to older adult clients. Many mutual assistance associations or cultural affiliations, such as the Khmer Community, Asian Counseling Services, Croatian Cultural Center, or Polish Club, provide programs for older adults to interact with young people and share cultural traditions. These cultural center programs, and similar church-affiliated programs, provide opportunities for older clients to receive affirmational support from their peers and to reinforce the cultural identities that restore self-esteem and dignity.

Other intergenerational programs support the involvement of older adults in the community and the educational system. These types of program include the Older American Volunteer Program, the Retired Senior Volunteer Program, and the Foster Grandparents Program. Intergenerational child care centers tap the resources of older volunteers in a community for the benefit of the younger generation of children in child care settings and school. The older participants benefit as well. Evaluations of multigenerational programs found that older volunteers had a high level of life satisfaction, including psychosocial adjustment and self-esteem (Iannuzzelli & England, 2000; Newman, 1983). Rather than concluding that a high level of life satisfaction could be attributed to participation in programs, research showed that volunteers may have already had a high level of life satisfaction. This suggests that older volunteers are a self-selected group of activists who demonstrate the active aging theory. Selected resources for practitioners working with older adult clients are included in Box 8-4.

| BOX 8–4 | SELECTED RESOURCES FOR NURSES WORKING WITH OLDER ADULT CLIENTS |

A Guide to Intergenerational Programs

> The National Association of State Units on Aging
> 600 Maryland Ave., S.W., West Wing, Suite 208
> Washington, DC 20024
> 202-898-2578

> The National Council on Aging, Inc.
> 600 Maryland Ave., S.W.
> Washington, DC 20024
> 202-479-1200
> www.ncoa.org

Additional Web Sites

U.S.

> Senior Net (www.seniornet.org). Book clubs and a forum on successful aging.
> National Senior Citizens Law Center (www.nsclc.org). Legal issues that affect the security and welfare of older persons of limited income.
> SeniorLaw Home Page (www.seniorlaw.com). Elder law, Medicare, Medicaid, rights of the elderly.
> National Association of Professional Geriatric Care Managers (www.caremanager.org).
> National Alliance for Hispanic Health (www.hispanichealth.org).
> Native Elder Health Care Resource Center (www.uchsc.edu/ai/nehrc/weblinks/index.htm).
> National Alliance for Caregiving (http://www.caregiving.org).
> Aging in Rurality (http://www.une.edu/com/othrdept/ahec/ruralaging/default.htm). Includes an interactive quiz and comparative information.

Canada

> Age of Reason (Canada) (www.wiredseniors.com/ageofreason)
> > Serves as a main internet resource center for users seeking information who are over 50 years old.
> Alzheimer's Society of Canada (www.alzheimer.ca/)
> > Provides information and support to caregivers and funds caregiving research to help those living with the disease.
> Canadian Association on Gerontology (www.cagacg.ca/)
> > The mission of this organization is the development of theoretical and practical understanding of individual and population aging through multidisciplinary research, practice, education, and policy analysis in gerontology.
> Information for Seniors—Revenue Canada (www.ccra-adrc.gc.ca/seniors/)
> > Revenue Canada's web page for seniors.
> Seniors Canada Online (www.seniors.gc.ca/index.jsp)
> > Offers key links to seniors-related Government of Canada information.

Some nurses working in community settings have more opportunities to be population-based practitioners. In a local health department, for example, the nurse may need to address and evaluate the cost effectiveness of day care programs, such as the On Lok program, that are options to long-term care placement of the frail older client. Advocates for community-based care, often nurses, argue that life satisfaction may be higher for clients and their family members in these programs. The Sault tribe in Sault Ste. Marie, Michigan, for example, administers a nutrition program with congregate and home-delivered meals to elders that helps maintain them in the community. The importance of volunteers in providing meals, transportation, and social support to complement the provision of professional services is expected to continue. Nurses may function as managers for home-based services that integrate volunteer services with professional assessment, intervention, and evaluation. A comparison of nurse roles in long-term care in international settings is included in Evidence-Based Practice 8–2.

Evaluating Services to Improve Delivery of Care

The nurse manager who evaluates the use of services by older clients can assess them for their cultural appropriateness and acceptability. Clients may be reluctant to use services because of the internal barriers, contextual barriers, and service barriers summarized in Box 8-5.

To overcome the barriers perceived by older clients, nurses can assume several approaches to interact effectively with older adults from diverse groups:

- Be sensitive to the life experiences and previous health care experiences of older clients.
- Listen attentively to the older client's experiences, complaints, and recollections.
- Listen to related conversations to assess for underlying depression.
- Elicit information about the older client's preferences for care, including diet and use of self-care remedies, and include them when appropriate.
- Identify and confirm available informal sources of support.

S U M M A R Y

A cultural approach to the older client recognizes that individuals are the products of, as well as participants in, a wider societal framework. Within this societal framework, the cultural backgrounds of older clients will influence their perceptions, behavior, and practices. Culture serves as a guide to the older client to determine what choices and actions are appropriate and acceptable. Within cultural groups, individual variation is evident in responses to both the physiologic signs and the psychosocial demands of increasing age. Older immigrant clients demonstrate that clients' views and perceptions may differ from those of family members and nurses. The differ-

EVIDENCE-BASED PRACTICE 8-2
Comparative Perspectives of Care for the Elderly

The authors used their observations and experiences as professionals, through commentary and related responses, to describe nurses' roles in the care of elderly clients in their respective countries. The comparative cross-cultural perspective reveals that Japan has the most rapidly aging society in the world, and Australia and Brazil have also projected high rates of growth of elderly populations. Japanese nurses are increasingly recognized as experts in long-term care, including client assessment and the management of chronic conditions. Australian nurses work on multidisciplinary teams providing specialized care for the aged. In Brazil, nurses are now developing roles and educational preparation in long-term care, because traditional family caregiving is diminishing for elderly patients and the need for trained professionals is increasing. Nurses in Turkey are being integrated into a national health plan that has a priority to plan and coordinate community-based care for the elderly. This cross-cultural comparison provides a perspective on the roles and educational preparation that nurses in the United States are acquiring in geriatric nurse practitioner and certification programs.

CLINICAL APPLICATION

- Nurses can be participant observers to self-assess the roles and functions that nurses implement in nursing facilities or in assisted living centers, and they can also identify the roles and the preparation that are needed to more fully meet the aging population's demands for services.
- Using a comparative perspective, nurses can appreciate that clients may have traditional cultural beliefs about long-term care and may have modified their expectations in relation to acquired cultural views on long-term care that come through their immigration or relocation.
- Nurses who become familiar with a comparative approach can practice viewing long-term care as outsiders to appreciate how older clients may view the range of services of in-home treatment, medication monitoring, and health assessments that are provided by nurses.

Tashiro, J. (1999). Long-term care for the elderly in Japan. *Image: Journal of Nursing Scholarship, 31,*(2), 133–134.

Beattie, E. R. A. (1999). Long-term care for the elderly in Australia. *Image: Journal of Nursing Scholarship, 31,*(2), 134–135.

de Barros, A. L. (1999). Long-term care for elders in Brazil. *Image: Journal of Nursing Scholarship, 31,*(2), 135–136.

Uyer, G. (1999). Long-term care for the elderly in Turkey. *Image: Journal of Nursing Scholarship, 31,*(2), 136–137.

ent attitudes, practices, and behaviors among older clients are the result of their heritage, experiences, education, acculturation, and socioeconomic status. Nursing care is not acceptable if it is based on the assumption that members of cultural groups are all the same. Instead, nursing care must be based on the assessment of individual differences in the variables that influence responses to illness and help-seeking behavior. Nurses who provide care in acute care settings or in the community often ask several questions as part of the nursing assessment:

BOX 8–5	**BARRIERS THAT IMPEDE DELIVERY OF SERVICES TO THE OLDER ADULT CLIENT**

Internal Barriers

Perception that there is no need for service
Lack of awareness of existing services
Inadequate knowledge needed to enroll in a service
Perception that one is not entitled to services
Desire to remain self-sufficient
Perception that providers are rude, address older clients in overly familiar terms, and interrupt the elderly

Contextual Barriers

Space: lack of private space for most interactions that occur in clinical settings
Position: embarrassing position of the client in relation to the health care provider
Technology overload: presence of signs, contact with many personnel
Sensory overload: printed instructions, verbal messages, visual cues, videotapes

Service Barriers

Accessibility to care (inconvenient transportation, hours of service)
Affordability of care (not covered by insurance)
Availability of services (practitioners, interpreters do not speak clients' languages)

1. Is the older adult isolated from culturally relevant supportive people, or is the older client enmeshed in a caring network of relatives and friends?
2. Has a culturally appropriate network replaced family members in performing some tasks for the older adult client?
3. Does the older adult expect family members to provide care, including nurturance and emotional support, that the family members are unable to provide?
4. Does language create a barrier in the older client's receipt of services from formal resources?

Older adult clients have often developed their own systems, including informal support, for coping with illness and the changes associated with aging. Nurses who work with older clients in a variety of settings need to assess who provides the affirmation and tangible support that maintains the older client at an optimal level of functioning. Formal resources may be used to sustain the informal support systems to promote the lifestyle preferred by the older client. Nurses need to recognize the expanded roles that the older client may have in his or her family as a caretaker of young grandchildren or other family members. Nurses caring for older adult clients should give attention to the client's family and social roles and develop care plans that maintain and restore the individual to his or her usual roles and patterns of activity. In the future, nurses will assess and work with more older clients as they progress along a continuum of services and through more than one type of residence in the community. By assessing the client's cultural background and available support resources, nurses will plan appropriate care that will help older clients to optimize their self-esteem and dignity based on the client's functional abilities, affective support, and affirmational support.

REVIEW QUESTIONS

1. What constraints and factors should be assessed and considered by the nurse who is developing a care plan for a recently discharged 80-year-old chronically ill man living in a downtown hotel?
2. As the nurse who does health assessments for frail older adults who attend a community comprehensive day program, what types of information are used to assess the cultural appropriateness of elderly Filipino and Chinese American clients' care plans?
3. The short-term subacute care unit where you are the nurse manager serves a multinational group of older clients who are admitted for orthopedic surgery. What cultural assessments do you teach the staff to use in identifying the needs of clients and their families?

CRITICAL THINKING ACTIVITIES

1. Many local communities offer exercise classes or an occupational health/physical activity session for community-based older adults. Many programs are day programs for older adults with some degree of impaired mobility or chronic health care problems. Request permission and plan to attend an activity as an observer and attentive listener. Through observation and, if possible, conversation with a participant, try to assess the levels of self-care possessed by session participants, and identify the types of assistance that these clients require to remain in the community.
2. As a case manager for a managed care organization, you receive many requests for authorization for in-home nursing services for older adults who have been discharged to their homes after hospitalization for acute illnesses or surgery. List the factors that you will consider and the types of data you will need to make an informed decision about the nursing and health-related services and the duration of services that the older client should receive while at home.
3. Maintaining continuity of care for the older client who may move from home to hospital to extended care facility and return to home is a challenge for nurses. As a community nurse assigned to the population of older adults in a low-income housing complex, your clients are often in different stages of

these transitions. You are asked by the housing agency and your health agency employer to develop care plans to maintain their self-sufficiency and safety while addressing the available sources of community support.

4. Some health care sites and skilled nursing facilities have developed intergenerational care centers that provide extended care for the older client and daily child care for a limited number of children. Determine whether your community offers such a program, and request permission to observe the interaction for a portion of a day. What can you infer from this observation about the needs of the older client for love, belongingness, and self-actualization?

5. Critical thinking: With your awareness that cultural traditions and life experiences influence many older adults to prefer independent living, what arguments would you develop as a home health care nurse to support extended government funding of home health services for older adults?

6. Critical thinking: Identify an issue that concerns you about care for older adults (such as cutbacks in chore services or coverage of prescription medications), and draft a letter to a local elected official.

• References

Angel, R. J., & Angel, J. L. (1997). *Who will care for us? Aging and long-term care in multicultural America.* New York: University Press.

Beattie, E. R. A. (1999). Long-term care for the elderly in Japan. *Image: Journal of Nursing Scholarship, 31*(2),134–135.

Beresford, L. (1997, January/February). New approaches to Alzheimer's disease. *Health Plan,* 77–82.

Bonura, D., Fender, M., Roesler, M., & Pacquaio, D. (2001). Culturally congruent end-of-life care for Jewish patients and their families. *Journal of Transcultural Nursing, 12*(3), 211–220.

Collins, C. E., Butler, F. R., Gueldner, S. H., & Palmer, M. H. (1997). Models for community-based long term are for the elderly in a changing health system. *Nursing Outlook, 45*(2), 59–63.

Cutillo-Schmitter, T. A. (1996). Aging: Broadening our view for improved nursing care. *Journal of Gerontological Nursing, 22*(7), 31–42.

de Barros, A. L. B. (1999). Long-term care for elders in Brazil. *Image: Journal of Nursing Scholarship, 31*(2),135–136.

Department of Health and Human Services Office of Disability, Aging and Long-Term Care Policy. (1997). Active aging: A shift in the paradigm. Available at: http://aspe.os.dhhs.gov/daltcp/reports/actaging.htm, June 9, 2001.

Elsner, R. J., Quinn, M. E., Fanning, S. D., Gueldner, S. H., & Poon, L. W. (1999). Ethical and policy considerations for centenarians—The oldest old. *Image: Journal of Nursing Scholarship, 31*(3), 24–28.

Federal Interagency Forum on Aging Related Statistics. *Older Americans 2000: Key indicators of well being.* Federal Interagency Forum on Aging Related Statistics. Washington, DC: U. S. Government Printing Office, August 2000.

Giarchi, G. C. (1996). *Caring for older Europeans: Comparative studies in 29 countries.* Aldershot, Hampshire, UK: Ashgate Publishing Limited.

Graber, D. R., & Kilpatrick, A. O. (2001). Health care organization and incentives under emerging models of elderly care. Available at: http://www.pamij.com/elderly/html, July 15, 2001.

Health Canada (1995, February). *Proceedings from the invitational symposium on continuing care/long-term care.* Available from: http://www.hc-sc.gc.ca/hppb/healthcare/qaehs/pubs/continuing_care/. Accessed: July 8, 2002.

Health Canada (1998). *Canada's seniors at a glance: Seniors are becoming a more diverse group.* Available from: http://www.hc-sc.gc.ca/seniors-aines/pubs/poster/seniors/page5e.htm. Accessed July 8, 2002.

Health Canada (1999). *Statistical report on the health of Canadians.* Available from: http://www.hc-sc.gc.ca/hppb/phdd/report/stat/eng/. Accessed July 8, 2002.

Health Canada (2002). *Canada's aging population.* Ottawa, ON: Author.

Heat and Stroke Foundation of Canada (1999, October). *The changing face of heart disease and stroke in Canada 2000.* Available from: http://www.hc-sc.gc.ca/hpb/lcdc/bcrdd/hdsc2000/pdf/card2ke.pdf. Accessed: July 8, 2002.

Iannuzzelli, J., England, E. M. (2000). The Relationship Between Activities of Daily Living and Life Satisfaction in the Elderly. ERIC Document Reproduction Service No. ED442977.

Kim, M. T., Juon, H. S., Hill, M. N., Post, W., & Kim, K. B. (2001). Cardiovascular disease risk factors in Korean American elderly. *Western Journal of Nursing Research, 23*(3),269–282.

Kunz, E., & Shannon, K. (1996). PACE: Managed care for the frail elderly. *American Journal of Managed Care, 11*(3), 301–304.

Lee, K. (2000). U*rban Poverty in Canada: A Statistical Profile.* Ottawa, ON: Canadian Council on Social Development.

Lewis, S., Messner, R. & McDowell, W. A. (1985). An Unchanging Culture. J*ournal of Gerontological Nursing, 11*(8), 21–26.

Markides, K. S. (1992). *A longitudinal study of Mexican American elderly health.* Washington, DC: National Institute on Aging.

Martin, J. C., & Panicucci, C. L. (1996). Health related practices and priorities: The health behaviors and beliefs of community-living black older women. *Journal of Gerontological Nursing, 22*(4), 41–48.

Moen, P., Dempster-McClain, D., & Williams, R. (1995). Pathways to women's well being in later adulthood: A life course perspective. Unpublished manuscript, Cornell University. In Cutillo-Schmitter, T. A. (1996). Aging: Broadening our view for improved nursing care. *Journal of Gerontological Nursing, 22*(7), 31–42.

Murashima, S., Zerwekh, J. V., Yamada, M., & Tagami, Y. (1998). Around-the-clock nursing care for the elderly in Japan. *Image: Journal of Nursing Scholarship, 30*(1), 37–41.

National Alliance for Caregiving and the American Association of Retired Persons. (1997). *Family caregiving in the United States: Findings from a national survey, June 1997.* Available at: http://www.caregiving.org/content/repsprods.asp

National LTC Resource Center. (1996, February). *Managed care handbook for the aging network.* Minneapolis, MN: University of Minnesota, National LTC Resource Center.

Newman, S. (1983). The Experience of Senior Citizen Volunteers in Intergenerational Programs in Schools and the Relationship to their Life Satisfaction (ERIC Document Reproduction Service No. ED263034).

Rodin, M. B., & Iris, M. (1998). Introduction: Applied anthropologists in aging. *Practicing Anthropology, 20*(2), 2–3

Schiavenato, M. (1997). The Hispanic elderly: Implications for nursing care. *Journal of Gerontological Nursing, 23*(6), 10–15.

Schoenberg, N. E. (1997). A convergence of health beliefs: An "ethnography of adherence" of African-American rural elders with hypertension. *Human Organization, 56*(2), 174–181.

Scribner, R. (1996). Paradox as paradigm—The health outcomes of Mexican Americans [Editorial]. *American Journal of Public Health, 86*(3), 303–305.

Statistics Canada (2000a). *Canadian seniors: A growing population.* Available from: http://www.hc-sc.gc.ca/seniors-aines/pubs/factoids/en/no1.htm. Accessed July 8, 2002

Statistics Canada (2000b). *Older seniors fastest growing group.* Available from: http://www.hc-sc.gc.ca/seniors-aines/pubs/factoids/en/no2.htm. Accessed July 8, 2002.

Spanish Speaking Elderly Council (RAICES). http://www.hispanicfederation.org/agencies/raices.htm. Accessed July 15, 2001.

Subgranon, R., & Lund, D. A. (2000). Maintaining caregiving at home: A culturally sensitive grounded theory of providing care in Thailand. *Journal of Transcultural Nursing, 11*(3), 166–173.

Sutherland, D., & Murphy, E. (1995). Social support among elderly in two community programs. *Journal of Gerontological Nursing, 21*(2), 31–38.

Tashiro, J. (1999). Long-term care for the elderly in Japan. *Image: Journal of Nursing Scholarship, 31*(2), 133–134.

U. S. Department of Commerce Economics and Statistics Administration. (1995). *Bureau of the Census statistical brief sixty-five plus in the United States.* Washington, D.C.: Bureau of the Census.

Uyer, G. (1999). Long-term care for the elderly in Turkey. *Image: Journal of Nursing Scholarship, 31*(2), 136–137.

Weissert, W., Lesnick, T., Musliner, M. Foley, K. (1997). Cost savings from home and community based services: Arizona's capitated Medicaid long term care program. *Journal of Health, Politics, Policy and Law, 22*(6), 1344–1348.

Yu, E. S., Kim, K., Liu, W. T., Wong, S. (1993) Functional abilities of Chinese and Korean elders in congregate housing. In C. M. Barresi & D. E. Stull (Eds.). *Ethnic elderly and long term care* (pp. 87–100). New York: Springer Publishing Company.

Zablocki, E. (2001). Social HMOs: An answer for an aging population. *Healthplan, 42*(4), 40–42.

3

Nursing in Multicultural Health Care Settings

CHAPTER 9

Creating Culturally Competent Organizations

Patti Ludwig-Beymer

KEY TERMS

Corporate culture
Cultural competence
Culturally competent
   organizations

Health disparities
Human resource frame
Organizational culture
Political frame

Structural frame
Symbolic frame
Transcultural nursing
   administration

OBJECTIVES

1. Demonstrate an understanding of how organizations can develop cultural competency.
2. Identify how health disparities can be decreased or eliminated.
3. Examine how organizations resolve conflict.
4. Evaluate organizational cultures.
5. Assess culturally competent initiatives taken by health organizations.

An individual's culture affects access to care and health-seeking behaviors, as well as perceived quality of care. In addition to understanding the culture of patients or clients, however, it is also essential to examine the culture of providers and organizations. The interplay of client, provider, and **organizational cultures** may create barriers, result in cultural conflicts, and even lead to a client's lack of trust or reluctance to access services.

Nurse leaders are recognizing the importance of transculturally based administrative practices (Andrews, 1998). According to the American Nurses Association Council of Cultural Diversity (1991), "[n]urse administrators must foster a climate in which nurses and other health care providers understand that provider-patient encounters include the interaction of three cultural systems." These three systems are the culture of the health care providers, the culture of the client, and the culture of the organizational setting.

Leininger (1996) defines **transcultural nursing administration** as "a creative and knowledgeable process of assessing, planning, and making decisions and policies that will facilitate the provision of educational and clinical services that take into account the cultural caring values, beliefs, symbols, references and lifeways of people of diverse and similar cultures for beneficial or satisfying outcomes" (p. 30). One very important role of nurse administrators is to ensure that organizational policies are culturally sensitive and appropriate and that they recognize the rights of individuals and families. Such policies should incorporate Leininger's (1991) decisions and actions of culture care preservation/maintenance, culture care accommodation/negotiation, and culture care repatterning/restructuring. Malone (1997) describes several strategies for improving organizational cultural competence. First, health care organizations must implement training that helps **corporate culture** to value and manage cultural diversity. Second, nursing administration must reward practice that values differences and is culturally appropriate and collaborative. Third, nursing should seek members who are culturally competent. Finally, nursing should recruit and hire members who are culturally diverse, to better reflect the demographics of the country.

This chapter serves to augment the current dialogue on creating **culturally competent organizations**. It begins by describing the need for culturally competent organizations, describing organizational culture, and providing a mechanism for assessing an organization's culture. Both the physical environment of care and the community context are considered. Finally, strategies for developing culturally competent initiatives and the role of health care providers in creating culturally competent organizations are described.

• THE NEED FOR CULTURALLY COMPETENT ORGANIZATIONS

Disparities in health have long been acknowledged. The National Institutes of Health (2000) define disparities in health as "differences in the incidence, prevalence, mortality, and burden of diseases and other adverse health conditions that exist among specific population groups in the United States." **Health disparities** have been documented in conditions such as cancer, diabetes mellitus, heart disease, infant mortality, overall mortality, and numbers of low-birth-weight babies, as well as others. Although death rates in the United States and Canada from cancer have generally declined, they remain higher for Blacks, have not decreased equally across racial and ethnic groups, and have increased in certain instances. For example, death rates for colorectal cancer, lung and bronchial cancer, and breast cancer have actually increased for American Indians and Alaskan Natives (Centers for Disease Control and Prevention, 2002).

Several studies suggest that members of minority racial and ethnic populations in the United States receive fewer invasive interventions related to cardiac disease, lung cancer, and renal transplants (Ayanian, Cleary, Weissman, & Epstein, 1999; Ayanian & Epstein, 2001; Einbinder & Schulman, 2000; King & Brunetta, 1999; Sheifer, Escarce, & Schulman, 2000). In addition, preventive services, such as infant immunizations, adult immunizations, and mammography, show disparities based on race and culture. Also, access to health care demonstrates variability in areas such as health insurance, prenatal care, doctor visits, and emergency department visits. Even in Canada, with it's National Health

Insurance Model, many individuals experience similar disparities in access to preventative services. Such disparities are often rooted in culture, race, geographic location, and socioeconomic status.

Disparities in access to and quality of primary care may be partially responsible for differences in health status among members of minority groups, although many other complex factors are undoubtedly involved.

Disparities in health cannot be explained wholly by disparities in income and health insurance coverage. For example, one study found that one half to three quarters of all disparities observed in 1996 would have remained even if racial and ethnic differences in income and health insurance had been eliminated (Weinick, Zuvekas, & Cohen, 2000). This implies that other factors may account for health disparities. Although these factors have not yet been identified, potential barriers that contribute to the disparities may be related to demographics, culture, and the health care system itself (potential barriers are summarized in Box 9-1). Culturally competent organizations are needed to address disparities in health within racial and ethnic groups.

According to the Office of Minority Health, **cultural competence** refers to the ability of health care providers and organizations to understand and respond effectively to the cultural and linguistic needs of patients (Office of Minority Health, 2000). Cultural competence encompasses a wide range of activities and considerations. It includes providing respectful care that is consistent with cultural health beliefs of the clients and family members. Competent interpreter services and programs to promote staff diversity are other ways in which health care organizations can increase cultural competence (Clancy & Stryer, 2001).

The identity of a group or organization is based on phenotype, culture, or any other characteristic that a group shares that sets it apart from others. The professional values espoused by nurses, for example, set us apart from other health care providers. Numerous boundaries exist in the health care professions; they may be based on gender, ethnic differences, class and hierarchy, licensure and certification, history, and tradition (Dreachslin, 1999).

Prejudice, racism, stereotyping, and ethnocentrism are present in all health care settings. The dominant subgroup is often ignorant of its own privilege. For example, services may be organized for the convenience of providers, and providers may be completely oblivious to the fact that inconvenient hours or locations are affecting the community members who seek services.

How, then, does an organization move toward cultural competency? A culturally competent organization is extremely complex. Within the health care setting, practitioners must be aware of the effects of culture on individual behaviors. A culturally competent organization, however, goes beyond this awareness and calls for an understanding of the interplay among organizational culture, professional culture, and community culture.

• ORGANIZATIONAL CULTURE

As nurses, we are familiar with the concept of culture, yet perhaps less familiar with organizational culture. Leininger defines organizational culture as the

BOX 9–1	POTENTIAL DEMOGRAPHIC, CULTURAL, AND HEALTH SYSTEM BARRIERS

Demographic Barriers

Age
Gender
Ethnicity
Primary language
Religion
Educational level and literacy level
Occupation, income, and health insurance
Area of residence
Transportation
Time and/or generation in the United States

Cultural Barriers

Age
Gender, class, and family dynamics
Worldview/perceptions of life
Time orientation
Primary language spoken
Religious beliefs and practices
Social customs, values, and norms
Traditional health beliefs and practices
Dietary preferences and practices
Communication patterns and customs

Health System Barriers

Access to care
Insurance and other financial resources
Orientation to preventive health services
Perception of need for health care services
Ignorance and/or distrust of Western medical practices and procedures
Cultural insensitivity and incompetence in providers
Lack of diversity in providers
Western versus folk health beliefs and practices
Poor doctor–patient communication
Lack of bilingual and bicultural staff
Unfriendly and cold environment

goals, norms, values, and practices of an organization in which people have goals and try to achieve them in beneficial ways (Leininger, 1996). Organizational culture encompasses an organization's preferred ways of accomplishing goals, determining priorities, and making decisions. These shared norms and expectations guide the thinking and behavior of the group members, and the shared values provide a sense of common direction and behavior. Organizations are subcultural systems with inherent values and beliefs, folklore, and language; these systems are organized in a hierarchy of authority, responsibilities, obligations, and functional tasks that are understood by members of the organization. Organizational culture affects not only people working in the institution, such as employees and volunteers, but also customers, such as physicians and patients. The social organization of hospitals and other health care facilities has a profound effect on patients, both directly through the care provided and indirectly through organizational policies and philosophy (Jones, Bond, & Cason, 1998).

Theories of Organizational Culture

Bolman and Deal (1997) describe four frames or perspectives in organizational culture that affect the way in which an organization resolves conflicts. The **human resource frame** strives to facilitate the fit between person and organization. When conflict arises, the solution considers the needs of the individual or group as well as the needs of the organization. The **political frame** emphasizes power and politics. Problems are viewed as "turf" issues and are resolved by developing networks to increase the power base. The **structural frame** focuses on following an organization's rules or protocols. This culture relies on its policies and procedures to resolve conflict. The **symbolic frame** relies on rituals, ceremony, and myths in determining appropriate behaviors.

To understand how these four perspectives will result in different outcomes, consider typical responses to the following situation. Hospital A is located on the border of two communities. One community is primarily Black. The other community is primarily Hispanic. The hospital has traditionally provided care to the Blacks and is well regarded by that community. The hospital has noted, however, that few members of the Hispanic community use its services. The hospital's board of directors realizes that, to survive, the hospital must expand its patient base. The approach to this challenge will vary based on the organization's culture.

Hospital leaders in a human resource perspective culture are likely to approach the situation by assessing the needs of both communities and the staff. For example, this type of hospital may convene focus groups with members of the Hispanic community to identify why the hospital's services are not used by that community. At the same time, the hospital will assess the Black community's perspective on the hospital's expanding its services and becoming a more inclusive organization. The hospital will also provide opportunities for staff members to provide input and to express their feelings about the goals of the organization. In the end, the hospital with a human resource perspective culture will reach a decision that balances the needs of all of these groups while enhancing the goal of expanding the patient base.

Hospital leaders in a political perspective culture will take a different approach. They will identify key "power" leaders in the Hispanic community. Perhaps they will invite a Hispanic leader to join their board of directors or serve in another advisory capacity, or ask a priest from a Hispanic congregation to serve as a hospital chaplain. In addition, they will actively recruit Hispanic physicians and other clinician leaders. They will build a Hispanic power base within the hospital and use it to reach out to the larger Hispanic community and expand the patient base.

Hospital leaders in a structural perspective culture will develop policies and procedures to attract more Hispanic patients. For example, they may make certain that all signage appears in both English and Spanish, or develop a policy that requires all patient educational materials to be available in both Spanish and English. They may require all staff to attend a session on Hispanic culture, and may strongly encourage or mandate Spanish-language training for key personnel.

Finally, hospital leaders in a symbolic perspective culture will use ceremony to meet their goal. They will make physical changes to the environment to attract more Hispanics. For example, they may create or alter a chapel, inviting a priest from a Hispanic congregation to say mass. They may display other religious symbols, such as a crucifix or a statue of Our Lady of Guadalupe, or alter their artwork to be more culturally inclusive. They may also include Hispanic stories and rituals in their internal communications. These leaders will draw on symbols and rituals that will make persons of Hispanic culture more comfortable in the hospital environment and that will attract a larger Hispanic patient base.

None of these organizational cultures are inherently good or bad, just different. Each presents both strengths and weaknesses, and more than one culture may exist in an organization. For example, an organization may be guided primarily by both human resource and symbolic perspectives.

Schein (1985) uses a tree analogy to describe organizational culture as having leaves, a trunk, and roots. Leaves represent the artifacts of the institution: what is seen and heard in the institution. Signage, statues and other decorations, pictures, décor, dress code, traffic flow, medical equipment, and visible interactions are all part of the visual "leaves." Audible "leaves" include languages spoken, stories, myths, and other conversations. The trunk represents an organization's values: what is good, what is right, and what is true. The roots represent an organization's assumptions. Assumptions define the culture of the organization, but because they are invisible, they may not be recognized. At times, the assumptions of an institution are ambiguous and self-contradictory, especially when an institutional merger or acquisition has occurred.

The basic premises of an organization, reflected in its mission statement, provide insight into the presence or absence of a commitment to providing culturally competent care. Organizations are well aware of the need to identify a consistent mission and set of values to guide their organizational culture. This need is especially present in merged organizations. For example, a large not-for-profit integrated health care delivery system was created as a result of the merger of two religiously affiliated organizations. The two organizations developed and agreed to a new mission statement as well as new values and philosophy (see Box 9-2) before the merger. Immediately after the merger, interdisciplinary teams from across the system came together to develop strategies for inculcating the mission, values, and philosophy into the practice settings.

BOX 9–2	MISSION, VALUE, AND PHILOSOPHY

Mission

The mission of Advocate Health Care is to serve the health needs of individuals, families, and communities through a wholistic philosophy rooted in our understanding of human beings as created in the image of God.

Values

The five values of Advocate Health Care serve as an internal compass to guide our relationships and actions: Compassion, Equality, Excellence, Partnership, and Stewardship

Philosophy

The philosophy of Advocate Health Care is grounded in the principles of human ecology, faith, and community-based health care. These principles arise from an understanding of human beings as whole persons in light of their relationship to God, themselves, their families, and the society in which they live. Through our actions we affirm these principles.

Courtesy of Advocate Health Care, Oak Brook, IL.

Organizational Culture and Employees

Organizations are aware of the impact of organizational culture on its employees. When filling positions, recruiters consider the "fit" between the organization and the potential employee, because a good "fit" results in better retention and satisfied employees. Nurses and other health care professionals are also taught how to determine whether an organization will match their personal values. For example, a nurse who wants to provide care in a culturally competent manner to lesbians and homosexuals will not be happy in a setting that openly engages in "gay bashing."

Culturally caring organizations are needed for nurses and other staff members, and humans need care to survive, thrive, and grow. Historically, however, organizations have made few attempts to nurture and nourish the human spirit. According to Leininger (1996), organizations need to incorporate universal care constructs, including respect and genuine concern for clients and staff.

An inclusive workplace is characteristic of a caring organization. Such a workplace, however, is not satisfied simply by a diverse workforce. An inclusive workplace reaches out beyond the organization by encouraging members of the workforce to become active in the community and participate in state and federal programs, working with the poor and with diverse cultural groups (Mor Barak, 2000).

An inclusive workplace goes beyond the golden rule of treating others as you wish to be treated yourself. Instead, such a workplace is receiver oriented and involves treating others as *they* wish to be treated, in what is sometimes called the platinum rule (Carnevale & Stone, 1995). Organizations with inclusive workplaces draw staff members who are committed to cultural competence and who value diversity and mutual respect for differences.

Although the impact of organizational culture on employees has been acknowledged, the impact of organizational culture on the community being served has received less attention. For years, hospitals and other health care organizations have espoused the view that "If we build it, they will come" (i.e., all that is needed is to offer the services). Now, health care services should be structured in ways to appeal to and meet the needs of various members of the community. Health care leaders recognize that cultural competence in organizations is essential if the organizations are to survive, grow, satisfy customers, and achieve their goals. Image is critically important for an organization's survival. A variety of factors are needed to move an organization toward cultural competence.

Assessing the Organizational Culture

Organizational culture can be assessed in numerous ways. Roizner (1996) identifies a checklist for culturally responsive health care services. Health care services are considered for their availability, accessibility, affordability, acceptability, and appropriateness. When the organizational culture is assessed by this model, it is important to consider these "five A's":

- Are the health services that are needed by the community readily available? In a community with rampant illicit drug use, for example, one should expect to find a variety of types of drug abuse prevention and treatment programs offered that are readily available to the local population.
- Are health care resources accessible? A pediatrician's office, for example, might need to expand its hours of operation to accommodate the schedules of working parents. Geographic location should be considered in terms of proximity to public transportation, traffic patterns, and available parking. Structural changes may also be needed to accommodate specific types of clients, such as those who use wheelchairs.
- Are the services affordable? Partnerships between public and private organizations may be needed to ensure that services are affordable. A sliding scale might be developed to accommodate the needs of people with diverse financial resources.
- Are the services acceptable? Providers need to carefully consider this question. Do community members who use the services perceive the services to be of high quality? Do community members value the services? Are the waiting rooms stark, dimly lit, or untidy? Is the furniture worn or the reading material frayed and outdated? Providers need to understand what makes services acceptable to the community they seek to serve. Community members may avoid a particular agency or institution because services are delivered in a noncaring and patronizing fashion.
- Are the services appropriate? Community members may not use services if they do not perceive that these services meet their needs. For example, community members who struggle with day-to-day survival with limited financial

and social resources may not use fitness classes. Programs that are disconnected from the daily life of community members constitute a recipe for failure.

Andrews (1998) provides an assessment tool for cultural change that examines demographic/descriptive data; strengths; community resources; continued growth; perspectives of patients, families, and visitors; institutional perspective; and readiness for change. This tool allows organizational leaders to assess the needs of the community they serve and to use their findings to guide strategic planning for the future.

Leininger's (1991) Theory of Culture Care Diversity and Universality is also helpful in assessing the culture of an institution. The culture care model may be used to conduct a cultural assessment of the organization, with dominant segments of the sunrise model identified. An example of such an assessment is provided in Table 9-1. Other cultural care assessment tools are available to assess the culture of an institution. This assessment is then compared with the values and beliefs of the groups who use the health care organization.

• THE PHYSICAL ENVIRONMENT OF CARE

Organizational leaders must assess the physical environment of care to determine barriers and potentially negative messages. A flow chart is a helpful tool for determining such barriers. For example, in an effort to provide comprehensive women's health programs in a caring fashion, organizational leaders may examine the steps for admission to a particular hospital for the delivery of a baby. To determine this, staff members may walk through this care process at their site, and then create a flow chart that outlines the steps. Staff members may be alert, in particular, for possible sources of confusion for parents at this highly stressful time. The flow chart can then be used to design changes in the environment that can be implemented to decrease barriers and improve services.

The physical environment should also be assessed. Approaching this assessment as a potential client is helpful, and a variety of factors should be considered. What message does organization send through its physical surroundings? How is the facility organized physically? How does the entryway present the culture of the organization to the public? Is the entrance warm and inviting? Is the signage prominent? What languages are presented on signs? Is the patient at a loss for where to go to give or receive information? Are amenities available to patients and their family members? Are the doors open or closed? Do people talk with one another, and what language(s) are spoken? What is the traffic pattern, and what is the general flow of traffic? Does the environment appear calm or turbulent? Are the staff members attentive and courteous?

A physical environment may send unintentional messages. Several years ago, I visited a birthing unit in a city hospital. The hospital's service area was undergoing tremendous changes, with a large influx from the Black, Hispanic, Indian, and Polish American communities. The birthing unit was beautifully and tastefully decorated with oak furniture and pastel prints. Every picture on

(Text continues on page 262)

TABLE 9–1	EXAMPLE OF LEININGER'S (1991) CULTURE CARE MODEL USED TO CONDUCT AN ORGANIZATIONAL ASSESSMENT IN A HYPOTHETICAL HOSPITAL	
FACTOR	**TYPES OF QUESTIONS**	**ASSESSMENT FINDINGS**
Environmental context	What is the general environment of the community that surrounds the organization? Socioeconomic status? Race/ethnicity? Emphasis on health? Living arrangements? Access to social services? Employment? Proximity to other health facilities?	Hospital A is in a low-income urban setting. The majority of residents in the area are Black, with a few Asians and Whites. A public housing complex is located within a few blocks of the hospital. The economy is depressed, and many are out of jobs. Drug abuse and alcoholism are rampant. Families are challenged to survive, and they tend to view disease prevention as unimportant. There is a short-term perspective on health, which is defined as being able to do normal activities. Several social agencies nearby provide assistance with food pantries. There are no other hospitals within a 5-mile radius.
Language and ethnohistory	What languages are spoken within the institution? By employees? By patients? How formal or informal are the lines of communication? How hierarchical? What communication strategies are used within the institution? Written? Poster? Electronic? Oral? "Grapevine"? How did the institution come to be? What was the original mission? How has it changed over the years?	Patients primarily speak English. Employees typically speak English, although Polish and Russian are heard, particularly among the housekeepers. The grapevine is alive and well at Hospital A. Although memos are circulated, verbal communication is prized throughout the institution. The president/chief executive officer, chief nurse executive, and chief medical officer all maintain an open-door policy in their offices. Posters are also used to communicate, especially in the elevators. Electronic communication via e-mail has not been successful because computer work stations are in short supply throughout the institution. Hospital A was founded by a Roman Catholic religious order of nuns in 1885. The original mission was to provide care to *(continues)*

258

| TABLE 9-1 | *(Continued)* | |

FACTOR	TYPES OF QUESTIONS	ASSESSMENT FINDINGS
		immigrants and the poor. Immigrants from many nations, including Ireland, Poland, Hungary, and Russia, originally inhabited the area. The mission is still to provide the highest quality of care to the poor and underserved, although that is becoming increasingly difficult financially.
Technology	How is technology used in the institution? Who uses it? Is patient documentation electronic? Is electronic order entry in place? Is cutting-edge technology in place in the emergency department, critical care units, labor and delivery, radiology, surgical suites, and similar units? Is electronic mail used? Is web-based technology embraced?	There are a few computer work stations on each nursing unit, which are primarily used by the clinical secretaries. Nurses do not document electronically, and physicians do not use electronic order entry. Hospital A received external funding several years ago to renovate their old emergency department (ED). The new ED has state-of-the art equipment, as do the critical care units. The labor and delivery area is cramped and overcrowded. Equipment is well worn. Similarly, the surgical suites are dated. The radiology department is scheduled for a major capital investment next year.
Religious/ philosophical	Does the institution have a religious affiliation? Are religious symbols displayed within the facility? By patients? By staff? Is the institution private or public? For-profit or not-for-profit?	Founded by a religious order, Hospital A is very clearly viewed as Roman Catholic. Outside, the hospital is marked with a large cross on its roof. Inside, a crucifix hangs in each patient room. A large chapel is used for daily mass. A chaplain distributes communion to patients and staff every evening. Nurses demonstrate a variety of religious symbols. One nurse is seen wearing a cross; another wears a Star of David. Patients adhere to a variety of faith traditions, including Southern Baptist and Black Muslim. Chaplains come from a *(continues)*

TABLE 9–1 *(Continued)*

FACTOR	TYPES OF QUESTIONS	ASSESSMENT FINDINGS
		variety of faith traditions and attempt to meet the needs of diverse groups.
Kinship and social factors	What are the working relationships within nursing? Between nursing and ancillary services? Between nursing and medicine? How closely are staff members aligned? Is the environment emotionally "warm" and close or "cold" and distant? How do employees relate to one another? Do they celebrate together? Turn to one another for support? Do employees get together outside of work?	RNs at Hospital A tend to be White and are often the children of immigrants. They are most often educated in associate degree or diploma programs. LPNs and aides tend to be Black. There is tension between the two groups especially as the role of the aide has expanded. Nurses tend to be somewhat in awe of physicians. Physicians' attitudes toward nurses range from respect to disrespect. Many physicians are angry about the erosion of their own careers. Units tend to be tight knit, with celebrations of monthly birthdays and recognition provided when staff members "go the extra mile." Nurses rarely socialize with one another outside of work. Staff nurses are middle-aged (mean age 42). Most of them commute from the suburbs to the hospital and are anxious to return home after their shift. On the other hand, many of the aides are from the immediate community, know each other, and socialize outside of work.
Cultural values	Are values explicitly stated? What is valued within the institution? What is viewed as good? What is viewed as right? What is seen as truth?	The institution clearly identifies its mission and strives to fulfill it in economically difficult times. Its stated values are collaboration and diversity. Although diversity training has been provided to managers, tensions still exist between work groups, particularly because the work force tends to be racially divided.
Political/legal	How politically charged is the institution? Where does the power rest within the institution? With medicine? With finance? With nursing?	Historically, Hospital A has been politically naïve. It has gone about its mission without regard to the external environment. Recently, the hospital has begun

(continues)

TABLE 9–1	(Continued)	

FACTOR	TYPES OF QUESTIONS	ASSESSMENT FINDINGS
	Is power shared? What types of legal actions have been taken against the institution? On behalf of the institution?	to lobby for better reimbursement for care provided under Medicaid. Institutional power rests with the strong medical staff and department chairs. Because the hospital is not academic, nurses are less likely to have advanced degrees.
Economic	What is the financial viability of the institution? Who makes the financial decisions? How do the salaries and benefits compare with those of competitors in the immediate environment?	Hospital A has a very low margin: 0.5%, compared with an industry standard of more than 2%. This means that little money is available for capital improvements, which results in less technology and some units being cramped. Community needs are considered, along with all financial decisions. People are valued, and salaries are kept competitive.
Educational	How is education valued within the institution? What type of assistance (financial, scheduling, flexibility) is provided for staff seeking advanced degrees? Does the institution provide education for medicine, nursing, and other professions? Are advanced-practice nurses utilized? What is the educational background of staff nurses? Nurse managers? Nursing leaders? How does this compare with education of other professional groups? With competing organizations?	Nurses tend to be educated at the associate and diploma levels. Although flexible scheduling and limited tuition reimbursement are provided, many nurses do not take advantage of the benefits because of the need to work extra shifts to ensure staffing and competing personal and family priorities. All nurse managers are required to have a BSN, and directors are required to have a master's degree. Nursing students from five different programs rotate through the institution. In addition, Hospital A has developed a relationship with one school of nursing and provides a summer preceptor program to those students. Faculty members are also employed during summers and holidays. Medical education is also provided at Hospital A: 150 residents and many third-year and fourth-year medical students rotate through the facility. The residents, while learning, also provide important service to the community, particularly through their clinic rotations.

the walls, however, showed a Caucasian family. This clearly sent a message of exclusivity rather inclusivity. When I brought this to the attention of the nurse manager, she was completely dumbfounded and quickly took steps to rectify the situation. Ethnocentrism and stereotyping were in play here, but it took an outsider to recognize this and bring it to recognition and resolution.

• A COMMUNITY CONTEXT

Health care institutions exist to provide care. A variety of factors, summarized in Box 9-3, contribute to mortality in the United States and Canada. Confronting these factors will require individual behavioral change, community change, social change, and economic change. Health care organizations cannot confront these complex factors in isolation but must partner with their communities to build trust in their institutions and meet the needs of their local communities.

Community partnerships may be configured in a variety of ways. Hospitals and health care systems usually articulate their desire to improve the health of the communities they serve. Historically, hospitals have fulfilled this mission through charity care, professional education and research in health care, community education programming, and community outreach (Pelfrey & Theisen, 1993). Recognition that true improvements in the health of a community require the focused efforts of the entire community is growing. Such improvement may occur only in partnerships with community members and other community organizations.

An ethnographic study of community (Davis, 1997) revealed five themes related to the experience of community caring. Of particular significance to this chapter are three themes: (1) reciprocal relationships and teams working together are central to building healthy communities; (2) education with a focus on prevention is key to enhancing health; and (3) understanding community needs is a primary catalyst for health care reform and change. The healthy communities program, with partnerships between communities and hospitals, is one example of this trend in health care. In a healthy

BOX 9–3	MAJOR CONTRIBUTORS TO MORTALITY IN THE UNITED STATES AND CANADA
	Tobacco use
	Poor diet and physical inactivity
	Microbial agents
	Toxins
	Firearms
	Sexual behaviors
	Motor vehicle accidents
	Illicit drug use
	Poverty
	Lack of access to medical care

communities program, health care professionals collaborate with surrounding communities to conduct community health assessments. In community mapping, staff collect a variety of data, including demographics,
health status, community resources, barriers, and enablers. Both strengths
and needs are identified from the perspective of the community. All these
data are then used collaboratively with communities to set priorities (an
example of such a community assessment is provided in Box 9-4). Data from

BOX 9–4	COMMUNITY ASSESSMENT EXAMPLE

By using the assessment of the communities served by Advocate Lutheran
General Hospital, one of Advocate Health Care's hospitals, and by analyzing data
from clinical practice, staff members realized that Hispanics made up an increasing proportion of the population and were the most frequently underserved population. As a result, a family practice physician initiated the idea for a community
center for health and empowerment. A coalition composed of individuals from
social services, health care agencies, schools, police, churches, businesses, city
government, and other community services also identified the Hispanic community as underserved. This group provided an etic, or outsider, view of the
Hispanic community.

To provide a local, or emic (insider), view, community members worked with
health care personnel to design and conduct a door-to-door community assessment. As described elsewhere (Ludwig-Beymer, Blankemeier, Casas-Byots, &
Suarez-Balcazar, 1996), Leininger's Theory of Cultural Diversity and Universality
served to guide the assessment. The assessment process involved 2 focus groups,
15 community interviewers, and 220 door-to-door interviews. In addition, 5 meetings, attended by 180 community members, were held to report the findings to
community members and solicit their input into the causes and retention of
strengths or resolution of needs. As a result, numerous task forces were formed
to preserve strengths or mediate needs.

Major strengths were identified as access to friends and families to socialize
and get support, prenatal and postnatal care, and pediatric care. Major needs
were identified as affordable housing, programs to help immigrants, Spanish-
speaking dentists, and activities for youth.

The community was involved in key decision making from the beginning,
including selecting the site for the center, choosing the name for the center, and
establishing a sliding scale for fees. The bilingual center provides primary health
care services, a Women-Infant-Children (WIC) program run by the county health
department, and a community empowerment program. A salaried community outreach worker coordinates the community empowerment program. In collaboration with businesses, churches, and city services, community members have
undergone training in group work and priority setting. Recently, monthly dental
services through a dental van were added at the center.

Activities for youth were identified as concerns in the community assessment. As a result, community members and center personnel have actively part-
nered with the park district, schools, churches, and the police to provide recreational activities for youth. The community also uses this as an opportunity to
celebrate their cultural heritage. Health promotion materials and activities are
also provided through collaboration.

these assessments are used to set priorities and guide the planning and implementation of key initiatives. These initiatives are most well accepted when they are sponsored by a variety of community organizations rather than by a single health care organization such as a hospital.

Conducting community assessments requires cultural awareness and sensitivity. Interpreting the data requires knowledge of the cultural dimensions of health and illness. Using the data to develop and implement programs in conjunction with the community requires the ability to plan and implement culturally competent care. The skill of a transcultural nurse or other culturally competent health care professional is invaluable in these situations.

• DEVELOPING CULTURALLY COMPETENT INITIATIVES

Once the basics, as previously outlined, are in place, it is possible to develop culturally competent initiatives. Many important factors must be considered in planning programs across cultural groups. Before a program is planned, a cultural assessment of the target population should be a routine component of the needs assessment process (Huff & Kline, 1999). In many cases, cultural competence must be demonstrated with multiple cultures simultaneously. For example, one hospital in the Chicago area provides care for individuals who speak 64 different languages. This calls for much effort and creativity on the part of patients, health care providers, and interpreters. Culturally competent initiatives must reach out to multiple cultural groups. In the case study below, the development and implementation of a culturally competent initiative are described.

CASE STUDY	9–1

Caring Health System is a not-for-profit integrated health system in a large midwestern city. Its 10 hospitals serve diverse clients in disparate geographic locations across a 50-mile area. Clients differ in multiple ways, including socioeconomic status, education, race, ethnicity, religion, language, and culture.

A constant, healthy tension exists within the system between doing things consistently across sites and meeting the highly individualized needs of the diverse populations served. Organizational leaders embrace Leininger's Theory of Culture Care. In particular, nursing leaders believe that nursing care must be congruent with the client's culture if nursing intends to promote the client's health and satisfaction.

Through a healthy community program at each hospital, the hospitals keep the system grounded in the reality of the clients. The healthy communities program, developed and staffed by nurses with community health backgrounds, is responsible for broadly defining community-based health promotion initiatives that address individual, social, and community factors. Their goal is to establish partnerships with community members and governmental and community organizations to ensure that everyone has access to the basics needed for health; that the physical environment supports healthy living; and that communities control, define, and direct action for health.

The nurses in the healthy community program bring together resources from settings both within and outside their system. For example, they work closely with other community-focused staff members, such as home care and parish nurses within the system. They also work with multiple external organizations, such as local health departments, government, religious institutions, community businesses, schools, and other health care entities. These nurses work specifically with the communities surrounding their facility. In this way, they acknowledge the specific needs of diverse groups. In addition, they meet to address areas of common concern across their sites. In this way, they uncover and articulate the needs that are universal across the system.

The healthy communities nurses use Leininger's Culture Care Diversity and Universality model in their practice. They use data gathered from cultural assessments to assist them in understanding the communities they serve. They consider environmental context, ethnohistory, language, kinship, culture values and lifeways, the political and legal system, and technologic, economic, religious, philosophic, and educational factors. They understand the interactions among the folk system, nursing care, and the professional systems. They also understand the importance of using the three culture care modalities: preservation/maintenance, accommodation/negotiation, and repatterning/restructuring.

Because of their community health backgrounds, the nurses are knowledgeable about disparities in health. The nurses also use data from a variety of sources, including hospital-specific data, census tract data, and health department data, to help them understand health and access disparities in their area. They also talk to community members and to health care providers to identify competing priorities. Using these processes, they might discover that their communities have not achieved the Healthy People 2010 goal of 90% full immunization for children by the age of two years.

To address the lack of immunizations, the nurses acknowledge that the issues that affect immunizations are multifaceted. The immunization schedule changes frequently and is quite complex. Even health care providers have difficulty interpreting it. Perhaps communication with parents has been sketchy and has been complicated by controversy. Immunizations may not be seen by parents as essential until they are mandated for entry into elementary school. Immunizations may not be easily accessible, available, and affordable. Parents may make decisions based on misinformation, rumor, or hearsay. The nurses know, however, that community members want to keep their children healthy and that immunizations have contributed greatly to reduced illness in individuals and better overall health for the community. They also know that community members prefer to have their children immunized in a consistent place, as part of an overall medical home.

Because the childhood immunization levels are suboptimal in the communities served by the health system's hospitals, childhood immunization is selected as a system-wide initiative. A group of clinicians is convened to implement a program with the goal of increasing immunization to the Healthy People 2010 goal of 90%. There is much discussion on the best way for increasing immunization rates, using a broad-based program. Both telephoned and mailed reminders are known to be effective in increasing immunizations in adults and children (Szilagyi et al., 2000). Because telephoned reminders are substantially more expensive than mailed reminders, the system opts to use mailed reminders.

Various materials are developed in both English and Spanish, and incentives are put into place to assist parents. Babies are automatically enrolled in the program when they are born in a system hospital. Mailings occur at regular intervals and include a personalized letter indicating what vaccines are due, a vaccine record, vaccine information statements, and a growth and development newsletter. Additionally, incentives are mailed to help keep the parents motivated to use preventive services. Materials are written at a sixth-grade level. All materials are reviewed for cultural congruity, and the illustrations include babies from various ethnic groups (Figure 9-1).

New materials are developed as needed, based on a continuous assessment of the needs of the parents. For example, reproducing all the materials in all the languages used by patients is too expensive, so a multiple-language brochure is developed in the 11 most common languages. The brochure explains the program and asks that non–English-speaking and non–Spanish-speaking families obtain help in translating the materials. In addition, after families express a major concern about the multiple injections required to keep their babies fully immunized and their babies' resultant distress and crying, a "calming strategies" flyer is developed (Figure 9-2).

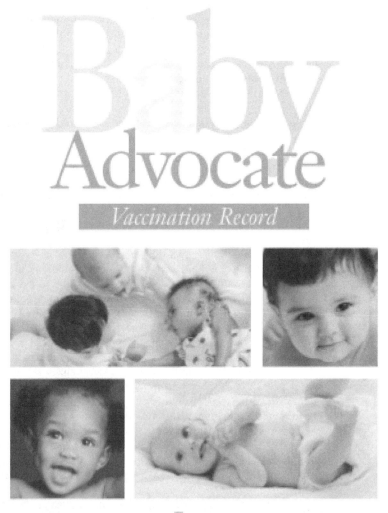

Figure 9–1. Vaccine schedule cover.

Baby Advocate *Calming* Strategies

✚ *Advocate Health Care*

Do you hate to take your baby for his vacciniation shots because he cries? Even though you know your baby needs the shots, do you delay taking her to her doctor because she fusses?

You are not alone. No one likes to see babies cry. On the other hand, we all know that sometimes a little pain is needed to prevent a lot of pain, illness and even potential death down the road.

We've identified some calming strategies you can use to help your baby after receiving baby shots or during other periods of crying. Try one or more of these suggestions:

1. Provide a monotonous background sound such as your humming voice or a tape of easy listening music.
2. Reduce visual, auditory and social stimulation. Dim lights, keep the room quiet.
3. Help your baby suck on his hand or a pacifier.
4. Swaddle your baby in a blanket, firmly but not tightly, with arms and legs flexed close to her body.
5. Hold your baby's hands in yours against his chest.
6. Rock your baby in a rocking chair and sing softly to her.
7. Hold your baby upright against your chest as you walk, rock or gently bounce him.
8. Lie your baby, tummy down, across your lap; stroke her back or sway your knees from side to side.
9. Stroke your baby's head in a rhythmical pattern.
10. Gently rock your baby in a cradled position.
11. Pick your baby up and hold her at your shoulder or in a cradled position.
12. Talk to your baby in a soft voice.
13. Put your baby in a Snugli or infant carrier to hold him close to your body.
14. Try changing your baby's position.

As always, talk to your baby's doctor for other advice if your baby doesn't console after you've tried these strategies.

If it's any consolation, school-age children who had recovered from the chickenpox were recently asked if they would rather have the disease or a shot to prevent the disease. Most of the children said they would rather have the shot! So even children know that the temporary discomfort is better than the longer pain and illness. Your baby is too young to express her preference. But you know what's best for your baby.

Figure 9–2. Calming strategies flyer.

In no way does the system-wide status of the initiative replace the need for site-specific actions. Instead, the system initiative augments additional activities implemented at specific hospitals to meet the needs of their diverse populations. For example, the healthy communities director at one hospital finds that the hospital has a very large Arabic-speaking population receiving care in its pediatric residency clinic, so clinic staff members do a mini-study to learn the barriers to immunizations in this population. They find that the group's members are well educated and want additional information. They find Arabic-language vaccine information statements on the Internet, print them, and make them available to all parents. In addition, they take the initiative to translate all materials into Arabic and provide them to parents at the clinic. And they make certain that staff members are prepared to discuss immunizations with the parents at every visit. The healthy community director also develops and provides a curriculum focusing on cultural aspects of immunizations for resident physicians.

At another hospital, the healthy communities director learns that financial barriers still exist among parents seeking immunizations for their children. She uses several strategies to overcome this barrier. First, she works with physicians and helps them enroll in the Vaccines for Children program, making vaccines available at no cost or low cost right in their offices. She also works with the staff in physicians' offices to enhance their role in fostering childhood immunizations. In addition, she works with the health department to provide monthly immunizations on site.

This case study focuses on one culturally competent program provided in a variety of communities. Additional programs, targeting the needs of other age groups, may also be envisioned. For example, adult immunizations are also an issue for many communities, so a program might be developed that focuses specifically on older adults and their immunization needs. Similarly, programs might be instituted to deal with other health issues of concern to community members. The case study demonstrates the importance of incorporating an understanding of culture in every aspect of an initiative. To design and implement an effective program, the cultural values of patients must be understood and addressed.

•THE ROLE OF INDIVIDUAL HEALTH CARE PROVIDERS IN CREATING CULTURALLY COMPETENT ORGANIZATIONS

All of us play a role in creating culturally competent organizations. Individual health care providers are at the core of helping an institution attain cultural competence. If they listen and attend carefully, health care providers have a valuable window directly into the world of their patients. They can take what they learn and escalate it as needed to improve the cultural responsiveness of their organization. Speaking the language can also be an advantage.

When health care providers fail to take the patient's culture seriously, they misinterpret the patient's value system and, by doing so, elevate their own value systems. This posture is culturally destructive (Dana, 1993) because it minimizes the other person's culture. A better approach is to take time to ask questions about what the patient prefers and to listen attentively. In the end, this will increase understanding, trust, collaboration, adherence, and satisfaction.

Even when serving a diverse patient base, health care providers can make a difference. At the University of California, San Diego, the assistant nurse manager of an oncology transplant unit created a special program that addresses the spiritual needs of terminally ill patients. She collected a variety of objects to bring comfort to the critically ill. In large wicker baskets, referred to as "love baskets," she places a variety of items, including spiritual texts that reflect individual patients' belief systems (Buddhist teachings, the Koran, Hindu prayers, the Torah, and the Bible translated into many different languages); CDs of ethnic music; religious items; aromatherapy products; and massage lotions. Nurses and family members can quickly use these items to provide a comforting atmosphere for patients. Patients, families, nurses, and physicians have given the baskets a positive evaluation (Gabriel, 2001).

SUMMARY

As with individuals, the quest for organizational cultural competence is a lifetime journey. There is always room for improvement. To be truly effective in improving patient care for all, health care services and social services that take cultural diversity into account must make an organizational commitment to cultural competence. Cultural competence cannot live in one or two nurses; it must be systemic. It must involve all layers of the organization: the policy making level, the administrative level, the management level, and the provider level. In addition, an organization must have a mutually beneficial relationship with the community it serves to achieve cultural competence. As such, organizations must reach out to community members.

REVIEW QUESTIONS

1. Critically describe the culture of a health care organization such as a local hospital or clinic.
2. Describe how the culture of the organization affects the quality of care provided.
3. Analyze the "frame" or perspective that an organization uses to resolve conflict.
4. Examine how an organization's culture influences or affects its employees.

CRITICAL THINKING ACTIVITIES

1. An excellent way to understand a culturally competent organization is to assess the organizational culture using the "five A's" described in this chapter. With some of your classmates, compare and contrast the availability, accessibility, affordability, acceptability, and appropriateness of the organization. Discuss what actions could be taken by the organization to increase its cultural competency.
2. Then, use a different approach to assess the cultural competency of the same organization. Use Leininger's (1991) Theory of Culture Care Diversity and Universality to assess the culture of the organization. Table 9-1 in this chapter provides an example of how Leininger's Culture Care Model can be used. Compare and contrast the values and beliefs of the organization with

the values and beliefs of the groups using the health care organization's services. What areas would be most problematic, and why?

3. Many members of ethnic or minority communities lack adequate access to care because they do not have adequate health insurance. Often, these individuals use the emergency rooms of city hospitals for episodic care. Assess the physical environment of an emergency room to determine potential barriers to culturally competent care. Develop a flow chart that outlines the steps a patient takes when he or she seeks care in an emergency room. Identify the changes that would decrease barriers and improve services if they were implemented.

• References

American Nurses Association Council on Cultural Diversity in Nursing Practice (1991). *Cultural diversity in nursing practice* [position statement]. Washington DC.

Andrews, M. M. (1998, October). A model for cultural change. *Nursing Management, 66,*62–64.

Ayanian, J. Z., Cleary, P. D., Weissman, J. S., & Epstein, A. M. (1999). The effect of patients' preferences on racial differences in access to renal transplantation. *New England Journal of Medicine, 341*(22), 1661–1669.

Ayanian, J. Z., & Epstein, A. M. (2001). Racial disparities in medical care. *New England Journal of Medicine, 344,*1443–1349.

Bolman, L. G., & Deal, T. E. (1997). *Reframing organizations: Artistry, choice, and leadership* (2nd ed.). San Francisco: Jossey-Bass Publishers.

Carnevale, A. P. & Stone, S. C. (1995). *The American mosaic: An in-depth report on the future of diversity at work.* New York: McGraw-Hill.

Centers for Disease Control and Prevention (2002). Recent trends in mortality rates for four major cancers, by sex and race/ethnicity—United States, 1990–1998. *Morbidity and Mortality Weekly Report, 51*(3), 49–53.

Clancy, C. M., & Stryer, D. B. (2001). Racial and ethnic disparities and primary care experience. *Health Services Research, 36*(6), 979–986.

Dana, R. H. (1993*). Multicultural Assessment Perspectives for Professional Psychology.* Boston: Allyn & Bacon.

Davis, R. N. (1997). Community caring: An ethnographic study within an organizational culture. *Public Health Nursing, 14*(2), 92–100.

Dreachslin, J. L. (1999). Diversity leadership. *Journal of Nursing Administration, 29*(6), 3–4, 21.

Einbinder, L. C., & Schulman, K.A. (2000). The effect of race on the referral process for invasive cardiac procedures. *Medical Care Research and Review, 57*(Suppl. 1), 162–180.

First NIH Working Group on Health Disparities (2000). Cited in Slideshow: The NIH Strategic Plan to Address Health Disparities, presented by Dr. Fuci to the Symposium on Challenges in Health Disparities in the New Millennium: A Call to Action, Washington DC, posted on www.niaid.nih.gov/director/healthdis.htm, accessed 2/12/02.

Gabriel, B. A. (2001, October). When physicians and patients "speak a different language": The difficult quest for cultural competency. *Association of American Medical Colleges Reporter, 11*(1), 8–9. Available from: http://www.hs-sc.gc.ca/fnihbdgspni/fnihb/chp/publications/second_diagnostic_fni.pdf; accessed July 8, 2002.

Health Canada (1999). *A second diagnostic on the health of First Nations and Inuit People in Canada.*

Huff, R. M., & Kline, M. V. (1999). The cultural assessment framework. In *Promoting health in multicultural populations: A handbook for practitioners.* Thousand Oaks, CA: Sage Publications.

Jones, M. E., Bond, M. L. & Cason, C. L. (1998). Where does culture fit in outcomes management? *Journal of Nursing Care Quality, 13*(1), 41–51.

King, T. E. & Brunetta, P. (1999). Racial disparities in rates of surgery for lung cancer. *New England Journal of Medicine, 341*(16), 1231–1233.

Leininger, M. (1991). *Culture Care Diversity and Universality: A Theory of Nursing Care.* New York: National League for Nursing Press.

Leininger, M. (1996). Founder's focus: Transcultural nursing administration: An imperative worldwide. *Journal of Transcultural Nursing, 8*(1), 28–33.

Ludwig-Beymer, P., Blankemeier, J. R., Casas-Byots, C., & Suarez-Balcazar, Y. (1996). Community assessment in a suburban Hispanic community: A description of methods. *Journal of Transcultural Nursing, 8*(1), 19–27.

Malone, B. L. (1997). Improving organizational cultural competence. In Dienemann, J. A. (Ed), *Cultural Diversity in Nursing: Issues, Strategies, and Outcomes.* Washington, DC: American Academy of Nursing.

Mor Barak, M. E. (2000). The inclusive workplace: an

ecosystems approach to diversity management. *Social Work, 45*(4), 339–353.

Office of Minority Health, Department of Health and Human Services. (2000). National standards on culturally and linguistically appropriate services (CLAS) in health care. *Federal Register, 65*(247), 80865–80879.

Pelfrey, S., & Theisen, B. A. (1993). Valuing the community benefits provided by nonprofit hospitals. *JONA, 23*(6), 16–21.

Roizner, M. (1996). *A practical guide for the assessment of cultural competence in children's mental health organizations.* Boston: Judge Baker's Children's Center.

Schein, E. H. (1985). *Organizational Culture and Leadership.* San Francisco: Jossey-Bass.

Sheifer, S. E., Escarce, J. J., & Schulman, K. A. (2000). Race and sex differences in the management of coronary artery disease. *American Heart Journal, 139*(5), 848–857.

Szilagyi, P. G., Bordley, C., Vann, J. C., Chelminski, A., Kraus, R. M., Margolis, P. A., & Rodewald, L. E. (2000). Effect of patient reminder/recall interventions on immunization rates. *Journal of American Medical Association, 284*(14), 1820–1827.

U.S. Department of Health and Human Services (2000). *Healthy People 2010.* Washington, DC: DHHS.

Weinick, R. M., Zuvekas, S. H., & Cohen, J. W. (2000). Racial and ethnic differences to and use of health care services, 1977 to 1996. *Medical Care Research and Review, 57* (Suppl. 1), 36–54.

CHAPTER 10

Transcultural Perspectives in Mental Health Nursing

Kathryn Hopkins Kavanagh

KEY TERMS

Acculturation

Assimilation

Culture-bound syndromes

Disease

Diversity

Diversity management

Explanatory models

Illness

Language of distress

Mental health

Somatization

OBJECTIVES

1. Provide a sense of mental health and mental illness as varying with culture, time, and place.
2. Relate issues related to mental health and mental illness as fully integrated into other aspects of living, health, and health care.
3. Realize the wide variability in expression of symptoms, interpretations, explanations, and expectations associated with phenomena related to mental health and mental illness.
4. Emphasize the potential that interactive processes and communication have for facilitating effective transcultural mental health care.
5. Suggest and use strategies to facilitate effective transcultural mental health care.

Given the fact that illness (unlike disease, which is physiologically based) is always socially constructed, there was a time when mental illness did not exist. People had problems and some were psychotic. But whether tolerated, pitied, shunned, or punished, and whether they lived out their years or died, the "mad" were more likely to be viewed as fools or possessed than ill. Eventually, with growing social consciousness, the mentally deranged were given refuge in asylums, where, isolated and in large part gratefully forgotten by society, they received at least a modicum of care and shelter (Conrad & Schneider, 1992).

Today, persons who are mentally ill are, for the most part, in the community. Community programs tend to emphasize basic, comprehensive, and preventive care (Matteson, 1995; Oakley & Potter, 1997), as well as crisis intervention and care management specific to client needs. At the same time, the aspects of health care systems that relate most closely to mental health tend to suffer from chronic neglect and lack of funding and support, largely because mental health care is not based firmly enough in biology or science to give it a high status in the culture of medicine. Most mentally ill individuals are not psychotic and therefore do not receive diagnoses of psychiatric diseases. Overall, other problems affecting **mental health** are far more numerous in today's society, such as severe stress, violence, anxiety, anger, mood disturbances (for example, depression, suicidal thoughts, or intense and prolonged grieving), confusion (related to aging, drug use, or other issues), and substance abuse. In a culture that tends to be oriented more toward consumerism than social interaction, people often have problems relating to others, sex, food, work, pain, chronic illness, and physical health problems. Spiritual distress also comes under the rubric of mental health.

The interrelatedness of mental health phenomena in everyday life with physical illness means that most mentally distressed and ill people are encountered in health care settings, both inpatient and outpatient, that are not labeled "psychiatric" or "mental health" (Gorman, Sultan, & Raines, 1996). This is particularly true in rural areas, where mental health resources may be scarce (Rohland, 1995). Wherever they occur today, nearly all services that support mental health are short term (Marmor, 1994). Meanwhile, the mentally ill often confront ongoing severe social and economic strains, while mental health needs and care resources are minimal and in flux (Billings, 1993; Gorman, Sultan, & Raines, 1996; Marmor, 1994; Oakley & Potter, 1997).

The challenge in providing appropriate and adequate psychiatric/mental health care is complicated by **diversity**. Each person learns, from those around him or her, one or more languages; ethical, religious, or other guidelines for living; and other meaningful and systematic ways of relating to a cultural orientation within society. That culture, in sum, is learned, transmitted, shared, integrated, both ideal and real, and constantly changing (Campinha-Bacote, 1997). Traditionally, ethnicity was the basis of such an orientation, but human diversity exists everywhere there are differences in age, sex, experience, socioeconomic status, social view, gender preference, race, and so on. Increasingly, in these postmodern times, traditional meanings of social categories give way to affinities for and allegiances to groups, meanings, and activities based on personal interest and preference (Kottak, 2000), rather than those passed along through family enculturation. It is important to keep in mind that transcultural nursing is limited to neither health care nor culture in the sense of ethnicity; it involves all human diversity in virtually all imaginable contexts.

The populations of the United States and Canada currently include large numbers of refugees and immigrants (Halli & Driedger, 1999; Lipson, 1996). Furthermore, both populations are changing continuously (Health Canada, 1999; Susser, 2001). The "browning of America" alludes to projections that by the middle of the 21st century, the average resident (as defined by Census Bureau statistics) will trace his or her ancestry to Africa, Asia, the Pacific Islands, or the

Hispanic or Arab worlds—or to a blend of widely disparate cultures—rather than to European roots (Henry, 1990). By 2050, one of every five Americans will be Hispanic (U.S. Census Bureau as cited by United States Department of Health and Human Services, 2001). Similar population trends exist in Canada. For example, the proportion of immigrants of Asian origin increased from 14% to 31% between 1981 and 1996 (Health Canada, 1999).

Given the complexity generated by such diversity, these nations are moving away from stereotyped "one-size-fits-all" expectations of medical treatment and nursing care. New themes related to diversity in mental health care are developing, such as advocacy and empowerment (Dunst, Trivette, & Deal, 1988; Rose & Black, 1985), participatory decision making, (Kavanagh & Kennedy, 1992), pluralism, multiculturalism (Christopher, 1999; Locke, 1992; Wali, 1992), mind/body holism (Anderson, 1996; Heiligenstein, 1999; Pert, Dreher, & Ruff, 1998), and increased emphasis on psychosocial issues in health and illness (Robert & House, 2000; Siegrist, 2000). Health care providers as well as clients are increasingly committed to recognizing the rights of individuals and affiliate groups (that is, the groups with which people identify or to which they reference themselves) as well as being involved in health care. This means that care is expected to meet the standards of the groups with which people are affiliated. Culturally competent nurses learn the effective use of cultural sensitivity, knowledge, and skills in meaningful cultural encounters (Campinha-Bacote, 1997).

This chapter discusses transcultural nursing as it relates specifically to psychiatric and mental health nursing. It presents a practical and flexible framework based on a balance of cultural awareness, sensitivity, knowledge, and skills (Kavanagh & Kennedy, 1992; Pedersen, 1988) (Figure 10-1). This model is premised on the value of respectful, open, mutual communication and collaborative relationships between nurses and clients. The medium for both collaborative treatment and **diversity management** is mutual communication. This approach portrays the client as someone more expert about his or her situation than the health care provider is, and from whom the nurse can learn to understand the situation as the client does. The culturally competent transcultural nurse has the ability to manage diversity effectively, when management of diversity is defined as helping each person to reach his or her full potential (Thomas, 1991).

A balance of cultural awareness, sensitivity, knowledge, and skills in the context of meaningful interaction allows nurses to link receptivity and sensitivity with knowledge of typical, expectable group patterns. Awareness, sensitivity, and knowledge, in combination with cultural assessment, communication, and other mental health nursing skills, can produce respectful, culturally acceptable, and effective nursing interventions for diverse peoples in specific, individual situations.

Cultural sensitivity is never enough. Limiting attention to awareness of issues and differences, and to sensitivity to their meaning and import, leaves the nurse powerless because he or she still lacks the knowledge and skills required to act knowingly on the issue. Knowledge of expectable cultural pat-

Figure 10–1. Transcultural nurses bring together sensitivity, knowledge, and skill to promote health and care for the mentally ill in culturally congruent ways.

terns provides starting places against which the reality of a given situation can be tested. Such knowledge differs from stereotypes, which lock out real evidence through acknowledgment of only that which was expected. Lack of sensitivity, knowledge, and skill may be involved when people are labeled "noncompliant," "problem patients," or too resistant or defensive to benefit from treatment or to recognize the value of the care being offered. It may be that the client's ideas (and their expression) about care and caring simply differ from those of the nurse.

• MENTAL ILLNESS AND MENTAL DISEASE

In many ways, health and illness are more central to transcultural psychiatric and mental health nursing than are mental diseases. Much of the counseling, therapy, and other care given by mental health professionals focuses on illness prevention and making everyday life better. The distinction between illness and disease is important. **Illness** emphasizes subjective behavioral, psychologic, sociocultural, and experiential dimensions of disorders. **Disease**, by contrast, pertains to chemical, physiologic, and other organic and objective phenomena related to sickness (Helman, 1990; McElroy & Jezewski, 2000; Tseng, 1997). Biologic disorders of memory, perception, and feeling surely exist, as do compensatory processes of rationalization and action that are strongly influenced by social and cultural factors (Kiev, 1972; Kleinman &

Seeman, 2000; Tseng & Streltzer, 1997). The rates of mental illness and of mental diseases do not seem to vary much among groups when social and economic factors are controlled for. There is no conclusive evidence that mental illness and disease rates vary with race or other intrinsic human characteristics, although they are clearly associated with low socioeconomic status, low educational level, separation, and loss.

Psychiatric Resources

Four fifths of the global population lives in non-Western, partially industrialized countries (Kottak, 2000), whereas most psychiatric resources are in Western and industrialized societies. The schizophrenias, manic-depressive disorders, major depressions, and anxiety disorders are thought to occur throughout the world, although diagnosis is difficult because the expression of symptoms varies so much with cultural differences. Depression anxieties and somatiform disorders (that is, the expressions of problems in physical rather than psychologic signs and symptoms) are probably most prevalent in the non-Western world (Kleinman, 1991). However, despite international epidemiologic and research efforts, at present there are no international centers focused on mental health treatment programs comparable to, for example, the World Health Organization. The global emphasis has been on physical health (Kleinman, 1991), although somatic disorders are interwoven with culture and with mental distress and illness (Chaplin, 1997; Kleinman & Seeman, 2000).

Every society has systems of beliefs and practices related to health care, and specific persons trained as healers. There are many places where biomedicine is not widely available and where most people depend on traditional healers, although they also exist (and are depended on) in modern westernized societies. Whereas shamans and traditional healers are often not very effective in treating chronic mental disorders, the outcome for some conditions tends to be more positive in societies where clients are not negatively stigmatized and are not alone with their problems. Where persons with mental illness are devalued, they are more likely to be demoralized and isolated, to feel dehumanized, and to curtail the development of potential support systems (Beiser, Waxler-Morrison, Iacono, Lin, Fleming, & Husted, 1987; Lipson & Steiger, 1996). The North American values of individualism and self-reliance further reinforce a tendency toward social isolation and alienation. Additionally, many individuals cross cultures, which requires special psychosocial resilience and adaptation (Kim & Gudykunst, 1988; McCubbin & McCubbin, 1988; Ory, Simons, Verhulst, Leenders, and Wolters, 1991; Tseng & Streltzer, 1997), both in everyday living and in health care.

Diagnosis: Problems with Normality and Abnormality

There is probably more variation among etiologic beliefs of mental health care professionals than is commonly acknowledged, but belief in relatively impersonal, environmental, and natural causation generally prevails. For a variety of reasons or simply by chance, parts, systems, families, or individuals take on characteristics that are assessed as dysfunctional. By contrast, members of many cultural groups believe illness is caused by a supernatural being (a deity or god), a nonhuman being (such as an ancestor, a ghost, or an evil spirit), or another human being (a witch or sorcerer) (Foster & Anderson, 1978). The sick person in such a case is viewed as a victim who is not responsible for his or her condition or its resolution.

The division of sickness into physical and mental categories is Western, although every society labels some behaviors as abnormal. The cultural assumption that mind and body are somehow separate, which is now increasingly challenged in terms of relationships between healing and the mind (Goleman & Gurin, 1993; Minson, 1999; Moyers, 1993; Pert, Dreher, & Ruff, 1998), has for several centuries strongly swayed Western ideas about normality and abnormality. What is considered "normal" and what is "abnormal" is always based on cultural perspective (Lock, 2000). Culture influences (that is, it shapes but does not determine) expression, presentation, recognition, labeling, explanations for, and distributions of mental illnesses (Evidence-Based Practice 10–1).

Interpretations of health and even of the overt signs of physical disease vary widely. Mental health and mental illnesses are more difficult than physical disorders to delineate because of the lack of readily observable, discrete, and organic phenomena. The symptoms of mental illness, dependent as they are on behavioral expression, vary because they depend on social definitions rather than physical measures. Assessment is based on the appropriateness of behaviors (for example, dress, posture, odor, gestures, speech, nonverbal communication, facial expression, and physical activity) that lack fixed standards and depend on context and social relationships to differentiate what is considered normal from what is viewed as abnormal. Although psychiatry is part of Western biomedicine, it deals with ambiguous areas of life, such as self and symbolic behavior, deviance and marginality, power and control (Fabrega, 1989; Frank, 2000).

Diagnoses involve social competence, which, to be sensitively evaluated, must be assessed against culture-specific criteria. Many cultures do not dichotomize normality and abnormality as rigidly as Western societies tend to, or even distinguish health from illness. These may be viewed as multidimensional, continual, and perhaps overlapping (Helman, 1990), with ideas about mental health and mental illness mixed with those about health and medicine in general (Joralemon, 1999). To members of such societies, concepts such as mental health have little meaning. The distinction between illness and health may be based on the ability to perform one's normal roles in society. A health care provider's diagnosis, prognosis, and treatment, based on imprecise and unobservable phenomena, may seem ludicrous.

The pattern used by a client to express concern or disorder is referred to as a **language of distress** (Helman, 1990). Close examination of how people interact and express themselves is essential in understanding relationships between psychiatric and social factors. The same phenomena (for example,

EVIDENCE-BASED PRACTICE 10–1
Mental Health Issues Among Vietnam Amerasians

Although the Vietnam War ended in 1975, its legacy remains a factor in the lives of the off-spring of American fathers and Vietnamese mothers. Currently, more than 21,000 Vietnam Amerasians and 50,000 of their accompanying family members reside in the United States. Research indicates that Amerasians from Vietnam tend to experience more psychologic distress and mental health risk factors during resettlement than do members of other refugee and immigrant groups. Although a variety of experiences both before and after migration strongly affect their current mental health, one of the most important predictors of adjustment is the fit between premigration expectations of life in the United States and the postmigration reality. A discrepancy between those often leads to higher rates of anxiety and depression.

CLINICAL APPLICATION

Be sensitive and attuned to symptoms of psychologic distress and mental health risk when providing care to Vietnam Amerasians who are resettling in the United States. Explore family and community support systems available to Vietnam Amerasians who seek health care services. Be cognizant of community resources and services for referral purposes.

Gently ask the Vietnam Amerasian refugee to describe his or her premigration expectations of life in the United States and to contrast that view with the reality encountered on migration to this country. Based on the discrepancies described, the nurse will be able to understand how well the person has adjusted to life in the United States.

Identify resources such as Vietnamese-speaking mental health professionals in your community or state. If these resources are not available locally in your community, are they available via telehealth/telemedicine sites?

Be knowledgeable about how symptoms are expressed and how they are perceived and treated by others in this cultural group.

Somatization likely occurs in this cultural group. Headaches, backaches, and stomachaches may reflect depression rather than an underlying physiologic cause. Although physiologic symptoms warrant careful examination, they may be a sign that the client needs a careful mental and emotional health evaluation.

Support family relationships, and encourage clients to engage in cultural practices that provide a connection to their Vietnamese cultural traditions.

Nguyen, M. N., & Organista, K. C. (1997). Vietnam Amerasians: Assimilation and adjustment problems in the United States. *Journal of Multicultural Social Work, 6*(1/2), 77–91.

visions and dream states, trance states, hallucinations, delusions, belief in spirits, speaking in "tongues," drug or alcohol intoxication, or suicide) may be judged normal or abnormal according to the settings and circumstances in which they occur (Conrad & Schneider, 1992). At times, cultural groups encourage altered states of consciousness that others may view as mental disturbances. However, because addictive substances (such as alcohol, tobacco, and opiates) in most societies were traditionally reserved for use during special times or rituals, widespread related health problems seldom occurred. Today, by contrast, the Western redefinition of addiction as disease (rather than as a primarily social, moral, or legal issue [Conrad & Schneider, 1992]) has made this a primary mental health concern.

How symptoms are expressed and how they are perceived and treated by others vary widely. Although psychotic disorders occur in every society, and the primary symptoms (that is, social and emotional withdrawal, auditory or visual hallucinations, general delusions, flat affect, mood changes, and insomnia) occur across cultures, the secondary features of these disorders are highly influenced by culture (Pang, 1995; Tripp-Reimer, 1984; Tseng & Streltzer, 1997). For example, in some groups, guilt and suicidal ideation do not accompany depression; in others they frequently do (Harrison, 1997). For some peoples, suicide is an acceptable escape from problems ranging from marital dissension, illness, sorcery, loneliness, and hopelessness to criticism from others (Farberow, 1975; Kral, 1998).

Analogously, among many groups, somatic (physical) rather than psychologic symptoms are prominent among depressed individuals; in others, such as middle-class European North Americans, psychologic "blues" prevail (Kleinman & Seeman, 2000). **Somatization** pertains to a preoccupation with physical symptoms that are thought to have a psychologic rather than a physical cause (Chaplin, 1997). Somatic symptoms that express psychologic distress occur at high rates, for example, among clients who are Hispanic (Escobar, 1987) or Chinese (Kleinman, 1988). It is not unusual for nurses to encounter clients who deny being depressed but describe having headaches, backaches, stomachaches, and other physical phenomena prompted by (and sometimes consciously associated with) sorrow and suffering.

The content of delusions and hallucinations also reflects cultural patterns. For instance, the content may be primarily psychologic, religious or spiritual, moral or social, naturalistic or supernatural, or physical or medical. In Western Ireland, psychiatric patients tend to have delusions of a religious nature (Scheper-Hughes, 1978), whereas schizophrenic persons in North America more often have persecution delusions involving electromagnetic or other secular, generically scientific phenomena (Helman, 1990; Oltmanns & Maher, 1988), believing perhaps that their toasters talk to them or that current from electric outlets is altering their thinking. Likewise, some people may associate sex with guilt, whereas others do not (Sanday & Goodenough, 1990; Bohannan, 1992). For example, middle-class European American criticism of sex and pregnancy outside of marriage among Blacks does not take into account the social history that made many women of color vulnerable to unwanted sexual activity and that, over time, helped some to redefine extramarital sex and pregnancy as events apart from moral apprehension. Despite considerable research evidence that married persons generally experience more positive mental health than the unmarried, too little research attention has been paid to Blacks to allow generalization to that group (Brown, 1996). As Lock (2000) points out, both "normal" and "abnormal" are interpretations that often become confounded with moral ideology.

Some conditions, such as posttraumatic stress disorder, can occur in various forms anywhere. Others, known as culture-bound syndromes, exist within specific cultural groups. Some conditions may represent labeling differences, as in China, where the term "neurasthenia" is widely used for symptoms produced by social stressors and may correspond to what Western medicine refers to as depression (Rin & Huang, 1989). Conditions fall into categories of folk illnesses that defy Western psychiatric identification, although they are very real to the persons experiencing them (McElroy & Jezewski, 2000; Pang, 1994). Examples of folk illnesses include fright or soul loss (*susto*), which is often associated by Hispanics with a sudden start or sneeze (Foster & Anderson, 1978). Various conditions thought to result from the evil eye (*mal ojo*) are believed to occur unintentionally when, for instance, a nurse fails to touch a child he or she has noticed or examined. Herbal remedies, rubbing, massage, and other physical manipulations by *curanderos* (*curanderas,* if they are women) are typical treatments. These may be used with home remedies (such as teas) or prayers and trips to religious shrines or charismatic folk healers to alleviate distress.

The United States and Canada have numerous folk illnesses, such as "nervous breakdown," that occur throughout the society. There are also **culture-bound syndromes**. Anorexia nervosa, for example, occurs only where food is abundant, although even there it takes various forms. Other culture-bound syndromes are seen more often in traditional, nonindustrialized societies and in immigrants from those societies. Despite the exotic nature of many of the classic culture-bound syndromes, it is useful to know of the existence of these ethnic conditions, or "reactive psychoses" (Yap, 1977). Several culture-bound syndromes are described in Box 10-1.

Misdiagnosis (for example, the overdiagnosis of antisocial disorders and psychoses and underdiagnosis of depressions [Brown, 1990]) is a major problem among members of groups that differ from the European North American, middle-class, Christian, and male orientation that dominates North American culture and medicine (Collins, Sorel, Brent, & Mathura, 1990; Pinderhughes, 1982; Secundy, 1992). An example of a commonly misdiagnosed folk illness is "falling out," a stress-relieving pattern of shaking and falling that typically occurs when sympathetic others are present; it is seen among Blacks, Haitians, Whites, and other southern United States ethnic groups (Gaines, 1992; Weidman, 1979). Adding to the complexity of psychiatric diagnosis is that despite the influence of culture in patterned psychologic and physical conditions, there are individual or idiosyncratic explanations and expressions of behavior.

Like any other field, psychiatry is not completely homogeneous. Sociocultural and cross-cultural approaches exist (Kleinman, 1988; Tseng & Streltzer, 1997) that extend the thinking of many psychiatric and mental health care providers to allow for cultural, social, and increasingly more holistic explanations of clients' behavior (*Expanding horizons of health care,* 2000).

BOX 10–1	**CULTURE-BOUND SYNDROMES AND VARIANTS**

Amok: an acute reaction resulting from hostility (Yap, 1977) and dissociative amnesia (Castillo, 1997). The term "running amok" comes from the frenzied lashing out associated with this syndrome.

Anorexia nervosa: an eating disorder associated in Western societies, but not in Eastern cultures, with fear of obesity (Gorman, Sultan, & Raines, 1996; Tseng & Streltzer, 1997).

Homophobia: an anxiety-related syndrome based on fear of homosexuals (Ficarrotto, 1990; Bernstein, 1997).

Malignant anxiety: acute anxiety states with panic and varying degrees of ego disorganization (Yap, 1977) that have been associated with criminality and loss of stable culture resulting from colonialism or other extreme societal disruption.

Pibloktoq: "Arctic hysteria" among polar Eskimos. Accounts are of bizarre, dramatized behavior, such as running naked through the snow (Parker, 1977).

Susto: a traumatic, anxiety-depressive state with psychophysiologic changes; "fright sickness" that results from such stimuli as a fall, a thunderclap, meeting some threat, or other frightening experiences. Susto causes anxiety, insomnia, listlessness, loss of appetite, and social withdrawal. This folk illness occurs throughout Latin America (Rubel, 1977; Uzzell, 1977).

Trance dissociation: possession syndromes occurring in various parts of the world with varying degrees of social sanction (Yap, 1977). This differs from primary schizophrenic reactions and is believed to be caused by disease, the loss of one's soul, or the invasion of a benign or evil spirit. In some circumstances it is viewed as a mystical state. Some American Indian vision quests result in altered states of consciousness similar to this.

Voodoo death: "magical" or sociocultural death that has been explained as a result of a "flight-or-fight" response, belief in the power of threat and suggestion, and the acceptance of hopelessness (Lex, 1977).

However, at the same time, the widely used series of *Diagnostic and Statistical Manuals of Mental Disorders* (American Psychiatric Association, 1994)—the "DSM-IV" and its previous versions—requires the surrender of many cultural insights (Conrad & Schneider, 1992; Eisenbruch, 1992). Works such as the DSM-IV (and now the DSM-V) organize symbolic and instrumental evidence of the forms of deviance that are considered medical concerns (Conrad & Schneider, 1992) and provide the medical community with administratively useful classifications for diagnosis and record keeping. However, despite varying cultural expressions of psychiatric problems, in less affluent countries than the United States and Canada, where library funds are particularly limited, the *Diagnostic and Statistical Manuals of Mental Disorders* standards tend to be used as the ultimate text on psychiatric diagnoses and categories (Eisenbruch, 1992; Littlewood, 1991). This seems contradictory to the evidence that although medical involvement in "madness" has been recorded for at least 2,000 years, the aspects of treatment and care that foster transcultural understanding emerge more as humanitarian reform than as biomedical accomplishment (Conrad & Schneider, 1992).

Socioeconomic Factors Influencing Mental Health

Social and environmental conditions often lead to mental health problems. Children and adolescents are vulnerable to the mental health effects of current social and economic conditions. Parenting styles vary greatly. Some parents, for example, may view "good parenting" as keeping a child safe, fed, and clean, but not including activities that stimulate cognitive, affective, and physical development. Substantial numbers of children and adolescents live in poverty, with severe mental health effects (Scheper-Hughes, 1987). Children and adolescents of every social class and ethnic background are vulnerable to sexual and physical abuse (Levinson, 1989). In the United States, children are likely to be exposed at a tender age to adult sexual roles and to violence through the mass media. High rates of depression are associated with problems in areas of family and personal relationships, finances, and general living conditions. Crime, drug use, and suicide are prevalent problems that may be associated with perceived limitations on hope (Harrison, 1997; Jackson, 1990; Poussaint, 1990).

Poverty and lack of social support also have implications for mental health. Although disorganized and dysfunctional families are not specific to the poor, the poor often have higher mortality and morbidity rates (Levinson, 1989) and access to relatively few treatment resources. Lower birth rates mean that elders have fewer adult children and kin as potential caregivers. Increased geographic mobility and separate living styles result in loose social networks and increased social alienation. Parents, particularly those who are single, are more alone with childrearing responsibilities in industrialized societies than is the case where extended families are more common and socialization responsibilities are shared with other adults. Immigration, globalization, and geographic change can lead to conflict between traditional and modern roles (Takeshita, 1997) and prompt new health concerns (Catalano & Pickett, 2000; Gutiérrez & Kendall, 2000). Similarly, increased divorce rates often disrupt the flow of personal support. Today, many members of groups that were traditionally cohesive find themselves isolated from culturally relevant support persons (Bond & Harvey, 1991; Lipson & Steiger, 1996) and are challenged to establish meaningful ties in merged, blended, or widely disparate families or support systems. Rapid increases in the populations of older adults have led to ethnogerontology: the study of relationships between culture and age and their impact on physical and mental well-being as elders' contexts, roles, prestige, and patterns of social interaction patterns (Ahmed, 1997; Dewit, Wister, & Burch, 1988; Estes & Linkins, 2000; Fry, 1990; Myerhoff & Simic, 1978; Oakley & Potter, 1997; Sokolovsky, 1985,1990).

Traumatic societal and personal events also affect mental health. Painful separations, torture, loss, sudden death, bereavement, uncertainty, and violence have made posttraumatic stress syndrome a general diagnostic category for persons of any age and any traumatic background (Eisenbruch, 1992; Schultz-Ross, 1997). Noninvasive expressive therapies such as therapeutic writing are increasingly used for treating posttrauma problems (Pennebaker, 1999). Although approaches to self-disclosure vary widely with cultural orientation (Francis & Pennebaker, 1992; Friedman, 1996; Pennebaker, Mayne, & Francis, 1997), the results have been positive among diverse groups. There is also increasing evidence that techniques borrowed from traditional Chinese medicine are useful in circumstances (such as treatment of drug addiction and intractable pain) in which Western biomedicine has not proved adequate to resolve mental health problems (Bensky & Gamble, 1993; Lao, 1999; Smith, Squires, Aponte, et al., 1982). Hypnosis is another form of treatment that is increasingly valuable in treating hard-to-manage psychosomatic conditions, such as obesity (Kirsch, Montgomery & Sapirstein, 1995; Levitt, 1993; Wickramaseker, 1999).

• MENTAL HEALTH BELIEFS AND PRACTICES OF SPECIFIC CULTURAL GROUPS AND SUBPOPULATIONS

In the early part of the 20th century, the goal was to Americanize the many peoples already in the United States, along with those who came from all over the world to make their homes in this country. They were expected to learn English and to become as much a part of the dominant culture as they could, which often meant compromising or even giving up their original cultures (Patterson, 2001; Scott, 2001). During this time, many minority groups in Canada also experienced similar pressures to assimilate. For example, to promote the incorporation of Indians into mainstream Canadian society, the Indian Act of 1876 defined nearly every aspect of Indian life and placed many restrictions on these people. Furthermore, until as recently as 1962, Canadian immigration policy favored European immigrants over those from Asia and other developing countries. This favoritism was based on the notion that immigrants from European countries could assimilate with greater ease and speed into mainstream Canadian Society (Li, 1999). Times have changed. As the new millennium opens, people from diverse ethnic and other backgrounds are expecting, demanding, and considered deserving of opportunities to preserve their various lifestyles, beliefs, and practices. Ethnicity and ethnic identity are viewed as relational and dialogic, multilayered and multifaceted, and dialectic in terms of the historical tension in the United States and Canada between cultural **assimilation** and cultural pluralism (Winkelman, 2001). Some people find the trend toward increased diversity (particularly recognition of ethnic, racial, and gender-oriented groups) threatening. Others view it as an opportunity to help North American society live up to its democratic ideals (Wali, 1992). In any event, this transition is occurring, and nurses must be prepared to care for this diverse population.

Many differences in mental health care needs are attributable to ethnic variation (Comas-Diaz & Griffith, 1988; Ho, 1987; Neighbors & Jackson, 1996), although it must be remembered that there is significant diversity within each group as well as between groups, and that many people cross groups, identifying with and belonging to several. Another important factor is that some peoples are very traditional in their views, whereas others are more acculturated and modern. There can be great variation within groups and even within families. Despite the limitations imposed because ethnic categories are not mutually exclusive in a diverse society, it is useful for transcultural nurses to be aware of the generalized patterns associated with those aggregates, who represent increasingly large proportions of the total population—but it must be remembered that the variability within each group is tremendous.

Blacks

Distinguished from others who come to the United States from the Caribbean islands or from Africa, Blacks today are very diverse. Centuries of discrimination in a predominantly "White" culture has perpetuated a focus on differences and leaves "Blacks" and "Whites" artificially divided and many people of color without access to culturally congruent mental health resources. Various ethnopsychiatric innovations have helped fill the need (Fontenot, 1994). More recent and more respectful mainstream mental health efforts have drawn attention to Black resilience and strengths, and away from association of difference with psychopathology (Neighbors & Jackson, 1996; Ruiz, 1990). Contemporary Blacks often remain enthusiastic about religion and spirituality, are characterized as adaptable and bicultural (that is, able to function in two worlds, one Black and one White, which requires considerable effort and energy), and typically value work and education despite a history of limited opportunity to acquire or use those institutions. Traditionally, strong networks extended beyond households to multiple collateral relationships. Expectations for culturally congruent care among Blacks generally include general concern for one another (the "brothers and sisters") (Leininger, 1984). In a society in which dark skin rendered people socially invisible for centuries (Baker, 2001), genuine respect and acknowledgment are essential to acceptable care (Evidence-Based Practice 10–2).

Black folk medicine, traditionally not separated into mental and physical components, contains elements of various origins (Fontenot, 1994; Snow, 1993). In addition to a strong and adaptive knowledge of the use of herbs, early 19th-century Haitian slaves rebelling against French masters brought with them a form of voodoo (a blend of European Roman Catholicism and African tribal religions with modified aspects of humoral pathology). This spread through the Protestant American south and assimilated practices from 17th- and 18th-century European occultism, probably because of the insistence on using English rather than African languages (Foster & Anderson, 1978). Reflecting its multiple origins, Black folk medicine today provides widely var-

EVIDENCE-BASED PRACTICE 10–2
Race and the History of Race Continue to Influence Relationships Today

Centuries of slavery, discrimination, and fear of unequal treatment by members of the dominant culture result in a collective psychology that requires special sensitivity, knowledge, and skills. Known as historical hostility, this phenomenon may be expressed as hostility, hopelessness, and a paranoid perception of discrimination in cross-racial encounters with health care providers. Members of Black and other groups may manifest such a response pattern, particularly if they are from cultures that were formerly oppressed by colonization.

Managing historical hostility starts with recognition that a client is both a unique individual and a member of a historically oppressed group. Although everyone deserves equal opportunities for culturally congruent care, care must also be specific to patterns of reaction and outlooks on reality. In psychiatry, as in the rest of health care, one size does *not* fit all! It is important to remember that there is a wide variation within any group. The effective transcultural psychiatric nurse realizes that the defensiveness known as historical hostility may or may not be manifested by clients. If it is anticipated, it can be recognized and managed. However, if it is expected, the nurse may project defensiveness that generates client resistance.

CLINICAL APPLICATION

Accept and work with the fact that some Black clients will be hostile toward White, middle-class health care professionals who are likely to be perceived (and to inadvertently behave) as privileged.

Recognize that although the client is a unique person with special attributes, he or she may also have patterns of reaction and outlooks that reflect a historical oppression. If hostility is recognized, it can be recognized and managed in the milieu of the therapeutic relationship.

Mental health professionals must be accepting and sensitive to cultural variations in their clients, and willing to explore clients' perceptions of "White" culture.

Cultural influences on stress and coping constitute important information for dealing with mental health problems, and these cultural influences should be understood by the culturally competent nurse.

Vontress, C. E., & Epp, L. R. (1997). Historical hostility in the African American client: Implications for counseling. *Journal of Multicultural Counseling and Development, 25,* 170–184.

ied terms and methods, including, for example, "root" medicine, "rootwork," "mojo," "conjuring," "voodoo," and "hoodoo." There remains a tendency to bring to the health care situation a mixture of somatic, psychologic, and spiritual problems (Capers, 1985; Snow, 1993).

In traditional Black belief systems, diseases may stem from causes that are natural or spiritual in nature (e.g., punishment for sins or violation of sacred beliefs) (Wood, 1989). The causes of disease may be viewed as natural (such as failure to protect the body against inclement weather) or unnatural (for instance, divine punishment for sin) and tend to represent a perspective that holds the world to be a dangerous and hostile place. The individual is traditionally viewed as being vulnerable to outside attack and dependent on outside help (Savitt, 1978; Snow, 1977, 1993). This perspective was reinforced by nearly three centuries of slavery and then another century of struggle for full rights.

North American Indians

There are more than 500 different Native American and Alaskan Native tribes and nations. Also referred to as American Indians, First Nations, Amerindians, or Indigenous Americans, and variously including or excluding Native Hawaiians, some indigenous groups in the United States are recognized by the federal government and others at only the state or local level (Brace & Nelson, 2001). Similarly, in Canada there are many different categories and titles applied to native peoples. For example, aboriginal peoples, North American Indians, and status and nonstatus Indians are terms commonly used in Canada to identify native peoples in both legal and social terms (Li, 1999). It is important to know individual and group preferences for being called Native American or North American Indian; there is no one correct label. Most native peoples with tribal affiliations identify with tribal names (for instance, Cree, Cherokee, Lakota, Mi'kmaq, or Navajo) rather than with the pan-Indian collective terms (Native American, Native Canadian, or North American Indian).

Most indigenous populations in the Americas shared a traditional orientation to being in the present (rather than to doing and to the future, which is more typical of European North Americans), to cooperation rather than competition, to giving rather than keeping, and to respect for age rather than youth (Attneave, 1982; Brant, 1990). Traditionally, the life cycle emphasizes rhythmic, natural phenomena aimed at a balance between living and working toward achieving Indian goals; self-development is never completed. Noninterference is valued, and behaviors that imply manipulation or control may be offensive (Biolsi, 2001; Brant, 1990) (Figure 10-2). The astute clinician makes sure that the North American Indian client is aware of the consequences of behavior but then leaves it to the individual to decide how to proceed. Silence and a conservative show of interest (including, for example, minimizing eye contact) are respectful, caring behaviors.

The potential for personal confusion is obvious in a situation where mainstream society devalues most of the concepts integral to traditional Native North American philosophies and ideologies. North American Indian ideas about health and illness place less emphasis on dysfunction of the body than is typical of biomedicine, and more on relationships within society. For many Indians, health typically denotes a special, balanced relationship between humankind and its physical, relational, and supernatural environment. Illness implies having fallen out of balance and harmony with the world.

Traditional self-care prevention measures may include religious or traditional magical elements (for example, burning herbs or candles, wearing

Figure 10–2. Cultural groups honor life stages in diverse ways. Here tobacco ties and sage, circular in form to reflect unity, mark a traditional Lakota grave.

amulets, reciting prayers, or making offerings) (McKenna, 1989). Although the prevalence of alcohol and drug use varies by tribe and by age within tribes (as it does within other groups, such as European North Americans, Latinos, and Blacks [Singer, 2001]), Native North Americans tend to have higher rates of alcoholism than those experienced by other groups. Associated phenomena include high suicide rates among the young, domestic (spouse and child abuse) violence (Baker, 1988; Myers, 1990; National Forum on Health, 1997), and homicide (Bell, 1990). However, many tribes today pride themselves on their increasing social pride, their tribal stability and sovereignty, and their rates of sobriety that are markedly higher than in the past.

Stress-producing socioeconomic situations accompanied by psychologic, cultural, and spiritual stressors lead to perceptions of loss and depression. Those who are least acculturated to White society and who have strong tribal identities often tend to have the fewest problems, whereas those living in two seemingly contradictory societies are greatly challenged. Group therapies with an emphasis on society have been found to be especially useful for treatment (Giago, 1984). Often they are family-network therapy and traditional Indian group talking (such as talking circles) and purification therapies such as ritual sweats (DuBray, 1992; Lewis, 1990; Manson, Walker, & Kivlahan, 1987; Vogel, 1970).

Hispanic Americans

Generally, the terms "Latino" and "Hispanic" refer to Spanish ethnicity, language skills, and ancestry, but they also imply significant cultural variation. Some common themes among Hispanic Americans include Roman Catholicism (although increasing numbers of Hispanics are turning to Protestant religions and Pentecostal sects), orientation toward extended family systems (which may include godparents [*compadres*] and other nonbiologic kin), distinctly different roles for men and women, a high value of respect for self and others, the priority of spiritual and humanistic over commercial values, clear hierarchy and patriarchy, and fairly common reliance on folk systems of medicine. Because Hispanic Americans tend to value being listened to and having time spent with them, task-oriented hurrying about is viewed as uncaring. Involvement, loving, and empathy are valued caring behaviors (Leininger, 1984). There is a wide variability in levels of **acculturation** (that is, integration into the mainstream European American system). Although the average Mexican American was born in the United States, and many members of other Hispanic groups are American by birth, numerous others are immigrants.

Latin American folk medicine, despite some variation by place and group, clearly reflects its humoral antecedents as well as Roman Catholic ritual and beliefs about supernatural influences. Many illnesses, whether predominantly physical or mental, are "hot" or "cold," based on a long tradition of humoral theory. These qualities do not refer to temperature but to symbolic properties. Ill persons are treated with medicines and foods of opposite characteristics. By understanding the hot/cold interpretations to which specific patients or groups ascribe, care and treatment regimens can be negotiated with patients within that framework.

Asian North Americans

North Americans of Asian ancestry represent numerous diverse cultures from Japan, China, Korea, India, the Philippines and other Pacific islands, and southeast Asia. Education and hard work have paid off for many Asian immigrants, although the "Asian success story" and assumptions of an extension of "White privilege" to Asian immigrants (Goode, 1998) fail to take into account that there are many poor Asian North Americans (despite relatively low rates of dependence on public assistance and welfare) and that a notable discrepancy between education level and income persists.

Strong Asian values generally involve harmonious interpersonal relationships, webs of obligation, and fear of shame (which is a social concept, in contrast to the Westernized notion of guilt, which is more individualized) (Waxler-Morrison, Anderson, & Richardson, 1990; Shon & Ja, 1982). The family and its honor are of great importance, and family sharing is a major construct in care. Respect—especially for family, elders, and those in authority—is seen as vital. Respect is expressed through recognition of family members and in listening to and valuing their input (Leininger, 1984; Waxler-Morrison et al., 1990).

Reciprocity and generosity are highly valued; disruptive and conflict situations are viewed as uncaring (Leininger, 1984).

Traditional Asian health care practices include such varied preventive strategies as worshiping gods and ancestors and striving for balance in all aspects of life (Burnside, 1988). The goal of balance also permeates all culturally congruent treatments. Asian societies share a tradition of Chinese medicine (which is more general than Western medicine because it has a single unifying theoretic basis and has been around for more than 4,000 years) as well as of shamanism. There is a strong reliance on Chinese medicine for specific problems and for prevention (Lao, 1999). Traditional healers draw on biologic, psychologic, social, and ecologic evidence to diagnosis conditions arising from disruptions in the client's life. For example, the patient's brain and body may be out of balance, and the patient's relationships with past lives, ancestors, and destiny may be disturbed in some way (Kuo & Kavanagh, 1994; Ratanakul, 1999). Inappropriate behavior may leave the patient vulnerable to problems stemming from traditional categories of brain collapse, ancestral vengeance, and interference from evil spirits and people. Communication is viewed as fundamental to the healer–patient relationship.

Traditional Chinese have characteristic ways of dealing with mental illness in the family, starting with a protracted period of intrafamilial coping with even serious psychiatric illness, followed by recourse to friends, elders, and neighbors in the community; consultation with traditional specialists, religious healers, or general physicians; and finally treatment from Western specialists. Although it may conflict with Western practices of multiple dosage in tablet or capsule form, many Asians prefer to use over-the-counter drugs that come in liquid form as well as in single doses, as was typical of liquid preparations in Chinese folk practices (Rempusheski, 1989). Others believe that only injections will be effective.

Like traditional Chinese medicine, with which it has much in common, classic Ayurvedic medicine is rooted in the mists of antiquity in the Indian subcontinent. Yoga, an important aspect of Ayurvedic medicine, promotes a balanced flow of energy that has great appeal to members of diverse groups, not only those from Asia.

For many Asian North Americans, the forces of tradition, with their holistic and complete (including mental health and stability) therapeutic systems, are entangled with those of modernization. Traditionally, most care has been provided within families despite the shame associated with mental illness; the strains and changes of recent urbanization and industrialization have led to increasingly diverse lifestyles and a need to discard stereotypes of well-satisfied, well-cared for, and respected ill persons and elders (Hirayama, 1985–86; Lee, 1985–86; Moon & Pearl, 1991) (Evidence-Based Practice 10–3).

Middle Eastern Cultural Groups

In recent decades, the United States and Canada have experienced an influx of peoples from Middle Eastern and Northern African cultures. This has increased the traditionally Judeo-Christian North American awareness of the

EVIDENCE-BASED PRACTICE 10–3
Mental Health Care for Asian and Pacific Islander Americans

Demographically, the category "Asian and Pacific Islander Americans" includes more than 40 different cultural groups. What they share in common is either ancient or recent roots in Asia. Asians are so often described as "model" or "successful" minorities that actual problems experienced by individuals, families, and subgroups may be overlooked or minimized. Levels of acculturation vary widely. The families of some Asian Americans have been in the United States for four or more generations; others may be new immigrants. Generally, more acculturated peoples tend to higher levels of mental health-seeking behaviors. Ancestral values and language patterns also differ greatly. Training to increase cultural competence is important for mental health practitioners.

CLINICAL APPLICATION

Explore with the client just how he or she views himself or herself culturally. For example, how does the individual client "name" his or her culture?

Ask the client to describe his or her culture for you and to explain cultural characteristics for your benefit.

Understand that by the act of seeking mental health care, your client is probably more acculturated than others of the same cultural group.

Organize a training session at your work site, and invite members of the local Asian and Pacific Islander communities to come and talk with you about themselves and their cultures.

Sandhu, D. S. (1997). Psychocultural profiles of Asian and Pacific Islander Americans: Implications for counseling and psychotherapy. *Journal of Multicultural Counseling and Development, 25,* 7–22.

complex cultural beliefs, values, and lifeways of members of predominantly (but not exclusively) Islamic societies. Despite considerable cultural diversity among Middle Eastern peoples (Meleis, Lipson, & Paul, 1992), generally shared value orientations include Moslem (Muslim or Islamic) submission and obedience to God and prescribed rituals of prayer and washing. Strict concepts of what is allowed and forbidden (that is, clean and unclean, good and bad) impose important dietary and other rules that should be verified and accommodated as much as possible in health care situations. Class, status, education, modesty, and emotional expression are generally valued. Patriarchy and the centrality of religion typify Middle Eastern social and familial organizations. Elders are honored, gain in status, and, interestingly, tend not to experience the senility common in more youth-oriented cultures (Luna, 1989).

Oriented traditionally to the present, some Middle Easterners may not value making plans, because the future is seen as neither uncertain nor preordained but as something that one accepts with fatalistic grace (Jalali, 1982; Waxler-Morrison et al., 1990). Nursing research indicates that Egyptian, Yemeni, Iranian, Armenian, and Arab immigrants who are more traditional in social integration, cultural attitudes, and family orientation tend to have less positive morale than those who are more acculturated (Meleis, Lipson, & Paul, 1992).

Since the terrorist attacks on the World Trade Center in New York City and the Pentagon in Washington, D.C., on September 11, 2001, many Arab Americans have experienced a backlash of bias, distrust, and hate crimes. Such a backlash can negatively affect their mental health. In response, many Arab Americans have been active in helping dispel negative images of their culture and in educating the public about Islam and the contributions of Arab Americans to American life. Many Americans have also shown an increased interest in learning about Islam and its history.

• THE APPEAL OF ALTERNATIVE SYSTEMS

Folk and popular systems of health care continue to serve, to a greater extent than is often recognized by mental health (or other health) personnel, to smooth harsh cultural gaps between traditional societies and the predominant North American systems. They are available in every North American city, do not require going to unfamiliar places or being seen by people who are strangers, and are readily understandable to someone socialized to the group. Folk systems are also simply organized, relative to biomedical health care systems, and relatively devoid of intimidating and invasive testing, technology, lengthy history taking (which often seems irrelevant to patients and families), and dubious diagnostic procedures designed to rule out rather than ascertain specific phenomena. Interpersonal, social, and kinship relationships are emphasized in traditional or folk systems of healing, rather than the isolated individual. Traditionally, a focus on groups has minimized the discomfort associated with unaccustomed attention to individuals outside the context of the family.

Traditional systems of understanding illness and healing are experienced as more humanistic than scientific, and are usually less mechanized, less urbanized, and less intellectualized than is biomedicine, with its focus on fixing dysfunctional components, limits in access and expectations regarding use, and dependence on rationality and efficiency to such an extent that emotional needs may be overlooked. For example, in some traditional cultures, the person who is mentally ill is labeled as "possessed by the devil." Because this disturbance and society's labeling are associated with the culture's religious system, the appropriate healing or "cure" is to include the religious leader in an attempt to cast out the devil through the use of prayer or other religious intervention, such as exorcism.

The use of psychiatric resources may be discouraged by professionals' intolerance for magical and religious orientations and practices, which is common when science and systems of symbolic beliefs and faith compete.

However, multiple systems of healing may be used while the professional system is simply not aware of the pluralistic practices. Interest in traditional healing beliefs and practices is in no way limited to immigrant or indigenous groups. Today, North Americans of every ethnic heritage are expressing an increased interest in alternative or complementary health and healing traditions.

• CULTURALLY COMPETENT NURSING CARE FOR CLIENTS WITH MENTAL HEALTH CONSIDERATIONS

Transcultural nurses use many ways of understanding to move beyond the rigidity of trying to fit diverse experiences, interpretations, and expectations into a few ready-made (but culture-bound) categories. All cultural groups share time-honored systems of health beliefs and practices; it is often nurses who can interpret expectations between groups. Sensitive cultural interviews are required to know who clients are. Nursing, to provide culturally congruent care, attends to relationships between the self and others; between mental illness and such phenomena as poverty, suffering, violence, chronic illness, and aging; between the cultures of nursing and psychiatry and those of our clientele; and between nursing ethics and the provision of appropriate care. When nurses and clients come from different cultural backgrounds, accurate diagnosis, treatment, and care depend on time-consuming special knowledge and skills (Benner, Tanner, & Chesla, 1996; Lipson & Steiger, 1996; Westermeyer, 1987).

Transcultural nursing may involve collecting information about specific cultures; acquiring a culturally acceptable ally or advocate for the client and/or a cultural consultant for the nurse; working with a translator; learning clients' behavioral, attitudinal, and cognitive norms; or ensuring that only culturally fair psychometric tests are used (Geller, 1988). Standardized tests are appropriate only when they are properly modified to fit a client's cultural heritage and experiences. Some transcultural nurses view culture brokering (bridging, linking, or mediating between groups that differ in background or orientation) as part of their roles (Jezewski, 1990, 1993; LaFargue, 1985). Ideally, this is done with information from the client's perspective; the nurse serves merely to facilitate the opportunity to be heard. Other transcultural nurses define their responsibility more in terms of expediting situations in which clients can do their own negotiating.

Because psychopathology occurs at roughly the same rate in every society (Hughes, 1990; Tseng & Streltzer, 1997; World Health Organization, 1973), it stands to reason that a transcultural perspective is essential to appropriate mental health and psychiatric nursing care. The value of psychiatry is questionable if cultural relevance is limited to middle-class Europeans and European North Americans (Kleinman, 1988). In its current thinking, ethnopsychiatry, which involves culture-specific constructions of psychiatric systems (Devereux, 1980), attempts to move beyond the assumption that Western ways of understanding and treating psychiatric conditions are universally applicable. Instead, mental health and mental illness are understood within the cultural contexts in which they develop (Gaines, 1992; Tseng & Streltzer, 1997). Nursing faces the same challenge; ethnonursing methods foster understanding of care-related phenomena from the perspectives of the people who experience the culture and the phenomena (Leininger, 1991).

It is essential for clients to feel accepted if they are to share with health care providers what they believe and practice outside the biomedical system. This will not happen if clients are left to assume that their beliefs and activities are not of interest to health care providers or will be rejected by them. It may be important, however, to know what the patient or client believes and does to minimize the possibility of harm from treatments or medicines that interact disadvantageously with those of the alternative systems. Although it is dangerous to assume that all indigenous approaches are innocuous, many practices are harmless, whether or not they are effective cures. Often treatments (and the contexts in which they are experienced) provide valuable psychologic support and, because of that contribution, should not be discouraged.

Assumptions that coping patterns of clients and patients are or should be similar to those of nurses (and others socialized to the health care system) can simplify care. However, differences may be overlooked in efforts to avoid time-consuming complications. The risk involved in such behavior is that clients and health care providers may work with different strategies or toward dissimilar goals. The nurse, for example, may hurry to include all items relevant to health promotion for high-risk clients, when it is the nurse's presence and the time spent with them that the clients value, rather than the information.

The two largest consumer groups of mental health care today are the chronically, seriously mentally ill and the aged. New care management and case management strategies are making significant inroads with both populations. The field of geropsychiatric nursing will require more and more skilled psychiatric nurses in the future, for work with both the elderly and their caregivers. Nurses are increasingly involved in rehabilitative training, resocialization programs, partial hospitalization centers, and support groups in addition to one-to-one relationships. Hospital admissions have become increasingly brief, despite increased acuity and the management problems that it presents. Most clients with diagnoses of chronic schizophrenia and other major psychiatric illnesses can receive maintenance care psychotropic drugs in community and ambulatory settings (Franks & Faux, 1990). Psychiatric and mental health nurses function as liaisons among clients, health care facilities, and families (Baldwin, 1993). As such, they can facilitate effective integration of multiple belief systems, or they can impose preset expectations that lead to interventions oriented toward the practitioner's and health care system's values and goals rather than the client's.

Nurses sometimes question how they can learn all the relevant characteristics of the clients they care for (they cannot, and they should not try) and why they should know about group patterns when it is individuals with whom they work. The important task is to ascertain a client's cultural orientation and what it means to him or her (or them, given that many nurses work with fam-

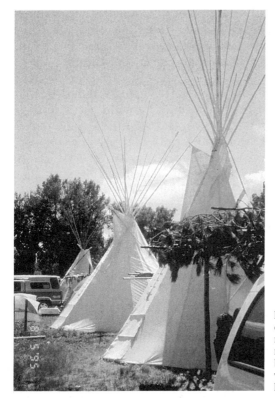

Figure 10–3. Traditional peoples bring cultures together in contemporary life in many ways. Ideally, individuals with more than one cultural affiliation can bring parts of each culture together without conflict. Tipis at a Lakota Nation Powwow, Pine Ridge, South Dakota.

ilies or other groups). It is not a matter of matching clients to their reference groups, but of learning about and understanding the actual relationships involved. It is, for example, more useful and accurate to ask "How is this client Norwegian or Lutheran?" than to ask "How Norwegian or Lutheran is this client?" (see Figure 10–3.)

The former question allows comparison of the answer against the expectable patterns (that is, generalizations about Norwegians and Lutherans), whereas the latter question seeks a match between the client and stereotypic standards for his or her reference groups. Always, easy stereotypes should be avoided: "Chinese do this and Latinos do that." Stereotypes simply cannot be depended on to work effectively. Although every group has discernible patterns that help distinguish it from other groups, most individuals also express beliefs or traits that do not match the group norm. One may be very traditional in one aspect and quite modern in others. When people are ill, they sometimes become more traditional in their expectations and thinking. There is also significant variation within and between groups. Knowledge of the group is valuable inasmuch as it provides a set of realistic expectations. However, only by learning about the individual or family at hand can the clinician understand in what ways the group patterns are meaningful.

Before 1950, psychiatric services in the United States were provided primarily at state hospitals (Mollica, 1983). Today, most patients hospitalized in the United States with a primary psychiatric diagnosis are treated in general hospitals, and many of them occupy beds scattered throughout various areas rather than in designated psychiatric units (Gorman, Sultan, & Raines, 1996; Summergrad, 1991). Likewise, many of Canada's large tertiary care psychiatric facilities have closed, and psychiatric patients now receive care in alternative institutional and/or community-based settings. This means that many nurses who do not particularly identify with care of the mentally ill are exposed to that population. Another reason it is important for nurses to be culturally sensitive, knowledgeable, and skillful is that they are instrumental in the export of mental health concepts to other societies (e.g., Stanley, 1993). Nurses educated in the United States and Canada work throughout the world, as well as with people who come to North America from elsewhere. We must be aware of our potential as communicators of more than we intend.

Assessment

The realization that perspectives are shaped by specific values and beliefs rooted in specific cultures and subcultures allows objective assessment of diverse practices that people use to promote health and cope with illness. Whether or not they are understood, people have reasons for their behavior. They may, for example, refuse to have blood drawn because of a belief that it could be used for sorcery or, as was traditionally believed in Asian societies, that blood contains the personality. It does not make sense to risk personality loss or disruption through exchange of blood or other organs. On the other hand, it may make sense for clients to alter their medication dosages when they believe that the "big" European North American physicians who prescribe medicines are likely to order too large a dose for someone of smaller stature (Goode, 1993). Likewise, the appreciation that one person's "superstition" may be someone else's firmly held explanation or belief allows the culturally competent nurse to objectively consider the behavior associated with that belief for its own merit, neutrality, or harm. Automatic discrediting of ideas or practices because they are unfamiliar, "old-fashioned," or not scientific risks the alienation of clients as well as the loss of potentially useful resources (Evidence-Based Practice 10–4).

Cross-Cultural Communication

The crux of transcultural psychiatric/mental health nursing is communication, the style of which varies greatly with the culture involved. Some of these differences are quickly evident, as is the contrast that appears when mental health practitioners expect a degree of openness, verbosity, self-disclosure, emotional expression, and insight that reflect the dominant Western culture (Tripp-Reimer, 1984; Young, 1988) rather than the client's orientation, which may be very different. Groups also vary widely in their ideas about appropriate stance, gestures, language, listening styles, and eye contact. Traditional Asian, Blacks, Native North Americans (Wood, 1989), and Appalachian people (Tripp-Reimer, 1984) typically consider direct eye contact inappropriate and disrespectful.

EVIDENCE-BASED PRACTICE 10-4
There Are Many Views of the History of Psychiatric and Mental Health Care

Oral histories have been collected as data for several books on the history of psychiatric and mental health nursing. Interviews of staff or former staff reveal opinions, attitudes, feelings, and practices of care. One wonders why the recollections of former patients are not collected as well as those of the staff. However, it is race and ethnicity that the author addresses, noting that "Differences of ethnic origin, surprisingly, do not seem to have been much discussed, in spite of the many different nationalities of nurses working at various times in the hospital" (p. 493). Russell speculates that the notable racial mix among both nurses and physicians may have facilitated tolerance and acceptance within the setting. Although that may be the case, other research has suggested that race, ethnicity, and gender issues may actually be avoided in psychiatric settings (Kavanagh, 1991). Culturally competent nurses realize that diversity-related issues can play important parts in communication, relationships, mental health, and mental illness. It is questionable, therefore, whether a care setting can truly be therapeutic if such issues are not openly and comfortably discussed.

CLINICAL APPLICATION

Issues related to diversity-such as race, ethnicity, and gender-must be identified, and health care professionals must make an effort to move beyond such issues. They can best do this by openly identifying the issues and discussing them with colleagues. Such a discussion calls for openness and sensitivity with other health care providers as well as with clients.

Russell, D. (1997). An oral history project in mental health nursing. *Journal of Advanced Nursing 26*, 489–495.

With the increasingly complex variety of languages used in the United States and Canada (Statistics Canada, n.d.; Urciuoli, 2001), the creation of linguistic boundaries is often prompted by the belief that there is a single standard English that should be used. Because language differences can cause mental health treatment to take much longer and be more complicated than treatment for English-speaking patients (Sherer, 1993), it is sometimes tempting to use the most readily available person to facilitate the process. However, dependence on family members (or unprepared others, such as a passing janitor or available food handler) to translate may only complicate the situation. Particularly when the patient and translator are not of the same sex, class, or age, the use of inappropriate translators may result in new problems being fabricated to avoid stating the real ones in front of the individual solicited to translate. It is important when using a translator to communicate with the client with a mental health condition that extra time be allowed to discuss the client's responses. For example, the nurse might want to ask the translator to be alert to nonverbal cues, such as body language, eye contact, or other behavior that would provide helpful information. Although linguistic assistance is vital, further difficulties arise when some translators interpret rather

BOX 10–2	**INFORMATION BOX**

AT&T's Language Line Services offers translations in nearly 150 languages. Call (800) 752-6096 to learn more about this service. You might want to share the information you learn with the local mental health facility.

than directly translate what the client says. The nurse unfamiliar with the language may not realize whose views are being expressed (Box 10-2).

Transcultural nursing care of mental health patients requires four primary transcultural communication skills (Kavanagh & Kennedy, 1992; Pedersen, 1985, 1988) (Figure 10–4). The first is the ability to understand and state an issue or problem as it is perceived from the client's perspective. It is important that sincere (not patronizing) interest be taken in the client's views and experiences, and that they be taken seriously. The second and third skills involve recognizing and reducing resistance and defensiveness, which directly impede the development of productive relationships between nurses and clients and further contribute to the basis for negative attitudes and labels such as "noncompliance." The fourth transcultural communication skill involves the recognition that everyone makes interactive mistakes from time to time.

Communicating with culturally diverse mental health patients requires testing stereotypes against reality. If one stereotypes all psychiatric patients

Figure 10–4. Effective cross-cultural communication skills are particularly important when caring for mental health patients. Developing lasting meaningful relationships across potential social barriers such as race contributes to improved communication.

EVIDENCE-BASED PRACTICE 10-5
"Lunatics" and the Moon: Nature and Madness, or Just a Phase?

For centuries (at least since Hippocrates posited the relationship some 2,500 years ago) people have associated increases in violence and aggression in psychiatric patients with the full moon. Over time, this came to be known as the Transylvanian effect. Research examined the use of seclusion in various phases of the moon as a way of investigating the relationship (if any) between the moon and madness. Seclusion, in various forms, is used universally for disturbed patients and in psychiatric settings for the control and management of violence and aggression. If the Transylvanian effect actually occurs, there should be a demonstrable relationship between lunar cycles and the use of seclusion. Although staff members may use seclusion when they fear that they or others may be in danger and thus may be hypervigilant during the full moon (whether or not the moon has any effect on patients' behavior), no such correlation was found between the full moon and use of seclusion for the mentally ill.

CLINICAL APPLICATION

Seclusion, in various forms and used universally for centuries, may be used appropriately when mental health professionals believe they are in danger from a client's violent and aggressive behavior.

Violent behavior in clients is sometimes triggered by such factors as noncompliance with medication, stress, or other events in the clients' environment, rather than the full moon.

Mason, T. (1997). Seclusion and the lunar cycles. *Journal of Psychosocial Nursing, 35*(6), 14–18.

as dangerous, for example, the generalization does not accurately represent the high proportion of patients who are not (Evidence-Based Practice 10–5). When cognition and affect are impaired by mental illness, communication can be especially time-consuming and complex, although it is no less important. Assumptions must be avoided. Unusual use of language may, for example, represent cultural differences rather than thinking or hearing impairments, although those explanations might also be valid. The skilled communicator learns how to identify and bridge differences.

Mutual communication involves awareness and knowledge of social process, and sensitivity to and recognition of barriers to acceptance and sharing, as well as skill in communication techniques. Whereas the functional utility of words and gestures have communicative value to all involved (Choi, Kim & Choi, 1993), most important is the ability to empathize—that is, to understand others' beliefs, assumptions, perspectives, and feelings (Pedersen, 1985, 1988). The effective communicator learns to acquire and to understand, to the greatest extent possible, multiple perspectives. Tolerance and acceptance of others' attitudes, beliefs, and behaviors, and the willingness to expose oneself as interested but still learning sensitivity, knowledge, and skills are important strategies.

Self Reflection and Awareness

Learning to understand the cultures of clients requires learning about your own cultural orientation and about yourself. "The one who would change others must himself be changed" (Milio, 1970). The culture of the nurse interacts with those of clients. It is important to realize that culture includes the values and norms learned in the process of becoming a nurse (or a member of any other group) as well as those associated with ethnicity, age, class, or gender background. Understanding who we are requires close examination of one's own orientation to recognize where one's own sense of personal and social identity comes from and how it was formed. Ask yourself what kind of person you were socialized to be, and how your social identity has changed and is changing. Culture is never static.

Such self-knowledge is critical to realizing which cultures or groups one tends to favor or avoid, and which groups one negatively or unrealistically positively stereotypes. Such blind spots (that is, biases) can keep one from considering, for example, that a "nice, middle-class grandmother" might also be a much conflicted lesbian woman who is addicted to cocaine. Each of us has attitudinal limitations that obscure facts from our consideration and vision. With whom do you feel strange and uncomfortable, and why? How do your concerns and biases affect who gets care and what type of care you give? It is well known that there are cultural preferences among mental health care providers for clients who are young, attractive, verbal, intelligent, and successful (also known as YAVIS) (Wilson & Kneisl, 1983), whereas those who are considered quiet, unattractive, old, indigent, different, and stupid (that is, the QUOIDS) often get less attention.

Commitment to transcultural nursing assumes the recognition and value of human dignity, cultural relativism (that is, the idea that all perspectives deserve respectful consideration) as an acceptable and preferred philosophy, willingness to alter personal behavior in response to the cross-cultural interactive process, and willingness to monitor personal resistance and defensiveness. Consider how you feel about those criteria.

People may avoid professional mental health care because of incompatible values and beliefs, poverty, social stresses that occur among special populations but are not well understood by professionals, language barriers, lack of education, social isolation, stigma, bureaucratic barriers, and the unequal distribution of services. It is crucial that the nursing process be examined from the cultural perspectives of health care providers *and* consumers to maximize appropriate use and quality of care. Then, care can be provided by informed practitioners in ways that are perceived as both acceptable and appropriate (Evidence-Based Practice 10–6).

Culture-Specific Care

It may be tempting to avoid close examination of basic values and beliefs because they seem amorphous, complex, or too intimate. However, a grasp of the concepts of normality, abnormality, ethnocentrism, relativism, pluralism,

EVIDENCE-BASED PRACTICE 10–6
Urban/Rural Differences Are Important Too

When major depressive disorders occur in rural areas where few professional mental health treatment resources exist and clients may be hard to access and treat, effective psychosocial interventions must be adapted for specific populations. A primary care setting providing screening, diagnostic care, brief treatment, and follow-up care can produce a significant reduction in symptoms, improved functional ability of clients, and programs of relapse prevention. This was done in the rural Piedmont area of the South by training generalist nurses with psychoeducational skills to work with a culturally competent advanced practice psychiatric nurse and by designing a program for specific care needs. Field testing and evaluation of the program for rural women in the area studied indicated that a combination of self-care skills (including self-assessment, stress reduction, and health behavior modification) and minimum psychiatric resources can create a promising and powerful partnership.

CLINICAL APPLICATION

Rural clients can be treated effectively in primary care settings in their own communities. These services should include screening and diagnostic and brief treatment services. Follow-up services can be provided as needed. This model has been shown to improve the functional ability of clients and reduce their symptoms.

Nurses can be trained to provide culturally competent psychiatric services in rural areas.

Self-care skills that can be taught to rural women include self-assessment, stress reduction, and health behavior modification. These practices can decrease symptoms in clients who live in hard-to-access rural areas.

Hauenstein, E. J. (1997). A nursing practice paradigm for depressed rural women: The women's affective illness treatment program. *Archives of Psychiatric Nursing, 1,* 37–45.

---

stereotyping, prejudice, and discrimination provides a basis for understanding how society handles differences in attitude and behavior. Social ranking (that is, social stratification) and its consequence, social inequality, affect human experience, opportunities, and the availability, acceptability, and use of mental health care resources.

It is a myth that treating people differently because of racial, religious, ethnic, cultural, gender, or other characteristics implies prejudice and discrimination. That is an overused excuse to avoid dealing with issues that are part of social process. On the other hand, treating everyone the same in the name of justice is equally insensitive, because it too denies differences that matter to people. Failure to acknowledge diversity denies meaningful variations in real life experience. It is not necessarily irrational for the individual who has been discriminated against because of his or her skin color or language, or the woman who has been raped, to feel paranoid. On the other hand, it is painful to have one's experience (including the identity affiliations that help us understand who we are) discredited or made to seem unimportant, and situations do not go away simply because they are ignored or avoided. The sense of distancing and pain remain, and aspects of the issues may eventually surface.

In trying to satisfy the basic needs of his or her client, the transcultural nurse asks: "What do you expect (or want) the nurse to do for you?" (McKenna, 1989). In other words, "How do you want to be cared for?" Culturally congruent nursing care decisions and actions have the potential to intervene in three ways: cultural care preservation, accommodation, and repatterning (Leininger, 1988).

The need for cultural maintenance or preservation is demonstrated in Case Study 10-1. The second mode of nursing intervention involves assisting clients to negotiate or adapt new cultural ways (Leininger, 1988). As nurses become sensitive to the complex factors that influence clients' responses to care, they learn to negotiate. This mode of intervention is illustrated in Case Study 10-2. A third approach to intervention involves culturally acceptable and appropriate care that enables change to new or different behavioral patterns that are meaningful, satisfying, and beneficial (Leininger, 1988). Changing a person's view of events requires altering the meaning of the situation (Pesut, 1991). However, the need for such restructuring is less common than that for cultural preservation and negotiation, and it involves only partial behavioral repatterning. Those cultural attributes that are useful are preserved, as described in Case Study 10-3.

Ideologic Conflict in Psychiatric/Mental Health Nursing

A growing awareness of the changing and complex nature of illness, the influence of social context, and the importance of holistic perspectives can leave

CASE STUDY	10–1

A student from New Zealand came to a university mental health clinic describing chronic headaches, sleeplessness, and inability to focus on his school work. He explained that the onset of these symptoms coincided with his father's death, about which he did not learn until it was too late to return for the burial rites. Owing to his failure to be there when his mother especially needed his support, a relative "pointed a bone" at him, and that action, he believed, resulted in his present problems. A thorough assessment did not produce additional reasons for the young man's somatic complaints, decreased academic achievement, and social discomfort.

Fortunately, a clinician was located who had previously worked in the South Pacific, and she made herself available to work with both the clinic staff and the disturbed student. Together they delineated the problem, worked to understand what it would take to alleviate it, and participated in an adapted ceremony that allowed the client to believe that the effect of the bone-pointing had been neutralized. The student was at peace with the knowledge that no fault of his had caused him to miss his father's funeral. He knew that further amends for the social transgression could wait until after the successful completion of his studies. This would allow him to serve his affiliation group more effectively than would his premature return as an academic failure.

CASE STUDY	10–2

Maria, a 15-year-old Mexican American girl, was referred to the mental health clinic after a suicide attempt. Her school attendance was sporadic, her grades were poor, and she was depressed. Both parents worked outside the home, and her older brothers had moved out, leaving her as primary caretaker for several young siblings. Although she had been dating a boy for several months, her parents planned to send her to Mexico to marry a man they knew there. Soon after she argued with her family about her household chores and her future, her boyfriend ended their relationship, and the school threatened to suspend her for nonattendance. Maria cut her wrists. Verbalizing her identity and role confusion, guilt over her rejection of her family's expectations, and anger at their rejection of her viewpoint, she intensely resented her parents' and the school authorities' expectations and her limited choices.

Individual and family therapy with mental health clinical nurse specialists helped negotiate a realistic and acceptable plan that would keep Maria in school (thus increasing her life choices later) while helping her bridge the gap between traditional and more modern ways. In a group with other young women, Maria was empowered by sharing and learning that there were aspects of her culture and her circumstances that she could accept, reject, ignore, and change. She had a voice and choices that she could learn to affirm.

---

nurses in a quandary when the dominant model in psychiatry focuses on organic and genetic factors as underlying causes of mental disease (Finkler, 2000; Lutzen, 1990). For some, psychiatry's realignment toward biology, high-tech brain scans, and powerful new drugs, along with a reorientation away from staff–patient relationships and toward objective observation and documentation, threatens to minimize the importance of the patient as a person or at least to risk the sacrifice of communication and understanding to cold, hard documentation (Goode, 1988). This substitution of psychiatric materialism for

---

CASE STUDY	10–3

In an urban program designed to strengthen family processes, families were encouraged to spend social time in the program's community center. When parents were confronted in writing (as well as with oral reprimand) with the program's expectation that there would be no hitting on the premises, several families stopped coming. It was not until the staff realized the parents' need to learn alternative ways to set limits for children that those families began to feel comfortable at the center.

For many program participants, physical recourse was the only mode of discipline with which they were familiar; the no-hitting policy had been interpreted as meaning "no discipline." Parents had to learn alternative ways of dealing with disciplinary issues and with stress, and children eventually learned that their parents would be consistent in their nonphysical limit setting, that punishments would correlate with the transgression, and that the expression of caring was not limited to physical evidence. With repatterning over time, meaningful verbal and other nonphysical ways of disciplining were modeled, learned, and implemented.

humanism may lead nurses who are surrounded by others who think differently to question their ability and worth (Arena & Page, 1992), to resent psychiatry's role in social control (Brown, 1989; Morrison, 1990), or to accuse mental health nursing of a lack of critical examination of its own ideology and of those hegemonic psychiatric beliefs and practices imposed on their practice from medicine (Hopton, 1997; Horsfall, 1997).

Ideologic conflict is not new in psychiatric/mental health care and continues to shadow nurse–physician and nurse–client relationships (Kavanagh, 1988, 1991). Continued frustration with a plethora of phenomena, many of them (such as poverty and discrimination) beyond the scope of conventional medical treatment, confront public psychiatric/mental health systems. Despite the medicalization of mental health, nurses often feel that they must balance structural requirements (which may conflict) with operationalizing knowledge of care and therapy (which may be ambiguous), all the while communicating with persons who may communicate not only in culturally diverse ways but also abnormally (Bunch, 1983). All of this occurs in a society that is ambivalent toward individuals who exhibit unpopular differences. Nurses must continue to explore diverse models of caring and attend closely to the practices they actually use (Figure 10-5).

Implications for Transcultural Mental Health/Psychiatric Nursing Practice

As a practical science of caring (Bottorff, 1991), nursing strives to use strategies that lead to positive outcomes. How does the nurse incorporate cultural beliefs

Figure 10–5. Being an applied profession with a humanistic ethic, nursing grapples with tension between the outsider (etic) values of the nursing and medical subcultures (which neglect the dominant society) and an insider (emic) view reflecting the values of individuals, families, communities, and other affiliation and cultural groups for whom nurses advocate. Transcultural nursing helps bring emic perspectives together with the etic.

and practices into daily practice? Key points for the transcultural mental health nurse are summarized here, using Diekelmann's (1991, 1994, 1995) framework of "concernful practices" (Kavanagh, Absalom, Beil, & Schliessmann, 1999).

Welcoming, Gathering, and Accepting

Welcoming, gathering, and *accepting* involve creating effective relationships and establishing open communication. The nurse's role is to suggest illness prevention and health maintenance practices, as well as treatment strategies that fit with and reinforce clients' cultural beliefs and practices. Understand clients' desire to please and their motivations to comply or not to comply. Often "noncompliance" occurs because clients are trying to preserve their own priorities ("Culture clash," 1996; Morrison, 1990). Understand relationships between clients and authority, health care institutions and bureaucracies. Whenever possible and appropriate, involve significant others and leaders of relevant local groups. Confidentiality is important, but ethnic and other leaders know the issues and can often suggest acceptable interventions. Try to make the setting comfortable. Consider colors, sound, atmosphere, scheduling expectations, seating arrangements, pace, tone, and other environmental variables. Be prepared for the fact that children go everywhere with members of some cultural groups, as well as with families who do not have options because of economic limitations; include them.

Knowing, Connecting, and Staying

Knowing, connecting, and *staying* involve finding meaningful ways in which clients, families, and others can contribute their own cultural input and goals, while both patterns and variations are recognized. As nurses become more mindful of managing their own diversity, questions initiated by "Why don't they . . .?" are gradually balanced with "Why do we . . .?" often prompting ongoing discussion of various approaches and perspectives. Becoming more aware of the potency of cultural expectations as well as personal choices, all participants in cross-cultural relationships find themselves consciously setting priorities and considering options regarding what to accept, reject, ignore, or try to change.

Presencing, Attending, and Staying Open

Presencing, attending, and *staying open* are confounded with time, which continually frustrates modern health care and nursing. Routinization and efficiency are valued by the dominant culture, whereas caring, connecting, and learning take time. Visiting, sharing stories, and many other simple encounters are useful strategies for learning what care and caring mean to the client and family. Understand what members of the cultural or subcultural group consider "caring," both attitudinally and behaviorally. Ask what they would like and expect to have happen. Acquire basic knowledge about cultural values, health beliefs, and traditional health-related practices common to the group you are working with. Learn about expectations for personal hygiene, rest and sleep, ideas about health and illness, communicating and eating (Rempusheski, 1989). Language and food are important symbols; respect and use them. Also know the folk illnesses and remedies common to the cultural group with which you are working. Inquire about over-the-counter and folk remedies being used; research indicates that up to 80% of treatments used by clients are not reported because health care professionals do not ask about them (Wood, 1989). Build on cultural practices, reinforcing those that are positive; do not discredit any beliefs or practices unless you know for sure that specific practices are harmful.

Creating a Place and Keeping Open Possibilities

Creating a place and *keeping open possibilities* entail working to establish caring relationships and increasing sensitivity to our own implicit understandings and expectations. Present yourself with confidence. Shake hands if it is appropriate. Ask how clients prefer to be addressed. Allow them to choose seating for comfortable personal space and culturally appropriate eye contact. Avoid assumptions about where people come from; let them tell you. Most people are pleased when others show sincere interest in them. Strive to gain the other's trust, but do not resent it if you do not get it. Avoid body language that may be offensive or misunderstood—which may involve some research and surprises. Determine the patient's level of fluency in English, and arrange for an interpreter if one is needed. Speak directly to the client, even if an interpreter is present. Choose a speech rate and style that promotes understanding and demonstrates respect for the client. Avoid jargon, slang, and complex sentences. Do not expect clients to share your medical orientation. Use open-ended questions or questions phrased in several ways to obtain information, but be aware that some groups do not consider direct questions to be polite. Invite individuals to tell you stories about themselves and their problems. Determine the patient's English reading ability before using any written materials.

Safeguarding, Preserving, Advocating, and Protecting

Safeguarding, preserving, advocating, and *protecting* guide awareness that people tend to see what they expect to see, and that stereotypes narrow vision by ignoring variations that occur naturally. Learning about diversity and caring involve recognizing and replacing stereotypes with informed, expectable patterns that serve merely as starting points for inquiry and comparison. Advocacy roles require cultural sensitivity, knowledge, and skill—including a willingness to examine personal values and those of the subcultures of nursing and biomedicine, as well as those of other individuals and cultural groups. Negotiate goals that are explicit and realistic. Check for the client's understanding and acceptance of recommendations. Be patient; do not expect rapid change. Be sensitive when describing or writing about groups. Present a generally comprehensive perspective that emphasizes the positive over the negative. Relate social organization, structure, and process to each group's unique history. Acknowledge the diversity that occurs within as well as between and among groups. Beware of literature that uses models of deviance or pathologic conditions rather than unbiased and fair information about groups. There is much of value to be found in both classic and modern literature, but it must be used critically, owing to the propensity for bias.

Engendering Mutuality and Community

The need for *engendering mutuality* and *community* reflects ways in which health care providers and clients come together, get to know and value differences as well as commonalities, and form flexible, open, and creative relationships and caring communities. Avoid stereotypes by sex, age, race, ethnicity, socioeconomic status, and other characteristics. Remember that cultural generalizations may not differ much from stereotypes and may lead to prejudice if they are not open to being revised, that some people do not like having ethnic labels attached to them and wish to "be treated like everyone else," that culture is not restricted to people of color, that differences within groups may be greater than differences between groups, and that our own attitudes and blind spots may be more important than those of clients in terms of outcome. Understand your own cultural values and biases. Emphasize the positive points and strengths of health beliefs and practices. Be respectful of values, beliefs, rights, and practices. Express interest in and understanding of other cultures without being judgmental. Some ideas may conflict with your own or with your determination to make changes, but every group and individual wants respect above all else. Show respect, especially for male clients, even if it is the female clients or children you are particularly interested in. Men are often decision makers about health care.

Letting Be and Letting Go

Transcultural mental health nursing also necessitates an additional genre of practices that constitute *letting be* and *letting go* to expedite openness to learning. Learn to appreciate the richness of diversity as an asset rather than viewing it as a hindrance to communication and effective intervention. Honor the uniqueness of clients and their dignity and worth. Attempt to establish caring relationships that can overcome any cultural misstep, and strive to help clients obtain their self-determined goals, to learn clients' **explanatory models** (Kleinman, 1988), and to get to know yourself as an effective transcultural nurse.

REVIEW QUESTIONS

1. How has the interpretation of mental health and mental illness changed with time?
2. Describe three ways in which diversity influences mental health and mental illness.
3. How are culture and mental health integrated into other aspects of living?
4. Describe ways in which interactive processes and communication facilitate effective transcultural mental health care. How might interactive processes

and communication erect barriers to effective transcultural mental health care?

5. Describe seven strategies that nurses can use to facilitate effective transcultural mental health care.

CRITICAL THINKING ACTIVITIES

1. Write a story or a narrative about a personal experience you have had or observed in which a cultural misunderstanding occurred. Critically evaluate and discuss how you felt as an observer and how you suppose the others involved in the situation felt. Discuss how the situation might have been more effectively managed.

2. Having a family member with a severe mental illness often poses a strain on the entire family. Ask someone who has a family member with a psychiatric diagnosis to share his or her story. Critically analyze what the situation has been like for the family. An excellent model or example for this is *Imagining Robert (my brother, madness, and survival): A memoir* by J. Neugeboren (1997).

3. A great activity for pulling together cultural sensitivity, knowledge, and skills for effective transcultural mental health nursing involves interviewing someone from a culture significantly different from your own. After getting to know the person and some background, practice your communication skills to ask about ideas and practices related to mental health and illness. Then delve into the literature about that person's affiliation or cultural group(s). Whether your interviewee is from Tibet, gay, or a century old, consider (and discuss with classmates) how what you have read fails to represent (or successfully represents) the individual that you interviewed.

4. Compile a list of the groups that you affiliate with and in which you feel you are an "insider." Then list several groups with which you are not affiliated and where you would feel an "outsider." As honestly and comprehensively as you can, critically analyze why you are comfortable with some groups and not with others. If possible, get an insider's perspective of the group(s) to which you do not belong. Critically analyze the traits and attributes with which you might be comfortable (or uncomfortable). Evaluate the strengths and vulnerabilities of each group.

5. Psychiatric symptoms typically reflect the cultural orientation of the mentally ill individual. How would you manage the following situation? You realize that your next-door neighbor, a retired European North American electrical engineer, has lined the interior walls of his house with aluminum foil to protect himself against the "beams" from the neighbors on the other side of him, who are immigrants from another country and speak little English. What assessment strategies would you use to distinguish the mental health issues from confounding social and cultural issues?

6. Role play is an effective strategy for developing cultural competence. With three colleagues, simulate a cultural encounter in which each of you takes a different role: one is the client, one is the nurse who does not know what

the client's cultural background is, one is a backup for the client and can say the things that the client is thinking but might hesitate to articulate, and one is the backup person for the nurse and provides ideas for questions or approaches when the nurse is stumped. Each person can see and hear each of the others as they role-play encounters that are as realistic as possible. (Adapted from Pedersen, 1985, 1988; Kavanagh & Kennedy, 1992).

7. Effective communication involves listening attentively to people, accepting and acting on what they say, ensuring that all communication can be understood by everyone, being trustful and sincere, acting in socially and culturally appropriate ways, and regularly advising others about what is happening (Stringer, 1996). Discuss with someone you consider culturally competent how each of these criteria contributes to understanding in mental health settings.

8. The attacks on the World Trade Center and the Pentagon on September 11, 2001, have left a lasting impact on America's mental health. Discuss, in both societal and personal terms, how threats such as terrorism and other violence pose hazards to positive mental health and challenge effective coping. In what ways has society been positively as well as negatively affected?

• References

Ahmed, I. (1997). Geriatric psychopathology. In W.-S. Tseng & J. Streltzer (Eds.) *Culture and psychopathology* (pp. 223–240). New York: Brunner/Mazel.

American Psychiatric Association. (1994). *Diagnostic and Statistical Manual—Fourth Edition (DSM-IV)*. Washington, DC: American Psychiatric Association.

Anderson, R. (1996). *Magic, science, and health: The aims and achievements of medical anthropology.* Fort Worth, TX: Harcourt Brace.

Arena, D. M., & Page, N. E. (1992). The impostor phenomenon in the clinical nurse specialist role. *Image, 24*(2), 121–125.

Attneave, C. (1982). American Indians and Alaskan Native families: Emigrants in their own homeland. In M. McGoldrick, J. K. Pearce, & J. Giordano (Eds.), *Ethnicity and family therapy* (pp. 55–83). New York: Guilford Press.

Baker, F. M. (1988). Afro-Americans. In L. Comas-Diaz & E. E. H. Griffith (Eds.), *Clinical guidelines in cross-cultural mental health* (pp. 151–181). New York: John Wiley & Sons.

Baker, L. D. (2001). The color-blind bind. In I. Susser & T. C. Patterson (Eds.), *Cultural diversity in the United States: A critical reader* (pp. 103-119). Malden, MA: Blackwell.

Baldwin, A. (1993, February). Psychiatric liaison nursing: A ready help in organizational change. *American Nurse*, p. 14.

Beiser, M., Waxler-Morrison, N., Iacono, W. G., Lin, T-Y., Fleming, J. A. E., & Husted, J. (1987). A measure of the "sick" label in psychiatric disorder and physical illness. *Social Science and Medicine, 25*(3), 251–261.

Bell, C. C. (1990). Black-black homicide: The implications for black community mental health. In D. S. Ruiz (Ed.), *Handbook of mental health and mental disorder among black Americans* (pp. 192–207). New York: Greenwood Press.

Benner, P., Tanner, C. A., & Chesla, C. A. (1996). *Expertise in nursing practice: Caring, clinical judgment, and ethics.* New York: Springer.

Bensky, D., & Gamble, A. (1993). *Chinese herbal medicine: material medica.* Seattle: Eastland Press.

Bernstein, D. M. (1997). Anxiety disorders. In W.-S. Tseng & J. Streltzer (Eds.). *Culture and psychopathology* (pp. 46—66). New York: Brunner/Mazel.

Billings, C. (1993, February). The "possible" dream of mental health reform. *American Nurse*, pp. 5, 9.

Biolsi, T. (2001). Contemporary Native American struggles. In I. Susser & T. C. Patterson (Eds.), *Cultural diversity in the United States: A critical reader* (pp. 175–189). Malden, MA: Blackwell.

Bohannan, P. (1992). *We, the alien: An introduction to cultural anthropology.* Prospect Heights, IL: Waveland.

Bond, J. B., & Harvey, C. D. H. (1991). Ethnicity and intergenerational perceptions of family solidarity. *International Journal of Aging and Human Development, 33*(1), 33–44.

Bottorff, J. L. (1991). Nursing: A practical science of caring. *Advances in Nursing Science, 14*(1), 26–39.

Brace, C. L., & Nelson, A. R. (2001). The peoplings of the Americas: Anglo stereotypes and Native American realities. In I. Susser & T. C. Patterson, Eds., *Cultural diversity in the United States: A critical reader* (pp. 46–56). Malden, MA: Blackwell.

Brant, C. C. (1990). Native ethics and rules of behavior. *Canadian Journal of Psychiatry, 35,* 534–539.

Brown, D. R. (1990). Depression among blacks: An epidemiological perspective. In D. S. Ruiz (Ed.), *Handbook of mental health and mental disorders among black Americans* (pp. 71–93). New York: Greenwood Press.

Brown, D. R. (1996). Marital status and mental health. In H. W. Neighbors & J. S. Jackson (Eds.), *Mental health in black America* (pp. 77–94). Thousand Oaks, CA: Sage.

Brown, P. (1989). Psychiatric dirty work revisited: Conflicts in servicing nonpsychiatric agencies. *Journal of Contemporary Ethnography, 18*(2), 182–201.

Bunch, E. H. (1983). *Everyday reality and the psychiatric nurses: A study of communication patterns between the schizophrenic and the psychiatric nurse.* Oslo, Norway: Gyldendal Norsk Forlag.

Burnside, I. M. (1988). *Nursing and the aged.* New York: McGraw-Hill.

Campinha-Bacote, J. (1997). Understanding the influence of culture. In J. Haber, B. Krainovich-Miller, A. L. McMahon, & P. Price-Hoskins (Eds.). *Comprehensive psychiatric nursing* (5th ed., pp. 75—90). St. Louis: C. V. Mosby.

Capers, C. F. (1985). Nursing and the Afro-American client. *Topics in Clinical Nursing, 7*(3), 11–17.

Catalano, R., & Pickett, K. E. (2000). A taxonomy of research concerned with place and health. In G. Albrecht, R. Fitzpatrick, & S. Scrimshaw (Eds.), *Handbook of social studies in health and medicine.* London: Sage.

Chaplin, S. L. (1997). Somatization. In W.-S. Tseng & J. Streltzer (Eds.). *Culture and psychopathology* (pp. 67–86). New York: Brunner/Mazel.

Choi, S.-C., Kim, U., & Choi, S.-H. (1993). Indigenous analysis of collective representations: A Korean perspective. In U. Kim and J. W. Berry (Eds.), *Indigenous psychologies: Research and experience in cultural context* (pp. 193–210). Newbury Park, CA: Sage.

Christopher, J. C. (1999). Situating psychological well-being: Exploring the cultural roots of its theory and research. *Journal of Counseling & Development, 77,* 141–152.

Collins, J. L., Sorel, E., Brent, J., & Mathura, C. B. (1990). Ethnic and cultural factors in psychiatric diagnosis and treatment. In D. S. Ruiz (Ed.), *Handbook of mental health and mental disorder among black Americans* (pp. 151–165). New York: Greenwood Press.

Comas-Diaz, L., & Griffith, E. E. H. (Eds.). (1988). *Clinical guidelines in cross-cultural mental health.* New York: John Wiley & Sons.

Conrad, P., & Schneider, J. W. (1992). In *Deviance and medicalization: From badness to sickness.* Philadelphia: Temple University Press.

Culture clash: Working with a difficult patient. (1996). *American Journal of Nursing, 96*(11), 58.

Devereux, G. (1980). *Basic problems of ethnopsychiatry.* Chicago: University of Chicago Press.

Dewit, D. J., Wister, A. V., & Burch, T. K. (1988). Physical distance and social contact between elders and their adult children. *Research on Aging, 10*(1), 56–79.

Diekelmann, N. (1991). The emancipatory power of the narrative. In R. H. Schaperow (Ed.). *Curriculum revolution: Community building and activism* (pp. 41–62). New York: National League for Nursing Press. Pub. No. 15–2398.

Diekelmann, N. (1994). Madison, WI: Advanced Nursing Institute for Heideggerian Hermeneutical Studies, University of Wisconsin-Madison.

Diekelmann, N. (1995). Narrative pedagogy: Caring, dialogue, and practice. Madison, WI: Advanced Nursing Institute for Heideggerian Hermeneutical Studies, University of Wisconsin-Madison.

DuBray, W. H. (1992). *Human services and American Indians.* Minneapolis: West Publishing.

Dunst, C., Trivette, C., & Deal, A. (1988). *Enabling and empowering families.* Cambridge, MA: Brookline Books.

Eisenbruch, M. (1992). Toward a culturally sensitive DSM: Bereavement in Cambodian refugees and the traditional healer as taxonomist. *Journal of Nervous and Mental Disease, 180*(1), 8–10.

Escobar, J. I. (1987). Cross-cultural aspects of the somatization trait. *Hospital and Community Psychiatry, 38*(2), 174–180.

Estes, C. L., & Linkins, K. W. (2000). Critical perspectives on health and aging (pp. 154–172). In G. Albrecht, R. Fitzpatrick, & S. Scrimshaw, Eds., *Handbook of social studies in health and medicine.* London: Sage.

Expanding horizons of healthcare: Five year strategic plan, 2001–2005. National Center for Complementary and Alternative Medicine, National Institutes of Health, U.S. Department of Health and Human Services, 25 September 2000.

Fabrega, H. (1989). An ethnomedical perspective of Anglo American psychiatry. *American Journal of Psychiatry, 146,* 588–596.

Farberow, N. L. (1975). Cultural history of suicide. In N. L. Farberow (Ed.), *Suicide in different cultures* (pp. 1–15). Baltimore: University Park Press.

Ficarrotto, T. J. (1990). Racism, sexism, and erotophobia: Attitudes of heterosexuals towards homosexuals. *Journal of Homosexuality, 19,* 111–116.

Finkler, K. (2000). *Experiencing the new genetics: Family and kinship on the medical frontier.* Philadelphia:

University of Pennsylvania Press.

Fontenot, W. L. (1994). *Secret doctors: Ethnomedicine of African Americans*. Westport, CT: Bergin & Garvey.

Foster, G. M., & Anderson, B. G. (1978). *Medical anthropology*. New York: John Wiley & Sons.

Francis, M. E., & Pennebaker, J. W. (1992). Putting stress into words: Writing about personal upheavals and health. *American Journal of Health Promotion, 6,* 280–287.

Frank, G. (2000). *Venus on wheels: Two decades of dialogue on disability, biography, and being female in America*. Berkeley: University of California Press.

Franks, F., & Faux, S. A. (1990). Depression, stress, mastery, and social resources in four ethnocultural women's groups. *Research in Nursing and Health, 13,* 283–292.

Friedman, M. J. (1996). PTSD diagnosis and treatment for mental health clinicians. *Community Mental Health Journal, 32,* 173–189.

Fry, C. L. (1990). Cross-cultural comparison of aging. In K. F. Ferraro (Ed.), *Gerontology: Perspectives and issues.* New York: Springer.

Gaines, A. D. (1992). *Ethnopsychiatry: The cultural construction of professional and folk psychiatries*. Albany: State University of New York Press.

Geller, J. D. (1988). Racial bias in the evaluation of patients for psychotherapy. In L. Comas-Diaz & E. E. H. Griffith (Eds.), *Clinical guidelines in cross-cultural mental health* (pp. 112–134). New York: John Wiley & Sons.

Giago, T. (1984). *Notes from Indian country* (Vol. 1). Pierre, SD: State Publishing Company.

Goleman, D., & Gurin, J. (1993). M*ind body medicine*. Yonkers, NY: Consumer Reports.

Goode, E. E. (1988, March 21). How psychiatry forgets the mind. *U.S. News and World Report, 56–58.*

Goode, E. E. (1993, February 15). The cultures of illness. *U.S. News and World Report, 74–76.*

Goode, J. (1998). The contingent construction of local identities: Koreans and Puerto Ricans in Philadelphia. *Identities, 5,* 33–64.

Gorman, L. M., Sultan, D. F., & Raines, M. L. (1996). *Davis's manual of psychosocial nursing for general patient care*. Philadelphia: F. A. Davis.

Gutiérrez, E. C. Z., & Kendall, C. (2000). The globalization of health and disease: The health transition and global change. In G. Albrecht, R. Fitzpatrick, & S. Scrimshaw (Eds.), *Handbook of social studies in health and medicine* (pp. 84–99). London: Sage.

Harrison, P. (1997). Suicidal behavior. In W.-S. Tseng & J. Streltzer (Eds.). *Culture and psychopathology* (pp. 157–172). New York: Brunner/Mazel.

Hauenstein, E. J. (1997). A nursing practice paradigm for depressed rural women: The women's affective illness treatment program. *Archives of Psychiatric Nursing, 1,* 37–45.

Health Canada (1999). Canadian research on immigration and health. Available at: MACROBUTTON HtmlResAnchor http://www.hc-sc.gc.ca/iacb-dgiac/nhrdp/metropolis/cirh_pdf_index_e.htm. Accessed November 23, 2001.

Heiligenstein, E. (1999, April 1). Balancing patient needs: Prescriptions for mental health. *The Integrative Medicine Consult, 1*(6): 54.

Helman, C. G. (1990). *Culture, health and illness*. London: Wright.

Henry, W. A. (1990, April 9). Beyond the melting pot. *TIME,* pp. 28–29.

Hirayama, H. (1985—86). Public policies and services for the aged in Japan. *Journal of Gerontological Social Work, 9,* 39–52.

Ho, M. K. (1987). *Family therapy with ethnic minorities.* Newbury Park, CA: Sage.

Hopton, J. (1997). Towards a critical theory of mental health nursing. *Journal of Advanced Nursing, 15,* 492–500.

Horsfall, J. (1997). Psychiatric nursing: Epistemological contradictions. *Advances in Nursing Science, 20*(1): 56–65.

Hughes, C. (1990). Ethnopsychiatry. In T. M. Johnson & C. F. Sargent (Eds.), *Medical anthropology: A handbook of theory and method* (pp. 133–148). New York: Greenwood Press.

Jackson, J. J. (1990). Suicide trends of blacks and whites by sex and age. In D. S. Ruiz (Ed.), *Handbook of mental health and mental disorder among black Americans* (pp. 95–109). New York: Greenwood Press.

Jalali, B. (1982). Iranian families. In M. McGoldrick, J. K. Pearce and J. Giordano (Eds.), *Ethnicity and family therapy* (pp. 289–309). New York: Guilford Press.

Jezewski, M. A. (1990). Culture brokering in migrant farm worker health care. *Western Journal of Nursing Research, 12,* 497–513.

Jezewski, M. A. (1993). Culture brokering as a model for advocacy. *Nursing and Health Care, 14*(2), 78–85.

Joralemon, D. (1999). *Exploring medical anthropology.* Boston: Allyn and Bacon.

Kavanagh, K. H. (1988). The cost of caring: Nursing on a psychiatric intensive care unit. *Human Organization, 47*(3), 242–251.

Kavanagh, K. H. (1991). Invisibility and selective avoidance: Gender and ethnicity in psychiatry and psychiatric nursing staff interaction. *Culture, Medicine and Psychiatry, 15,* 245–274.

Kavanagh, K. H., & Kennedy, P. H. (1992). *Promoting cultural diversity: strategies for health care professionals.* Newbury Park, CA: Sage.

Kavanagh, K.H., Absalom, K., Beil, W., & Schliessmann, L. (1999). Connecting and becoming culturally competent: A Lakota example. *Advances in Nursing Science, 21*(3), 9–31.

Kiev, A. (1972). *Transcultural psychiatry.* New York: Free Press.

Kim, Y. Y., & Gudykunst, W. B. (1988). *Cross-cultural adaptation: Current approaches.* Newbury Park, CA: Sage.

Kirsch, I., Montgomery, G., & Sapirstein, G. (1995). Hypnosis as an adjunct to cognitive-behavioral psychotherapy: A meta-analysis. *Journal of Consult Clinical Psychology 63*(2), 214–220

Kleinman, A. (1988). *Rethinking psychiatry: From cultural category to personal experience.* New York: Free Press.

Kleinman, A. (1991, March 28). "The future psychiatry." Baltimore, MD: Special Department of Psychiatry Grand Rounds, University of Maryland Medical System.

Kleinman, A., & Seeman, D. (2000). Personal experience of illness. In G. Albrecht, R. Fitzpatrick, & S. Scrimshaw, Eds., *Handbook of social studies in health and medicine* (pp. 230–242). London: Sage.

Kottak, C. P. (2000). *Anthropology: The exploration of human diversity.* Boston: McGraw-Hill.

Kral, M. J. (1998). Suicide and the internalization of culture: Three questions. *Transcultural Psychiatry 35*(2), 221–233.

Kuo, C-L., & Kavanagh, K. H. (1994). Chinese perspectives on culture and mental health. *Mental Health Nursing, 15*(6), 551–567.

LaFargue, J. (1985). Mediating between two views of illness. *Transcultural Nursing, 7,* 70–77.

Lao, L. (1999). Traditional Chinese medicine. In W. B. Jonas & J. S. Levin, Eds., *Essentials of complementary and alternative medicine* (pp. 277–313). Philadelphia: Lippincott Williams & Wilkins.

Lee, J. J. (1985–86). Asian American elderly: A neglected minority group. *Journal of Gerontological Social Work, 9,* 103–116.

Leininger, M. (1984). Transcultural interviewing and health assessment. In P. B. Pedersen, N. Sartorius, & A. J. Marsella (Eds.), *Mental health services: The cross-cultural context* (pp. 109–133). Beverly Hills, CA: Sage.

Leininger, M. M. (1988). Leininger's theory of nursing: Cultural care diversity and universality. *Nursing Science Quarterly, 1*(4), 152–160.

Leininger, M. M. (1991). Ethnonursing: A research method with enablers to study the theory of culture care. In M. M. Leininger (Ed.), *Culture care diversity and universality: A theory of nursing* (pp. 73–117). New York: National League for Nursing Press. Pub. No. 15–2402.

Levinson, D. (1989). *Family violence in cross-cultural perspective.* Newbury Park, Sage.

Levitt, E. E. (1993). Hypnosis in the treatment of obesity. In J. W. Rhue, S. J. Lynn, & I. Kirsch, Eds., *Handbook of clinical hypnosis* (pp. 511–532). Washington, DC: American Psychological Association.

Li, P. S. (Ed.)(1999). *Race and ethnic relations in Canada* (2nd ed.). New York: Oxford University Press.

Lewis, Thomas. (1990). *Medicine men: Oglala Sioux healing.* University of Nebraska, Lincoln, NE.

Lex, B. (1977). Voodoo death: New thoughts on an old explanation. In D. Landy (Ed.), *Culture, disease and healing: Studies in medical anthropology* (pp. 327–332). New York: Macmillan.

Lipson, J. G. (1996, fourth quarter). Come all peoples of the earth. *Sigma Theta Tau International Reflections, 9*–10.

Lipson, J. G., & Steiger, N. J. (1996). *Self-care nursing in a multicultural context.* Thousand Oaks, CA: Sage.

Littlewood, R. (1991, April). DSM-IV and culture: Is the classification valid? Paper presented at the NIMH/American Psychiatric Association meeting, Pittsburgh, PA.

Lock, M. (2000). Accounting for disease and distress: Morals of the normal and abnormal. In G. Albrecht, R. Fitzpatrick, & S. Scrimshaw, Eds., *Handbook of social studies in health and medicine* (pp. 259–276). London: Sage.

Locke, D. C. (1992). *Increasing multicultural understanding: A comprehensive model.* Newbury Park CA: Sage.

Luna, L. J. (1989). Transcultural nursing care of Arab Muslims. *Journal of Transcultural Nursing, 1*(1), 22–26.

Lutzen, K. (1990). Moral sensing and ideological conflict. *Scandinavian Journal of the Caring Sciences, 4*(2), 69–76.

Manson, S. P., Walker, R. D., & Kivlahan, D. R. (1987). Psychiatric assessment and treatment of American Indians and Alaskan Natives. *Hospital and Community Psychiatry, 38*(2), 165–173.

Marmor, T. R. (1994). *Understanding health care reform.* New Haven: Yale University Press.

Mason, T. (1997). Seclusion and the lunar cycles. *Journal of Psychosocial Nursing 35*(6), 14–18.

Matteson, P. S. (1995). *Teaching nursing in the neighborhoods: The northeastern university model.* New York: Springer.

McCubbin, H. I., & McCubbin, M. A. (1988). Topologies of resilient families: Emerging roles of social class and ethnicity. *Family Relations, 37,* 247–254.

McElroy, A., & Jezewski, M. A. (2000). Cultural variation in the experience of health and illness. In G. Albrecht, R. Fitzpatrick, & S. Scrimshaw, Eds., *Handbook of social studies in health and medicine* (pp. 191–209). London: Sage.

McKenna, M. A. (1989). Transcultural perspectives in the nursing care of the elderly. In J. S. Boyle & M. M. Andrews (Eds.), *Transcultural concepts in nursing care.* Glenview, IL: Scott, Foresman.

Meleis, A. I., Lipson, J. G., & Paul, S. M. (1992). Ethnicity and health among five Middle Eastern immigrant groups. *Nursing Research, 41*(2), 98–103.

Milio, N. (1970). *9226 Kercheval: The storefront that did not burn.* Ann Arbor: University of Michigan Press.

Minson, R. (1999). Integrating mind/body medicine into

conventional practice. *The Integrative Medicine Consult 1*(15), 144.

Mollica, R. F. (1983). From asylum to community. *New England Journal of Medicine, 308*(7), 367–373.

Moon, J.-H., & Pearl, J. H. (1991). Alienation of elderly Korean American immigrants as related to place of residence, gender, age, years of education, time in the U.S., living with or without children, and living with or without a spouse. *International Journal of Aging and Human Development, 32*(2), 115–124.

Morrison, E. F. (1990). The tradition of toughness: A study of nonprofessional nursing care in psychiatric settings. *Image, 22*(1), 32–38.

Moyers, B. (1993). *Healing and the mind.* New York: Doubleday.

Myerhoff, B. G., & Simic, A. (Eds.). (1978). *Life's careers–aging: Cultural variations on growing old.* Beverly Hills, CA: Sage.

Myers, L. J. (1990). Understanding family violence: An Afrocentric analysis based on optimal theory. In D. S. Ruiz (Ed.), *Handbook of mental health and mental disorder among black Americans* (pp. 183–189). New York: Greenwood Press.

National Forum on Health (1997). *The need for an aboriginal health institute in Canada: The situation of aboriginal peoples.* Ottawa, ON: Health Canada Communications. Available at: http://wwwnfh.hc-sc.gc.ca/publicat/finvol2/aborig/situat.htm. Accessed February 7, 2002.

Neighbors, H. W., & Jackson, J. S. (1996). *Mental health in black America.* Thousand Oaks, CA: Sage.

Neugeboren, J. (1997). *Imagining Robert (my brother, madness, and survival): A memoir.* New York: William Morrow.

Nguyen, M. N., & Organista, K. C. (1997). Vietnam Amerasians: Assimilation and adjustment problems in the United States. *Journal of Multicultural Social Work, 6*(1/2), 77–91.

Oakley, L. D., & Potter, C. (1997). *Psychiatric primary care.* St. Louis: C. V. Mosby.

Oltmanns, T. F., & Maher, B. A. (1988). *Delusional beliefs.* New York: John Wiley & Sons.

Ory, F. G., Simons, M., Verhulst, F. C., Leenders, F. R. H., & Wolters, W. H. G. (1991). Children who cross cultures. *Social Science and Medicine, 32*(1), 29–34.

Pang, K. Y. C. (1994). Understanding depression among elderly Korean immigrants through their folk illnesses. *Medical Anthropology Quarterly, 8*(2), 209–216.

Pang, K. Y. (1995). A cross-cultural understanding of depression among elderly Korean immigrants: Prevalence, symptoms and diagnosis. *Clinical Gerontologist 15*(4), 3–20.

Parker, S. (1977). Eskimo psychopathology in the context of Eskimo personality and culture. In D. Landy (Ed.), *Culture, disease and healing: Studies in medical anthropology* (pp. 349–358). New York: Macmillan.

Patterson, T. C. (2001). Class and historical process in the United States (pp. 16–28). In I. Susser & T. C. Patterson (Eds.), *Cultural diversity in the United States: A critical reader.* Malden, MA: Blackwell.

Pedersen, P. (Ed.). (1985). *Handbook of cross-cultural counseling and therapy.* Westport, CT: Greenwood Press.

Pedersen, P. (Ed.). (1988). The three stages of multicultural development: Awareness, knowledge, and skill. In *A handbook for developing multicultural awareness* (pp. 3–18). Alexandria, VA: American Association for Counseling and Development.

Pennebaker, J. W. (1999). The effects of traumatic disclosure on physical and mental health: The values of writing and talking about upsetting events. *International Journal of Emergency Mental Health* (Winter) Vol. 1, No. 1, pp. 9–18.

Pennebaker, J. W., Mayne, T. J., & Francis, M. E. (1997). Linguistic predictors of adaptive bereavement. *Journal of Personality and Social Psychology 72*, 863–871.

Pesut, D. J. (1991). The art, science, and techniques of reframing in psychiatric mental health nursing. *Issues in Mental Health Nursing, 12*(9), 9–18.

Pinderhughes, E. (1982). Afro-American families and the victim system. In M. McGoldrick, J. K. Pearce, & J. Giordano (Eds.), *Ethnicity and family therapy* (pp. 108–122). New York: Guilford Press.

Pert, C. B., Dreher, H. E., & Ruff, M. R. (1998). The psychosomatic network: Foundations of mind-body medicine. *Alternative Therapies, 4*(4): 30–41.

Poussaint, A. F. (1990). The mental health status of black Americans, 1983. In D. S. Ruiz (Ed.). *Handbook of mental health and mental disorder among black Americans* (pp. 17–52). New York: Greenwood Press.

Ratanakul, P. (1999). Buddhism, health, disease, and Thai Culture. In H. Coward & R. Ratanakul (Eds.), *A cross-cultural dialogue on healthcare ethics* (pp. 17–33). Waterloo, ON: Wilfrid Laurier University Press.

Remen, R. N. (1996). *Kitchen table wisdom: Stories that heal.* New York: Riverhead Books.

Rempusheski, V. F. (1989). The role of ethnicity in elder care. *Nursing Clinics of North America, 24*(3), 717–724.

Rin, H., & Huang, M. (1989). Neurasthenia as nosological dilemma: Special issue: Neurasthenia in Asian cultures. *Culture, Medicine and Psychiatry, 13*(2), 215–226.

Robert, S. A., & House, J. S. (2000). Socioeconomic inequalities in health: Integrating individual-, community-, and societal-level theory and research. In G. Albrecht, R. Fitzpatrick, & S. Scrimshaw, Eds., *Handbook of social studies in health and medicine* (pp. 115–135). London: Sage.

Rohland, B. (1995). A survey of utilization of psychiatrists in community mental health centers in Iowa. *Psychiatric Services, 46*, 81–3.

Rose, S. M., & Black, B. L. (1985). *Advocacy and empowerment: Mental health care in the community.* Boston: Routledge & Kegan Paul.

Rothenberg, P. S. (1988). *Racism and sexism: An integrated study.* New York: St. Martin's Press.

Rubel, A. J. (1977). The epidemiology of a folk illness. In D. Landy (Ed.), *Culture, disease and healing: Studies in medical anthropology* (pp. 119–129). New York: Macmillan.

Russell, D. (1997). An oral history project in mental health nursing. *Journal of Advanced Nursing, 26,* 489–495.

Ruiz, D. S. (Ed.). (1990). *Handbook of mental health and mental disorder among black Americans.* New York: Greenwood Press.

Sabatino, F. (1993, May 20). Culture shock: Are U.S. hospitals ready? *Hospitals,* pp. 23–28.

Sanday, P. R., & Goodenough, R. G. (Eds.). (1990). *Beyond the second sex: New directions in the anthropology of gender.* Philadelphia: University of Pennsylvania Press.

Sandhu, D. S. (1997). Psychocultural profiles of Asian and Pacific Islander Americans: Implications for counseling and psychotherapy. *Journal of Multicultural Counseling and Development 25,* 7–22.

Savitt, T. L. (1978). *Medicine and slavery: Blacks in the New World.* Urbana: University of Illinois Press.

Scheper-Hughes, N. (1978). Saints, scholars, and schizophrenics: Madness and badness in Western Ireland. *Medical Anthropology, 2,* 59–93.

Scheper-Hughes, N. (1982). Recent works in cultural psychiatry. *Medical Anthropology Newsletter, 13*(3), 1–2, 6–11.

Scheper-Hughes, N. (Ed.). (1987). The cultural politics of child survival. *Child survival* (pp. 1–29). Dordrecht, Holland: D. Reidel.

Schultz-Ross, R. A. (1997). Violent behavior. In W.-S. Tseng & J. Streltzer (Eds.). *Culture and psychopathology* (pp. 173–189). New York: Brunner/Mazel.

Scott, E. M. (2001). The roots of U.S. inequality. In I. Susser & T. C. Patterson, Eds., *Cultural diversity in the United States: A critical reader* (pp. 155–174). Malden, MA: Blackwell.

Secundy, M. G. (1992). *Trials, tribulations, and celebrations: African-American perspectives on health, illness, aging and loss.* Yarmouth, ME: Intercultural Press.

Sherer, J. L. (1993, May 20). Crossing cultures: Hospitals begin breaking down the barriers to care. *Hospitals,* 29–31.

Shon, S. P., & Ja, D. Y. (1982). Asian families. In M. McGoldrick, J. K. Pearce, & J. Giordano (Eds.), *Ethnicity and family therapy* (pp. 208–228). New York: Guilford Press.

Siegrist, J. (2000). The social causation of health and illness. In G. Albrecht, R. Fitzpatrick, & S. Scrimshaw, Eds., *Handbook of social studies in health and medicine* (pp. 100–114). London: Sage.

Singer, M. (2001). Health, disease and social inequality. In I. Susser & T. C. Patterson (Eds.), *Cultural diversity in the United States: A critical reader* (pp. 76–100). Malden, MA: Blackwell.

Smith, M. O., Squires, R., Aponte, A., et al. (1982). Acupuncture treatment of drug addiction and alcohol abuse. *American Journal of Acupuncture, 10*(2), 161–163.

Snow, L. F. (1977). Popular medicine in a black neighborhood. In E. H. Spicer (Ed.), *Ethnic medicine in the southwest* (pp. 19–95). Tucson, AZ: University of Arizona Press.

Snow, L. F. (1993). *Walkin' over medicine.* Boulder, CO: Westview.

Sokolovsky, J. (1985). Ethnicity, culture and aging: Do differences really make a difference? *Journal of Applied Gerontology 4*(1), 6–17.

Sokolovsky, J. (Ed.). (1990). *The cultural context of aging: Worldwide perspectives.* New York: Bergin & Garvey.

Stanley, S. (1993, February). Bringing mental health care to Russia. *American Nurse,* pp. 12, 14.

Statistics Canada (n.d.) 1996 Census nation tables: Population by knowledge of official language. Available at: MACROBUTTON HtmlResAnchor http://www.statcan.ca/english/Pgdb/People/Population/demo19a.htm. Accessed November 16, 2001.

Stringer, E. T. (1996). *Action research: A handbook for practitioners.* Thousand Oaks, CA: Sage.

Summergrad, P. (1991). General hospital impatient psychiatry in the 1990s: Problems and possibilities. *General Hospital Psychiatry, 13,* 79–82.

Susser, I. (2001). Cultural diversity in the United States. In I. Susser & T. C. Patterson (Eds.), *Cultural diversity in the United States: A critical reader* (pp. 3–15). Malden, MA: Blackwell.

Takeshita, J. (1997). Psychosis. In W.-S. Tseng & J. Streltzer (Eds.), *Culture and psychopathology* (pp. 124–138). New York: Brunner/Mazel.

Thomas, R. R. (1991). *Beyond race and gender: Unleashing the power of your total work force by managing diversity.* New York: American Management Association.

Tripp-Reimer, T. (1984). Cultural diversity in therapy. In C. M. Beck, R. P. Rawlins, and S. R. Williams (Eds.), *Mental health–psychiatric nursing: A holistic life-cycle approach* (pp. 381–398). St. Louis: C. V. Mosby.

Tseng, W.-S. (1997). Overview: Culture and psychopathology. In W.-S. Tseng & J. Streltzer (Eds.). *Culture and psychopathology* (pp. 1–27). New York: Brunner/Mazel.

Tseng, W.-S., & Streltzer. J. (1997).Integration and conclusions. In W.-S. Tseng & J. Streltzer (Eds.), *Culture and psychopathology* (pp. 241–252). New York: Brunner/Mazel.

United States Department of Health and Human Services. (2001). *Healthy people 2000.* Arlington, VA: CACI Marketing Systems.

Urciuoli, B. (2001). The complex diversity of language in the United States. In I Susser & T. C. Patterson (Eds.),

Cultural diversity in the United States: A critical reader (pp. 190–205). Malden, MA: Blackwell.

Uzzell, D. (1977). Susto revisited: Illness as strategic role. In D. Landy (Ed.). *Culture, disease and healing: Studies in medical anthropology* (pp. 402–408). New York: Macmillan.

Vogel, V. J. (1970). *American Indian medicine.* Norman: University of Oklahoma.

Vontress, C. E., & Epp, L. R. (1997). Historical hostility in the African American client: Implications for counseling. *Journal of Multicultural Counseling and Development, 25,* 170–184.

Wali, A. (1992). Multiculturalism: An anthropological perspective. *Report from the Institute for Philosophy and Public Policy* (University of Maryland College Park), *12*(1), 6–8.

Waxler-Morrison, N., Andrews, J., & Richardson, E. (1990). *Cross-cultural caring: A handbook for health professionals in Western Canada.* Vancouver, BC: University of British Columbia Press.

Weidman, H. (1979). Falling out: A diagnostic and treatment problem viewed from a transcultural perspective. *Social Science and Medicine, B13*(2), 95–112.

Westermeyer, J. (1987). Clinical considerations in cross-cultural diagnosis. *Hospital and Community Psychiatry, 38*(2), 160–165.

Wickramaseker, I. (1999). Hypnotherapy. In W. B. Jonas & J. S. Levin (Eds.), *Essentials of complementary and alternative medicine* (pp. 120–138). Philadelphia: Lippincott Williams & Wilkins.

Wilson, H. S., & Kneisl, C. R. (1983). *Psychiatric nursing.* Reading, MA: Addison-Wesley.

Winkelman, M. (2001). Ethnicity and psychocultural models. In I. Susser & T. C. Patterson (Eds.), *Cultural diversity in the United States: A critical reader* (pp. 281–301). Malden, MA: Blackwell.

Wood, J. B. (1989). Communicating with older adults in health care settings: Cultural and ethnic considerations. *Educational Gerontology, 15,* 351–362.

World Health Organization. (1973). *The international pilot study in schizophrenia.* Geneva, Switzerland: WHO.

Yap, P. M. (1977). The culture-bound reactive syndromes. In D. Landy (Ed.), *Culture, disease and healing: Studies in medical anthropology* (pp. 340–349). New York: Macmillan.

Young, J. C. (1988). Rationale for clinician self-disclosure and research agenda. *Image, 20*(4), 196–199.

Culture, Family, and Community

Joyceen S. Boyle

OBJECTIVES

1. Use cultural concepts to provide care to families, communities, and aggregates.
2. Understand the necessary components of a cultural assessment of an aggregate group.
3. Explore interactions of community and culture as they relate to concepts of community-based practice.
4. Analyze how cultural factors influence health and illness of groups.
5. Critically evaluate potential health problems and solutions in refugee and immigrant populations.
6. Assess factors that influence the health of diverse groups within the community.

An understanding of culture and cultural concepts enhances the nurse's knowledge and facilitates culturally competent nursing care in **community settings.** Currently, many nurses practice in community settings with clients from a wide variety of cultural backgrounds, and this trend is expected to increase, with more nurses moving from acute-care institutions to community settings. In addition, it is predicted that cultural diversity will increase in the United States and Canada. Trends in the health care delivery system as well as an increased emphasis on health promotion and disease prevention have influenced nurses to make changes in their nursing practice. Concepts such as partnership, collaboration, empowerment, and facilitation now form the basis for community-based nursing practice with individuals, families, and **aggregates** in the community. However, a word of caution is in order. Just because services are provided in a community setting does not mean they are community based. **Community-based services** "require active involvement of clients and communities in assessing the needs for care, designing service programs, implementing interventions, and evaluating outcomes" (National Institute of Nursing Research, 1995, p. 2).

Community-based services are built on collaboration and partnerships between community leaders, consumers, and providers. When community residents are involved as partners, community-based services are more likely to be responsive to locally defined needs, are better used, and are sustained through local action. Federal, state, and provincial agencies as well as private foundations are increasingly requiring broad-based public and private collaboration and partnerships as prerequisites for funding of community-based services (Flynn, 1997; National Institute of Nursing Research, 1995). This implies a sustained collaboration between the public and private sectors as well as the people most directly affected by a health concern or problems (Huff & Kline, 1999).

Community-based services are complex and often fragile. They require a high level of nursing knowledge and skills in working with and relating to different individuals and groups. In many instances, the complexity is increased when clients and their families come from diverse cultures. Nurses must understand how to help persons from various cultures work with community leaders and health care providers to form partnerships that are responsive and can structure health care in ways that are culturally sensitive and appropriate. It is often the cultural factors that determine whether a particular population or group will choose to participate in community-based health services. There is always a need for continuing communication among health care providers and community residents that is characterized by mutual understanding and respect.

In this chapter, the terms **community nursing**, **community-based nursing**, and **community health nursing** are used interchangeably, even though they have different meanings in some settings and in different contexts. Whether the nurse is employed as a community health nurse in a health department or practices in a community-based setting, he or she needs the ability to provide culturally competent care. The practice of nursing in a community setting requires that nurses be comfortable with clients from diverse cultures and the broader socioeconomic context in which they live. In the current health care climate of economic restraints, the health care industry has focused on cost effectiveness, but such a focus is tempered with positive outcomes. Care that is not congruent with the client's value system is likely to increase the cost of care because it compromises quality. Furthermore, members of diverse cultural groups, such as officially designated minority groups in the United States, tend to experience more health problems than do members of the general population. This was the impetus for targeting the four ethnic minority groups in *Healthy People 2000* (U.S. Department of Health and Human Services, 1990) and *Healthy People 2010* (U.S. Department of Health and Human Services, 2000), because cultural diversity must be respected and taken into account by health care professionals. Equally important, we must address the stark disparities that exist in health status between minority groups and the wider North American society. Indeed, reducing inequities is the number one health challenge identified in Canada's *Framework for Health Promotion* (Health Canada, 2001, October 11).

•OVERVIEW OF CULTURALLY COMPETENT NURSING CARE IN COMMUNITY SETTINGS

Nurses practice in many setting within the community, including worksites, schools, health care program sites, churches, and the community itself (Figure 11-1). The use of **cultural knowledge** in community-based nursing practice begins with a careful assessment of clients and families in their own environments. Cultural data that have implications for nursing care are selected from clients, families, and the environment during the assessment phase and are discussed with the client and family to develop mutually shared goals.

Community nurses are particularly challenged when they frequently encounter clients and families who must change behaviors and living pat-

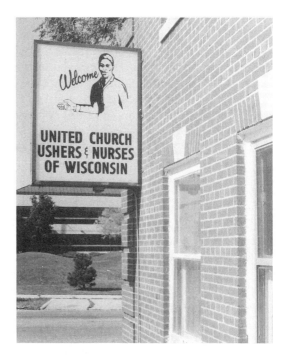

Figure 11–1. Some Black churches are organized to meet health, social, and emotional needs of church members.

terns to maintain health or promote wellness. Nursing interventions based on cultural knowledge help clients and families to adjust more easily and assist nurses to work effectively and comfortably with all clients, especially those from different cultural backgrounds. An appreciation of cultural factors enhances family support of the client and the family's acceptance of nursing goals that have been developed collaboratively with the client and family.

Cultural data are important in the care of all clients; however, in community nursing, they are a prerequisite to successful nursing interventions. Community nursing is practiced in a community setting, often in the home of the client, and frequently requires more active participation by the client and family. Usually, the client and family must make basic changes in lifestyle, such as changes in diet and exercise patterns. Cultural competence requires that the nurse understand the family lifestyle and value system, as well as those cultural forces that are powerful determinants of health-related behaviors. This competency assists the client and family to plan and cope with changes in activities of daily living. Nurses often monitor clients with chronic diseases or other health problems over a long time, and nursing interventions must include aspects of counseling and education as well as anticipatory guidance directed toward helping clients and families adjust to what may be lifelong conditions. Nursing care must take account of the diverse cultural factors that will motivate clients to make successful changes in behavior, because improvement in health status requires lifestyle and behavioral modifications.

Transcultural nursing practice improves the health of the community as well as the health of individual clients and families. Additional considerations of the nurse who is involved in community-focused planning are the health needs of populations at risk. Special at-risk groups can be found in all communities: the homeless, the poor, persons with HIV/AIDS and/or tuberculosis, refugees, prison populations, and even the elderly are groups at risk for decreased health status. From a community standpoint, an understanding of culture and cultural concepts will increase the skill and abilities of the nurse to work with diverse groups within the community. Identification of high-risk groups and appropriate community-based strategies to reduce health risks requires considerable knowledge about cultural and ethnic groups and their place in the community.

Consider, if you will, what problems might arise if one were to design a health program for a community composed primarily of Hmong who recently arrived in the United States or Canada. Certainly language would be a major problem, but so could many other cultural differences, from nuances in communication to differences in beliefs of what constitutes health and illness, as well as treatment and cure. A failure to understand and deal with these differences would have serious implications for the success of any health or nursing intervention. Nurses who have knowledge of, and an ability to work with, diverse cultures are able to devise effective community interventions to reduce risks that are consistent with the community, group, and individual values and beliefs of community members.

• A TRANSCULTURAL FRAMEWORK

A distinguishing and important aspect of community-based nursing practice is the nursing focus on the community as the client (Clark, 1996; Stanhope & Lancaster, 2000). Effective community nursing practice must reflect accurate knowledge of the causes and distribution of health problems and of effective interventions that are congruent with the values and goals of the community. An epidemiologic model is used by the community nurse to collect, organize, and analyze information about high-risk groups that are encountered in community practice.

An **epidemiologic model** emphasizes human biology, environment, lifestyle, and the health care system; however, with modifications, the nurse can use this model to collect cultural data that influence the health of the community (Clark, 1996). The epidemiologic model focuses on the community or on aggregate groups rather than on individuals or families. Using a cultural overlay with the epidemiologic model enhances nurse–community interactions in numerous ways.

Identifying Subcultures and Devising Specific Community-Based Interventions

A transcultural framework for nursing care helps the nurse to identify **subcultures** within the larger community and to devise community-based interventions that are specific to community health and nursing needs. In the multicultural societies of the United States and Canada, it is common to speak of "the Black community," "the Hispanic community," or "the Francophone community." We might also speak more broadly of "the immigrant community" or of other unique groups within or near a local community. A cultural focus allows this variety and facilitates data collection about specific groups based on their health risks. A cultural/epidemiologic framework facilitates a view of the community as a complex collective yet allows for diversity within the whole. Interventions that are successful in one subgroup may fail with another subgroup of the same community, and often the failure can be attributed to cultural differences or barriers that arise because of these differences.

Identifying and Analyzing Various Components of the Community

Transcultural concepts often are useful in identifying and analyzing various components of the community, such as social structure and religious and political systems. A cultural approach allows the nurse to identify **cultural health care systems**, which are made up of individuals who experience illness as well as those who provide care for them. Anderson and MacFarlane (2000) suggest that each cultural health care system can have as many as three recognized sectors, most commonly referred to as popular, folk, and professional. We often forget that alternative systems and **alternative therapies** exist side by side with the professional system. How individuals organize themselves to meet group and individual needs is important information for community nurses. An assessment of whether social institutions such as churches and schools meet the health, social, and emotional needs of their members, and of whether the health and political systems are responsive to the needs of all citizens, can sometimes pinpoint critical needs and identify gaps in care. Cultural traditions within a community often determine the structure of community support systems as well as how resources are organized and distributed.

Identifying the Values and Cultural Norms of a Community

A transcultural framework is essential to the community nurse's identification of the values and cultural norms of a community. Although values are universal features of all cultures, their types and expressions vary widely, even within the same community. Values often serve as the foundation for a community's acceptance and use of health resources or a group's participation in community-based intervention programs to promote health and wellness. Just as nurses share data and collaborate with clients and families to establish mutually acceptable goals for nursing care, the community-based nurse works with the community or aggregates within the community to plan community-focused health programs. In addition to forming partnerships with communities, the community nurse considers the influences of social, economic, ecologic, and political issues. Many if not all community health issues are directly and profoundly affected by larger policy issues. These larger policy issues are, in turn, influenced by the wider national and/or international culture.

• CULTURAL ISSUES IN COMMUNITY NURSING PRACTICE

The need for nurses to be sensitive to clients who are culturally different is increasing as we become more aware of the complex interactions between health care providers and clients and of how these interactions might affect the client's health. The material in this section will assist nurses to be aware of cultural factors that affect health, illness, and the practice of nursing in community settings. Several cultural assessment tools or guides are available that provide comprehensive frameworks to guide the nurse in the assessment of cultural factors in the care of individuals, families, and groups (Stanhope & Lancaster, 2000; Spector, 2000; Huff & Kline, 1999). The majority of cultural assessment guides are oriented to individuals and occasionally to families. Only a few have the comprehensive view necessary for assessing cultural factors for intervention at the community level. Because individual clients and their families constitute larger communities, nurses who work in community settings must understand cultural issues as they relate to individuals and families as well as communities. We shall begin with a discussion of cultural influences on individuals and families before moving to a discussion of cultural factors within communities.

Cultural Influences on Individuals and Families

When assessing individuals and families, the community health nurse should carefully examine the following:

1. Family roles, typical family households and structure, and dynamics in the family, particularly communication patterns and decision making
2. Health beliefs and practices related to disease causation, treatment of illness, and the use of indigenous healers or folk practitioners and other alternative therapies
3. Patterns of daily living, including work and leisure activities
4. Social networks, including friends, neighbors, kin, and significant others, and how they influence health and illness
5. Ethnic, cultural, or national identity of client and family, e.g., identification with a particular group, including language
6. Nutritional practices and how they relate to cultural factors and health
7. Religious preferences and influences on well-being, health maintenance, and illness, as well as the impact religion might have on daily living and taboos arising from religious beliefs that might influence health status or care
8. Culturally appropriate behavior styles, including what is manifested during anger, competition, and cooperation, as well as relationships with health care professionals, relationships between genders, and relations with groups in the community.

A cultural assessment of individuals and families includes all the preceding factors. This list is by no means exhaustive; rather, it is presented as a guide for community nurses as they assess cultural aspects of individuals and families.

Cultural values shape human health behaviors and determine what individuals will do to maintain their health status, how they will care for themselves and others who become ill, and where and from whom they will seek health care. Families have an important role in the transmission of cultural values and learned behaviors that relate to both health and illness. It is in the family context that individuals learn basic ways to stay healthy and to ensure the well-being of themselves and their family members.

One commonality shared by members of functioning families is a concern for the health and wellness of each individual within the family, because the family has the primary responsibility for meeting the health needs of its members. The nurse not only must assess the health of each family member but also must define how well the family can meet family health needs. Just how well families function in relation to this will determine how, when, and where interventions will take place; by whom; and what the specific approach to the family will be. A cultural orientation assists the nurse in understanding cultural values and interactions, the roles that family members assume, and the support system available to the family to help them when health problems are identified.

The family is usually a person's most important social unit and provides the social context within which illness occurs and is resolved and within which health promotion and maintenance occur. Most **traditional health beliefs and practices** promote the health of the family because they are generally family and socially oriented. Frequently, traditional beliefs and practices reinforce family cohesion. Some values are more central and influential than others; given a competing set of demands, these central values will typically determine a family's priorities. In families that adhere to traditional cultural values, the family's needs and goals often will take precedence over an individual's needs and goals (Friedman & Ferguson-Marshalleck, 1996). A culturally competent nurse can recognize and use the family's role in promoting and maintaining health. This requires an appreciation of the family context in health and illness and how this varies among diverse cultures. Box 11-1 provides some ideas on how to develop the cultural competence and sensitivity that is necessary for successful health promotion programs for diverse cultural groups.

BOX 11–1	DEVELOPING CULTURAL COMPETENCE TO PROMOTE HEALTH IN DIVERSE CULTURAL GROUPS

- Learn about the history of the cultural group or diverse population with which you are working. For example, an understanding of Black culture would not be complete without considering the effect of slavery on this group of Americans.
- Make an effort to understand the cultural values beliefs and ways of life of the community.
- Incorporate as many of the traditional values, beliefs, and ways of life into the design and use of any educational materials. Whereas Chinese American teenagers might prefer a comic book in English, their grandparents might prefer a health magazine in the Chinese language.
- Become familiar with the appropriate verbal and nonverbal communication patterns within the group as well as many of the communication nuances that are contextual in nature. An example might be that a traditional Afghan woman would never speak to a strange man outside of her own kinship circle.
- Become familiar with beliefs and practices related to religion, gender, food preferences, and other related cultural differences that might lead to the quick success or failure of a health program. Be aware that the most effective health programs are those that foster community ownership and involvement.
- Spend as much time as possible within the community, attending local events. Examples might be churches, school programs, fairs, and meetings with leaders. Taking an intervention into the community rather than having the community come to the intervention might be more effective over time.
- Seek the community's input and feedback for any health program that is planned for the community. Be aware that the use of peer educators from within the community has been found to be effective in delivering health promotion programs to diverse communities.

Adapted from R. M. Huff & M. V. Kline (1999). *Promoting health in multicultural populations.* Thousand Oaks, CA: Sage.

Cultural Factors Within Communities

In addition to identifying and meeting the cultural needs of clients and families, the community health nurse must consider social and cultural factors on a community level to respect cultural values, mobilize local resources, and develop culturally appropriate health programs and services. Important cultural factors include demographics in the United States and Canada; cultural diversity in communities; subpopulations in the United States and Canada; refugee and immigrant populations, with special consideration given to Afghan refugee communities; maintenance of traditional cultural values and practices; and access to health and nursing care for diverse cultural groups.

Demographics and Health Care

During the 21st century, the United States and Canada will face enormous demographic, social, and culture change. North America is becoming more diverse, not less so, and thus it is incumbent on nurses to be prepared to respond appropriately. Since the 1980s and 1990s, there has been a steady growth in cultural diversity in the United States and Canada. The health status of individuals in the United States differs dramatically across cultural groups and social classes. Certain populations groups in the United States face greater challenges than the general population in accessing timely and needed health care services (Lurie, 1997; Shi & Singh, 2001). Major indicators such as morbidity and mortality rates for adults and infants show that the health status of minority Americans in the United States is substantially worse than that of White Americans. The same holds true for differences in social class: health status is worse among those who live in poverty. Similarly, in Canada, older people, the unemployed, welfare recipients, single women supporting children, and minorities such as Native Canadians and immigrants have a higher chance of experiencing poor health (Health Canada, 2001). Lack of economic resources predisposes individuals, families, and communities to major difficulties in accessing appropriate health care. Thus, community nurses must assess groups within the community in a very sensitive manner; often those characteristics that we assume are related to the group's culture may be caused by poverty instead.

Cultural Diversity Within Communities

The United States and Canada have many diverse cultures as a result of their history of immigration by a variety of cultural and ethnic groups to both countries and because of the indigenous populations of Native Americans and Alaskans and, for the United States, the Native Hawaiians. If current immigration trends continue, the United States will consist of an even greater variety of cultural groups. If present immigration patterns and policies hold, (nearly a million people every year could be admitted in several categories), then a possible 30 million people could be added between 1990 and 2030, contributing further to the number and diversity of the population (U.S. Bureau of the Census, 1998). Although broad cultural values are shared by most people in this country, a rich diversity of cultural orientations does exist, including those with considerable variations in health and illness practices. The same immigration trends are similar for Canada. For example, population projections imply that by the year 2036, 90% of Canada's population growth will be the result of immigration (Halli & Driedger, 1999).

Subcultures in the United States and Canada

Subcultures are fairly large aggregates of people who, although members of a larger cultural group, have shared characteristics that are not common to all members of the culture and that enable the subculture to be thought of as a distinguishable group (Saunders, 1954). Many newcomers are actually relatives of United States and Canadian citizens or are new immigrants, adding numbers to the original subculture. Obviously, there can also be diversity within each subculture. Hispanic culture as a group includes Mexican North Americans, Puerto Ricans, Cubans, and Central and South Americans, and there is diversity within each of these groups as well.

Certain geographic areas of the country such as Appalachia can be singled out as containing subcultures. Persons born and reared in the South or in New York City can often be identified by their language and mannerisms as members of a distinct subculture. We used to believe that the United States had a "melting pot" culture in which new arrivals gave up their former languages, customs, and values to become Americans. It is now agreed that the "melting pot" or "blending" concept may not be appropriate, at least not for everyone. A more accurate metaphor would be to view the United States and Canadian populations as consisting of a rich and complex tapestry of colors, backgrounds, and interests (Figure 11-2).

Refugee and Immigrant Populations

Immigrants are persons who voluntarily and legally immigrate to Canada and United States to live. Immigrants come of their own choice, and most plan to eventually become citizens of their new host country. Of course, many persons also come to the United States and Canada illegally. Although terms differ for these persons, usually they are referred to as illegal immigrants. Evidence-Based Practice 11–1 discusses the health issues and problems encountered by Afghan refugee women. **Refugee** is a special term that is used for groups of persons who come to this country under special legal processes, usually requiring congressional action. By definition, refugees are persons escaping persecution based on race, religion, nationality, or political stance (Isajiw, 1999; Scanlan, 1983). Table 11–1 shows other terms that are used to refer to persons who are in the process of moving to another country or of leaving their birthplace or a country in transition.

Perhaps the most well-known group of refugees is made up of persons who came to the United States from Southeast Asia after the Vietnam War. Most often, refugees are fleeing war, famine, and other social upheavals. They are fleeing for their lives and safety rather than personally choosing to leave their homeland. The term "refugee" and the status of an individual who is a refugee have legal meanings and designations that differ from those of ordinary immi-

Figure 11–2. Communication between people from different cultures can help to breakdown misunderstandings, stereotypes, and other cultural barriers. Immigrants from other cultures have contributed much to enrich American culture.

grants. Another classification of newcomers is that of **asylee**—persons who come to a particular country seeking political asylum from some sort of persecution in their home country. These various types of classification—immigrant, refugee, asylee, or illegal immigrant—often determine the rights of individuals, for example, the granting of work permits, or the types of social and health services that newcomers may access.

EVIDENCE-BASED PRACTICE 11–1
Afghan Women's Health

Afghan citizens began leaving their war-torn country in 1979. Afghans remain among the world's largest refugee population, with northern California being home to some 20,000 refugees. Afghan culture is strongly patriarchal even in the United States, and this has caused considerable family conflict for young women. Women face problems with access to health care because of cultural emphasis on modesty; their care is complicated by their lower status and men's gatekeeping. Older women avoid preventive care such as mammograms and Papanicolaou smears because of embarrassment. Lack of health education is especially problematic; many older Afghan women have little or no formal education. The problem of wife abuse is of much concern in this population. Health education can be accomplished in a culturally sensitive and appropriate manner.

CLINICAL APPLICATION

1. Afghan women will be more comfortable with female providers, i.e., female nurse practitioners, physician assistants, or physicians.
2. Nurses who are culturally competent can interpret mainstream health culture to Afghans and Afghan culture to health care providers.
3. Health education can be successful if presented appropriately. It can best be accomplished in small groups of women who know one another, meeting face to face, teaching in their own language. It is important to have plenty of pictures and time to ask questions as well as to socialize, perhaps over a cup of tea.
4. Sex education in the schools is more culturally acceptable if it is conducted privately and separate classes are held for boys and girls. Parents' permission for their children to attend the classes is important, and an Afghan adult should be present.
5. Wife battering is an extremely sensitive issue in this patriarchal society, where men consider it their right and duty to physically discipline their wives. Health care professionals must approach this problem with considerable caution and sensitivity. Afghan women who advocate for other women should be asked for advice on how to approach this concern.

Lipson, J. G., Hosseini, M. A., Kabir, S., Omidian, P. A., & Edmonston, F. (1995). Health issues among Afghan women in California. *Health Care for Women International, 16*(4), 279–286.

The United States and Canada have grown and achieved their success as nations of immigrants and foreigners. Immigration is a continuing phenomenon in these countries. For example, between 1981 and 1996, more than 3 million persons came legally to the United States from Mexico (U.S. Immigration and Naturalization Services, 1997). Many recent immigrants and refugees are not acculturated to prevailing Western norms of health beliefs or behaviors. Many arrive with scant economic resources and must learn English and become economically self-sufficient as quickly as possible. Certain factors such as settlement patterns or living near friends or family, communication networks, social class, and education have helped many immigrants maintain their cultural traditions. Meleis (1997) noted that such communities provide

TABLE 11–1	TERMS USED FOR INDIVIUALS RESIDING IN A COUNTRY WHO ARE NOT CITIZENS
Illegal immigrant	A person who is in a country without the appopriate documentation and permission
Immigrant	A person who comes to a country to take up permanent residence
Refugee	A person who is escaping persecution based on race, religion, nationality, or political persuasion
Emigrant	A person departing from a country to settle elswhere
Emigre	A person forced to emigrate for political reasons
Asylee	A person seeking political asylum from persecution in his or her home country
Temporary stay migrant	A person who moves to another country with the intention of staying there for only a limited time, usually for occupational reasons

support for newcomers and opportunities for cultural continuity, because these ethnic communities reflect the identities of the home countries. At the same time, belonging to such a community tends to set immigrants and refugees apart and isolate them from the larger community. For example, newcomers from Mexico realize that they need to learn English to get better jobs, but they often join expanding Latino communities where most residents speak Spanish. Learning English well enough to obtain employment in the English-speaking world is difficult, and it is to their credit that most immigrants do learn English and make significant contributions to their new country. Nevertheless, where immigrants live and how they participate should remain individual choices and privileges, rather than prescribed options.

In addition to the legal entrance of immigrants and refugees, many other persons seeking political asylum have entered the United States and Canada from all over the world. Often, those seeking asylum or those who enter the country both legally and illegally are at considerable risk for health and social problems (Aroian, 1993; Health Canada, 1999a). In addition to language and employment barriers, they have few economic resources, some have experienced rapid change and traumatic life events, their coping abilities have been overwhelmed, and few resources are available to assist them. Immigrants in general, whether they are here legally or illegally, have special health risks.

Special Considerations: Cultural Factors Affecting an Afghan Refugee Community

*Afghans fled their country beginning in 1978 after a coup d'etat by the communist faction of the Afghan government, which was followed by an invasion from the Soviet Union. Although the Soviets left Afghanistan in 1989, continued

*The author thanks Juliene G. Lipson, RN, PhD, FAAN, for her assistance and contributions to the sections in this chapter about Afghan refugees.

fighting between political groups and the deprivations of war reduced Afghanistan's population from 15.5 million to 8 or 9 million people. Lipson (1991) pointed out that a decade ago, Afghans were the largest group of refugees in the world. Pakistan was host to 3.4 million, Iran had 2.2 million, and a third group of countries, including the United States, hosted 100,000 Afghans. This huge displacement of Afghans began before or during the Soviet invasion of Afghanistan and the fierce fighting that followed. Then, a radical fundamentalist Islamic group, the Taliban, gained control of the Afghan government in 1996 and imposed its harsh view of Islamic law on the population (McGeary, 2001). This has included the severe repression of women, including seclusion and veiling as well as other extreme measures, such as forbidding the education of women and prohibiting them from occupational pursuits or working in public places. Several years of famine and natural disasters have further worsened the conditions in this country, long one of the poorest in the world. Afghans have continued to leave their country in spite of restrictions on their migration and resettlement that have been imposed by neighboring countries and Western countries, including the United States. The number of Afghans fleeing their country has greatly accelerated after the September 11, 2001, terrorist attack in the United States and the subsequent antiterrorist campaign focused on the Taliban forces in Afghanistan.

In particular, Afghan refugees and immigrants have undergone stressful, traumatic, and even catastrophic experiences such as war, torture, refugee camps, death of family members, and loss of homeland. Obviously, under such circumstances, the experiences associated with fleeing one's country of birth can produce psychologic stress (Lipson, 1993). However, trying to make a new life in their host country can also be very stressful. Factors such as unemployment, decreased family income, changes in lifestyle, lack of ability to speak English, culture conflict, and separation from family and loved ones continue to add to stress and decrease the quality of life for many Afghan refugees (Lipson & Omidian, 1997).

Many studies have indicated that many Afghan refugees experience posttraumatic stress disorder, which follows a psychologically traumatic event outside of the range of usual human experiences. The symptoms may include nightmares, depression, withdrawal, hopelessness, sleep disorders, and other somatic complaints (American Psychiatric Association, 1987). The terrorism of September 11, 2001, and its association with Afghanistan has only added to the stress faced by Afghan refugees living in the United States, such as bias and hate crimes, and pain at the further destruction of their country. However, Afghan activists are redoubling their efforts on behalf of women's rights and in educating the public about Afghanistan and Islam.

TRADITIONAL AFGHAN CULTURE

Traditional culture in Afghan was strongly patriarchal and was divided among tribal, political, social class, and ethnic lines. These political divisions continue and are often intensified by the high levels of stress as Afghans attempt to cope with life in the United States. Traditional customs include arranged marriages, often between first cousins; polygyny when affordable (as many as four wives);

and a patriarchal family system (Lipson & Omidian, 1992). Women are usually fairly young when they marry and have less education than men. Marriage and childbearing are the only acceptable roles for women. There are considerable variations, given that Afghan family life is in transition. Women do not usually socialize with men outside the family. Afghan women remain in the home and socialize only with other women within the extended family; however, many women work to help support the family, and some educated women are activists in the community. Despite social class and generational variations, family life is the core of Afghan culture. A key difference between Afghan and American culture is family interdependence versus individualism. For traditional Afghans, family obligations always come before anything else. Lipson and Omidian (1992) reported that culture conflict is central to difficulties in adjustment.

CHARACTERISTICS OF AN AFGHAN REFUGEE COMMUNITY

A community assessment of a refugee community requires that the nurse assess cultural factors such as **kinship**, religious practices, family roles and patterns, language use, and cultural health beliefs and practices. Obviously, other parameters of a community assessment such as population trends, environment, industry, education, recreation, and health care services are important also. However, the composition of refugee or other ethnic communities requires that nurses study and interpret cultural data and understand how these data influence health and wellness. DeSantis (1997) has observed "that interventions that are not built on an understanding of the concept of culture will always limit the effectiveness of nursing (p. 184)."

Although Afghans share nationality and religion, the community is strongly heterogeneous and divisive in politics, social class, ethnicity, and region as well as urban or rural origin in Afghanistan (Lipson, 1991). Afghans often appear to be divided and disorganized along the traditional lines of politics, social class, and urban or rural origin. Lack of community cohesion is not unusual, because Afghans are organized by kinship and the extended family. Barth (1987) observed that these divisions reflect Afghanistan's traditional tribal social structure. Lipson and Miller (1994) and Lipson and Omidian (1997) found that the Afghan community is further divided along gender and generational lines—the experiences of men, women, and the children who have grown up in the United States are strikingly different from those of their elders. Thus, any attempt to bring health care services to the community or to address some of the community's health problems must take into account the tremendous diversity within the whole community. Further complicating this situation are several languages. Most Afghans speak Pashto or Dari (Farsi/Persian), but other languages are also spoken. Elderly women, in particular, are illiterate in their own language (Lipson, Omidian, & Paul, 1995).

The Afghan Family

Family life is at the core of Afghan culture. Although many health care professionals are familiar with strong family systems among United States and Canadian families, they still cannot comprehend the differences and the profound influence of Afghan family life on psychologic well-being. Lipson & Miller

(1994) reported that what Western psychiatrists call **enmeshment** (and is labeled as abnormal by American culture) is normal family behavior for Afghans. Afghans tend to socialize almost exclusively with extended family members, and this can cause cultural conflict when they live in the United States because there may be geographic distances between the family members, thus making frequent visiting very difficult. Afghan culture supports dependence on family members, whereas North American culture emphasizes independence and individualism. Extended family obligations, especially to parents and older siblings, take precedence over all other responsibilities, including affiliation with one's spouse, work responsibilities, and certainly one's own preferences and needs. Extended families may average 50 to 70 individuals and are contained within a tribal unit of 1,000 or more. The main social events are related to family obligations such as engagement parties and weddings. In traditional families, these parties can be very elaborate and occur over several days and nights.

Afghan Women's Roles

Most Afghans are staunch Muslims. Although the role of women is changing, women tend to socialize almost exclusively with other women. They experience conflict over women's freedom, conflict between maintaining traditional values and becoming Americanized, role overload from adding new American roles to Afghan roles, a lack of suitable spouses for single women, and parenting difficulties.

Lipson and Miller (1994) reported that there are generational differences in changes in women's roles. For example, elderly women, who are often widows, appear the most stressed and unhappy. They are socially isolated because their grown children and grandchildren work outside the home or are at school. Many women, especially if they are of late middle age or older, do not speak English and are essentially homebound; they miss the constant visiting and support from kin that they experienced back home in Afghanistan. Traditionally, the status of women in Afghanistan increased with age, but this has not been the case in the United States, and elderly women tend to dwell on past traumatic experiences, to be depressed, and to experience numerous psychosomatic symptoms (Lipson & Miller, 1994). There are variations in Afghan family life after families have relocated to the United States. Thus, it is important to carefully assess each situation rather than making assumptions based on stereotypes.

Middle-aged Afghan women, like other women refugees, have experienced profound role changes. In traditional Islamic culture, a woman's proper place is in the home. However, in the United States, it has been necessary for many Afghan women to work outside the home. Professional Afghan women at first have difficulty obtaining employment in their accustomed profession, and often they have been able to obtain only low-status jobs in the United States. As women's roles have changed, their husbands have often reacted with frustration. Some men have begun to drink heavily or abuse family members, increasing the stress and pressure on women and families.

Single status is viewed as unnatural. As previously stated, women marry at a fairly young age. However, finding an appropriate spouse has been difficult for some young Afghan women. Many Afghan men believe that women who have lived in the United States have been contaminated by American ideas and thus are not properly submissive to their husbands. Unmarried women live with parents or siblings; it would be extremely rare for a young woman to live alone. There are no role models for single women. Teenaged girls are also caught in a bind. Daughters who do not maintain modest behavior are perceived as destroying the family's reputation. Traditional Afghans perceive the dress, makeup, behavior, speech, and freedom of American teenagers as improper and even immoral. Young Afghan women who have spent several years in the United States, exposed to a culture that views women in quite a different way, are not always willing to marry traditional Afghan men.

Afghan parents frequently worry about their children as they are exposed to American culture at school and on television. Sex, violence, and other controversial aspects of American life are pervasive and difficult to avoid. Children tend to acculturate more rapidly than their parents, learning English more quickly and, in general, adapting to new social roles and gender identities as well as establishing roots in American culture. This does not imply that Afghan childhood is free from conflict. On the contrary, the cultural clash between generations can be profound, given that Afghan parents are often adamantly opposed to many of the American cultural beliefs and behaviors their children have acquired. This is often a source of great conflict and dissension.

HEALTH CARE FOR AFGHAN REFUGEE COMMUNITIES

Case Study 11-1 describes an Afghan refugee family struggling with the difficulties of adjusting to a new and different life. The case study serves as the basis for this discussion on health care for Afghan refugee communities.

Careful assessment of cultural backgrounds and individual factors can help nurses anticipate and work with difficulties experienced by refugees with regard to seeking health care. The Andrews/Boyle Cultural Assessment Guide used in this text is recommended for use with clients and their families or even whole communities. Because this assessment is quite comprehensive, the following topics, adapted from Lipson & Meleis (1983), are suggested to provide minimum information for the nurse to plan culturally competent care.

- Length of time the client and family have been here, and where the client was brought up. Not only is the country important, but rural and urban differentiation may also be important.
- Language spoken in the home, and language skill in English.
- Nonverbal communication style.
- Religious practices.
- Ethnic affiliation or identity
- Family roles and how they are influenced by the resettlement experience
- Social support or networks in the new country.

Assessment of these factors would assist the nurse in planning health care for the Abduls and other Afghan families. Mental health services, preventive care,

CASE STUDY	11–1

The Abdul family came to the United States in 1990 after an extended stay in a refugee camp in Pakistan. Like other Afghan refugees, they experienced difficulty fleeing Afghanistan and lost family members in the war and turmoil that engulfed their home country. They came to California because they had relatives in the San Francisco Bay area and knew of the Afghan community there. Even though they have lived in the United States for more than 10 years, they still struggle with the difficulties of adjusting to a new and different life. Resettlement and adjustment in the United States have not been easy for them. Although they appreciate the safety they have experienced in this country, they believe that the quality of life was better in Afghanistan, where they had fresher food, more exercise and social support, and no pollution (Lipson, Omidian, & Paul, 1995).

Many of the health problems experienced by both Mr. and Mrs. Abdul can be traced to significant stressors of migration. Mr. Abdul was a successful businessman in Afghanistan. He has worked only intermittently in the United States and, as could be predicted, he has experienced considerable stress related to work problems, loss of property, and loss of status. Like many Afghans in the United States, the Abduls have received welfare assistance, and Mr. Abdul was reluctant to forfeit this income for a minimum-wage job with few or no benefits. Mr. Abdul has struggled to learn English, and as his English-language ability has improved he has been able to find more satisfactory employment. Mr. Abdul is not aware that he is hypertensive because he has not seen a physician for several years. Like all refugees and immigrants, Mr. Abdul has experienced difficulties with access to health care, insurance problems, and the need for translation and transportation.

Mrs. Abdul has been relatively isolated at home with the children. In Afghanistan, she would have lived very close to family members, and she would have spent a great deal of time visiting with them. Without the social support and interaction of her family, she feels very lonely and has experienced some depression, which is not uncommon in refugee women. Like many other Afghan refugee women, Mrs. Abdul would seek and accept health care only from a woman physician or nurse. Cultural barriers often inhibit such health practices as breast self-examination and Papanicolaou smears. Mrs. Abdul does not talk about such intimate matters with her husband or even with another woman. The lack of social interaction with other women relatives makes her vulnerable not only to social isolation but also to the lack of health information that would be shared among women in a traditional culture. She is reluctant to make friends with strangers, even if they are other Afghan women. She misses the constant visiting and social interaction characteristic of life back in Afghanistan. Although many Afghan men and women had horrific experiences in the war and the escape from Afghanistan, many others like the Abdul family are adjusting to life in the United States and are coping as well as possible with their past experiences. Their lives are not stress free by any means, but the Abduls and other refugees have demonstrated considerable strength in adjusting to traumatizing experiences and the stress of adapting to life in the United States.

Mr. and Mrs. Abdul worry a great deal about their children, a boy aged 16 years and a girl aged 14 years. They are worried about raising their children in American society. The parents are distressed by what they see on television and are shocked by the explicit sex and violence portrayed in the media. They are offended by public demonstrations of affection between men and women. And, as Lipson (1991) indicated, like other Afghan refugees, the Abduls are concerned because their children are served pork in school lunch rooms and are exposed to poor role models. The Abduls fear that schools often teach disrespect for parents and encourage sexual freedom through sex education.

The teenaged girl, Rahima, like other young Afghan girls, is torn between traditional values, which emphasize socializing only with families, and behaving like her American peers. Although her father is pleased that she can receive an education in the United States, he is worried that she might wear lipstick and short skirts like her American classmates. Rahima sometimes is resentful because her brother has more freedom than she does to visit friends, play sports, and participate in other activities outside the home and away from parents.

News from Afghanistan through the media, the telephone, and direct communication with friends and family members is a source of great stress for Afghans in the United States. Many Afghans have cable television and can monitor television news from Middle Eastern countries. The powerful effect of news and the events in Afghanistan in the wake of the terrorist attacks on the United States cannot be overstated. The Abdul family is upset and distressed about the news from their country and the family members who remain there. They are equally worried about what might happen to them as Afghans living in the United States, and they fear repercussions and stigmatization related to their cultural and ethnic identity.

---

and health education needs were identified as important in an Afghan community health survey conducted by Lipson, Omidian, & Paul (1995). Stress is a significant problem for the Abdul family and is not uncommon in other Afghan families. Stress is related to the refugee experience and also to inadequate income, work-related problems, and loss of culture and tradition. Lipson, Omidian, & Paul (1995) reported in their community survey of Afghan health that many Afghans were reluctant to seek mental health services because of fear of stigma—of "being crazy"—as well the lack of health insurance and the existence of few Dari/Pashto-speaking therapists. The lack of mental health services is a grave concern in refugee communities and should be addressed by creative and innovative solutions. Afghan men like Mr. Abdul are reluctant to seek mental health services. He is reluctant to admit that he needs such services, his income is limited, and his health insurance will not pay for psychiatric services even if they were available from a professional who spoke his own language.

Preventive care in the areas of dental health, breast self-examination, mammography, and Papanicolaou smears are important for Mrs. Abdul. Surveys have shown that many Afghans are not aware of the risks of smoking, overweight, and hypertension (Lipson, Omidian, & Paul, 1995). Many barriers to good preventive care are environmental and social rather than cultural. Constraints are based on Afghan refugees' language, economic, occupational, and transportation problems. Mrs. Abdul is not likely to seek these personal health care services on her own initiative and would not be likely to talk about them with other women unless they were family members. Health care professionals must learn sensitive ways of broaching these subjects and helping Afghan clients access culturally appropriate care. Health care professionals, especially women physicians and nurses, should design outreach programs that consider problems in access to and lack of language-appropriate and culturally sensitive health care. Many Afghan women would not be comfortable with a male physician; perhaps female nurse practitioners and/or midwives could be used in culturally specific settings.

Health education, including information about access to care, is always important in planning services for refugee communities. Many Afghans do not use health education services, not necessarily because of cultural barriers but because of difficulties with access, the need for translation and transportation, and the desire for women health care providers, as well as other barriers. Lipson, Omidian, & Paul (1995) reported that Afghans wanted information on dealing with stress, heart health, nutrition, raising children (particularly adolescents) in the United States, aging in the United States, and diabetes. They requested that health education be delivered in lectures via television or through face-to-face lectures, written brochures, or videotapes in their own language.

Health services, from the beginning, should include bicultural health care providers on their staff. Community health workers could be trained to serve as interpreters and translators. Lipson (1991) cautions against using family members as interpreters because of divisions along age and gender lines. The health care provider's gender is especially important for Afghan women, who will not feel comfortable with male doctors or nurses and may avoid health care altogether if female care providers are not available. Obviously, non-Afghan care providers must be knowledgeable about the refugees' experiences and background, cultural and social factors, and other unique aspects of this population. Health education is especially important for this community; however, barriers to care are often environmental and social. Afghans need access to language-appropriate and culturally sensitive health care; according to one study (Lipson, Omidian, & Paul, 1995), they prefer to receive such information in a group or social setting.

The traditional or classic definition of community tended to use a geographic boundary, such as a village, town, or urban settlement like a city. This sense may be conveyed somewhat in terms such as Little Havana, Little Kabul, and Little Saigon, but such designations do not really convey the nature or quality of the immigrant experience, which tends to cross geographic boundaries and does not remain the same as in the home country. The sense of shared displacement or uprootedness that serves to unite and distinguish the immigrant community from other groups or communities is quite profound and cannot be ignored (DeSantis, 1997).

Immigrant communities have often been reduced to a psychoemotional phenomenon. Immigrants are seen as dominated by the psychoemotional experiences and consequences of relocation. This view, according to DeSantis (1997), focuses on the primacy of the individual rather than the community and thus prescribes psychiatric treatment rather than addressing the sociocultural and economic barriers at the macro level. It is at the macro level that transcultural health care providers must be engaged if they are to be effective participants in building healthy refugee communities.

Maintenance of Traditional Cultural Values and Practices

An important aspect of transcultural nursing is the collection of cultural data and the assessment of traditional values and practices and how they are maintained over time. The processes of **assimilation** and **acculturation** can be briefly defined as those ways in which individuals and cultural groups adapt and change over time. Yet, at the same time, both individuals and groups may be resistant to some changes and retain many traditional cultural traits. Hispanics are the largest cultural/ethnic group in the United States, and in several large American cities, they constitute large percentages of the population. Obviously, in these ethnic communities, it is easier to speak Spanish and to maintain other traditional cultural practices. Because traditional health beliefs and practices influence health and wellness, it is important for the nurse to understand the degree to which clients, families, and communities adhere to traditional health values and how nursing practice should reflect those values. Spector (2000) suggests that a person's health care and behavior during illness may well have roots in that person's traditional belief system. Unless community health nurses understand the traditional health beliefs and practices of their clients and communities, they may intervene at the wrong time or in an inappropriate way.

Many factors influence the likelihood that clients, families, and communities will maintain traditional health beliefs and practices. For example, the length of time a person lives in the new host country will influence factors such as language and the use of media such as radio and television. The ability to speak English and to communicate with members of the majority culture is crucial to acculturation. The size of the ethnic or cultural group is also important; obviously, if the group is small, individuals from that group are more likely to be exposed to outsiders and will not spend all their time within their own group or community.

Generally, children acculturate more quickly because they are exposed to others through schooling and learn cultural characteristics through that association. The need to work outside the household often exposes women from traditional cultures to others of the majority culture; thus, they learn English more quickly than if they remain isolated at home. When individuals from other cultures seek health care in their Western host country, they become familiar with its health care system. This does not necessarily mean that they comply with all health advice, but contact with the system decreases anxiety and confusion, and individuals are more likely to seek care again. In addition, if individuals or groups have distinguishing ethnic characteristics such as skin color, they may be more isolated because of discrimination and thus retain traditional values, beliefs, and practices over a longer time.

Some factors that influence the likelihood that clients, families, and communities will maintain traditional health beliefs and practices are shown in Box 11-2.

Access to Health and Nursing Care for Diverse Cultural Groups

Members of diverse cultural groups, especially those who are poor, face special problems in accessing health and nursing care. Access to care is often determined by economic and geographic factors. Community nurses who focus on the care of aggregates face the challenge of promoting the health of populations

BOX 11–2	FACTORS INFLUENCING TRADITIONAL BELIEFS AND PRACTICES

1. Length of time in the new host country.
2. Size of the ethnic or cultural group with which an individual identifies and interacts.
3. Age of the individual. As a general rule, children acculturate more rapidly than adults or seniors.
4. Ability to speak English and communicate with members of the majority culture.
5. Economic status. For example, if the family economic situation necessitates that a Salvadoran woman work outside the home, she may learn English more quickly than if she remains within the household and speaks only Spanish with her family members.
6. Educational status. In general, higher levels of education lead to faster acculturation.
7. Health status of family members. If individuals and their families seek health care in their host country, they begin to "learn the system," so to speak. This does not mean that they comply with all health advice by any means, but contacts with the system should decrease anxiety and confusion.
8. Individuals and groups who have distinguishing ethnic characteristics, such as skin color, may be more isolated because of discrimination and thus may retain traditional values related to health beliefs and behavior.
9. Intermarriage. Ethnic intermarriage is associated with a greater loss of traditional ethnic identity.
10. Rigidity or flexibility of the host society. This refers to the extent to which the host society is willing to allow members of different ethnic groups, along with their traditions and practices, into their structure, culture, and identity.

with new causes of mortality (such as HIV/AIDS) and underserved populations who are more likely to experience health problems. Certain cultural groups have faced discrimination and poverty, and their ability to access care has been compromised. Sensitivity to cultural factors has often been lacking in the health care of traditional communities and identified minority groups. In addition to economic status and discriminatory factors that limit access to care, geographic location plays an important role. Many rural areas lack medical personnel and the variety of health facilities and services that are available to urban populations. For example, Native Americans, living in sparsely settled and isolated reservations in the western part of the United States, must travel long distances over primitive roads to obtain health care services. Many individuals from culturally diverse backgrounds seek the services of health care professionals who speak their language. When this is not possible, they are reluctant to seek care or may not understand the importance of following medical advice.

Another common and significant factor that limits access to health services is a lack of understanding by clients of how to use health resources. This lack of understanding may be due in part to cultural factors. Often this lack of understanding means that members of diverse cultural groups are less able to adequately cope with health problems than are other members of the community. Nurses can develop sensitivity to diverse groups within communities and reach out to them with culturally specific health programs. Some important factors that nurses must take into account for culturally appropriate community-based care are shown in Box 11-3.

• ASSESSMENT OF CULTURALLY DIVERSE COMMUNITIES

A **cultural assessment** may be directed toward individual clients to assess their cultural needs (Leininger, 1991) (see also the Andrews/Boyle Transcultural Nursing Assessment Guide). In general, all successful cultural assessments have at their foundation extensive data to help them better understand and address the specific health needs and interests of their target populations. Individual cultural assessments are accomplished through the use of a systematic process. In community health nursing, the community is considered the client, and several schemas have been proposed to help nurses assess the community (Stanhope & Lancaster, 2000; Lowry & Martin, 2000). A community nursing assessment requires gathering relevant data, interpreting the data base (including problem analysis and prioritization), and identifying and implementing intervention activities for community health (Schuster & Goeppinger, 2000). Although the community nursing assessment focuses on a broader goal, such as improvement in the health status of a group of people, it is important to remember that the characteristics of people are what give every community its uniqueness. These common characteristics, which influence norms, values, religious practices, educational aspirations, and health and illness behavior are frequently determined by shared cultural experiences. Thus, adding the cultural component to a community nursing assessment strengthens the assessment base. Box 11-4 highlights four basic principles of cultural assessment, as suggested by Clark (1996).

Nurses have become interested in using cultural data in nursing care. Leininger (1978) presented assessment domains within which to seek data to understand culture and later (Leininger, 1991) developed a tool to assess

BOX 11–3	**FACTORS TO CONSIDER IN THE NURSING CARE OF CULTURALLY DIVERSE GROUPS**

1. Lack of employment opportunities and finances for health care services
2. Different traditional belief systems as well as different norms and values
3. Lack of cultural sensitivity on the part of social service and health care workers
4. Lack of bilingual personnel or staff members or the lack of interpreters to assist clients and care providers
5. Rapid changes in the U.S. health care system, where clients are "lost" in the gaps between agencies and services
6. Inconvenient locations or hours that preclude clients from accessing care
7. Lack of understanding, trust, and commitment on the part of health care providers

BOX 11–4	BASIC PRINCIPLES OF CULTURAL ASSESSMENT

1. **All cultures must be viewed in the context in which they have developed.** Cultural practices develop as a "logical" or understandable response to a particular human problem, and the setting as well as the problem must be considered. This is one reason why environmental and/or contextual data are so important.
2. **The underlying premises of the behavior must be examined.** For example, the Hispanic client's refusal to take a "hot" medication with a cold liquid is understandable if the nurse is aware that many Hispanic patients adhere to hot/cold theories of illness causation. There is often a range or spectrum of illness beliefs, with one end encompassing illnesses defined within the Western biomedical model and the other end firmly anchored within the individual culture (Huff, 1999). Obviously, the more widely disparate the differences between the biomedical model and the beliefs within the cultural group, the greater the potential for encountering resistance to biomedical interventions.
3. **The meaning and purpose of the behavior must be interpreted within the context of the specific culture.** An example would be the close relationship that is often seen in Hispanic cultures between mother and son; such an intense relationship might be viewed as abnormal in European American families.
4. **There is such a phenomenon as intracultural variation.** Not every member of a cultural group displays all the behaviors that we might associate with that group. For instance, not every Hispanic client will adhere to hot/cold theories of illness, and not every Hispanic mother will have a close personal relationship with her son. It is only by careful appraisal of the assessment data, and validation of the nurse's assessment with the client and family, that culturally competent care can be provided.

clients' cultural patterns by broadly looking at lifeways. Inherent in most definitions of culture is the concept of shared cultural backgrounds or a way of life or a **worldview**. Thus, the concept of culture may be more easily applied to a community or group of persons than to an individual. An overview of selected cultural components is presented in Table 11-2. These components can be used to assess diverse cultural groups within a community. For example, using these components, a cultural assessment of the Navajo would provide the data detailed in Box 11-5.

• COMMUNITY NURSING INTERVENTIONS

Cultural Competence in Health Maintenance and Health Promotion

Leininger (1978, 1995) suggested that cultural groups have their own culturally defined ways of maintaining and promoting health. Pender (1987) suggested that "health promoting behaviors can be understood only by considering persons within their social, cultural, and environmental contexts"

TABLE 11–2	**COMPONENTS OF THE CULTURAL ASSESSMENT**
CULTURAL COMPONENT	**DESCRIPTION**
Family and kinship systems	Is the family nuclear, extended, or "blended"? Do family members live near by? What are the communication patterns among family members? What is the role and status of individual family members? By age and gender?
Social life	What is the daily routine of the group? What are the important lifecycle events such as birth, marriage, and death? How are the educational systems organized? What are the social problems experienced by the group? How does the social environment contribute to a sense of belonging? What are the group's social interaction patterns? What are its commonly prescribed nutritional practices?
Political systems	Which factors in the political system influence the way the group perceives its status vis-à-vis the dominant culture, i.e., laws, justice, and cultural heroes? How does the economic system influence control of resources such as land, water, housing, jobs, and opportunities?
Language and traditions	Are there differences in dialects or language spoken between health care professionals and the cultural group? How do major cultural traditions of history, art, drama, etc. influence the cultural identity of the group? What are the common language patterns in regard to verbal and nonverbal communication? How is the use of personal space related to communication?
Worldview, value orientations, and cultural norms	What are the major cultural values about the relationships of humans to nature and to one another? How can the groups' ethical beliefs be described? What are the norms and standards of behavior (authority, responsibility, dependability, and competition)? What are the cultural attitudes about time, work, and leisure?
Religion	What are the religious beliefs and practices of the group? How do they relate to health practices? What are the rituals and taboos surrounding major life events such as birth and death?
Health beliefs and practices	What are the group's attitudes and beliefs regarding health and illness? Does the cultural group seek care from indigenous health (or folk) practitioners? Who makes decisions about health care? Are there biologic variations that are important to the health of this group?

(p. 16). Community nurses who have direct access to clients in the context of their daily lives should be especially aware of the importance of cultural knowledge in promoting and maintaining health, because the promotion and maintenance of health occurs in the context of everyday lives rather than in

(Text continues on page page 343)

Family and Kinship Systems

- Often an extended family that consists of an older woman and her husband and unmarried children, together with married daughters and their husbands and unmarried children.
- The Navajo (or other North American Indians) have many unique categories of relatives.
- Descent is traced through the mother.
- Head of household is the husband, although the wife has a voice in decision making.
- Children are highly valued and are given responsibilities to make decisions about themselves.
- There is prestige with age as long as the elderly person can function independently.

Social Life

- The earth and nature are valued; the individual should be in harmony with nature; this thought is interwoven with daily activities.
- Cooperation with others, rather than competition, is a cultural value.
- Lifecycle events are marked by special rituals; for example, the Blessing Way ceremony takes place shortly after the birth of a child.
- Like many other indigenous people, the Navajo have high rates of alcoholism, suicide, domestic violence, and homicide. Currently, abuse of drugs and HIV disease are becoming more common.
- Tribal and family ties are strong and contribute to a sense of belonging to a social group.
- Educational opportunities are often limited because of an inferior school system.
- Diet is often high in carbohydrates and fats; staple foods are corn, mutton, and fried bread.

Political Systems

- The system of tribal government was imposed by Whites.
- Poverty and high rates of unemployment are overriding concerns.
- The extended family has an economic as well as a social function.
- Control of resources (land, water) has been problematic, given the role of the U.S. Government.
- Improving housing, sanitation, and work opportunities are major goals.
- A major problem is making deteriorated lands productive in an underpopulated region.

Language and Traditions

- Younger Navajo speak English. Reading, writing, and speaking English are taught in all the schools. Many elderly Navajo speak little or no English.
- There are many homonyms in the Navajo language: words that have identical sounds but different meanings. The Navajo language is very specific.
- Periods of silence during communication show respect.
- Nonverbal communication is a high art form among the Navajo, and silence is highly respected. There may be little eye contact. Direct and prolonged eye contact is considered extremely rude and intrusive.

(continued)

BOX 11–5

COMPONENTS OF A CULTURAL ASSESSMENT APPLIED: NATIVE AMERICAN (NAVAJO) *(Continued)*

- There is a lack of need for personal space.
- The group has a history of oppression from the White dominant group.
- The "Long Walk" (a forced move of 300 miles to Fort Sumner in 1863) was a major calamity for the Navajo and remains a poignant chapter in cultural history that reinforces Native American culture and identity.

Worldview, Value Orientations, and Cultural Norms

- In all North American Indian cultures, interactions on all levels contain the fundamental element of respect. Respect is how one presents himself or herself to the world and how one acts, and is tied to being Indian or Native American.
- The xbasic nature of human beings is neither good nor bad; both qualities exist in each person.
- Nature is more powerful than human beings.
- Individual success is not valued as highly as providing security to the extended family.
- The traditional Navajo views on the relationship of human beings with other human beings are both individualistic and collateral.
- The integrity of the individual must be respected. There is respect for the choice of an individual (even a child's decision is respected).
- There is also pressure for a Navajo to consider the extended family's welfare when making decisions.
- Time orientations are not strict; work and productivity are valued.

Religious Ideology

- Religion enters every phase of the traditional Navajo life, and an important emphasis is on curing illness.
- Many important Navajo ceremonies may be used with illness; theology and medicine are difficult to separate in traditional Navajo culture.
- Earth and nature are a part of the Navajo's cosmology, and health is viewed as harmony with the universe.
- Many Native Americans, including some Navajo, are members of the Native American Church.
- Peyote may be used in religious curing rituals to restore natural harmony. Peyote ceremonies may be conducted by special medicine men, known as Roadmen, who charge for their services.
- Certain individuals who are able to cause sickness in others may practice witchcraft.

Health Beliefs and Practices

- Health is a reflection of a correct relationship between human beings and the environment. Health is associated with good, blessing, and beauty, all of which are valued in life.
- All ailments, both physical and mental, are believed to have supernatural aspects. The Navajo frequently use both their traditional health care system, including traditional health care practitioners, and the modern health care system.

(continued)

BOX 11–5	COMPONENTS OF A CULTURAL ASSESSMENT APPLIED: NATIVE AMERICAN (NAVAJO) *(Continued)*

- There are two major types of traditional health care practitioners. The first is the diviner or diagnostician. Different methods, such as star gazing or hand trembling, are used to identify the cause of an illness. Then, once the cause of the illness has been determined, the individual seeks the second kind of practitioner, the singer, who provides the treatment that counters the cause of the disease and restores harmony.
- Different types of ceremonials as well as herbal medicines and traditional remedies may be used. Infants are placed in cradleboards, which have both traditional and religious significance.
- Cornmeal may be used in healing ceremonies.
- Women herbalists may prescribe herbs for specific and general reasons.

Health Concerns

- Unintentional injuries and violence reflect the combined efforts of living conditions, environment, and behavior. All told, North American Indians have much higher death rates from alcoholism, tuberculosis, diabetes, accidents, suicide, pneumonia, influenza, and homicide (Indian Health Service, 1999; National Forum on Health, 1997).
- Suicide is the second leading cause of death among Indian adolescents. Nearly half (44.6%) of emotionally distressed adolescents have attempted suicide, compared with 16.9% of youths in general (Division of General Pediatrics and Adolescent Health, 1992). In Canada, between 1986 and 1990, the suicide rate in aboriginal children 10 to 19 years old was five times the rate in non-Indian children (Canadian Institute for Child Health, 1994).
- Fetal alcohol syndrome and domestic violence, both related to alcohol abuse, are common problems.
- The rate of fetal alcohol syndrome is six times that in other Americans. Alcohol-related mortality is four times that in the nation as a whole, and traumatic injury related to alcohol and substance abuse is a leading cause of death (U.S. Department of Health and Human Services, 1993).
- Heart disease and malignant neoplasms are leading causes of death for American Indians (Spector, 2000). Very similar health patterns and concerns are found among North American Indians living in Canada.
- Obesity, hypertension, and diabetes are also health concerns in Native North American groups.
- Mortality in adults from infectious diseases is twice that in the general population, and tuberculosis remains a pressing health problem (U.S. Department of Health and Human Services, 1992; National Forum on Health, 1997). In fact, tuberculosis was 475% greater in American Indians than in the U.S. population (U.S. Department of Health and Human Services, 1997).
- Reservations remain poor and often are geographically isolated. Geographic access to health care is of concern.

Adapted from Spector, 2000; Huff & Kline, 1999; Phillips & Lobar, 1990; Boyle, Szymanski, & Szymanski, 1993; Huttlinger & Tanner, 1994; Bell, 1994; Clark, 1996; Kluckhohn & Leighton, 1974.)

the doctor's office or in a hospital. The range of cultural influences on health maintenance and promotion is considerable. Major cultural issues and considerations must be addressed before health maintenance and promotion programs are implemented for culturally diverse groups.

First, it is very important to involve local community leaders who are members of the cultural group being targeted, to promote the acceptance of health promotion programs. Such a leader, for example, might be the pastor of a Black Church in the rural south. The nurse must also be sensitive to cultural differences in leadership styles. For example, the pastor may not speak in favor of the health education program from his or her pulpit but might choose instead to work through more informal networks. Roberson (1985) found that religious beliefs influenced health choices in her study of Black health beliefs and practices. In addition to local community leaders, it is important in the planning process to involve those who are most affected by the health-related problem. Those involved in the planning and participating in the program's activities should likewise participate in its evaluation. Collaboration between the planner and the participants is often the key to success in community-based health programs (Kline, 1999).

Second, family members, churches, employers, and community worksites need to be involved in supporting a health education program by the use of networks that already exist. For example, a health education program about mammography and breast self-examination can be established at a work site that employs mostly women. A display could be set up in the cafeteria, dining room, or other accessible site. Women could peruse the educational material during breaks or after lunch.

Third, health messages are more readily accepted if they do not conflict with existing cultural beliefs. If the nurse plans to talk about prevention of teenage pregnancy to mothers and daughters at a local conservative church, he or she could discuss these plans in advance with some of the mothers and the pastor, and ask for ways to strengthen the church's support of abstinence programs. This is not the appropriate time to focus on contraception methods but to be sensitive to the group's religious values.

Fourth, language barriers and cultural differences are a very real problem in many larger United States and Canadian cities. Local volunteers should be used to disseminate messages in their own language and to help organize and present information that is culturally appropriate and understood by community members. The health care professional should not be afraid to ask for help and suggestions, and should make it a point to find educational material such as brochures or videotapes in the appropriate language.

Last of all, sensitivity is essential to meeting health needs that exist within diverse cultural groups. For example, HIV/AIDS is spreading rapidly in some Hispanic and Black populations and is associated with intravenous drug use, violence, and the spread of crack cocaine use. In addition, the root causes of poverty and unemployment should be examined, and programs that improve overall economic status of culturally diverse communities should be developed. Culturally relevant treatment programs should be implemented. Many minority women who seek treatment programs for cocaine addiction encounter barriers that seem insurmountable. Treatment programs are not available in many areas, and child care facilities are not provided, even in day treatment programs. Thus, a young mother living in a rural area with children would not be able to find a treatment center that meets her needs. If she seeks admittance to a residential treatment program, she might have to agree to place her children in foster care.

Family Systems

Because the family is the basic social unit, it provides the context in which health promotion and maintenance are defined and carried out by family members within culturally diverse communities. The nurse can recognize and use the family's role in altering the health status of a family member and in supporting lifestyle changes. This requires an appreciation of the role of the family in diverse culture groups. Black families, for example, may demonstrate interchangeable roles for their male and female members, extended ties across generations, and strong social support systems, including the Black church, all of which can be tapped by a community health nurse to activate health and wellness in families (Andrews & Bolin, 1993; Spector, 2000; Boyle, Ferrell, Hodnicki, & Muller, 1996).

Coping Behaviors

Culturally diverse clients often have distinct behaviors to cope with illness as well as to maintain and promote health. These behaviors may be traced to the health–illness paradigms that were discussed earlier in Chapter 4. Beliefs about hot and cold, yin and yang, harmony and balance may underlie actions to prevent disease and maintain health. Community nurses who understand their clients' cultural values and beliefs can assess their understanding of health and illness. These assessment data serve as the basis for planning health guidance and teaching strategies that focus on incorporating cultural beliefs and practices in the nursing care plan. It seems likely that clients in the process of coping with illness and seeking help may involve a network of persons, ranging from family members and select lay persons to health care professionals.

Seeking social support is often seen as a means of coping. It is now evident that social support varies widely across people, cultural groups, and circumstances. For example, Hill, Hawkins, Raposo, and Carr (1995) examined the relations among coping strategies of Black mothers, their exposure to community violence, and their interpersonal victimization. Their findings indicated that coping strategies are used differently, depending on the amount of violence within the sociocultural context and the education and financial resources of the mothers. Other studies of coping behaviors during an illness of a family member (Stewart, 1994; Picot, 1995) also show that interactions may differ remarkably at any one time during the illness, depending on intrapersonal, interpersonal, and environmental factors. Certainly, nurses working with multicultural populations will want to learn and understand how coping styles are used by individuals and family members.

Lifestyle Practices

Cultural influences have a significant impact on such health-promoting factors as diet, exercise, and stress management. Community health nurses should assess the implications of diet planning and teaching to clients and family members who adhere to culturally prescribed practices concerning foods. Some cultural groups believe that certain foods maintain or promote health. Some foods often are restricted during illness, just as there are "sick foods"—special dishes served to an ill person, such as the proverbial chicken soup. Cultural preferences determine the style of food preparation and consumption, the frequency of eating, the time of eating, and eating utensils. Milk is not always considered a suitable source of protein for Native Americans, Hispanics, Blacks, and some Asians because of their relatively high incidence of lactose intolerance.

Nurses who work with culturally different clients must evaluate patterns of daily living as well as culturally prescribed activities before they suggest forms of physical activity or exercise to clients. Exercise is often defined in terms of White middle-class values. Not everyone has access to the tennis court at a local country club, and many individuals would not feel comfortable in such surroundings or in aerobics classes regardless of the setting. Although stereotyping is possible, some Black men might feel more comfortable playing basketball after work. Tribal dancing has become popular on some reservations for Native North Americans. Helping clients plan physical activities that are culturally acceptable is only the first step in implementing a program of physical activity. Health Canada offers online guidelines for developing individual physical activity programs appropriate for a wide variety of lifestyles and circumstances. The URL for this website is www.paguide.com

Another aspect of lifestyle that must be understood for the successful promotion of health and wellness is the manner in which culturally different clients manage stress. Stress management is learned from childhood through our parents, our social group, and our cultural group. Smoking and/or chewing tobacco are often used to manage stress. Persons who choose to smoke greatly increase the risk of the development of heart disease and cancer. Debates currently rage about smoking in public places and the use of tobacco.

In addition, environmental tobacco smoke—that is, smoke that nonsmokers are exposed to from smokers—poses a risk of lung cancer and asthma to the nonsmoker (Cookfair, 1991). The use and abuse of alcoholic beverages are also related to lifestyle practices. Families coping with multiple stressors often feel overwhelmed by the challenges of everyday living, and individuals within families may develop dysfunctional ways of coping such as alcohol abuse and domestic violence. Although many of these lifestyle practices are not associated with a group's culture per se, they are often found in groups whose members do not have appropriate options and/or alternatives and who are poor and unable to access employment and educational opportunities.

Many cultural groups tend to express psychologic distress through somatic symptoms, and some studies have found that women are at high risk for depression and somatic complaints. Depressed women report more physical complaints, increased disability, increased functional limitations, and increased use of health care services than do nondepressed women (Betrus, Elmore, & Hamilton, 1995). Indeed, for many immigrants and refugees, stress-related disorders such as posttraumatic stress disorder are relatively common. The presence of large numbers of families with altered family processes and unhealthy lifestyles within the community may create problems for all members of the larger community or society. The nurse who works in community settings will frequently encounter these families and is in an ideal position to care for them, to act as their advocate, to refer them to appropriate care, and, in effect, to improve the health of the community at large.

The nurse may find that in some cultural groups such as Mexican Americans, traditional healers, such as *curanderas,* can be helpful for persons with some emotional or psychologic disorders. In addition, health professionals such as physicians, dentists, and nurse practitioners may be more acceptable if they share the same ethnic heritage as the client. In some aggregate ethnic settings, such as the Chinatowns in San Francisco and Toronto, there are practitioners of traditional Chinese medicine as well as Western medicine, acupuncturists, neighborhood pharmacies, and herbalists, which are available to meet the diverse needs of that particular neighborhood.

Cultural Competence in Primary, Secondary, and Tertiary Preventive Programs

Nurses working in community settings use health-related concepts that are identified with the practice of community health nursing. Concepts such as "community as client" and "population-focused practice" were discussed briefly in the first sections of this chapter. Another concept of importance to community nurses is that of **levels of prevention**. Preventive care, consisting of primary, secondary, and tertiary activities, is directed toward high-risk groups or aggregates within a community setting. **Primary prevention** is composed of activities that prevent the occurrence of an illness, a disease, or a health risk. The preventive actions take place before the disease or illness occurs. **Secondary prevention** involves the early diagnosis and appropriate treatment of a condition or disease. **Tertiary prevention** focuses on rehabilitation and the prevention of recurrences or complications. The major aim of community-based preventive programs is to reduce the risk for the population at large rather than to prevent illnesses in specific individuals. As long as preventive actions are directed toward a given population rather than toward individuals, there is a chance of altering the general balance of forces so that although not all will benefit, many will have a chance to avoid illness. This last section of this chapter discusses the use of cultural knowledge to plan community nursing interventions for diverse cultural groups at the primary, secondary, and tertiary levels of prevention.

Primary Prevention: Prenatal Services in a Mexican American Community

OVERVIEW OF THE HEALTH CONCERN

For some time now, it has been recognized that adequate prenatal care helps to reduce infant mortality. With this in mind, public health agencies have tried to improve maternal and infant services to high-risk populations. In the 1980s, a special government report on minority health reported that only 58% of Mexican American mothers begin prenatal care in the first trimester, less than that for Blacks or non-Hispanic women (Heckler, 1985a). The neonatal mortality rate appeared good for Mexican American babies; but still, by 1995, fewer Hispanic mothers began their prenatal care during the first trimester than did mothers of certain other ethnic origins (73.7% for Hispanic mothers versus 84.7% for White mothers and 82.1% for Asian and Pacific Islander mothers) (Health, United States, 1995). Berry (1999) suggested that cultural factors such as a strong extended family support system and the preservation of traditional beliefs and values might influence pregnancy outcomes in Hispanic mothers.

The risk factors of pregnancy include age (both extremes), parity, and low socioeconomic status. Many women of Mexican American origin fall in these categories; a high-risk group of great concern is the pregnant adolescent. A program of primary prevention would focus on preventing infant mortality and other health problems in young Mexican American mothers and their infants. Nursing care must be broadly focused, providing some specific services but also helping clients access other resources in the community. Information can be provided through media campaigns geared to the Mexican American community, informing women of available services and how to access them. Spanish radio shows that play popular music might be a good avenue for advertising prenatal services. Culturally related factors that might prevent Mexican American women from obtaining care early in their pregnancies include the factors discussed below.

Access to Care

There are various reasons why Mexican Americans might not seek care during pregnancy. Cost is often a factor, and in many areas of the country, Mexican Americans have tended to belong to poorer socioeconomic groups (Heckler, 1985a, 1985b). The community health nurse can provide information about community resources and help clients access care early in pregnancy by referral to appropriate agencies. Nearly all states now provide programs that provide funds and services for low-income pregnant women.

Cultural Views About Modesty

Any prenatal program that serves Mexican American women may be underused unless consideration is given to some Mexican American women's extreme modesty and reluctance to be examined by male health care providers. The use of female nurse practitioners and midwives is ideal for this population. In addition, some consideration should be given to incorporation of the traditional *parteras* (lay midwives) into the preventive educational services, if that is deemed appropriate.

Language Barriers

It is absolutely essential in a prenatal program for a Mexican American population that the majority of health care professionals in the program be bilingual. If that is impossible, interpreters must be employed to facilitate the professional services. All prenatal classes should be offered in Spanish and English. This sometimes means that two classes must be offered concurrently; many Mexican American women speak predominantly either Spanish or English and would choose the class where they understand the language. The availability of health education material in Spanish is critical to reinforce teaching and anticipatory guidance. In Berry's study (1999) of Mexican American women and prenatal care, the key informants who were bilingual spoke only Spanish within their homes because they did not want their children to forget their heritage.

Cultural Views of Motherhood and Pregnancy

Some evidence indicates that women of Mexican American culture may adhere to different value orientations and cultural views of motherhood and pregnancy than those found in mainstream American culture (Burk, Wieser, & Keegan, 1995). The Mexican American culture traditionally values motherhood, and young women are encouraged to prepare themselves for this role. In most traditional cultures, motherhood is the appropriately defined role for women, and there are few alternatives. White (1985) found that pregnant Mexican American women viewed their growing bodies as feminine, softening, and beautiful. Community health nurses, nurse practitioners, and professional midwives are in important positions to help pregnant women prepare for motherhood and its associated responsibilities. Understanding and reinforcing the approved cultural views of pregnancy may be helpful for clients because trust and mutual goal setting can thus develop more rapidly.

Traditional Pregnancy-Related Folk Beliefs of Mexican Americans

Many Mexican Americans adhere to traditional beliefs and practices related to pregnancy and childbirth. Additionally, children are greatly valued and are desired soon after marriage. As in many other cultures, Mexican Americans consider pregnancy, birth, and the immediate postpartum period as a time of great vulnerability for women and their newborns. Some traditional beliefs and practices related to pregnancy and childbirth are shown in Box 11-6.

Mexican American Cultural Networks

Traditionally, the family is very important in Mexican American culture, and nursing care should be family focused. The most important social structural factor in the Mexican American culture is family and kinship ties. These ties often go beyond the family to a wide network of kin. Bauwens and Anderson (1992) observed that a Mexican American is expected to turn first to the family for help; if preventive services are to be effective, they must tap these kinds

BOX 11–6	**SELECTED BELIEFS AND PRACTICES OF PREGNANCY AND CHILDBIRTH IN TRADITIONAL MEXICAN AMERICAN CULTURE**

- Avoid strong emotions such as anger and fear during pregnancy.
- Cool air is dangerous during pregnancy and should be avoided.
- Bathe often during pregnancy; be active so that the baby will not grow too big and hinder delivery.
- Eat a nutritious diet; "give in" to food cravings.
- Massage is helpful to place the baby in the right position for birth.
- Don't raise your arms above your head or sit with your legs crossed during pregnancy, because it will cause knots in the umbilical cord.
- Moonlight should be avoided during pregnancy, especially during an eclipse, because it will cause a birth defect.
- After delivery, a 40-day period known as *la diet* or *la cuarentena* is observed. Certain activities and foods are restricted.
- Chamomile tea will relieve nausea and vomiting in pregnancy.
- Heartburn can be treated with baking soda.
- Laxatives and purges may be used to "clean" the intestinal tract.

of cultural networks to ensure the support of community residents in preventive programs in their neighborhoods that involve family members, neighbors, or friends. Health care professionals face challenges such as language barriers, literacy levels, socioeconomic and educational levels, cultural backgrounds, and other subtle differences when they work with the varied Hispanic groups in the United States.

USING CULTURAL COMPETENCE AT THE PRIMARY LEVEL OF PREVENTION

Certain high-risk behaviors during pregnancy, such as smoking, using drugs, consuming alcohol, and maintaining poor nutritional habits, should be targeted by the community health nurse for change. Although there is no set rule of thumb, a Mexican American mother-to-be may respond to suggestions for change if she is convinced that her behavior will cause harm to her baby. Family and social support groups in Mexican American culture can also be helpful and supportive to expectant mothers wishing to make lifestyle changes. Some researchers have found that pregnant Latin women will attempt to stop smoking and will be successful with the help, support, and assistance of their families. Evidence-Based Practice 11–2 provides an example and offers clinical applications for nursing practice.

Prenatal services should go beyond the birth of the baby to include information about breastfeeding and family planning services. Traditionally, some health care professionals have assumed that family planning services will not be accepted in a Mexican American population because of religious opposition and *machismo*—the need of the man to prove his manhood by having children or to believe in the biologic superiority of men. However, it may be that Mexican American men as well as women are interested in family planning and are concerned about the number of children they can support. This issue

EVIDENCE-BASED PRACTICE 11–2
Cigarette Smoking and Pregnant Latinas

Because cigarette smoking is harmful to pregnant women and their babies, most pregnant women make some smoking changes through cessation or reduced smoking. This study described cigarette smoking and smoking cessation experiences of pregnant Latinas who participated in focus groups. Smoking was described as a personal resource to deal with stress and as a social activity that facilitated interactions with family and friends. Many women described concern for their babies related to their smoking. The women related that the men in their lives disapproved of women smoking. Although the addictive properties of cigarette smoking impeded the cessation process, women reported that the support of others was a key element for success. Examination of the data in the context of cultural values revealed family involvement in Latinas' smoking behavior during pregnancy as powerful, unique, relevant, and consistent with the cultural values of allocentrism and familism. This finding provides a substantive base from which smoking cessation programs, tailored for pregnant Latinas, can be developed and implemented.

CLINICAL APPLICATION

1. Involve family members such as mothers, sisters, and husbands in smoking cessation programs, because they provide important support to Hispanic women.
2. Smoking cessation messages and educational programs in Hispanic cultures should be targeted to families rather than to individuals.
3. Pregnancy is a time when many women are concerned for their babies' health and will be more committed to quit smoking.

Pletsch, P. K., & Johnson, M. A. (1996). The cigarette smoking experiences of pregnant Latinas in the United States. *Health Care for Women International, 17,* 549–562.

should be validated with individual clients and their spouses. During *la cuarentena,* the 40 days after the birth of the baby, women kin of the new mother often help with infant care, household tasks, and preparation of special foods for the mother (Berry, 1999).

Strategies for promoting breastfeeding should be identified and encouraged. For example, educational levels, family experiences with breastfeeding, the husband's attitude, the need to return to work, and feelings of embarrassment have been associated with infant feeding choices among Mexican American women (Young & Kaufman, 1988). These factors need to be explored with individual women to help them make the best choices for themselves and their babies.

Secondary Levels of Prevention: Type II Diabetes and Native Americans

OVERVIEW OF THE HEALTH CONCERN

Non–insulin-dependent diabetes (NIDD), or type II diabetes, is seen commonly among some Native North Americans, and certain tribes have extremely high rates of the disease, 154% higher than those for other groups in the United

States (Hodge & Fredericks, 1999). In Canada, the prevalence of diabetes among aboriginal peoples is at least three times that of the general population (Health Canada, 1999b). By all accounts, the high rate of diabetes in Native North American groups is a leading health concern, because diabetes is a leading cause of outpatient visits at Indian Health Service facilities. Further, Indian deaths resulting from renal failure alone were reported to be 290% higher than the national average in the United States (U.S. Department of Health and Human Services, 1993). Similarly, in Canada, an aboriginal person is up to 12 times more likely to have diabetic nephropathy than is a nonaboriginal person (Health Canada, 199b).

The reasons for the epidemic of type II diabetes among some Native North Americans are not clear. It is believed that some Native North American tribes have an underlying genetic propensity for the disease that is triggered by changes in dietary practices, a sedentary lifestyle, and increasing obesity (Neel, 1962; West, 1978; Young, 1994). These factors have been complicated by social conditions such as poverty as well as by problems of compliance or lack of adherence to medical regimens (Huse, Oster, Kildeen, Lurey, & Coldez, 1989).

Because of the high rate of diabetes on some reservations, numerous secondary preventive services that focus on early diagnosis and treatment have been initiated. Many of them are modeled after programs that have been successful with White middle-class North Americans. Culturally related factors that could influence the success of secondary preventive programs for diabetes among some Native North Americans are shown in Box 11-7. Readers are cautioned that validation of beliefs and practices should always take place with individual clients and families, and stereotyping (thinking that all Native North Americans are the same) should be avoided.

Using Cultural Competence at the Secondary Level of Prevention

Nursing interventions at the secondary level of prevention should focus on the implementation of healthful lifestyle changes that will ultimately decrease the complications of diabetes. Most of these are related to what health professionals call diet and exercise, but what is appropriate for Native North American culture is an emphasis on health and a healthy lifestyle.

Emphasize health and a healthy lifestyle rather than negative factors such as control of diabetes, prevention of complications, weight reduction, and exercise. The choice of words, as well as the emphasis, is important. For example, when teaching the client and family about diabetic diets, the nurse can substitute the word "nutrition" for "diet," thus removing the negative perceptions and leading to a nursing plan that emphasizes substitution rather than deprivation. Substituting fruits for candy bars and packaged pastries, whole grains for potato chips or doughnuts, and vegetables for sugared snacks will improve nutritional status and lead to a healthier lifestyle. Special traditional foods, even fried bread, can be eaten on special occasions, and other types of bread can be substituted during regular meals.

Health education can be oriented toward individual clients and directed toward the family rather than provided in an impersonal clinic situation.

BOX 11–7	BELIEFS AND PRACTICES RELATED TO DIABETES FOUND IN SOME NATIVE NORTH AMERICANS

Nutritional Practices

- Diets are high in calories, carbohydrates, and fats.
- Sharing communal meals is a common and valued cultural practice.
- Some groups have a high incidence of obesity.
- Food preparation often adds fats and calories.
- Snack foods (potato chips, carbonated beverages, prepackaged pastries) are common.
- High intake of alcohol seriously compromises the treatment of diabetes.

Activity Levels/Fitness Practices

- Sedentary lifestyles have become common.
- Many reservations lack recreational facilities.
- Formal exercise activities are associated with the White man's culture and are not thought to be appropriate for Native North Americans.

Beliefs and Values Related to Diabetes

- Ideal body image favors a heavier physique, and weight gain is considered normal; thinness is a cause for worry and concern.
- Concept of "control of one's body," i.e., weight, glucose levels, blood pressure, may conflict with values and norms of Native North American culture. For example, Native North American clients may be uncomfortable with comparison of individual performance against others or against the norms and standards of biomedical care.
- Many Native North Americans are uncomfortable with discussing or exposing private body functions, such as providing urine samples or blood testing in a public situation.
- Illness is a personal and unpleasant topic, and Native North American clients may be uncomfortable when asked to talk about it.
- Diabetes is a "White man's disease"; Native North Americans did not have diabetes until Whites came to this continent.
- The term "diabetic" may be offensive to some, and the label "diabetic clinic" may discourage clients from seeking health care services.
- White health professionals may be viewed with some suspicion and distrust, given the history of cultural contact between Whites and Native North Americans.
- Because diabetes is so common in some tribal groups, there is a fatalism about the disease, especially if a family member already has diabetes.
- Beliefs and health practices surrounding diabetes may vary according to the Native North American tribe.

Physical activities that are culturally congruent can be encouraged; again, the value of health and a healthy lifestyle should be stressed over exercise and weight reduction. Physical activities that are congruent with overall lifestyle and cultural context will be easier to incorporate into daily living situations.

Usually, the Native North American family system is an extended family that includes several households of closely related kin. Family members become exceedingly important during times of crisis because they are a source of support, comfort, assistance, and strength. The importance of cultural ties with kin and other members of the reservation community always must be considered in planning for early diagnosis and treatment programs. It is in this context (family and community) that clients are encouraged and supported not only to seek care but also to institute lifestyle changes that are congruent with cultural practices and that will enhance the health status of all members of the family and, ultimately, the tribal community.

Serious behavioral and social problems contribute to the high risk factors in North American Indian groups. Suicide rates are rising, and deaths resulting from homicide, accidents, and injuries have resulted in increased Indian mortality. Newer threats to Indian health such as cancer, diabetes, nutritional diseases, and other illnesses caused by changing behaviors and environment contaminants are on the rise. These problems contribute significantly to death and disease (Hodge & Fredericks, 1999).

Tertiary Levels of Prevention: Hypertension and Blacks

OVERVIEW OF THE HEALTH CONCERN

Blacks are a highly heterogeneous group and display considerable variation in health beliefs and behaviors. For the most part, this section will discuss a more traditional, rural Black culture, and the reader is advised to validate beliefs and behaviors with individual clients and communities.

Hypertension is a major risk factor for heart disease and stroke. Mean blood pressure levels are higher in Blacks than in European Americans, with a marked excess in Blacks. A decade ago, in a government study on minority health, Heckler (1985a) stated that "hypertensive Blacks were at least as likely as Whites of the same sex to be treated with antihypertensive medication and nearly as likely to have their blood pressure controlled" (p. 110). Heckler also noted that from 1968 to 1982, stroke mortality in Blacks declined 5%, and coronary heart disease also had decreased dramatically.

Control of hypertension has certainly been one factor responsible for this improvement. It is critical that efforts to treat hypertension in Black populations be continued. Unfortunately, appropriate care often has been complicated by discrimination, poverty, and limited access to care.

The goal of tertiary prevention is to reduce disability and prevent complications from developing. A major aim of nursing care in the implementation of tertiary activities is to help clients adjust to limitations in daily living, to increase their coping skills, to control symptoms, and in general to minimize the complications of disease by reducing the rate of residual damage in a given population. Cultural factors that should be considered in tertiary prevention programs for Blacks are shown in Box 11-8.

| BOX 11–8 | CULTURAL FACTORS TO CONSIDER IN PLANNING TERTIARY PREVENTION FOR A TRADITIONAL BLACK POPULATION |

Language

Black communication concepts and patterns can be identified and used in community education programs.

Cultural Health Beliefs

Good health comes from good luck.
Health is related to harmony in nature.
Illnesses are classified as "natural" or "unnatural."
Illness may be God's punishment.
Maintenance of health is associated with "reading the signs," i.e., phase of the moon, seasons of the year, position of the planets.

Cultural Health Practices

The use of herbs, oils, powders, roots, and other home remedies may be common.

Cultural Healers

Older woman ("old lady") in the community who has a knowledge of herbs and healing.
Spiritualist who is called by God to heal disease or solve emotional or personal problems.
Voodoo priest/priestess who is a powerful cultural healer who uses voodoo, bone reading, etc. to heal or to bring about desired events.
Root doctor who uses roots, herbs, oils, candles, and ointments in healing rituals.

Time Orientation

May be present-time oriented, which makes preventive care more difficult to implement and maintain.

Nutritional Practices

Soul food takes its name from a feeling of kinship among Blacks and may be served at home, provided at church dinners, or served at home-style restaurants.
Diets may reflect traditional rural southern foods such as greens, grits, corn bread, and chick peas.

Economic Status

Blacks account for many persons in the lower socioeconomic strata in American society.

(continued)

BOX 11–8	**CULTURAL FACTORS TO CONSIDER IN PLANNING TERTIARY PREVENTION FOR A TRADITIONAL BLACK POPULATION** *(Continued)*

Educational Status

High aspirations for education, but socioeconomic status and other complex factors limit educational opportunities.

Family and Social Networks

Often strong extended family networks with a sense of obligation to relatives.

Self-concept

The importance of race has been a continual issue for the self-identity of Blacks.

Impact of Racism

Unfortunately, racism is still present, and a negative perception of the Black's skin color by health professionals will seriously interfere with efficacious health care.

Religion

Black churches have tremendous influence on the daily life of their members because they serve as a source of spiritual and social support.
The Black church acts as a caretaker for the cultural characteristics of Black culture (Roberson, 1985).

Biologic Variations

There is a high incidence of lactose intolerance and lactase deficiency; this has implications for diet planning if Black clients cannot tolerate milk or milk products.
There is a higher prevalence of hypertension among Blacks than among Europeans. Sickle cell anemia is more common among Blacks.

Adapted from Bloch, B. (1983). Nursing care of black patients. In M. S. Orque, B. Bloch, & L. S. Monroy (Eds.). *Ethnic nursing care: A multicultural approach, pp. 81–113.*
St. Louis: C. V. Mosby; and Andrews, M. M., & Bolin, L. (1993). The African American community. In J. M. Swanson & M. Albrecht (Eds.). *Community health nursing: Promoting the health of aggregates, pp. 443–458.* Philadelphia: W. B. Saunders.

USING CULTURAL COMPETENCE AT THE TERTIARY LEVEL OF PREVENTION

Community nurses have demonstrated competence in the management of community hypertension programs. Although these programs are vital to the early diagnosis and management of hypertension, they also include a component that focuses on helping clients manage a chronic disease—an aspect of tertiary prevention. The community should be involved in every aspect of community-based programs. The goals, objectives, and interventions of the services should reflect the felt needs of the target group. Hypertension programs should reflect the values, beliefs, and interests of the community to which they are targeted.

Community health nurses are in the advantageous position of assessing clients and families in their own homes and neighborhoods. This provides an understanding of the daily life situation faced by clients that other health care professionals often lack. Community health nurses can bring this understanding to bear on helping clients with tertiary preventive activities.

SUMMARY

Cultural concepts related to community health nursing practice were discussed. A framework for providing culturally sensitive nursing care was introduced to help nurses and other health professionals provide care to individuals and groups with diverse cultural backgrounds. These frameworks help nurses use cultural knowledge in assessing, planning, and implementing nursing care. This chapter explored the role of the family in transmitting beliefs and practices concerning health and illness. Cultural diversity within communities was addressed, and various subcultures within the United States and Canada, including refugees and immigrants, were discussed. A community case study of Afghan refugees was provided. Special concerns related to refugee populations were described. Cultural data about traditional Afghan culture were related, and examples of culturally competent care were provided.

Cultural concepts were explored as they relate to the community at large. A cultural assessment was described as an integral component of a community nursing assessment. A selected cultural assessment of the Navajo (Native North American) people was presented as an example to provide cultural data that assist nurses in providing culturally sensitive nursing care to individuals and groups. Culturally competent nursing interventions for community health maintenance and health promotion were presented. Preventive care in the community is of particular importance to community health nursing. The use of cultural knowledge in primary, secondary, and tertiary levels of prevention was introduced. Examples of cultural diversity and levels of prevention were described to illustrate how cultural knowledge can be used in community health nursing practice.

REVIEW QUESTIONS

1. Describe four cultural concepts, and discuss how they can be used to provide transcultural nursing care to families and aggregates.
2. Describe an example of how cultural factors influence the health of an aggregate group within the community. How do cultural factors influence illness levels in an aggregate group?

3. List the major cultural considerations in implementing preventive pro- grams for culturally diverse groups. How can cultural considerations be used to identify barriers and facilitators for preventive programs?
4. Identify special health considerations in immigrant groups within the com- munity.
5. Describe an approach to primary preventive health care for several cultural groups, i.e., Hispanics, Blacks, Amish, and Laotians.
6. Describe secondary and tertiary programs targeting hypertension for eld- erly Chinese North Americans.
7. Describe similarities and differences between folk and scientific health care systems. Give an example of each.

CRITICAL THINKING ACTIVITIES

1. Describe sociocultural factors and their impact on health care for a cultural group within your community. Evaluate the access to, availability of, and acceptability of various health care services. Is this cultural group at risk? Why?
2. Conduct a community cultural assessment of a group within your commu- nity. Critically analyze the cultural knowledge and/or information that should be considered when planning care for the group. Use the outline provided in Table 11-2 to identify and collect cultural assessment data, i.e., family and kinship, social life, political systems, language, worldview, reli- gious behaviors, health beliefs and practices, and health concerns. Compare and contrast the assessment of other groups in your community.
3. For a cultural group in your community, develop a program plan or inter- vention that has components of primary, secondary, and tertiary preven- tion.
4. Attend religious services at a church, temple, mosque, synagogue, or place of worship to learn about a religion different from your own. Assess how each church meets the unique needs of its congregation.
5. Identify alternative health care practitioners within your community. Which subcultures do they serve? Describe the kinds of care that they offer to residents.

• References

American Psychiatric Association. (1987). *Diagnostic and statistical manual of mental disorders* (3rd ed., rev.). Washington, DC: American Psychiatric Association.

Anderson, E. T., & McFarlane, J. M. (2000). *Community as partner: Theory and practice in nursing* (3rd ed.). Philadelphia: Lippincott Williams & Wilkins.

Andrews, M. M., & Bolin, L. (1993). The African-American community. In J. M. Swanson & M. Albrecht (Eds.). *Community health nursing: Promoting the health of* *aggregates (pp. 433–458)*. Philadelphia: W. B. Saunders.

Aroian, K. J. (1993). Mental health risks and problems encountered by illegal immigrants. *Issues in Mental Health Nursing, 14,* 379–397.

Barth, F. (1987). Cultural Wellsprings of Resistance in Afghan Islam. In R. Klass (Ed.) *Afghanistan: the great game revisited* (pp. 187–202). Boston: Freedom House.

Bauwens, E., & Anderson, S. (1992). Social and cultural influences on health care. In M. Stanhope & J. Lancaster (Eds.). *Community health nursing: Process and health, practice for promoting* (3rd ed., pp. 91–108). St. Louis, MO: C. V. Mosby.

Bell, R. (1994). Prominence of women in Navajo healing beliefs and values. *Nursing and Health Care, 15,* 232–240.

Berry, A. B. (1999). Mexican American women's expressions of the meaning of culturally congruent prenatal care. *Journal of Transcultural Nursing, 10,* 203–212.

Betrus, P. A., Elmore, S. K., & Hamilton, P. A. (1995). Women and somatization: Unrecognized depression. *Health Care for Women International, 16,* 287–297.

Bloch, B. (1983). Nursing care of black patients. In M. S. Orque, B. Bloch, & L. A. Monrroy (Eds.). *Ethnic Nursing Care: A Multicultural Approach, pp. 81–113.* St. Louis, MO: C. V. Mosby.

Boyle, J. S., Ferrell, J., Hodnicki, D., & Muller, R. (1996). Going home: African American caregiving for adult children with human immunodeficiency virus disease. *Holistic Nursing Practice, 11,* 27–35.

Boyle, J. S., Szymanski, M. T., & Szymanski, M. E. (1993). Improving home health care for the Navajo. *Nursing Connections, 5*(4), 3.

Burk, M. E., Wieser, P. C., & Keegan, L. (1995). Cultural beliefs and health behaviors of pregnant Mexican American women: Implications for primary health care. *Advances in Nursing Science, 17*(4), 37–52.

Clark, M. J. (1996). Care of the community or target group. In M. J. Clark (Ed.). *Nursing in the community* (2nd ed., pp. 389–421). Stamford, CT: Appleton & Lange.

Cookfair, J. M. (1991). *Nursing process and practices in the community.* St. Louis, MO: C. V. Mosby.

DeSantis, L. (1997). Building healthy communities with immigrants and refugees. *Journal of Transcultural Nursing, 9,* 20–31.

Flynn, B. C. (1997). Are we ready to collaborate for community based health services? *Public Health Nursing, 14*(3), 135–136.

Friedman, M. M., & Ferguson-Marshalleck, E. G. (1996). Sociocultural influences on family health. In S. M. Hanson & S. T. Boyd, *Family Health Care Nursing: Theory, Practice, and Research,* pp. 81–98. Philadelphia: F. A. Davis.

Halli, S. S. & Driedger, L. (1999). Immigrant Canada: Demographic, economic, and social challenges. Toronto: University of Toronto Press.

Health Canada (1999a). Canadian research on immigration and health. Available at: http://www.hc-sc.gc.ca/iacb-dgiac/nhrdp/metropolis/cirh_pdf_index_e.htm. Accessed November 23, 2001.

Health Canada (1999b). Diabetes in Canada: Diabetes and aboriginal peoples. Available at: http://www.hc-sc.gc.ca/hpb/lcdc/publicat/diabet99/d12_e.html. Accessed November 30, 2001.

Health Canada (2001, October 11). Achieving health for all: A framework for health promotion. Available at: http://www.hc-sc.gc.ca/english/care/achieving_health.html. Accessed November 23, 2002.

Health, United States, 1995, p. 119. Division of Health and Utilization Analysis. Division of Vital Statistics and Health, United States, 1999.

Heckler, M. M. (1985a). *Report of the Secretary's Task Force on Black and Minority Health:* Vol. I: Executive summary. Washington, DC: U.S. Department of Health and Human Services.

Heckler, M. M. (1985b). *Report to the Secretary's Task Force on Black and Minority Health, Vol.2: Crosscutting Issues in Minority Health.* Washington, DC: U.S. Department of Health and Human Services.

Hill, H. M., Hawkins, S. R., Raposo, M., & Carr, P. (1995). Relationship between multiple exposures to violence and coping strategies among African-American mothers. *Violence and Victims, 10* (1), 55–71.

Hodge, F. S., & Fredericks, L. (1999). American Indian and Alaska Native populations in the United States. In R. M. Huff & M. V. Kline (Eds.), *Promoting health in multicultural populations (pp. 269–289).* Thousand Oaks, CA: Sage.

Huff, R. H. (1999). Cross-cultural concepts of health and disease. In R. M. Huff & M. V. Kline (Eds.), *Promoting health in multicultural populations (pp. 23–40).* Thousand Oaks, CA: Sage.

Huff, R. M. & Kline, M. V. (1999). *Promoting Health in Multicultural Populations.* Thousand Oaks, CA: Sage.

Huse, D. M., Osler, G., Kildeen, A. R., Lurey, M. T., & Coldez, G. A. (1989). The economic costs of non-insulin dependent diabetes mellitus. *Journal of the American Medical Association, 8,* 391–406.

Huttlinger, K. W., & Tanner, D. (1994). The peyote way: Implications for culture care theory. *Journal of Transcultural Nursing, 5,* 5–11.

Indian Health Service, 1999. *Comprehensive care program for American Indians and Alaska Natives, pp. 34–35, 43.* Washington, DC: U.S. Public Health Service.

Isajiw, W. W. (1999). *Understanding diversity: Ethnicity and race in the Canadian context.* Toronto: Thompson Educational Publishing, Inc.

Kline, M. V. (1999). Planning health promotion and disease prevention programs in multicultural populations. In R. M. Huff & M. V. Kline (Eds.), *Promoting health in multicultural populations (pp. 73–102).* Thousand Oaks, CA: Sage.

Kluckhohn, C., & Leighton, D. (1974). *The Navaho.* Cambridge, MA: Harvard University Press.

Leininger, M. (1978*). Transcultural nursing: Concepts, theories and practices.* New York: John Wiley & Sons.

Leininger, M. (1991). Leininger's acculturation health care assessment tool for cultural patterns in traditional and nontraditional lifeways. *Journal of Transcultural Nursing, 2*(2), 40–42.

Leininger, M. (1995). Teaching transcultural nursing in undergraduate and graduate programs. *Journal of Transcultural Nursing, 6*(2), 10–26.

Lipson, J. (1991). Afghan refugee health: Some findings and suggestions. *Qualitative Health Research, 1,* 349–369.

Lipson, J. (1993). Afghan refugees in California: Mental health issues. *Issues in Mental Health Nursing, 14,* 411–423.

Lipson, J. & Meleis, A. (1983). Issues in health care of middle eastern patients. *Western Journal of Medicine, 139*(6), 854–861.

Lipson, J. & Miller, S. (1994). Changing roles of Afghan refugee women in the U.S. *Health Care for Women International, 15,* 171–180.

Lipson, J., Omidian, P., & Paul, S. (1995). Afghan health education project: A community survey. *Public Health Nursing, 12,* 143–150.

Lipson, J., & Omidian, P. (1997). Afghan refugee issues in the U.S. Social environment. *Western Journal of Nursing Research, 19*(1), 110–126.

Lipson, J., & Omidian, P. (1992). Afghan refugees: Health issues in the United States. *Western Journal of Medicine, 157,* 271–275.

Lowry, L. W., & Martin, K. S. (2000). Organizing frameworks applied to community health nursing. In M. Stanhope & J. Lancaster, *Community Health Nursing: Promoting Health of Aggregates, Families and Individuals* (5th ed., pp. 202–225). St. Louis, MO: C. V. Mosby.

Lurie, N. (1997). Studying access to care in managed care environments. *Health Services Research, 322,* 691–701.

McGeary, J. (2001, October 1). Afghanistan: The Taliban troubles. *Time*, pp. 36–43.

Meleis, A. I. (1997). Immigrant transitions and health care: An action plan. *Nursing Outlook, 45,* 42.

National Forum on Health (1997*). The need for an aboriginal health institute in Canada.* Available from: http://wwwnfh.hc-sc.gc.ca/publicat/finvol2/aborig/idxabo.htm. Accessed November 30, 2001.

National Institute of Nursing Research (1995). *Community-based health care: Nursing strategies.* Bethesda, MD: U.S. Department of Health and Human Services.

Neel, J. V. (1962). Diabetes mellitus: A "thrifty" genotype rendered detrimental by progress. *American Journal of Human Genetics, 14,* 353–362.

Phillips, S., & Lobar, S. (1990). Literature summary of some Navaho child health beliefs and rearing practices within a transcultural nursing framework. *Journal of Transcultural Nursing, 1,* 13–20.

Pender, N. J. (1987). Health and health promotion: Conceptual dilemmas. In M. E. Duffy & N. J. Pender (Eds.), *Proceedings of a Wingspread Conference: Conceptual Issues in Health Promotion, (pp. 7–23).* Indianapolis: Sigma Theta Tau International, Honor Society of Nursing.

Picot, S. J. (1995). Rewards, costs, and coping of African American caregivers. *Nursing Research, 44,* 147–152.

Roberson, M. H. B. (1985). The influence of religious beliefs on health choices of Afro-Americans. *Topics in Clinical Nursing, 7*(3), 57–63.

Saunders, L. (1954). *Cultural differences and medical care: The case of the Spanish speaking people of the southwest.* New York: Russell Sage Foundation.

Scanlan, J. (1983). Who is a refugee? Procedures and burden of proof under the Refugee Act of 1980. *In Defense of the Alien, 5,* 23.

Schuster, G. F. & Goeppinger, J. (2000). Community as client: Using the nursing process to promote health. In M. Stanhope & J. Lancaster (Eds.). *Community health nursing: Process and practice for promoting health* (5th ed., pp. 306–329). St. Louis, MO: C. V. Mosby.

Shi, L. & Singh, D. A. (2001). Health services for special populations. In L. Shi & D.A. Singh (Eds.), *Delivering health care in America: A systems approach (pp. 412–465).* Gaithersburg, MD: Aspen.

Spector, R. E. (2000). *Cultural diversity in health and illness* (5th ed.). New York: Appleton-Century-Crofts.

Stanhope, M., & Lancaster, J. (2000). *Community health nursing: Promoting health of aggregates, families and individuals* (5th ed.). St. Louis, MO: C. V. Mosby.

Stewart, B. M. (1994). End-of-life family decision-making from disclosure of HIV through bereavement. *Scholarly Inquiry for Nursing Practice: An International Journal, 8,* 321–352.

U.S. Bureau of the Census—The Official Statistics. (1998). Country of origin and year of entry into the U.S. of the foreign born, by citizenship status. Available at: http://www.bis.census.gov/cps/pub/1998/for_born.htm.

U.S. Department of Health and Human Services (1990). Healthy People 2000. National Health Promotion and Disease Prevention Objectives. Washington, DC: US Government Printing Office.

U.S. Department of Health and Human Services (1992). Trends in Indian Health. Rockville, MD: Indian Health Service.

U.S. Department of Health and Human Services. (1993*). Healthy people, 2000 review.* Washington, DC: U.S. Government Printing Office.

U.S. Department of Health and Human Services, 2000. Healthy people 2010. National health promotion

& disease prevention objectives. Available at: http:www.health.gov.healthypeople/document, July, 2002.

U.S. Immigration and Naturalization Service. *Statistical yearbook of the Immigration and Naturalization Service, 1996.* Washington, D.C: U.S. Government Printing Office, 1997.

U.S. Department of Health and Human Services. (1997). *Comprehensive health care program for American Indians and Alaska Natives.* Rockville, MD: U.S. Public Health Service, Indian Health Service.

West, K. (1978). *Diabetes in American Indians: Advances in metabolic disorders.* New York: Academic Press.

White, V. (1985). *The experience of pregnancy among Hispanic women.* Unpublished master's thesis, University of Utah, Salt Lake City, Utah.

Young, K. (1994). *The health of Native Americans.* New York: Oxford University Press.

Young, S. A., & Kaufman, K. (1988). Promoting breast-feeding at a migrant health center. *Journal of the American Public Health Association, 78,* 523–525.

CHAPTER 12

Cultural Diversity in the Health Care Workforce

Margaret M. Andrews

KEY TERMS

Attitude change
Barriers
Bigotry
Collectivism
Conflict
Corporate culture
Cross-cultural communication
Cultural diversity
Cultural self-assessment
Cultural values
Discrimination
Dress code
Emic
Ethnoviolence

Etic
Etiquette
Facilitators
Family obligations
Formal attitude change
    approach
Group dynamics approach
Hatred
Human relations
Hygiene
Individual cultural self-assess-
    ment
Individualism
Moral and religious beliefs

Multicultural workforce
Multicultural workplace
Organizational climate
Organizational cultural self-
    assessment
Prejudice
Race relations
Racism
Resistance to change
Role
Social amnesia
Time orientation
Transcultural nursing
    administration

OBJECTIVES

1. Analyze past, present, and future trends in the racial and ethnic composition of the health care workforce.
2. Identify the cultural meaning of work and its influence on the corporate culture and organizational climate of health care organizations.
3. Critically examine the manner in which hatred, prejudice, racism, discrimination, and ethnoviolence manifest themselves in the health care workplace.
4. Critically analyze the cultural origins of conflict in the health care workforce.
5. Evaluate strategies for promoting effective cross-cultural communication and preventing conflict in the multicultural workplace.
6. Examine the process and content of cultural self-assessment for nurses and for health care organizations, institutions, and agencies.

The U.S. Department of Health and Human Services (2001) reports that 13.4% of the 2,696,540 registered nurses in the United States come from racial/ethnic minority backgrounds (Table 12–1), an increase of 10.3% since 1996. With the exception of American Indian and Alaskan Native nurses, all minority groups tracked in the national survey showed increases. Reflecting the multicultural approach of the United States Census, the 2000 survey gave nurses the option of categorizing themselves as multiracial for the first time. Between 1996 and 2000, the percentage of men in the total population of registered nurses rose from 4.9% to 5.4% (U.S. Department of Health & Human Services, 2001).

When both initial and post–registered nurse education are examined, Asian, Native Hawaiian, Pacific Islander, and Black nurses are more likely than White and Hispanic nurses to have at least baccalaureate preparation. Similar findings prevail for graduate education among the racial and ethnic minorities, with 11.1% of Black registered nurses holding master's or doctor's degrees, compared with 10.4% of White nurses, 10.2% of Hispanic nurses, and 5% of Asian nurses (U.S. Department of Health & Human Services, 2001).

The three most common employment settings for registered nurses in the United States are hospitals (59.1%), public/community health centers (18.3%), and ambulatory care (9.5%). More minority nurses than White nurses reported being currently employed in nursing (86.4% compared with 81%), and minority nurses were more likely to work full time than were their White counterparts (86% compared with 70%). Although fewer than 4% of licensed nurses in the United States are foreign educated, this represents more than 74,000 nurses (U.S. Department of Health & Human Services, 2001).

At nearly 8%, the proportion of foreign-educated nurses working in Canada is almost double that in the United States (Canadian Institute for

TABLE 12–1	RACIAL/ETHNIC DIVERSITY AMONG REGISTERED NURSES IN THE UNITED STATES						
	BLACK (NON-HISPANIC)	HISPANIC	ASIAN	AMERICAN INDIAN ALASKA NATIVE	NATIVE HAWAIIAN/ PACIFIC ISLANDERS	WHITE	TWO OR MORE RACIAL BACK-GROUNDS
N	133,041	54,861	93,415	13,040	5,393	2,396,490	32,358
%	4.9	2	3.5	0.5	0.2	86.6	1.2

Figures total less than 100% because some nurses chose not to report their racial/ethnic background.

Source: U.S. Department of Health and Human Services, Bureau of Health Professions (2001). The registered nurse population. National sample survey of registered nurses, March 2000. Washington, DC: U.S. Government Printing Office.

Health Information, 2000). Nevertheless, Canada continues to have less diversity in its nursing workforce than does the United States. For example, data from the 1996 Canadian Census indicate that only 9.4% of registered nurses employed in Canada identify themselves as members of a visible minority (Data Development Section, Labor Branch, Human Resources Development Canada, 1998). There are also slightly fewer male nurses in Canada (4.8% of the registered nurse workforce) than in the United States (5.4% of the registered nurse workforce). However, as in the United States, the number of male registered nurses employed in Canada is on the rise (Canadian Institute for Health Information, 2000).

In both Canada and the United States, there continues to be an increasingly diverse workforce. According to the Bureau of Labor Statistics (U.S. Department of Labor, 2002), the net rate of growth between 1986 and 2000 in the United States labor force of Hispanic women (85%), Asian women (83%), Hispanic men (68%), Asian men (61%), Black women (33%), and Black men (24%) will outpace the net rate of growth of White women (22%) and White men (minus 9%). Similarly, Canada has witnessed vast increases in occupational and social mobility opportunities for practically all ethnic groups since the end of World War II (Isajiw, 1999).

The emerging United States and Canadian workforces are dramatically different from those in former times. In many health care settings there is diversity in race, ethnicity, religion, age, sexual orientation, and national origin. Recent strides in the women's movement have called attention to important gender differences and the manner in which changing societal roles of both men and women influence relationships in the **multicultural workplace**. The interrelationship between culture and the physical, mental, and emotional handicaps and disabilities of some health care workers must also be considered in the complex web called the **multicultural workforce**.

Women have historically constituted the majority of personnel in nursing and in many allied health disciplines. For the past two decades, women and members of racially and ethnically diverse groups have made significant inroads into health professions that were once overwhelmingly the province of White men. The largest gains for most culturally diverse groups, however, occurred during the mid- to late 1970s. Since that time, with the exception of Asians and Hispanics, **cultural diversity** in the health care fields has been relatively stable.

• THE CHALLENGES AND OPPORTUNITIES OF A GROWING MULTICULTURAL POPULATION AND HEALTH CARE WORKFORCE

A significant number of the United States and Canadian national health goals for the year 2000 and beyond involve specific objectives for improving the health status of members of the panethnic minority groups identified by both countries' federal governments, particularly those with low incomes. Meanwhile, culturally diverse cohorts of children, women of childbearing age, and the elderly are expected to grow, exacerbating the need for culturally competent providers of health care.

Since 1972 there has been an explosion in the numbers of people migrating to the United States and Canada, both with and without legal documentation. Overall, 9%, or 26.5 million people in the United States (U.S. Census Bureau, 2000) and 17.4%, or 4.9 million people in Canada (Health Canada, 1999) are foreign-born residents. The top 10 countries of origin for the foreign-born population in the United States are Mexico (27%), Philippines (5.5%). China and Vietnam (3.7% each), Cuba (3.6%), India (3.2%), El Salvador (2.9%), Dominican Republic (2.6%), Great Britain (2.5%), and Korea (2.3%) (U.S. Census Bureau, 2000). In Canada, the largest number of immigrants (close to 60%) comes from Asia. The remaining immigrants to Canada come mainly from Central and South America, the Caribbean and Bermuda, the United States, and Eastern Europe (Isajiw, 1999).

Because the health care workplace is a microcosm of the changing demographic patterns in society at large, the growing diversity among nurses and other members of the health care team frequently poses challenges and opportunities in the multicultural work setting (Case Studies 12–1 through 12–6).

CASE STUDY 12–1

When a Black patient was admitted to a small rural hospital with predominantly White staff and patients, nurses from one shift would include "Black male" in their report to the oncoming shift. When one of the few Black nurses began using "White male" or "White female" in her report, she was accused of "having an attitude" and "trying to instigate racial trouble."

CASE STUDY 12–2

When informed that a patient was requesting medication for pain, a Lutheran nurse of German heritage responded to a fellow nurse, "She's just a Jewish princess who complains about pain all the time." A Jewish laboratory technician overheard the remark and demanded to know what the nursing supervisor was going to do about the "blatant anti-Semitism" on the unit.

CASE STUDY 12–3

A slightly built Black male nurse asked to meet with the operating room nurse manager about a surgeon who had recently immigrated from Russia. The nurse complained, "Dr. Ivanovich keeps asking me why I became a nurse. He asks very personal questions about my sexual orientation and wants to know if I'm 'queer.' I consider this a hostile work environment and refuse to scrub for his surgical cases any more."

CASE STUDY	12–4

After receiving a report on a critically ill victim of a motor vehicle accident, Dr. Juan Valdez-Rodriguez, the physician on call, asked for the patient's name. The reporting nurse said, "I don't know. Martinez, Hernandez, something like that. You'll recognize him when you see him—just another drunk Mexican who ran his pickup truck into a tree." Upon entering the examination room, the physician immediately recognized the victim as his cousin.

CASE STUDY	12–5

A nurse entered into a conversation with a Chinese American food service worker. Ms. Chin remarked that for the past 4 days she had been asked to be the interpreter for an elderly Chinese man on one of the units where she delivers food. "I don't want to offend the nurse manager who asked me to translate, but it is not right for a younger woman to speak for an older man. It is not our custom. Besides, my supervisor scolded me for being so slow to do my work. She thinks I have become lazy. Would you talk to the nurse manager for me?"

CASE STUDY	12–6

Mrs. Patel, a native of India, was a nurse manager in a small rural hospital that had difficulty attracting qualified professional staff. Mrs. Patel told her supervisor that she must "take some time off" because of a family emergency in her homeland. When the supervisor inquired about the details, he learned that Mrs. Patel already had purchased a nonrefundable airline ticket with a return flight in 6 weeks. Mrs. Patel's husband was the chief executive officer for the town's major industry and chairman of the hospital's board of directors.

• TRANSCULTURAL NURSING ADMINISTRATION

According to Leininger (1996), **transcultural nursing administration** refers to "a creative and knowledgeable process of assessing, planning, and making decisions and policies that will facilitate the provision of educational and clinical services that take into account the cultural caring values, beliefs, symbols, references, and lifeways of people of diverse and similar cultures for beneficial or satisfying outcomes" (p. 30). Transcultural nursing administrative perspectives are essential for survival, growth, satisfaction, and achievement of goals in the multicultural workplace (Gooden, Porter, Gonzalez, & Mims, 2001; Lambert & Nugent, 1999; Mateo & Smith, 2001; Parsons & Reiss, 1999; Schmeiding, 2000).

In the contemporary health care industry, nurse administrators necessarily focus their time and energy on issues such as cost–benefit outcomes, downsizing, territorial struggles with members of other disciplines, appropriate use of technology, and other important topics. With increasing frequency, nurse administrators are realizing the critical importance of transculturally based administrative practices that positively influence cost–benefit and quality outcomes. With the increasing diversity among members of the health care workforce, nurses are challenged to develop and practice a new kind of administration known as transcultural nursing administration.

• CULTURAL PERSPECTIVES ON THE MEANING OF WORK

The earliest recorded ideas about work refer to it as a curse, a punishment, or a necessary evil needed to sustain life. People of high status did not work, whereas slaves, indentured servants, and peasants worked. In contemporary society, the concept of work must be considered in its historical and cultural context. Cultural views about caring for the sick also must be considered, because such care may be perceived as a divine calling for those with supernatural powers (some African tribes), a religious vocation (some ethnic Catholic groups), or an undignified occupation for lower-class workers (some Arab groups such as Kuwaitis and Saudi Arabians).

Cultural norms influence a staff member's consideration of group interest as opposed to individual interests in the multicultural workplace. Scholars have identified two major orientations embraced by people: individualism and collectivism. With **individualism**, importance is placed on individual inputs, rights, and rewards. Individualists emphasize values such as autonomy, competitiveness, achievement, and self-sufficiency. Most English-speaking and European countries have individualist cultures.

Collectivism entails the need to maintain group harmony above the partisan interests of subgroups and individuals. In collectivist cultures, values such as interpersonal harmony and group solidarity prevail. A staff member whose ethnic heritage is Asian or South American is likely to be influenced by collectivism. Amish and Mennonite groups also are considered collectivist cultures.

One of the most notable distinctions between people from individualist and collectivist cultures is the meaning of work. Individualists work to earn a living. People are expected to work; they need not enjoy it. Leisure or recreational activities frequently are pursued to alleviate the monotony of work. People from individualist cultures tend to dichotomize work and leisure. Individualist concepts of work reflect an orientation toward the future.

It also is useful to understand cultural differences about appropriate and desired behavior in the workplace. People from most individualist cultures are typically achievement oriented. Stereotypically, they want to do better, accomplish more, and take responsibility for their actions. They tend to develop personality traits such as assertiveness and competitiveness that facilitate these goals. In many collectivist cultures, however, qualities such as commitment to relationships, gentleness, cooperativeness, and indirectness are valued.

Some researchers have suggested that the motivation strategies of Japanese managers must appeal to the Japanese worker's sense of loyalty, commitment, and group orientation, whereas the motivation strategies of North American managers must appeal to the worker's sense of contract, rules, and individuality. Although some individuals have a combination of the two qualities, most staff members will display either an individualistic or a collectivistic orientation in the workplace. Nurses in leadership positions need to recognize the fundamental value system embraced by their staff members to understand why they behave as they do at work.

• CORPORATE CULTURES AND SUBCULTURES

Health care organizations are minisocieties that have their own distinctive patterns of culture and subculture. One organization may have a high degree of cohesiveness, with staff working together like members of a single family toward the achievement of common goals. Another may be highly fragmented, divided into groups that think about the world in very different ways or that have different aspirations about what their organization should be. Just as individuals in a culture can have different personalities while sharing much in common, so can groups and organizations. This phenomenon is referred to as **corporate culture**. Corporate culture is a process of reality construction that allows staff to see and understand particular events, actions, objects, communications, or situations in distinctive ways. These patterns of understanding help people cope with the situations they encounter and provide a basis for making behavior sensible and meaningful.

Shared values, beliefs, meaning, and understanding are components of the corporate culture. The corporate culture is established and maintained through an ongoing, proactive process of reality construction. It is an active, living phenomenon through which staff members jointly create and recreate their work place and world. One of the easiest ways to appreciate the nature of corporate culture and subculture is to observe the day-to-day functioning of the organization. Observe the patterns of interaction among individuals, the language that is used, the images and themes explored in conversation, and the various rituals of daily routine. Historical explanations for the ways things are done will emerge in discussions of the rationale for certain aspects of the culture.

The corporate culture metaphor is useful because it directs attention to the symbolic significance of almost every aspect of organizational life. Structures, hierarchies, rules, and organizational routines reveal underlying meanings that are crucial for understanding how organizations function. For example, meetings carry important aspects of organizational culture, which may convey a sense of conformity and order or of causal informality. The environment in which the meetings are held reflects the formality or informality of the organization.

Box 12–1 poses several questions that might be considered in the determination of the corporate culture of a health care organization, institution, or agency. The answers to the questions will provide a beginning understanding of the corporate culture of the organization.

BOX 12–1	DETERMINING CORPORATE CULTURE

It is useful to pose the following questions when determining the corporate culture of an organization.

- Does the person presiding over the group stand or sit?
- Does the presider encourage discussion among group members or engage in a monologue?
- Are group members encouraged to express opinions freely, or is there pressure to silence those who express opposing points of view?
- How do group leaders and members dress?
- What message does the institutional dress code convey about the acceptance of cultural diversity?
- Do policies allow for cultural expressions in clothing, accessories, hair style, and related areas?
- Although most institutions require employees to wear identification badges or name tags, what flexibility does the individual have for self-expression and expression of cultural identity and affiliation?

Health care work environments are social settings that encompass many elements of a social system. It is useful to distinguish between the **organizational climate** of the work environment and the corporate culture. According to Flarey (1993), the organizational climate usually measures perceptions or feelings about the organization or work environment. The corporate or organizational culture, on the other hand, is what its members share—beliefs, values, assumptions, rituals—often unconsciously. Culture provides the community, the sameness, and the consensus that makes those people unique and special.

•NEGATIVE ATTITUDES AND BEHAVIORS IN THE MULTICULTURAL WORKPLACE

Hatred, prejudice, bigotry, discrimination, racism, and violence represent negative attitudes or behaviors in the multicultural workplace, which must be considered. The formation of attitudes and strategies for changing these attitudes must also be considered.

Hatred

In some organizations, the use of racial, ethnic, sexual, and other derogatory remarks signals a disturbing underlying problem in the workplace. Why does hatred exist in the workplace? Although the reasons are complex and interconnected, some contributing factors include the early socialization of children to cultural and gender stereotypes, personal experiences (or lack of them) with people from diverse backgrounds, and exposure to negative societal attitudes.

According to Henderson (1994), **hatred** in the workplace is exacerbated during times of rapid immigration, periods of economic recession or depression, and high unemployment. Competition for sexual partners also is cited as a cause for hatred. Hatred can be the cause of tremendous hostility in the workplace. In some organizations, technology is used to transmit derogatory remarks electronically to individuals or targeted groups by e-mail or fax. Sites on the Internet that allow free expressions of hatred have proliferated. Those responsible justify their actions by citing either the Canadian Charter of Rights and Freedoms or the United States Constitution's First Amendment rights to freedom of expression.

Prejudice, Bigotry, and Discrimination

The term **prejudice** refers to inaccurate perceptions of others. Prejudice results in conclusions that are drawn without adequate knowledge or evidence. All people are prejudiced for or against other people. Prejudices in the community at large are acted out in the workplace. **Bigotry** connotes narrow-mindedness and an obstinate or blind attachment to a particular opinion or viewpoint. The bigot blames members of out-groups for various misfortunes. In their efforts to make expedient decisions, bigots react to concepts rather than to people.

Whereas prejudice and bigotry refer to attitudes, **discrimination** refers to behaviors and is defined as the act of setting one individual or group apart from another, showing a difference or favoritism. Discriminatory behaviors, not attitudes, constitute the majority of intergroup problems. Although there are many laws against discriminatory behaviors, especially in the workplace, there are none against prejudice or bigotry (Henderson, 1994).

The nurse in Case 12–1, who points out in the report that the patient is Black, may not have any conscious discriminatory intent. By departing from the usual practice of not mentioning race, however, she makes a statement that race is a variable that needs to be mentioned. In turn, this gives an opportunity for prejudices in the minds of the other nurses to surface. Keeping people of color exploitable is a foundation of racial inequality.

Contrary to popular writings, prejudices in the workplace are not limited to Black–White conflicts and confrontations. There is prejudice against various members of the workforce, including women, older workers, individuals with disabilities, foreign-born workers, and White workers.

In Case 12–2, the nurse's characterization of the patient experiencing pain as a "Jewish princess" is a transparently anti-Semitic remark. The ability to control the lives of people is a psychologic aspect of nursing that is often unconsciously manifested. The nurse in the case study may be exercising a certain degree of power over the patient, knowing that she is at the nurse's mercy for the relief of her pain. It also may reflect an underlying "scientific racism," i.e., that there are biologic differences between certain groups. The nurse may believe that there are different pain thresholds among persons of diverse backgrounds and that Jewish patients tend to have a relatively low tolerance for pain.

As discussed in Chapter 13 (Transcultural Aspects of Pain), the nurse's own ethnic background, religious affiliation, and personal experience with pain may contribute to her perceptions of the patient's need for pain relief. Although the nurse may be using "scientific racism" to rationalize her beliefs that a patient is requesting more pain relief than the average person, there is no excuse for the racist reference to her patient as a "Jewish princess." The nurse's racism adversely affects not only the patient but also a fellow nurse and a laboratory technician. The racial slur is an example of an implicit cue passed on to others, in which the nurse perpetuates both prejudice against and stereotypes about Jewish people. The laboratory technician is likely to view the nurse, and perhaps by extension the entire multicultural workplace, as being hostile to Jews.

Prejudice is also based on sexual orientation, as illustrated in Case 12–3. The Black nurse expresses his concern with the hostile work environment created by the imposing Russian surgeon, who asks inappropriate questions about his sexual orientation. Because the offender is a recent immigrant, he may be unaware of cultural differences concerning appropriate topics for discussion in the workplace—though it is doubtful that his behavior would be widely accepted in a Russian operating room setting, either. Furthermore, the surgeon may have a limited English vocabulary and/or may be unaware of the negative connotation of the slang term "queer." These explanations for the surgeon's inappropriate behavior in the workplace do not excuse him; rather, they are offered as factors worthy of the nurse manager's consideration in an attempt to address the problem.

Racism

Racism implies that superior or inferior traits and behavior are determined by race. Racism connotes prejudice and discrimination. To understand racism in the workplace, distinctions need to be made among (1) institutional structures and personal behavior, and the relationship between the two; (2) the variation in both degree and form of expression of individual prejudice; and (3) the fact that racism is merely one form of a larger and more inclusive pattern of ethnocentrism that may be based on various factors, both racial and nonracial (Henderson, 1994; Williams & Rucker, 2000).

Racism is caused by a complex web of factors, including ignorance, apathy, poverty, historic patterns of discrimination against particular groups, and social stratification. According to Brown (1973), society "is racially divided and its whole organization...promotes racial distinctions" (p. 8). With this frame of reference, racial bias and discrimination have been built into most United States and Canadian institutions, and every citizen is a product of institutional racism. According to Henderson (1994), "What is commonly called racism is part of the larger problem of ethnic identification, of power and powerlessness, and of the exploitation of the weak by the strong....What most writers commonly call **race relations** should be properly understood in the larger context of **human relations**" (p. 21) (emphasis added).

In the multicultural workplace, the expression of negative attitudes and behaviors by people toward others according to their identification as members of a particular group is of particular concern. The expression of these attitudes and behavioral patterns is learned as part of the cultural process. Negative group attitudes and destructive group conflicts are less likely to arise when employees treat each other as individuals and respond to each other on the basis of individual characteristics and behaviors (Williams & Rucker, 2000).

In Case 12–4, the nurse's remark "just another drunk Mexican" is an example of a stereotype that may have an element of truth in it but is nevertheless inaccurate. Although it is true that the majority of motor vehicle accidents are alcohol related, and that in this hospital a large proportion of those involved are Mexican Americans, it is untrue that all Mexican American men are alcoholic. By overgeneralizing in this way, the nurse fails to assess important information about the individual person and depersonalizes him through the stereotype. The nurse's apparent insensitivity to Dr. Valdez-Rodriguez' ethnic heritage is appalling. The pathos of the situation is further realized when the physician learns that "just another drunk Mexican" accident victim is his cousin.

According to Schwartz and Sullivan (1993), selective mistreatment, often in the absence of adequate social support, undermines the work experiences of individuals who are identified with groups that are the targets of discriminatory behavior. The career potential of staff from diverse backgrounds is frequently undermined by the relative lack of access to informal networks and mentors and by the expectation that these persons will assimilate into organizational cultures that are often intolerant of the cultures with which these staff members identify. These manifestations of discrimination can be expected to undermine the functioning of the health care organization. Paradoxically, the victims of mistreatment are often the perpetrators as well. The victim of mistreatment may, in turn, mistreat others. One explanation for this phenomenon is that people are likely to experience a form of internalized oppression as a result of low self-esteem.

According to Holmes (1994), Blacks, Hispanics, and Asians resent one another almost as much as they do Whites. This raises doubt about the strategy of merely hiring more minorities. Unless there is systematic training to help all staff members accept each other, conflicts of racial and ethnic origin will increase (Henderson, 1994). On the other hand, a critical analysis of the percentages of managers in health care by race and ethnicity suggests that there are serious inequities. Moore and Jensen (1997) report that only 1% of the top executives among the 5 million United States hospital workers are members of minorities. These data are supported by U.S. Census Bureau (1995) data in which the following racial and ethnic diversity among managers is reported: 85.9% White, 9% Black, and 5.1% Hispanic. Similar hierarchies of ethnic inequality also exist within the Canadian labor market (Lautard & Guppy, 1999).

Violence in the Workplace

Although not all hatred leads to violence, there is a significant increase in the number of attacks on gays, anti-Semitic incidents, and reported cases of **ethnoviolence.** According to Henderson (1994), Blacks, Hispanics, homosexual men, and Jews are the primary targets of hate crimes, many of which occur in the workplace. Although it is impossible to protect all employees and patients from violence in health care settings, reasonable steps must be taken to protect those believed to be at risk. Verbal threats and/or assaults by or against staff members should not be tolerated.

Health care administrators have a moral imperative to take reasonable steps in ensuring the physical safety of staff, patients/clients, and visitors. The institution's security officers and/or local police should be notified whenever violence is threatened. Some institutions require staff and visitors to pass through a metal detector when entering the premises, whereas others have posted security officers at entrances to ensure that only authorized persons are admitted. In extreme cases, it may be necessary to obtain a court order to prohibit an individual or group from the premises or to establish a safe perimeter so patients and staff may have safe access to the facility.

In recent years, attorneys representing health care institutions have sometimes found it necessary to obtain a court order to ensure a safe work environment during times of racial, ethnic, religious, and social discord. Unfortunately, some demonstrators with strong convictions have violated others' civil liberties and engaged in violent acts against those who disagree with their point of view. The shooting of staff at clinics where abortions are performed is an extreme example of hatred that has resulted in violence. This violence is caused by a complex web of interconnected factors, including religious, moral, ethical, social, political, and cultural differences.

Formation of Attitudes

Attitudes are learned, not innate. Researchers have found that as children grow older they tend to forget that they were instructed in attitudes by their parents and significant other people. Around the age of 10, most children regard their attitudes toward people from different cultural backgrounds as being innate. Seldom do they recall being coached. **Social amnesia** develops, and elaborate rationalizations are presented to account for learned attitudes (Henderson, 1994).

The superiority or inferiority of a group (versus an individual) is usually less obvious than an individual's behavior. Most staff bring their cultural baggage to work with them, and they are molded and shaped by peer pressure. The values, behaviors, and customs of those in the out-group are labeled as strange or unusual. As children, many staff learned to reject people who were culturally different and to view differences as being synonymous with inferiority. In the insightful words of Carl Jung (1968):

"We still attribute to the other fellow all the evil and inferior qualities that we do not like to recognize in ourselves, and therefore have to criticize and attack him, when all that has happened is that an inferior soul has emigrated from one person to another. The world is still full of *betes noir* and scapegoats, just as it formerly teemed with witches and werewolves" (p. 65).

Changing Attitudes

Although some argue that the focus should be on behavior change rather than **attitude change**, others maintain that hatred, prejudice, bigotry, racism, discrimination, and ethnoviolence begin with an individual's attitudes toward certain groups. Staff members' attitudes can be changed in several ways, but they require commitment by all levels of management within an organization. They also require a certain degree of openness and receptivity by the individual.

Efforts to change staff members' attitudes about people from culturally diverse groups should center on communication. Several approaches have been used by organizations. The first, called the **formal attitude change approach**, is based on learning theories: on the assumption that people are rational, information-processing beings who can be motivated to listen to a message, hear its content, and incorporate what they have learned when it is advantageous to do so. There is an actual or expected reward for embracing diversity.

The second, known as the **group dynamics approach** assumes that staff members are social beings who need culturally diverse coworkers as they adjust to environmental changes. The amount of change depends on people's attitudes toward diversity, their attention to the message and to the communicator, their understanding of the message, and their acceptance of the message. Acceptance of diversity is likely to be enhanced by activities that provide tangible rewards for staff. It is seldom enough for top management to urge staff members to embrace diversity as a moral imperative.

• CULTURAL VALUES IN THE MULTICULTURAL WORKPLACE

Cultural values frequently lie at the root of cross-cultural differences in the multicultural workplace. Values form the core of a culture. Time orientation, family obligations, communication patterns (including etiquette, space/distance, touch), interpersonal relationships (including long-standing historic rivalries), gender/sexual orientation, education, socioeconomic status, moral/religious beliefs, hygiene, clothing, meaning of work, and personal traits exert influences on individuals within the multicultural health care setting.

What is the importance of learning about the values of people from diverse cultural groups?

Values exert a powerful influence on how each person behaves, reacts, and feels. In the multicultural workplace, values affect people's lives in four major ways. Values underlie *perceived needs, what is defined as a problem, how conflict is resolved,* and *expectations of behavior.* When cultural values of individual staff members conflict with the organizational values or those held by coworkers, challenges, misunderstandings, and difficulties in the workplace become inevitable. You must use these inevitable conflicts as opportunities to foster cross-cultural understanding among staff members from diverse backgrounds and to enhance cross-cultural communication (Gooden et al., 2001; Ivancevich & Gilbert, 2000; Lambert & Nugent, 1999; Mateo & Smith, 2001).

Cultural Perspectives on Conflict

The term **conflict** is derived from Latin roots (*confligere*, "to strike against") and refers to actions that range from intellectual disagreement to physical violence. Frequently, the action that precipitates the conflict is based on different cultural perceptions of the situation. According to some social scientists, when participants in a conflict are from the same culture, they are more likely to perceive the situation in the same way and to organize their perceptions in similar ways.

By examining proverbs used by members of various cultural groups, it is possible to better understand differences in the way conflict is viewed. Table 12–2 summarizes selected proverbs that relate to conflict and its resolution. The dominant culture's proverbs emphasize that people should behave assertively and deal with conflict through direct confrontation. Other cultures—particularly collectivist groups—may promote avoidance of confrontation and emphasize harmony (e.g., Native North Americans, Alaskan Natives, Amish, and Asians). The culture-based choices that lead people in these opposite directions are a major source of conflict in the workplace.

Many people from individualist cultures view conflict as a healthy, natural, and inevitable component of all relationships. People from many collectivist cultures, on the other hand, have learned to internalize conflict and to value harmonious relationships above winning arguments and "being right." To many people of Native North American and Asian descent, conflict is not healthy, desirable, or constructive. In the Arab world, mediation is critical in resolving disputes, and confrontation seldom works. Mediation allows for saving face and is rooted in the realization that all conflicts do not have simple solutions.

The assertive, confrontational, direct style of communicating is characteristic of people from individualistic cultures, whereas the cooperative, conciliatory style is a more collectivist or Eastern mode of managing conflict. When attempting to influence others during a disagreement, for example, nurses from China, Japan and other collectivist cultures may use covert conflict prevention strategies to minimize interpersonal conflicts. Nurses from individualistic cultures are more likely to rely on the overt confrontation of ideas and argumentation by reason.

In Case 12–5, the Chinese food service worker demonstrates the cultural value for harmonious relationships, indirect communication, and nonconfrontational resolution of conflict. The nurse manager has inadvertently placed Mrs. Chin in an awkward position by violating Chinese norms concerning gender and age. In traditional Chinese culture, it is inappropriate for a younger person to speak for an older one and for a female to speak for a male. Serving as an interpreter for the elderly Chinese man has been uncomfortable for both Mrs.

TABLE 12-2	CROSS-CULTURAL PERSPECTIVES ON PROVERBS AND CONFLICT	

PROVERB	VALUE
Dominant Culture	
The squeaky wheel gets the grease.	Aggressiveness Direct confrontation
Tell it like it is.	Direct confrontation Honesty even if it hurts the other
Take the bull by the horns.	Direct confrontation
Shoot first, ask questions later.	Aggressiveness Direct confrontation Protection of individual rights (versus good of the group)
Might makes right.	Aggressiveness Dominance
Japanese	
The nail that sticks out gets hammered.	Not calling attention to oneself Going along with the group Harmony and balance
Senegalese	
Misunderstandings do not exist; only the failure to communicate does.	Strive to understand the other's point of view Harmony and balance is normal state, not conflict and confrontation
Zen	
He who knows does not speak, and he who speaks does not know.	Listen to the other's side during conflict Silence
Arab	
The hand of Allah is with the group. Haste comes from the devil.	Primacy of group good (versus individual) Patience Conflict resolution takes time

Chin and the patient. Mrs. Chin's value for harmonious relationships in the workplace prevent her from speaking directly to the nurse manager and food service supervisor about the problem. By involving the staff nurse as an intermediary with the nurse manager, she is attempting to convey her dissatisfaction with the situation in a nonconfrontational, indirect, and polite manner. She also attempts to avoid appearing like a complaining, disgruntled employee who is unwilling to cooperate with other workers. For these reasons, she is reluctant to bring the problem to her food service supervisor's attention. She believes that she must please those in authority, foster harmonious relationships, and avoid direct confrontation if she is to be a valuable employee of the hospital.

Cultural Origins of Conflict

Let's examine some cultural values and the manner in which they may result in conflict in the multicultural workplace. The origins of cultural conflict result from influences on the organization and on individuals. As indicated in Figure 12–1, political, economic, technologic, and legal factors influence the corporate culture and the organizational climate of both organizations and their employees. For organizations owned and operated by religious groups, religious influences must be considered. For example, in a hospital owned and operated by a Roman Catholic religious order, abortions, tubal ligations, and other gynecologic procedures may be prohibited. Factors such as educational background, socioeconomic status, culture, moral and religious beliefs, and personal traits of employees must also be considered when determining the cultural origins of conflict. Staff members contribute to the perception that values are in conflict. Although there are many conflicting values that underlie problems, the following areas will be explored in the remainder of this chapter: Cultural perspectives on family obligations, personal hygiene, cross-cultural communication (including etiquette and touch), clothing and accessories, time orientation, interpersonal relationships (including historic rivalries between groups), gender/sexual orientation, and moral and religious beliefs (including dietary practices).

Cultural Perspectives on Family Obligations

Although family is important in all cultures, the constellation (e.g. nuclear, single-parent, extended, same-sex), emotional closeness among members, social

Figure 12–1. Origins of conflict in the multicultural health care setting.

and economic commitments among members, and other factors vary cross-culturally. Both staff nurses and those in administrative positions frequently report difficulty with requests from nurses of diverse cultural backgrounds that pertain to **family obligations**.

Some nurses from different cultures have been labeled as uncommitted to their work and/or disinterested in their nursing careers because family is a higher priority than job or career. The so-called appliance nurse has long been recognized among members of the dominant culture as well. Given that it is highly unlikely (and undesirable) that the nurse manager will be successful at changing fundamental family-related values, the most useful approach is to focus on the problematic behavior. For example, if excessive absenteeism is the undesirable behavior, the nurse manager should arrange for a face-to-face meeting in which the problematic behavior is discussed. In addition, the use of peer pressure by coworkers also can be helpful in changing the undesirable behavior as fellow workers communicate to the individual why his or her behavior is troublesome. It is generally useful to identify the reason(s) for the excessive absenteeism and to explore culturally appropriate strategies for resolving the problem, such as use of the natural social support that is culturally expected of extended family members. The solution is seldom simple, as the following case analysis illustrates.

In Case 12–6, Mrs. Patel, the nurse manager from India, reflects the high value placed on family relationships and obligations when she tells her supervisor that she plans to absent herself from work for 6 weeks to help with a family emergency in India. Although she has a large extended family in India, she believes that it is her duty to be present during this family crisis. By purchasing a nonrefundable airline ticket, she has demonstrated her resolve. The significant community influence exerted by Mrs. Patel's husband in this small rural community and his position in the hospital hierarchy further complicate the situation. The nursing supervisor is posed with an awkward dilemma because Mrs. Patel is not entitled to 6 weeks' vacation, nor has she adequately planned to cover her unit's needs during her absence. The 6 weeks that she has requested exceed the leave time permitted by hospital policy, yet she is legally entitled to this abscence by the U.S. Family Medical Leave Act. Canadian provinces have Employment Standards Acts, which govern Family Responsibility Leave. Such leaves grant employees leaves of abscence without pay of 3 to 10 days during the 12 calendar month period. More generous Family Responsibility Leaves are sometimes negotiated in Collective Agreements developed between individual employers and union representatives. By allowing Mrs. Patel to be gone for 6 weeks, the supervisor would need to shift the burden to other nursing staff members, who will need to adjust their workloads. Granting authorized leave would set a precedent that may leave the hospital vulnerable if other staff members decide to make similar requests for extended time off. Because of Mr. Patel's powerful influence in both the hospital and the community, the nursing supervisor is well aware of the external pressures that are likely to be exerted on him from multiple sources both inside and outside the hospital. In this decision-making process, the supervisor must consider the cultural, ethical, legal, social, and economic dimensions of the situation from the perspectives of both the institution and the employee.

The value of independence from the family, for example, is highly valued by many from the dominant cultural groups in the United States and Canada, but it ranks very low in the hierarchy of people from most Middle Eastern and Asian cultures. In the latter groups, the family is highly valued, and the individual's lifelong duties toward the family are explicit. Thus, absence from work for family-related reasons may be considered legitimate and important by workers from some cultures but may be perceived as an unnecessary inconvenience to the supervisor. For example, a Mexican American staff member may submit a last-minute request for vacation time to visit with a distant cousin who has unexpectedly arrived in town after traveling a great distance. The Mexican American staff member thinks, "What a great opportunity to develop a stronger relationship with a distant member of my mother's family. How nice that cousin Juan has traveled so far to see me. I've been thinking about making a trip to Mexico next year, so perhaps I can stay with Juan during my visit. Surely my nurse manager understands how important family relationships are to Mexican Americans and will be able to rearrange the unit schedule to accommodate my request." The nurse manager may think, "What's wrong with these Mexican American staff? Don't they want to work? This vacation request means that I'll have to redo the schedule for the entire unit. If I permitted everyone to submit last-minute vacation requests, I'd go crazy. What's the big deal about a distant cousin coming to visit, anyway?"

Ideas about the importance of anticipating and controlling the future vary significantly from culture to culture. Whereas some staff members place a high priority on planning for retirement, accumulating sick days, and purchasing insurance, others, particularly recent immigrants with family obligations in their homelands, may be more concerned with current obligations and living in the present. Similarly, some workers in high-risk jobs will participate actively in preventive immunization programs aimed at hepatitis and influenza, whereas others bewilder managers by saying, "What will be, will be. I can't spend time worrying about something that may or may not happen in the future."

Cultural Perspectives on Personal Hygiene

Another value that influences behavior is found in the proverb "cleanliness is next to godliness." This proverb highlights the value for cleanliness, including an obsession with eliminating or minimizing natural bodily odors—as evidenced by the plethora of deodorants, douches, body lotions, mouthwashes, and the like with hundreds of different fragrances. Members of the dominant culture sometimes have difficulty with staff members from other cultures who are not unduly bothered by body odors and see no reason to refrain from masking nature's original smells. In some cases, the staff member may come from a country in which water is scarce and bathing is restricted. Other staff members may be following religious or cultural practices that prohibit bathing during certain phases of the menstrual cycle, after the delivery of a baby, and at other times. Nurse managers and other supervisors frequently find the sensitive topic of **hygiene** difficult to discuss with staff from diverse cultural backgrounds.

Cross-Cultural Communication

Underlying the majority of conflict in the multicultural health care setting are issues related to effective **cross-cultural communication**, verbal and/or nonverbal. Even when one is dealing with staff members from the same cultural background, it requires administrative skill to decide whether to speak with someone face to face, send an electronic or paper memorandum, contact the person by telephone, or opt not to communicate about a particular matter at all. The nurse must exercise considerable judgment when making decisions about effective methods for communicating with staff members and patients/clients from diverse cultural backgrounds, considering a sense of timing, tone and pitch of voice, choice of location for face-to-face interactions, and related matters (Figure 12–2). Communication difficulties caused by differences in language and accent become compounded on the telephone. It is sometimes necessary to counsel recent immigrants from non–English-speaking countries to refrain from giving or receiving medical orders by telephone until their English language skills have developed (Gooden et al., 2001; Lambert & Nugent, 1999; Parsons & Reiss, 1999).

In the United States, approximately 32 million people (14% of the total United States population) speak languages other than English. In rank order, the most frequently spoken languages are Spanish (54%), French (6%), German (5%), Italian (4), and Chinese (4%). In Canada, 68% of the total population speak English most often, 24% speak French most often, and the remaining 8% (2.1 million people) speak other languages most often. In rank order, the most frequently spoken languages in Canada other than English and French include Chinese (430,000 people), Italian (288,000), Portuguese (153,000), Spanish (145,000), and German (134,000) (Isajiw, 1999). It is estimated that the United States will continue to attract about two thirds of the world's immigration and that 85% of the immigrants will come from Central and South America (U.S. Census Bureau, 2000). Immigration rates to Canada are also predicted to remain proportionately high, with approximately 250,000

Figure 12–2. Effective cross-cultural communication among staff is necessary to ensure optimal patient care. (Copyright B. Proud)

BOX 12–2

STRATEGIES TO PROMOTE EFFECTIVE CROSS-CULTURAL COMMUNICATION IN THE MULTICULTURAL WORKPLACE

- Pronounce names correctly. When in doubt, ask the person for the correct pronunciation.
- Use proper titles of respect: "Doctor," "Reverend," "Mister." Be sure to ask for the person's permission to use his or her first name, or wait until you are given permission to do so.
- Be aware of gender sensitivities. If uncertain about the marital status of a woman or her preferred title, it is best to refer to her as Ms. (pronounced mizz) initially, then ask how she prefers to be called at the first opportunity.
- Be aware of subtle linguistic messages that may convey bias or inequality, for example, referring to a white man as Mister while addressing a Black female by her first name.
- Refrain from Anglicizing or shortening a person's given name without his or her permission. For example, calling a Russian American "Mike" instead of Mikhael, or shortening the Italian American Maria Rosaria to Maria. The same principle applies to the last name, or surname.
- Call people by their proper names. Avoid slang such as "girl," "boy," "honey," "dear," "guy," "fella," "babe," "chief," "mama," "sweetheart," or similar terms. When in doubt, ask people if they are offended by the use of a particular term.
- Refrain from using slang, pejorative, or derogatory terms when referring to persons from ethnic, racial, or religious groups, and convey to all staff that this is a work environment in which there is zero tolerance for the use of such language. Violators should be counseled immediately.
- Identify people by race, color, gender, and ethnic origin only when necessary and appropriate.
- Avoid using words and phrases that may be offensive to others. For example, "culturally deprived" or "culturally disadvantaged" imply inferiority, and "non-White" implies that White is the normative standard.
- Avoid cliches and platitudes such as "Some of my best friends are Mexicans" or "I went to school with Blacks."
- Use language in communications that includes *all* staff rather than excludes some of them.
- Do not expect a staff member to know all the other employees of his or her background or to speak for them. They share ethnicity, not necessarily the same experiences, friendships, or beliefs.
- Communications describing staff should pertain to their job skills, not their color, age, race, sex, or national origin.
- Refrain from telling stories or jokes demeaning to certain ethnic, racial, age, or religious groups. Also avoid those pertaining to gender-related issues or persons with physical or mental disabilities. Convey to all staff that there will be zero tolerance for this inappropriate behavior. Violators should be counseled immediately.
- Avoid remarks that suggest to staff from diverse backgrounds that they should consider themselves fortunate to be in the organization. Do not compare their employment opportunities and conditions with those people in their country of origin.
- Remember that communication problems multiply in telephone communications because important nonverbal cues are lost and accents may be difficult to interpret.
- Provide staff with opportunities to explore diversity issues in their workplace, and constructively resolve differences.

immigrants being admitted each year (Kalbach & Kalbach, 2000). Box 12–2 suggests strategies for promoting effective cross-cultural communication in the multicultural workplace.

CULTURAL PERSPECTIVES ON TOUCH

Differences in behavioral norms in the multicultural workforce are often inaccurately perceived. Typically, people from Asian cultures are not as overtly demonstrative of affection as are Whites or Blacks. Generally they refrain from public embraces, kissing, and loud talking or laughter. Affection is expressed in a more reserved manner. Whites and Blacks may be perceived as boisterous, loud, ill-mannered, or rude by comparison. In some cases, staff members from different cultures may send messages through their use of touch that are not intended. Special attention to male–female relationships is warranted in the multicultural workplace. In general, it is best to refrain from touching staff members of either sex unless necessary for the accomplishment of a job-related task, such as the provision of safe patient care. For nurses who tend to be more tactile, it is important to consciously refrain from placing one's hand on another's arm or shoulder, as frequently happens during ordinary conversation. For a further discussion of this topic, see Chapter 2.

CULTURAL PERSPECTIVES ON ETIQUETTE

Values frequently underlie cultural expectations of behavior, including matters of **etiquette**, the conventional code of good manners that governs behavior. For example, some people from Hispanic, Middle Eastern, and African cultures expect the nurse manger to engage in social conversation and to establish personal and social rapport before giving assignments or orders for the day's work. In developing interpersonal relationships, a high value is placed on getting to know about a person's family, personal concerns, and interests before discussing job-related business. The nurse manager's reluctance to engage in self-disclosure about personal matters may leave the impression that he or she is uncaring and is not interested in the staff member. These behaviors by the manager are not conducive to building productive, harmonious relationships and may be misunderstood by staff members from diverse backgrounds. Similarly, some cultures value formal greetings at the start of the day or whenever the first encounter of the day occurs—a practice found even among close family members. For example, it is important to say, "Good morning, Mr. Okoro. There has been a change in your patient's insulin orders" rather than immediately "getting to the point" without recognizing by name the person to whom you are speaking (Lambert & Nugent, 1999; Parsons & Reiss, 1999).

Cultural Perspectives on Clothing and Accessories

Most health care institutions have a **dress code** or policy statement about clothing and accessories worn by staff in various parts of the facility (e.g., delivery room, operating room, specialty units). It is important to review these documents periodically from a cultural perspective. For example, modification of the dress code may be necessary to accommodate Hindu women dressed in saris, Sikh men who wear turbans, Amish and Mennonite women who wear bonnets and men who wear straw or black felt hats, Muslim women and Roman Catholic nuns who cover their heads with veils, and Arab men who wear kaffiyehs. Special consideration may need to be given to some Blacks and others who wear jewelry and other accessories in their hair, particularly when the hair is braided.

Cultural Perspectives on Time Orientation

In some cases, cultural differences in **time orientation** create difficulty in the workplace. This may manifest itself when staff members from diverse cultures are tardy, take excessive time for breaks, and fail to complete assignments within the expected time frame. These differences may be interrelated with the cultural meaning of work, religious practices, and cross-cultural communication issues. It is important to be explicit in the job-related expectations about punctuality, schedule for breaks, and time allotted for assignments.

If a staff member develops a pattern of tardiness, the reason(s) should be explored. Although a uniform standard of punctuality needs to be applied to all staff members, it may be useful to listen to the staff member's explanation and ask what he or she thinks will rectify the problem. The reasons for problems with punctuality may range from child care to car repair needs. Solutions may include the mobilization of cultural resources, such as using extended family members to look after dependents, or networking with coworkers who might be able to recommend a reliable auto mechanic. It is important to listen attentively without rendering judgment or dictating solutions that the person has not agreed to (Ivancevich & Gilbert, 2000).

It is sometimes useful to divide an assignment into subtasks with specific time lines for each activity. If the staff member has difficulty completing the assignment within the allotted time, it is important to follow up with a discussion of the reasons why there were problems. This follow-up discussion should be conducted in a positive, proactive manner and viewed as an opportunity to promote cross-cultural communication, not as a punitive or disciplinary measure.

Cultural Perspectives on Interpersonal Relationships

AUTHORITY FIGURES, PEERS, SUBORDINATES, AND PATIENTS/CLIENTS

As indicated in Figure 12–3, there are cultural differences in interpersonal relationships involving authority figures, peers, subordinates, and patients/clients. To examine, these cultural differences, consider the following example. Dr. Kelly, an Irish American physician, gave an order for vital signs to Kim Li, a Chinese American nurse. The nurse perceived the order as unnecessary (but not harmful) to the patient, i.e., she thought the physician was requesting vital signs more frequently than was warranted by the patient's condition. Nurse Li refrained from questioning the physician or negotiating with him out of respect for his position of authority and the value she placed on maintain-

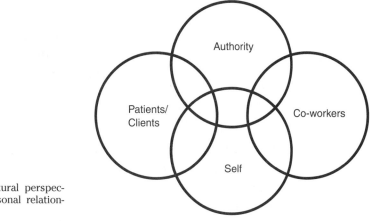

Figure 12–3. Cultural perspectives on interpersonal relationships.

ing harmony in the relationship. Nurse Li said nothing and carried out the physician's order.

At the change of shift, the charge nurse became angry because she concurred with the assessment that Dr. Kelly had ordered vital signs too frequently and thought Nurse Li should have confronted the physician about the order. Nurse Li intentionally chose to avoid questioning Dr. Kelly's order because she perceived him as an authority figure and wanted to foster harmony and balance. In her cultural value system, causing conflict through direct confrontation would be perceived negatively. She would have experienced lowered self-esteem and "loss of face" if she had been responsible for causing disharmony in the nurse–physician relationship. The charge nurse, on the other hand, perceived the physician as a colleague whose respect would be earned by assertive, direct communication with him.

LONG-STANDING HISTORIC RIVALRIES

Some historians refer to the 1900s as the century of war. At any given moment, there was armed conflict between two or more nations or between factions within nations. On occasion, the multicultural workplace becomes a battleground, where long-standing historic rivalries and more recent geopolitical differences are reenacted in the form of interpersonal conflict between two or more staff members. After ruling out other potential sources of conflict, it may be worth examining the ethnic heritage and national origins of staff members for possible reasons. For example, the nurse manager may observe a pattern of strained relationships between an Israeli physician and Palestinian physicians, nurses, laboratory technicians, physical therapists, and other health care providers. Similar observations may be made concerning staff members from countries known to be rivals, such as North and South Korea, Russia and Afghanistan, Iran and Iraq, India and Pakistan, and so forth.

Cues that may signal underlying historic rivalries include (1) the expression of high levels of emotional energy when a staff member is interacting with a person from a rival group when the topic does not seem to warrant it; (2) sudden, uncharacteristic behavior changes when the staff member is in the presence of a person from the rival group, e.g., an ordinarily cordial staff member unexpectedly becomes acrimonious for no apparent reason; (3) the repeated expression of strong opinions about historical, political, and current events involving rival nations or factions; and (4) inappropriate attempts to persuade others to adopt the staff member's partisan views about the rivalry.

Cultural Perspectives on Gender and Sexual Orientation

Women have historically constituted the majority of personnel in nursing and in many allied health disciplines. Currently, women constitute 94.6% of the nursing profession in the United States (U.S. Department of Health and Human Services, 2001) and 95.2% of the nursing profession in Canada (Canadian Institute of Health Information, 2000). Although Chapter 2 provides information about gender and sexual orientation, a few remarks about issues in the multicultural workplace will be made here. The complex interrelationship between gender and culture has been studied extensively. In the health care setting, nurses of both genders may face the biases and preconceptions of physicians, fellow nurses, and other health care providers. The issue is further complicated by cultural beliefs about relationships with authority figures and cross-national perspectives on the status of various health care disciplines. For example, in many less developed nations, nursing is a low-status occupation. In some oil-rich Arab countries (e.g., Saudi Arabia, Kuwait), care for the sick is carried out by health care providers who are hired from abroad for the purpose of caring for the bodily needs of the sick—an activity that is considered unacceptable in its cultural context.

Men in nursing and other health care disciplines dominated by women continue to struggle as minority members of their professions (Figure 12–4). In the multicultural health care workplace, both men and women face the gender biases that exist in society. These issues frequently emerge in verbal and nonverbal communication and in interpersonal relationships. Our language also betrays covert gender biases and preconceptions. For example, the expression "male nurse" is sometimes used, but seldom does one hear about the "female nurse" because that term is considered redundant and unnecessary. An extensive analysis of workplace issues concerning gay, lesbian, and bisexual staff members is beyond the scope of this text, but these types of diversity must be considered in the multicultural workplace.

Cultural Perspectives on Moral and Religious Beliefs

In some circumstances, **moral and religious beliefs** may underlie conflicts in the multicultural workplace. Consider the following dilemmas:

- A nurse who believes that it is morally wrong to drink alcohol refuses to carry out a physician's order for the therapeutic administration of alcohol as a sedative/hypnotic or to administer medicines with an alcohol base (e.g., cough syrup).

Figure 12–4. Although women historically have comprised the majority in nursing, men make significant professional contributions. In considering diversity inthe multicultural workplace, the role of men in nursing must be included along with an examination of racial, ethnic, religious, and other types of differences. (Copyright B. Proud)

- A nurse who believes that humankind should not unleash the power of nuclear energy refuses to care for cancer patients undergoing irradiation.
- A Roman Catholic nurse working in the operating room refuses to scrub for abortions, tubal ligations, vasectomies, and similar procedures because of religious prohibitions.
- A Jehovah's Witnesses nurse refuses to hang blood or counsel patients concerning blood or blood products.
- A Seventh-Day Adventist nurse who cites biblical reasons for following a vegetarian diet is unwilling to conduct patient education involving diets that contain meat.
- Muslim and Jewish staff members express concern that the hospital cafeteria fails to serve foods that meet their religious requirements.

These moral and religious issues reflect the diversity that characterizes staff members in the health care workplace. The challenge is to balance the health care needs and rights of patients with the moral and religious beliefs of health care providers. In some instances, it may be impossible to provide the services demanded by the organization's mission statement if all nurses refuse to engage in a particular activity. There may be legal implications for refusing to provide patients with certain services, e.g., those related to reproductive health. In the clinical world, the options available to accommodate the diverse moral and religious beliefs of staff members frequently depend on the size of the organization, the moral and religious proclivities of workers, the attitudes and beliefs of managers, the organizational climate, fiscal constraints, and other factors. The challenge faced by nurse managers is to balance the conflicting moral and religious beliefs of diverse groups with the achievement of organizational goals. This must be accomplished in a manner that is respectful of the moral and religious beliefs of staff members.

• CONFLICTING ROLE EXPECTATIONS: STAFF EDUCATED ABROAD

Many graduates of foreign nursing programs are currently practicing as registered nurses in the United States and Canada. The majority of these nurses practicing in the United States were educated in the Philippines; a markedly increased number have come from Asia and the British Commonwealth countries, the United Kingdom, Ireland, Australia, New Zealand, and Canada in recent years. In Canada, the majority of foreign-educated nurses come from the United Kingdom, the Philippines, and the United States (Canadian Institute for Health Information, 2000). Similar trends prevail for foreign-educated physicians, laboratory technicians, and other health care providers in the United States and Canada.

Role is defined as the set of expectations and behaviors associated with a specific position. Considerable research has been conducted on the patient sick role and on the roles of nurses, physicians, and other health care providers. Furthermore, it is suggested that persons entering the United States or Canada from a similar culture (e.g., Australia, England, Ireland) with English as the primary language may experience a lesser degree of culture shock than someone from a more diverse culture. For example, it is suggested that staff members from Australia or the United Kingdom will experience less difficulty with cultural adjustment to the United States or Canada than will persons from the Near and Middle East, Asia, or Africa, where language, religion, dress, and many other components of culture may be markedly different. Although social scientists speculate that people from similar cultures are more readily able to relate to one another, health care providers must be able to transcend cultural differences and to recognize that there are differences in role expectations.

Discrepancies in role expectations tend to create intrapersonal and interpersonal conflict. For example, nurses in Taiwan, the Philippines, and many African nations expect the families of patients to participate significantly in caregiving during the patient's hospitalization. All aspects of personal hygiene are provided by family members, who may be encouraged to remain with the patient around the clock, often sleeping on the floor or in uncomfortable lounge chairs.

In many countries, nurses have considerably expanded roles and their scope of practice is correspondingly broader. For example, in Nigeria it is clearly stated by the Board of Nursing and Midwifery that nurses diagnose and treat common illnesses such as malaria, typhoid, cholera, tetanus, and similar maladies. To graduate from a nursing program in the Philippines, nursing students must deliver a minimum of 25 babies unassisted and also assist at major and minor surgical procedures. In Haiti, nurses routinely start intravenous lines, perform episiotomies, and repair lacerations. In the mastery of technical skills, recent graduates of many foreign nursing programs have logged a considerable number of hours of clinical experience, often as apprentices mentored by experienced nurses who serve as their clinical faculty.

Some British and Irish nurses perceive United States and Canadian nurses as "junior physicians," second-guessing and anticipating therapy. Many perceive that in Great Britain and Ireland, nurses have greater freedom in ordering nursing modalities without a physician's orders. For example, decubitus ulcer care, ambulation, dressings, and nutritional therapy are all nurse-initiated activities based on nursing assessment. British and Irish nurses also expect that the nursing role includes activities that are defined by United States and Canadian nurses as nonnursing activities. For example, in many British hospitals, nurses are expected to clean patients' units after discharge and prepare them for the next admission.

In many nations, nurse midwives are primarily responsible for obstetric care. In some ways, the United States and Canada are anomalous with so much emphasis on the medically dominated specialty of obstetric medicine. Viewing childbirth as a medical problem, rather than a normal physiologic process, reveals an underlying philosophic difference between the United States and Canadian health care delivery systems and those in other nations. Some nurses who have been educated abroad are both nurses and midwives; thus, the transition to the medically dominated United States and Canadian models may leave them feeling underutilized and confused about the roles of the obstetrician and the maternal-child nurse or nurse midwife.

Because of the shortage of qualified health care providers in many less developed countries, there usually are fewer interdisciplinary differences about the nature and scope of practice for various health care disciplines. There are also various categories of licensed and unlicensed health care providers who contribute to the overall health and well-being of people in countries around the world. For example, there are feldspars in the former Soviet Union, barefoot doctors in China, and herbalists in nearly every nation.

• CULTURAL ASSESSMENT IN THE MULTICULTURAL WORKPLACE

Cultural self-assessment in the multicultural workplace focuses on (1) staff members and their beliefs about multiculturalism in the workplace (**individual cultural self-assessment**) or (2) the entire or particular unit or division of a health care organization, institution, or agency (**organizational cultural self-assessment**).

Individual Cultural Self-Assessment

As indicated in Chapter 1, it is important for nurses to be aware of their own ethnocentric tendencies. This is best accomplished when individuals review

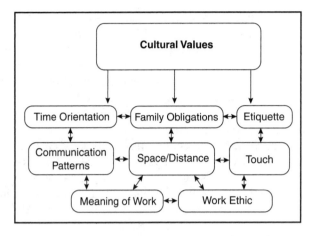

Figure 12–5. Influence of cultural values in the multicultural workplace

their cultural attitudes, values, beliefs, and practices. Figure 12–5 shows the importance of cultural values in the workplace, and Table 12–3 contains the individual cultural assessment instrument, which is one instrument used for gathering cultural data about staff members and their beliefs about multiculturalism in the workplace. By gathering responses to the individual cultural assessment instrument, nurse managers can identify staff perceptions about diversity issues and determine what management strategies might be useful.

(Text continues on page 392.)

TABLE 12–3	**INDIVIDUAL CULTURAL ASSESSMENT INSTRUMENT**				
	STRONGLY AGREE	AGREE	NO OPINION	DISAGREE	STRONGLY DISAGREE
1. Open acknowledgment and/or general discussion of cultural diversity occurs in my work environment.	1	2	3	4	5
3. Multicultural education or awareness programs are emphasized in my work environment.	1	2	3	4	5
5. I have personally experienced communication or interaction difficulties with a manager because of my ethnic, cultural, gender, or racial values.	1	2	3	4	5

(continued)

TABLE 12–3	*(Continued)*				
	STRONGLY AGREE	**AGREE**	**NO OPINION**	**DISAGREE**	**STRONGLY DISAGREE**
7. Coworkers in my work environment tend to "hang out" during lunch or breaks with workers from the same cultural background.	1	2	3	4	5
9. Members of my own culture are participants on existing work committees or task forces that help set direction for the work environment.	1	2	3	4	5
11. In my work environment, I have access to work-related growth and development opportunities like my coworkers.	1	2	3	4	5
13. In my work environment, coworkers communicate verbally and/or through body language in ways that demean my culture or race.	1	2	3	4	5
15. All workers in my work environment are held to the same standards of job performance regardless of gender, race, or cultural background.	1	2	3	4	5
17. Staff in my work environment are more successful if they share the same cultural values and ancestry as the manager.	1	2	3	4	5
19. When bicultural or multicultural conflict occurs in my work	1	2	3	4	5

(continued)

TABLE 12–3	*(Continued)*	STRONGLY AGREE	AGREE	NO OPINION	DISAGREE	STRONGLY DISAGREE
	area, cultural, gender, and racial influences are openly discussed as part of the conflict resolution steps.					
	2. It is important that openness and general discussion of cultural diversity take place in my work setting.	1	2	3	4	5
	4. Multicultural education and awareness program emphasis is important in my work environment.	1	2	3	4	5
	6. It is important that various cultural values are understood and respected by all managers working in a multicultural environment.	1	2	3	4	5
	8. It is important for management to facilitate work and to plan culturally mixed social activity for the workers and my work environment.	1	2	3	4	5
	10. It is important for management to ensure that the cultures of all workers in my work environment are represented on work committees.	1	2	3	4	5
	12. It is important for managers to recognize and encourage growth opportunities equally for all workers.	1	2	3	4	5

(continued)

TABLE 12–3	*(Continued)*				
	STRONGLY AGREE	**AGREE**	**NO OPINION**	**DISAGREE**	**STRONGLY DISAGREE**
14. It is important for managers to work with staff to increase sensitivity to cultural values and perceptions that will help to reduce or eliminate racial and cultural barriers.	1	2	3	4	5
16. It is important for managers to have systems to identify and analyze which employees receive promotions and growth experiences, and to consider biases that influence performance standards so that they are achievable for all groups of staff.	1	2	3	4	5
18. It is important for the administration to recognize, reward, and value the managers who successfully promote, manage, and retain a harmonious multicultural work force.	1	2	3	4	5
20. It is important for managers to facilitate, promote, and participate in open dialogue about cultural influences and diverse perceptions that occur because of differences in ethnicity or gender.	1	2	3	4	5

Modified and used with permission. From Davis, P. D. (1995). Enhancing multicultural harmony. Nursing Management 26(7), 32D-32E © Springhouse Corporation.

EVIDENCE-BASED PRACTICE 12–1
Research on Actions by Nurse Managers that Enhance Multicultural Harmony

Health care managers have a responsibility to create harmony within the multicultural workforce at their institutions. Suggestions in the literature for managers' actions to deal effectively with cultural diversity may not agree with staff members' perspectives on the issue. The investigator introduced a quasi-experimental evaluation method that may be used as introductory work for research in multicultural workforce management. Using recommendations from the literature, the researcher asked 100 health care workers of various ethnic backgrounds, experience, and ages to complete a 20-item Likert-type instrument concerning management actions that create multicultural harmony in a hospital setting.

CLINICAL APPLICATION

The study findings indicate that staff members perceive equal growth opportunity, achievable standards, respecting values, and striving to eliminate barriers as important actions. Nurses will find that concrete issues of equity and fairness are more significant to members of the staff than awareness education and opportunities for social activities among staff from various cultural backgrounds. The researcher indicates that staff are looking for actions by managers, not rhetoric.

Davis, P. D. (1995). Enhancing multicultural harmony. Ten actions for managers. *Nursing Management 2*(7), 32A–32H.

A culturally diverse workforce should be a strength in meeting the needs of culturally diverse clients/patients and should be viewed as an asset. Nurse managers, however, need to release the cultural talents of this workforce.

After responding to the questions on the individual cultural assessment instrument, read Evidence-Based Practice 12–1, which summarizes a study in which the instrument was administered to staff nurses. Notice that the White, Black, Hispanic, and Asian nurses who participated in the study gave different responses, which indicates that perceptions of effective management actions vary according to the nurse's ethnic heritage.

Cultural Self-Assessment of Health Care Organizations, Institutions, and Agencies

Before engaging in a cultural self-assessment of a health care organization, institution, or agency, it is necessary to consider both content and process. Box 12–3 illustrates recommended content in a sample instrument. The instrument may be used to assess an entire organization, such as a hospital, a long-term care facility, a home health agency, or another institution, organization, or agency, or it may be modified for the assessment of a particular unit or division. For example, staff in the operating room, specialty units, home health care division, ambulatory care area, and so forth may perceive a need to

BOX 12–3	**CULTURAL ASSESSMENT OF AN ORGANIZATION, INSTITUTION, OR AGENCY**

Demographics/Descriptive Data

- What types of cultural diversity are represented by clients, families, visitors, and others significant to the clients? Indicate approximate numbers and percentages according to the conventional system already used for reporting census data.
- What types of cultural diversity are represented? What types of diversity are present among patients, physicians, nurses, x-ray technicians, and other staff? Indicate approximate numbers and percentages by department/discipline.
- How is the organization, institution, or agency structured? Who is in charge? How do you assess the administrators in terms of support for cultural diversity and interventions to foster multiculturalism?
- How many key leaders/decision makers within the organization, institution, or agency come from culturally diverse backgrounds?
- What languages are spoken by patients, family members/significant others, and staff?

Assessment of Strengths

- What are the cultural strengths or positive characteristics and qualities?
- What institutional resources (fiscal, human) are available to support multiculturalism?
- What goals and needs related to cultural diversity already have been expressed?
- What successes in making services accessible and culturally appropriate have occurred to date? Highlight goals, programs, and activities that have been successful.
- What positive comments have been given by clients and significant others from culturally diverse backgrounds about their experiences with the organization, institution, or agency?

Assessment of Community Resources

- What efforts are made to use multicultural community-based resources (e.g., anthropology and foreign languages faculty and students from area colleges and universities, community organizations for ethnic or religious groups, and similar resources)?
- To what extent are leaders from racial, ethnic, and religious communities involved with the institution (e.g., invited to serve on boards and advisory committees)?
- To what extent is there political and economic support for multicultural programs and projects?

Assessment of Weakness/Areas for Continued Growth

- What are the cultural weaknesses, limitations, and areas for continued growth?
- What could be done to better promote multiculturalism?

(continued)

BOX 12–3	**CULTURAL ASSESSMENT OF AN ORGANIZATION, INSTITUTION, OR AGENCY** *(Continued)*

Assessment from the Perspective of Clients and Families

- How do clients (and families/significant others) evaluate the multicultural aspects of the organization, institution, or agency? Do quality assurance data indicate that clients from various cultural backgrounds are satisfied/dissatisfied with care? Be specific.
- How adequate is the system for translation and interpretation? What materials are available in the client's primary language (in written and other forms such as audiocassettes, videotapes, computer programs)?
  Note: the literacy level of clients must be assessed.
- Are educational programs available in the languages spoken by clients?
- Are cultural and religious calendars used in determining scheduling for preadmission testing, procedures, educational programs, follow-up visits, or other appointments?
- Are cultural considerations given to the acceptability of certain medical and surgical procedures (e.g., amputations, blood transfusions, disposal of body parts, and handling various types of human tissue)?
- Are cultural considerations a factor in administering medicines? How familiar are nurses, physicians, and pharmacists with current research in ethnopharmacology?
- If a client dies, what cultural considerations are given during postmortem care? How are cultural needs associated with dying addressed with the family and others significant to the deceased? Does the roster of religious representatives available to nursing staff include traditional spiritual healers such as shamans and medicine men/women as well as rabbis, priests, elders, and others?

Assessment from an Institutional Perspective

- To what extent do the philosophy and mission statement support, foster, and promote multiculturalism and respect for cultural diversity? Is there congruence between philosophy/mission statement and reality? How is this evident?
- To what extent is there administrative support for multiculturalism? In what ways is support present or absent? Provide evidence to support this.
- Are data being gathered to provide documentation concerning multicultural issues? Are there missing data? Are data disseminated to appropriate decision makers and leaders within the institution? How are these data used?
- Are opportunities for continuing professional education and development in topics pertaining to multiculturalism provided for nurses and other staff?
- Are there racial, ethnic, religious, or other tensions? If so, try to objectively and nonjudgmentally assess their origins and nature in as much detail as possible.
- Are adequate resources being allocated for the purpose of promoting a harmonious multicultural health care environment? If not, indicate areas in which additional resources are needed.
- What multicultural library resources and audiovisual and computer software are available for use by nurses and other staff?

(continued)

BOX 12–3	**CULTURAL ASSESSMENT OF AN ORGANIZATION, INSTITUTION, OR AGENCY** *(Continued)*

- What efforts are made to recruit and retain nurses and other staff from racially, ethnically, and religiously diverse backgrounds? What other types of diversity (e.g., sexual orientation) are fostered or discouraged?
- How would you describe the cultural climate of the institution? Are ethnic/racial/religious jokes prevalent? Are negative remarks or comments about certain cultural groups permitted? Who is doing the talking and who is listening to negative comments/jokes?
- Are human resources initiatives pertaining to advertising, hiring, promotion, and performance evaluations free from discrimination?
- Are cultural and religious considerations reflected in staff scheduling policies for nursing and other departments?
- Are policies and procedures appropriate from a multicultural perspective? What process is used for reviewing them for cultural appropriateness and relevance?

Assessment of Need and Readiness for Change

- Is there a need for change? If so, indicate who, what, when, where, why, and how.
- Who is in favor of change? Who is against it?
- What are the anticipated obstacles to change?
- What financial and human resources would be necessary to bring about the recommended changes?

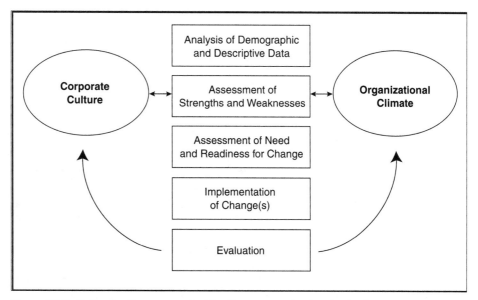

Figure 12–6. Cultural self-assessment of healh care organization, institution, or agency.

engage in an organizational self-assessment because of changing demographics in populations served or concerns with quality of care for diverse clients/patients. Figure 12–6 provides a schematic representation of the cultural self-assessment of a health care organization, institution, or agency.

The Process of Cultural Self-Assessment by Organizations, Institutions, and Agencies

Although the manner in which the cultural self-assessment is carried out will vary for each institution, organization, or agency and for different units or divisions within it, the process remains fundamentally the same. After identifying key staff members to lead the institutional cultural self-assessment process, the leaders should communicate the purpose of the cultural self-assessment to those who will be participating in it. It is important to involve grassroots members of the staff and to solicit input from the patient/client population served through interviews, focus groups, written surveys, or other methods. The process of cultural self-assessment by organizations, institutions, and agencies involves collecting demographic and descriptive data, identifying strengths and limitations, assessing the need and readiness for change, identifying community resources, evaluating the effectiveness of changes, and implementing any necessary revisions.

DEMOGRAPHIC AND DESCRIPTIVE DATA

As with any assessment, begin by gathering demographic and descriptive data. It is highly likely that some of these data have already been collected and stored centrally. If reports containing the necessary data are available, they should be reviewed and discussed by the group as part of the cultural assessment process. Data such as types and numbers of diverse patients/clients and staff members should be determined. There should be an assessment of the predominant languages spoken and of the effectiveness of the system being used for translation and interpretation.

STRENGTHS AND LIMITATIONS

After the data have been gathered, a team of key leaders should convene to critically review and analyze them. Because this will be an active working group, membership should be limited to approximately 12 people. If the group is larger, consideration should be given to division into smaller subgroups. The purpose of the review is to assess the strengths, limitations, and areas for continued growth in terms of promoting a harmonious multicultural environment for patients/clients and staff members of diverse backgrounds. It is important to identify strengths and limitations from both an **emic** (insider) and an **etic** (outsider) perspective (i.e., from the viewpoint of health care providers [insiders] and clients/patients, those significant to them, and visitors [outsiders]). For example, although the staff may believe the system is structured adequately to meet the needs of linguistically diverse persons, it would be important to compare that perception with the patients' and clients' point of view. From their perspective, examine the ways in which cultural aspects are part of the care provided. From the institutional perspective, critically examine the infrastructure for philosophic, fiscal, and human resources that reflect a commitment—or lack of one—to promoting harmony in the multicultural workplace. Throughout the process, comparative analyses are made between input from staff members and that from patients and clients to identify strengths and limitations.

NEED AND READINESS FOR CHANGE

Once the strengths and limitations have been identified, there should be an assessment of the need and readiness for change. If changes are needed, it is important to identify why, who, what, when, where, and how. Identify the fiscal and human resources that will be needed to bring about the recommended change(s).

Be sure to anticipate staff **resistance to change**. Determine who is likely to favor and oppose the proposed change, anticipate obstacles to it, and develop contingency plans. Different people will see different meanings in activities by organizations to become more culturally diverse. Members of the federal minority groups may see job opportunities, whereas White men may complain of reverse discrimination. Depending on the nature of the recommendation and the corporate culture of the organization, an action plan should accompany the recommendation, i.e., specifically what does the group believe ought to be done? Although most staff members will support the change, it is insufficient for nurse managers and supervisors to say, "A new law has been passed mandating diversity" or "Hospital policy requires diversity." Resistance can be expected to increase to the degree that staff members influenced by the changes have pressure on them to change, and it will decrease to the degree they are actively involved in planning diversity activities. Resistance can be expected if the changes are made on personal grounds rather than as requirements, sanctions, or policies. Finally, resistance can be expected if the organization culture is ignored. There are informal as well as formal norms within every organization. An effective change will neither ignore old customs nor abruptly create new ones. As with most change, timing is important.

COMMUNITY RESOURCES

In developing an action plan for change, be sure to assess the community resources available to assist with goal achievement. For example, it may be possible to invite leaders from ethnic communities to provide staff in-service programs aimed at increasing understanding of the health care needs of persons from diverse backgrounds. A second example might be to involve foreign-language faculty and students from area colleges and universities to assist with translation for linguistically diverse patients and clients. A final example might be to invite clergy to discuss health-related religious beliefs and practices (Parsons & Reiss, 1999). If organizational resources are limited, it may be possible to identify community-based resources that are available at low cost.

EVALUATION OF THE EFFECTIVENESS OF CHANGES
AND IMPLEMENTATION OF REVISIONS

After implementation of the recommended change(s), there should be an evaluation of their effectiveness, and revisions should be made as needed. In recognition of the rapid pace of change in contemporary health care, the process of institutional cultural self-assessment should be repeated at periodic intervals. Mateo and Smith (2001) note that although significant fiscal and human resources are expended by organizations in diversity initiatives, there is a need to be more diligent in monitoring and evaluating outcomes. They recommend the development of a grid that articulates goals, diversity initiatives, and outcome measures.

Promoting Harmony in the Multicultural Workplace

After conducting a cultural assessment of the health care organization, institution, or agency, the nurse will have data about the strengths and weaknesses; fiscal, human, and community resources; areas in which to pursue change; and readiness of the staff to engage in change.

As indicated in Box 12–4, there are **facilitators** and **barriers** to promoting harmony in the multicultural workplace. Facilitators include identification of the cultural values of the organization, institution, or agency; clear articulation of the mission statement and policies about diversity; zero tolerance for discrimination; effective cross-cultural communication; skill with conflict resolution involving diversity; and commitment to multiculturalism at all levels of management. The barriers that must be overcome include hatred, prejudice, bigotry, racism, discrimination, and ethnoviolence. Negative behaviors aimed at employees, clients/patients, their families, others significant to them, and other

BOX 12–4	PROMOTING HARMONY IN THE MULTICULTURAL WORKPLACE

Facilitators

Identification of cultural values of the organization, institution, or agency
Mission statement and policies about diversity
Zero tolerance for discrimination
Effective cross-cultural communication
Skill with conflict resolution involving diversity
Commitment to multiculturalism at all levels of management

Barriers

Hatred
Prejudice
Bigotry
Racism
Discrimination
(Negative attitudes or behaviors based on race, ethnicity, religion, gender, sexual orientation, national origin, class, handicap/disability)

visitors, based on race, ethnicity, religion, gender, sexual orientation, national origin, class, or handicap/disability should not be tolerated. All employees should be apprised that there will be zero tolerance for those who engage in negative behaviors, and management staff at all levels should be given the authority to impose sanctions when violations occur.

SUMMARY

Given the demographic composition of contemporary United States and Canadian societies, nurses will continue to find both challenges and opportunities as they practice nursing in multicultural health care settings. Microcosms of society at large, health care organizations, institutions, and agencies will consist of staff members from increasingly diverse backgrounds. It is important to remember that culture influences the manner in which people perceive, identify, define, and solve problems in the workplace. Among the complex and interrelated factors that must be considered when workplace diversity is addressed are cultural perspectives on values, the meaning of work, interpersonal relationships, cross-cultural communication patterns (including etiquette, touch, space/distance), gender and sexual orientation, moral and religious beliefs, hygiene, and clothing. Characteristics of the staff member such as individual preferences, biases and prejudices for and against certain groups, educational background, and previous experiences living and working in culturally diverse settings also must be considered.

Understanding cultural differences in the workplace and developing skill in conflict resolution will continue to be needed in transcultural nursing administration in the new millennium. The successful transcultural nurse administrator will behave respectfully toward others from diverse backgrounds and will implement policies that promote cultural understanding, knowledge, and skill in the workplace. Nurses in leadership and management positions will apply the principles of transcultural nursing to the multicultural workplace, just as they have done in the past to provide culturally competent and congruent care for clients and patients.

REVIEW QUESTIONS

1. Compare and contrast the concepts hatred, prejudice, racism, discrimination, and ethnoviolence. Critically examine the manner in which they may manifest themselves in the health care workplace.
2. What is meant by transcultural nursing administration? How is transcultural nursing administration useful for nurses who hold leadership positions in multicultural health care settings?
3. How do the cultural meanings of work embraced by staff from diverse cultures influence the corporate culture and organizational climate of contemporary health care institutions, organizations, and agencies?
4. Identify strategies to promote effective cross-cultural communication in the multicultural workplace.

5. Critically analyze the cultural origins of conflict that may arise in the health care workplace.

6. Review the process and content of cultural self-assessment by organizations, institutions, and agencies. What aspects of the change process must be considered during engagement in cultural self-assessment?

7. Identify facilitators and barriers to promoting harmony in the multicultural workplace.

CRITICAL THINKING ACTIVITIES

1. Using the guidelines in Box 12–3, conduct a cultural assessment of a health care organization, institution, or agency. Alternatively, you may use the guidelines to gather assessment data on a unit or department within a larger facility.

2. Ask at least 10 nurses working at a health care organization, institution, or agency (hospital, long-term care facility, prison, home health care agency, or related facility) if they would be willing to respond to the items found in the instrument in Table 12–3, Individual Cultural Assessment Instrument. Average the numeric responses for each of the 20 items to identify trends. Write a one-page summary of your findings that includes a critical analysis of the results. What do the responses tell you about the organizational climate and corporate culture that prevail within the health care facility?

3. Reflect on your personal experience with hatred, prejudice, bigotry, racism, discrimination, and/or ethnoviolence. Were you the victim or the perpetrator? How did you feel during the incident(s)? Discuss your responses with another member of the class, preferably someone from a different cultural background from your own.

4. From a cultural perspective, critically examine the dress code or policy statement about clothing and accessories that are permitted for staff at a health care organization, agency, or institution. How effectively does the code or policy address the widespread diversity that characterizes our contemporary health care workforce? Identify the strengths and limitations of the dress code or policy statement. What modifications or changes would you recommend to accommodate the attire worn by staff from diverse cultures?

5. Choose two of the six case studies presented at the beginning of the chapter, and analyze them from the perspective of a nurse manager. For the purpose of analysis, assume the role of nurse manager, and critically examine approaches you might use to change the negative attitudes and behaviors of those mentioned in the case studies.

• References

Brown, I. C. (1973). *Understanding race relations.* Englewood Cliffs, NJ: Prentice-Hall.

Canadian Institute for Health Information (2000). Supply and distribution of registered nurses in Canada, 2000 Report: Executive Summary. Available at: http://www.cihi.ca/Roadmap/RNPD/RNDB/pdf/ExecSum2000.pdf. Accessed March 19, 2002.

Data Development Section, Labor Branch, Human Resources Development Canada (1998). Workforce population showing Canadian citizen representation by employment equity occupations groups and unit groups for women, aboriginal peoples, and visible minorities. Available from: http://info.load-otea.hrdc-drhc.gc.ca/workplace_equity/downloads/separate/table05cit.pdf; accessed March 19, 2002.

Davis, P. D. (1995). Enhancing multicultural harmony. *Nursing Management, 26*(7), 32A–32H.

Flarey, D. L. (1993). The social climate of work environments. *Journal of Nursing Administration, 23*(6), 9–15.

Gooden, M. B., Porter, C. P., Gonzalez, R. I., & Mims, B. L. (2001). Rethinking the relationship between nursing and diversity. *American Journal of Nursing, 101,* 1, 63, 65.

Health Canada (1999). Canadian research on immigration and health. Available at: http://www.hc-sc.gc.ca/iacb-dgiac/nhrdp/metropolis/cirh_pdf_index_e.htm. Accessed November 23, 2001.

Henderson, G. (1994). *Cultural diversity in the workplace.* Westport, CT: Praeger.

Holmes, S. A. (1994, March 3). Survey finds minorities resent each other almost as much as they do whites. *New York Times,* A9.

Isajiw, W. W. (1999). *Understanding diversity: Ethnicity and race in the Canadian context.* Toronto, ON: Thompson Educational Publishing, Inc.

Ivancevich, J. M., & Gilbert, J. A. (2000). Diversity management: Time for a new approach. *Public Personnel Management, 29*(75), 75–92.

Jung, C. A. (1968). In G. Adler, *The Collected Works of Carl Jung* (Vol. 10). Princeton, NJ: University Press.

Kalbach, M. A., & Kalbach, W. E. (2000). *Perspectives on ethnicity in Canada.* Toronto: Harcourt Canada.

Lambert, V. A., & Nugent, K. E. (1999). Leadership style for facilitating the integration of culturally appropriate health care. *Seminars for Nurse Managers, 7*(4), 172–178.

Lautard, H. & Guppy, N. (1999). Revisiting the vertical mosaic: Occupational stratification among Canadian ethnic groups. In P. S. Li (Ed.), *Race and ethnic relations in Canada* (2nd ed., pp. 219–252). New York: Oxford University Press.

Leininger, M. M. (1996). Founder's focus. Transcultural nursing administration: An imperative worldwide. *Journal of Transcultural Nursing, 8*(1), 28–33.

Mateo, M. A., & Smith, S. P. (2001). Workforce diversity: Challenges and strategies. *Journal of Multicultural Nursing & Health, 7*(2), 8–12.

Moore, J. D., & Jensen, B. (1997). Unchanging face of health care: Diversity still hard to find in top executive rank. *Modern Healthcare, 27*(50), 30–34.

Parsons, L. C., & Reiss, P. L. (1999). Promoting collaborative practice with culturally diverse populations. *Seminars for Nurse Managers, 7*(1), 160–165.

Schwartz, R. H., & Sullivan, D. B. (1993). Managing diversity in hospitals. *Health Care Management Review, 18*(2), 51–56.

Schmeiding, N. J. (2000). Minority nurses in leadership positions: A call for action. *Nursing Outlook, 48,* 120–127.

U.S. Census Bureau (1995). Employed civilians by occupation, sex, race, and Hispanic origin: 1995. *Current population reports,* Section 13: Labor Force Employment and Earnings. Washington, DC: U.S. Government Printing Office.

U.S. Census Bureau (2000). *Current population reports,* P20–519. Washington, DC: U.S. Government Printing Office.

U.S. Department of Health and Human Services, Bureau of Health Professions (2001). *The registered nurse population: National sample survey of registered nurses.* Washington, DC: U.S. Government Printing Office.

Williams, D. R., & Rucker, T. D. (2000). Understanding and addressing racial disparities in health care. *Minority Health, 2*(1), 30–39.

4

Contemporary Challenges
in Transcultural Nursing

CHAPTER **13**

Transcultural Aspects of Pain

Patti Ludwig-Beymer

OBJECTIVES

1. Analyze the components responsible for pain perception.
2. Identify the universal aspects of the pain experience.
3. Compare and contrast expressions of pain by culture, gender, and type of pain.
4. Describe the views and attitudes about pain held by the nursing subculture.
5. Explain the rationale for nurses to identify their personal attitudes toward pain.
6. Illustrate the steps used in establishing a relationship with individuals experiencing pain.
7. Compare and contrast alternative practices in pain management.
8. Apply theoretic content to case studies.

Pain, a universally recognized phenomenon, is an important area of consideration in nursing practice. According to the American Pain Society, 50 million people in the United States, or one in five, have intractable pain (Lang & Pratt, 1994). Pain is a frequent and compelling reason for seeking health care and is a common result of many diagnostic, surgical, and treatment procedures. Chronic pain is now considered to be the most frequent cause of disability in the United States and in other industrialized nations. Chronic pain has often been mismanaged and has resulted in decreased quality of life, medical expense, lost work hours, and lawsuits. The elderly are at special risk for pain. One study found that 51% of nursing home residents reported pain every day (Ferrell & Ferrell, 1990), and other studies have reported that approximately 70% of elderly people living in the community experience some degree of pain regularly (Crook, Rideout, & Brown, 1984; Roy & Thomas, 1986; Sorkin, Rudy, Hanlon, Turk, & Steig, 1990). Even in acute care settings, pain may not be adequately treated, and the ethnicity of patients affects pain management (Todd, Samaroo, & Hoffman, 1993).

The management of pain is particularly important in nursing because nurses often encounter people either experiencing or anticipating pain. Of equal importance, pain management has traditionally been a nursing responsibility. Thus, nurses are in an ideal position to assess pain and to take action to alleviate it. Many nurses, however, may not be sufficiently prepared to care for patients in pain. Inadequacies in pain management may result from lack of knowledge about pain management and disease processes. Ferrell, Virani, Grant, Vallerand, and McCaffery (2000) surveyed 50 textbooks used in nursing education and found that pain constituted only 0.5% of the total text content. Pharmacologic management of pain was identified as a particular weakness.

Pain is a very private experience and is influenced by a variety of factors, as summarized in Table 13-1. Culture has long been recognized in nursing practice and research as a factor that influences a person's expression of and reaction to pain. Expectations about pain and its manifestations and management are embedded in a cultural context. The definition of pain, like that of health or illness, is culturally influenced. Zborowski (1952, 1969) has made perhaps the greatest contribution to our understanding of cultural responses to pain and the subjective nature of the pain experience (Evidence-Based Practice 13-1).

•DEFINITION OF PAIN

Definitions of pain are quite diverse, partly because of the complex nature of pain and partly because of the many different existing perspectives on pain. The term **pain** is derived from the Greek word for *penalty,* which helps to explain the long association between pain and punishment in Judeo-Christian thought. The medical profession has dominated our understanding of pain since the late 1800s. Consequently, pain has come to be defined as a sensation associated with real or potential tissue damage involving chemical disturbances along neurologic pathways. In the United States, the national guidelines on acute pain management define pain as an unpleasant sensory and emotional experience arising from actual or potential tissue damage or described in terms of such damage (U.S. Department of Health and Human Services, 1992).

However, pain is much more variable and modifiable than has previously been believed. Variations within and among people and cultures have been

TABLE 13–1	FACTORS THAT AFFECT EXPRESSIONS OF PAIN

FACTOR	EXPLANATION
Family	Experiences and attitudes of one's family affect response to painful situation.
Cultural group	Patterned attitudes toward pain behavior exist in every culture, and appropriate and inappropriate expressions of pain are thus culturally prescribed.
	Cultural responses to pain can be divided into two categories: stoic and emotive. Patients who are stoic are less likely to express their pain, whereas emotive patients are more likely to verbalize the expressions of pain.
Emotional factors	Perceived significance of pain affects response to pain.
Gender	Studies suggest that women tend to express distress and strain related to pain more openly and more often than men (Kleinman, 1988; Lawlis, Achterberg, Kenner & Kopetz, 1984; Encandela, 1993).
Spirituality and religious heritage	Studies suggest that spiritually focused or strongly religious people find meaning and expression for their pain through religious doctrines (Kotarba, 1983; Ohnuki-Tierney, 1984, Encandela, 1993).
Age	Specific biological and psychosocial factors influence elderly people's perceptions and experience of pain. Elderly people may believe that pain is a normal part of aging and should be tolerated, staff are too busy to hear complaints of their pain, and telling nurses about pain may result in further testing and expenses. The elderly may also be resigned to pain, ambivalent about the benefits of pain relief, and reluctant to express pain. (For further information, see Melding, 1991; Herr & Mobily, 1991; Hofland, 1992; Witte, 1989; and Yates, Dewar, & Fentiman, 1995.)

identified. Pain measurements are summarized in Table 13-2. These measurements include **sensation threshold, pain threshold, pain tolerance**, and **encouraged pain tolerance**. Stimuli that would produce intolerable pain in one person may be embraced by another. For example, in some cultures, initiation rites and other rituals involve procedures generally associated with severe pain, but the participants reportedly feel little or no pain (Melzack & Wall, 1983).

EVIDENCE-BASED PRACTICE 13–1
Zborowski's Classic Study of Pain

An anthropologist, Zborowski studied 103 patients on a Veterans Administration hospital medical-surgical unit using a variety of qualitative methods, including questionnaires, unstructured interviews, and direct observations. Data were collected from four cultural groups: Irish Americans, Italian Americans, Jewish Americans, and "Old American" (defined as third-generation Americans).

Zborowski compared pain interpretation, significance of pain, and other specific aspects of the pain experience, such as intensity, duration, and quality, across the four cultural groups. He found that Irish Americans had difficulty describing and talking about pain, showed little emotion with pain, deemphasized the pain, and withdrew socially when experiencing pain. Italian Americans were expressive in their pain and preferred the company of others when in pain. They tended to request immediate pain relief by any means possible and were generally happy when the pain was relieved. Like the Italian Americans, the Jewish Americans preferred company while in pain, sought relief from pain, and freely expressed their pain through crying, moaning, and complaining. However, the Jewish American men were skeptical and suspicious of the pain and were concerned about the implications of the pain. The "Old Americans" were precise in defining pain, displayed little emotion, and preferred to withdraw socially when in pain.

Clinical Application

Zborowski maintained that cultural traditions dictate whether to expect and tolerate pain in certain situations as well as how to behave during a painful experience. In addition, cultural groups expect individuals to conform to these culturally prescribed rules and norms. Despite some methodologic flaws, Zborowski's research remains the classic study of cross-cultural pain responses.

Zborowski, M. (1952). Cultural components in response to pain. *Journal of Social Issues, 8,* 16-30, and Zborowski, M. (1969). *People in Pain.* San Francisco: Jossey-Bass.

Pain perception, then, cannot be defined simply in terms of particular kinds of stimuli. Rather, pain is a highly personal experience, depending on cultural learning, the meaning of the situation, and other factors unique to the individual. Pain is subjective, occurring whenever the experiencing person says it does. The meaning of painful stimuli for individuals, the way individuals define their situation, and the impact of previous personal experiences all help determine the experience of pain (McCaffery & Pasero, 1999)

•CULTURALLY COMPETENT NURSING CARE FOR CLIENTS IN PAIN

Six helpful strategies for dealing with the client in pain are described below: identifying **personal attitudes**, creating an effective **nurse-client relationship**, establishing **nurse competence**, assessing pain, managing pain, and

TABLE 13–2	**MEASUREMENT OF PAIN**	
TYPE OF PAIN	**DEFINITION**	**IMPACT OF CULTURE**
Sensation threshold	Lowest stimulus that results in tingling or warmth	Research suggests that most people, regardless of cultural background, have a uniform sensation threshold
Pain threshold	Point at which the individual reports that a stimulus is painful	Cultural background appears to have some effect on this measure of pain
Pain tolerance	Point at which the individual withdraws or asks to have the stimuli stopped	Cultural background appears to have a strong effect on pain tolerance levels
Encouraged pain tolerance	Amount of painful stimuli an individual accepts when encouraged to tolerate increasingly higher levels of stimulation	Cultural differences have been documented

clarifying responsibility. Transcultural concepts are integrated into these strategies. When these strategies are not used, culturally insensitive care may result.

Identifying Personal Attitudes

Nurses bring their own attitudes about pain to each client interaction. Some research suggests that nurses, as part of a **nursing subculture**, have been socialized to have certain pain expectations, as summarized in Table 13-3. Nurses must understand and confront their own personal beliefs about pain and suffering. It is helpful for individual nurses to identify how they view, express, and manage their own pain. Nurses must also identify their beliefs about clients' expression of pain. The learner activities at the end of this chapter will assist nurses in this process. For example, is a nurse truly nonjudgmental or does the nurse prefer the patient to express pain stoically? Identifying personal cultural beliefs is the first step in recognizing how these beliefs may interfere with truly therapeutic nurse-client relationships.

Creating an Effective Nurse-Client Relationship

The issue of power and powerlessness always colors the relationship between the person in pain and the health care provider. Because pain is a wholly subjective experience that cannot be proved or verified, people in pain are at the mercy of the health care provider to whom they chose to disclose information

TABLE 13–3	THE NURSING SUBCULTURE: EXPECTATIONS ABOUT PAIN

EXPECTATIONS	DESCRIPTION
Silent suffering	Social customs and practices in society at large, particularly in health care, have been dominated by white Anglo-Saxon Protestants. Regardless of their ethnic backgrounds, most nurses have been somewhat influenced by these dominant values and beliefs. The majority of nurses in the United States and Canada are white, middle-class women who have been socialized to believe that self-control is better than open displays of strong feelings. Nurses may be socialized to place a high value on self-control in response to pain. (For further information, see Benoliel & Crowley, 1974; Acheson, 1988; and Howell, Butler, Vincent, Watt-Watson, & Stearns, 2000).
Ability to describe pain	Nurses expect people to be objective about the very subjective experience of pain. In clinical practice, nurses may expect a person experiencing pain to report it and give a detailed description of it, but to display few emotional responses to the pain.
Pain inferences	Individuals who are in frequent contact with people in pain may pain. Nurses may deny or downplay the pain they observe in others. Research suggests that the ethnic background of both the client and the nurses is an important determinant for inference of suffering caused by both physical and psychological distress. One study asked nurses from 13 countries to infer physical and psychologic pain for clients described in brief case studies. Nurses from these cultures differed markedly. Korean nurses inferred the highest level of psychologic distress, followed by Puerto Rican and Ugandan nurses. Nepalese, Taiwanese, and Belgian nurses inferred the least amount of psychological distress. Korean nurses also inferred the greatest amount of physical pain, followed by Japanese and Indian nurses. Nurses from Belgium, the United States, and England inferred the least amount of physical pain. (For further information, see Baer, Davitz, & Lieb 1970; Davitz & Davitz, 1975, Davitz & Davitz, 1981; Davitz, Sameshima, & Davitz, 1976; and Acheson, 1988.)

about their pain. The health care provider may decide to believe or disbelieve the person's account of pain, ignore it completely, or intentionally or inadvertently make it worse.

Thus, in nursing practice, it is important to establish an effective and supportive nurse-client relationship. The quality of the relationship may be as important as the pain-relieving skills or techniques used. The nurse should strive to create a relationship with the client that is characterized by genuineness, empathy, warmth, and respect. These caring behaviors constitute the essence of transcultural nursing. A positive relationship incorporates respect for the client and avoidance of stereotyping.

Respect Clients as Individuals

Nurses must respect clients as unique individuals and recognize that culture is an important aspect of that individuality. For example, nurses must recognize that clients hold a variety of beliefs about pain. In addition to recognizing the existence of different perspectives on pain, nurses must acknowledge that clients are entitled to their own belief systems.

Respect the Client's Response to Pain

Although personal values and cultural expectations differ, nurses must accept the rights of clients to respond to pain in the way they deem appropriate. Clients should never be made to feel ashamed of their responses to pain, even if the responses are not congruent with what nurses consider typical. Nurses need to remember that **pain expressions** vary widely and that no expression of pain is inherently good or bad.

The nurse who is aware of cultural differences and understands clients in terms of cultural backgrounds will respond effectively and appropriately to their needs. Such a nurse will not be disturbed by the emotional expressiveness of a client whose culture expects and encourages open expression of pain. Similarly, the sensitive nurse will not mistake the stoic attitude of a client from another culture for lack of pain.

Never Stereotype a Person on the Basis of Culture

Culture should never be used as a basis on which to stereotype an individual. Intragroup differences in pain perception and expression have been well documented in pain research (Wolff & Langley, 1977). When providing care, the nurse should take into account many aspects of the experience, including the pain itself, the client's culture, the psychologic aspects of the situation, and additional needs of the client. Expressions of pain vary widely within each culture, and nurses must anticipate and accept these variations.

Establishing Nurse Competence

Nurses must demonstrate and establish their competence for clients. The manner in which nurses present themselves and their care may greatly influence their reception. For example, research suggests that the status of the person who suggests that a treatment will be effective influences the extent to which individuals believe the suggestion (Neufeld, 1970). Clients should feel comfortable with both the technical and interpersonal skills of nurses. An important aspect of establishing credibility relates to the nurse's ability to provide culturally competent care.

Part of establishing interpersonal competence involves being available to the client who is experiencing pain. This may involve staying with the client, providing privacy to the client, or using ordinary touch as an adjunct to pain relief. Research findings indicate that nurses often provide "instrumental touch," such as dressing changes and technology-related touch. However, "caring touch" is essential for comforting clients, generating warmth, decreasing anxiety, diminishing pain and creating a bond (Figure 13-1).

In addition, nurses should not assume that they are the only people available to clients in pain. Involvement of family members in the nursing care may be helpful. Friends, volunteers, and other health care providers may also provide care and help relieve pain. The ideal caregiver is at least partially determined by culture. For example, a member of a particular culture may prefer a caregiver of the same gender. These restrictions should be respected and honored as much as possible.

Assessing Pain

According to Leininger (1991), the emic, or insider perspective, provides a true knowledge base for culturally congruent care. Perception is a crucial component of **pain assessment** and forms the basis of subsequent decisions about pain management. Nurses obtain the most useful results when they approach pain assessment not as a task but as an important interaction with the client. *Self-report is the single most reliable indicator of the existence and intensity of pain* (National Institute of Health, 1987). In practice, however, nurses tend to use other, less reliable measures for assessing pain. For example, McCaffery, Ferrell, and Pasero (2000) found that five of the six top factors identified by nurses as useful in assessing the patient's degree of suffering

Figure 13–1. Caring touch helps to create a bond between client and nurse and provides comfor ot the client. A reassuring handclasp uses touch to express concern and interest. (© Copyright B. Proud)

were influenced by the patient's culture. These factors include facial expression, position and movement, vocalization, request for relief, and verbalization. The danger in using these measures alone is that clients who do not show the expected signs of distress may be overlooked by nurses. Neither vital signs nor behavior can substitute for self-report of pain.

When people in pain realize that others do not believe the existence of their pain, they experience stress and increased pain intensity. Nurses need to try to understand how the client is experiencing pain and convey that understanding to the client. Because the word *pain* has so many different meanings and refers to such a variety of sensations, clarifying clients' experience of pain will be helpful for both nurses and clients. Assessing pain in the elderly presents additional challenges. Despite these challenges, however, the nurse is responsible for knowing the person's pain history and established coping mechanisms.

The assessment of pain has three major objectives. First, it allows the nurse to understand what the client is experiencing. Second, it evaluates the effect the experience of pain is having on the client. Third, it sometimes allows for a determination of the physical cause of the pain. The first two objectives are described in the next section. The third objective falls primarily within the domain of medicine rather than nursing and is therefore not addressed.

Understanding the Experience

To understand what the client is experiencing, the nurse seeks information about the location, duration, intensity, and type of sensation. The main task is to facilitate communication about what is being experienced. Cultural sensitivity (as described in Chapter 2) must always be a component of pain assessment. A variety of pain assessment tools have been developed and summarized (U.S. Department of Health and Human Services, 1992). Although they have different formats, they are meant to assess the same type of information. Many clients are able to use numbers to describe and rank their pain. Other clients may use poker chips, drawings, or words to describe their pain. A helpful tool for assessing pain in children is the Oucher Scale (Villarruel & Denyes, 1991). It allows children in pain to compare their pain intensity with pictures of children in pain. It is available in Caucasian, African American, and Hispanic versions (Beyer & Kuott, 1998).

The nurse must remember that pain expressions will vary among clients and even with the same client in different situation. For example, stress resulting from fear of cancer may result in an increased expression of pain. Clients experiencing chronic pain may display less intense nonverbal behavior relative to their pain than do clients experiencing acute pain. The absence of nonverbal pain behaviors such as grimacing and squinting, however, does not signify the absence of pain. Variations must also be acknowledged within cultures.

Evaluating the Effect

Often the most difficult aspect of pain assessment is evaluating the effect of the experience on the client. At the most fundamental level, the nurse should avoid dictating to clients what effect the pain "should" be having on them.

Instead, the meaning of the experience should come from the clients. An assessment of actual responses to pain should include gathering data on what a particular behavior means to each client.

A baseline understanding of the client and his or her response to pain is essential. The nurse needs to assess the type of interventions desired by the client. For example, does the client want traditional interventions, nurturing behaviors, psychologic support, physical interventions, or a combination of these interventions? The role of the family or social support network in providing these interventions should also be assessed. Children, too, should be asked about their preferred coping strategies for managing pain.

Managing Pain

Undertreatment of pain has been identified as a problem for many years. The Agency for Health Care Policy and Research has issued guidelines related to acute pain management in "recognition of the widespread inadequacy of pain management" (U.S. Department of Health and Human Services, 1992). Several studies (Cohen, 1980; Teske, Daut & Cleeland, 1983; Rankin & Snider, 1984) suggest that nurses' perception of pain does not coincide with the patients', which results in increased suffering for patients. In addition, Dudley and Holme (1984) found that nurses tended to infer a greater degree of psychologic distress than physical distress from pain. This may lead to inappropriate interventions, such as psychologic support without other pain interventions.

The administration of analgesia may differ by cultural group, and medications may be withheld from less vocal clients. For example, Streltzer and Wade (1981) studied postcholecystectomy pain in Whites, Hawaiians, and Asians. They found that nurses limited the amount of analgesia given to all groups and gave significantly fewer analgesics to Japanese, Filipino, and Chinese patients—those least vocal in the study.

Thus, it is important for nurses to take several active roles in pain management. First, the nurse must base his or her interventions on pain assessment rather than personal beliefs. Second, the nurse must intervene and obtain medical orders for analgesia when it is required by the patient.

Clarifying Responsibility

Responsibilities in pain relief should always be clarified with clients so that they know what they can do to achieve relief. For example, a member of a particular cultural group may consider it inappropriate to report having pain. The client may need permission to request pain relief. A simple statement such as "please tell me when your pain returns" may be all that is needed. This will allow the client to feel in control of the situation and involved in pain management. In addition, the nurse should assess how the client ordinarily copes with pain. This will identify some potentially effective therapeutic techniques, which are outlined later in this chapter. Above all, the nurse must be open to alternative forms of treatment.

Nurse-client collaboration is essential in pain management. Too often, nurses approach a situation as if they had all the answers. Clearly, this attitude is not helpful. Instead, the client should be involved in actively setting goals. The client should not be left alone to manage the situation. Similarly, the health team should not manage the client's condition without his or her input. Instead, health professionals and clients should work together to meet the challenge of pain. It is clearly the health professional's responsibility to elicit and evaluate cultural knowledge that can be used in pain management.

• CLINICAL APPLICATION

Several case studies are presented in this section to illustrate principles of pain management, using a transcultural nursing framework. It is important to emphasize the great variation that exists within cultures. Differences exist among individuals in any culture in terms of the perception and expression of pain. Nurses should avoid stereotyping patients or assuming that an individual will respond to pain in a certain way based on his or her culture.

Culturally Competent Nursing Care of a Black Adolescent with Sickle Cell Crisis

In this section, culturally insensitive and culturally competent nursing actions are presented for a client with sickle cell crisis. Additionally, detailed information on the specific physiology of **sickle cell pain** is presented. Case Study 13-1A highlights culturally insensitive nursing actions.

CASE STUDY	13–1A

Jamil Jones is a 13-year-old Black male with sickle cell disease. He has arrived in the emergency department writhing and screaming in pain. His grandmother is crying and shouting, "Why can't you help him? He's hurting!"

Jamil is well known in the emergency department; this is his second visit this month. Sometimes, in a very insensitive manner, health care providers refer to these patients as "frequent flyers," meaning that they frequently come to the emergency room. Staff members are frustrated with his frequent visits, and they express their concern that he is addicted to the pain medication. They also believe that the discharge education they provide is ignored, contributing to frequent crises.

In report, one nurse states: "Jamil's back. Same pain. Is he making it up? Why doesn't he do what we tell him to? He wouldn't have all these problems. He's failing school; he stays home all the time and just lies around. We'll get him stabilized and send him home with a prescription for pain medication. He'll probably sell the pain meds on the street. Might even be taking some street drugs. Who knows? No wonder he ends up back here so often."

Case Analysis

This interchange demonstrates a lack of understanding of two important aspects of care: sickle cell disease (SCD) and the cultural dynamics in play during family and professional interactions. It also portrays cultural stereotyping on the part of the nurse. Let's examine each of the nurse's statements.

SICKLE CELL PAIN

Sickle cell disease is an autosomal recessive inherited condition that occurs primarily the African American population. An estimated 50,000 Americans have the disease, and approximately 2.5 million people carry the sickle cell trait (Beyer, Platt, Kinney, & Treadwell, 1999). The disease is characterized by a defective hemoglobin molecule (HBS) that causes red blood cells to become sickle (crescent) shaped. This causes hemolysis and vaso-occlusion, with impaired circulation, inadequate oxygenation, pain, and tissue infarction. The disease is recurrent and unpredictable, causing physiologic and psychologic distress. The pain, triggered when misshapen blood cells create capillary blockages, is episodic and severe. In fact, the degree of pain has been compared to the pain of a myocardial infarction, although individuals with myocardial infarction typically receive more aggressive and immediate attention to prevent further infarction. The nurse needs to recognize and acknowledge that the pain associated with SCD is real, rather than minimizing it.

A basic understanding of the pathophysiology of vaso-occlusion is important for proper nursing care. Pain in SCD is very complex, requiring continuous adjustment of comfort measures, especially analgesics. Nursing care must incorporate multisystem assessments and interventions that are developmentally appropriate. Pain control, hydration, establishment of trust, and support of individual and family coping are needed to improve recovery and reduce long-term complications.

Pain is a common and important problem for children with SCD, but it has been undertreated and understudied. According to one study, most children are still in pain during crisis, despite receiving nalbuphine by intravenous infusion drip (Beyer, 2000). Another study found that 43% of children aged 4 to 18 reported intense pain levels during vaso-occlusive episodes; older children reported higher levels of pain than did younger children. The most frequently used pain management tools were acetaminophen with codeine, fluids, and ibuprofen. Self-care behaviors used by the children included the application of heat, sleeping, reading, and exercising. These interventions helped children to remain in their normal environment and experience some control over their disease (Conner-Warren, 1996).

Living with vaso-occlusive episodes is physically and psychosocially stressful for adolescents. They experience feelings of helplessness as a result of their interrupted lives and their feelings of being discounted by some individuals during a vaso-occlusive event. McLeod-Fletcher (1996) found that adolescents with SCD who believed they could control and decrease vaso-occlusive episodes used cognitive and behavioral coping strategies that were associated with positive adjustment. Adolescents engaged in a variety of behaviors to control the vaso-occlusive event. This allowed them to decrease the impact of the event, maintain a positive outlook for the future, and make a difficult situation tolerable. Psychologic approaches are commonly used in an attempt to improve coping ability in patients with SCD, but the outcomes have not been carefully studied or researched.

As a result of the treatment they receive, patients and families may feel distrustful, humiliated, intimidated, demoralized, frustrated, angry, and abused. The relationship between provider and patient may become adversarial. The lack of cultural understanding, and socioeconomic differences between provider and patient, may contribute to the problems.

SCHOOL ABSENCES AND DRUG ABUSE

Studies suggest that school absences are frequent in children with SCD and that standardized academic achievement is approximately one standard deviation below the normative mean for the broader population, with class grades below a C average (Eaton, Haye, Armstrong, Pegelow, & Thomas, 1995). The nurse should be aware of this issue and should not make light of the situation. Also, though drug abuse is a serious problem, there is no reason to suspect drug abuse in every African American male patient who arrives in the emergency department. This represents racial profiling: a severe type of stereotyping.

ADDICTION TO PAIN MEDICATIONS

It is important for patients, families, and clinicians to understand the differences among tolerance, dependence, and addiction. Tolerance and dependence are involuntary and predictable physiologic changes that develop with the repeated administration of narcotics. Tolerance occurs when larger doses are needed to obtain the same effect. Dependence exists if withdrawal symptoms occur when a narcotic is stopped abruptly. Addiction refers to marked psychologic and physiologic dependence on a substance, beyond voluntary control.

Emergency department physicians tend to overestimate addiction rates for individuals with SCD (Shapiro, Benjamin, Payne, & Heidrich, 1997). Waldrop and Mandy (1995) found that 8% of staff physicians, 17% of residents, and 13% nurses in an emergency department estimated that patients with SCD experiencing pain were opioid dependent. This is far in excess of estimates made regarding other populations of patients and may reflect stereotyping and prejudice. It could lead to the inappropriate withholding of pain medication from patients with SCD.

Delivering Culturally Competent Care

Although the emergency department staff cannot address all the issues outlined in the case study in an ongoing way, they can and should provide culturally competent care by acknowledging the pain, providing appropriate pain medication, assessing the usual coping strategies, providing assistance in using the pain strategies, and establishing trust.

ACKNOWLEDGMENT OF THE PAIN

Staff members must acknowledge that Jamil is an adolescent in pain. There is no denying that the vaso-occlusion in SCD is extremely painful. It has been estimated that 90% of hospital admissions among patients with SCD are for the treatment of acute pain (Ballas, 1998). The unpredictability of painful episodes adds to their discomfort. Rather than minimizing the experience, staff members must recognize the pain and encourage dialogue about it. Staff members must assess the location, duration, intensity, and type of pain.

Jamil will find the Oucher scale to be too childish, and he should therefore be encouraged to quantify his pain using numbers or words. This will help build a trusting relationship between Jamil and the nursing staff. It will also help family members know that their loved one is believed and is receiving competent care.

ASSESSMENT OF USUAL COPING STRATEGIES

In addition to assessing the pain, it is essential for the nurse to assess how Jamil typically copes with his pain. Because he is an adolescent, a sense of control or mastery over the experience is important. Coping strategies allow some measure of control. When the nurse asks Jamil how he has handled pain in the past, she helps him identify his own strengths and coping mechanisms.

APPROPRIATE PAIN MEDICATION

Rapid, accurate assessment of the patient's condition and prompt delivery of pain relief are essential. Pain medication should be based on Jamil's analgesic history and should be titrated in response to qualitative and quantitative pain assessment. Under no circumstances should the staff belittle or minimize Jamil's pain. Some individuals discount pain as a major stressor for adolescents with SCD during the vaso-occlusive event (McLeod-Fletcher, 1996). Instead, Jamil needs information on what he is receiving for pain and what he can expect from the medication.

PROVIDING ASSISTANCE IN USING THE COPING STRATEGIES

Although medications are important during the vaso-occlusive crisis, they do not constitute the only strategy that nurses should use for pain management. Jamil needs to be encouraged to use his coping strategies. His family and friends should also be involved. In addition, the nurse might select other strategies that have been found to be helpful by others with SCD. For example, when the pain is under control, Jamil could be encouraged to find out more about SCD and to share what he has learned with his care providers, who can confirm his understanding and acknowledge his mastery of information. Often, this will help mitigate the helplessness that is commonly felt by adolescents with SCD.

ESTABLISHMENT OF TRUST

The actions just described will help to establish a relationship of trust between Jamil, his grandmother, and the nursing staff. However, it is important to realize that trust will not develop immediately. Many members of the African American community are somewhat distrustful of health care providers and indeed of many organizations, institutions, and officials. Some of this distrust harkens back to atrocities committed in the name of research, such as the Tuskegee study that allowed African American men with syphilis to remain untreated for years. Some of the distrust is related to society at large. Shared group historical experiences and individual experiences with prejudice, discrimination, and racial profiling affect every interaction with institutions and individuals. Often, predominately White health care professionals are not aware of the degree of distrust. An understanding of the shared history of African Americans is helpful to health care providers. The nurse interacting with Jamil and his family needs to be aware of this dimension and must make every effort to be open, welcoming, and honest.

REFERRAL FOR FOLLOW-UP

Obviously, the emergency department staff can address only a small part of Jamil's care. Across the nation, emergency departments are inundated with patients, and they exist to provide acute care to very ill patients. However, the emergency department must be viewed as part of a continuum of care. Most likely, Jamil will be admitted to the hospital and then will be discharged to his home. Jamil cannot be allowed to fall between the cracks in our health care system. Instead, the hospital needs to be sure Jamil has appropriate follow-up care after discharge. This may include both medical and psychosocial follow-up care.

Case Revisited

Let's take another look at the case of Jamil Jones. Case Study 13-1B highlights culturally competent nursing care (Case Study 13-1B).

Culturally Competent Nursing Care of a Hospitalized Lebanese American Patient in Pain

This section presents the case of a hospitalized Lebanese American patient in pain to illustrate additional principles of pain management using a transcultural nursing framework (Case Study 13-2).

Let's examine what has occurred in this encounter. The nurse has assumed that Mrs. Abdullah will tell her when her pain returns. However, Reizian and Meleis (1986) suggest that Arab Americans have a present-time orientation to pain similar to that described in Italian Americans by Zborowski (1952, 1969). As such, Arab Americans tend to focus on the immediacy of the pain. Pain is viewed as unpleasant, to be avoided or controlled at all costs. Pain responses are private and are reserved for immedi-

CASE STUDY	13–1B

Jamil Jones is a 13-year-old Black male with sickle cell disease. He has arrived in the emergency department writhing and screaming in pain. His grandmother is crying and shouting, "Why can't you help him? He's hurting!"

Jamil is well known in the emergency department; this is his second visit this month. Staff members are frustrated by his frequent visits. Chris Brown, the nurse assigned to Jamil's care, understands that previous discharge planning has been unsuccessful. She wonders what she can do differently to help Jamil and his family.

Chris Brown begins by going immediately to Jamil's bedside. "I know you're in pain, Jamil," she says. "The doctor is ordering you something to manage your pain. The medicine you had last time seemed to work well. How does that sound to you?"

Jamil responds, "Yes—but hurry, please. It's worse than last time."

The nurse nods and turns to Jamil's grandmother. "I'll go get the medicine right away. In the meantime, Jamil might like to listen to some of his favorite music. Remember how that helped him last time? How does that sound, Jamil?"

Jamil states, "No, no, I don't want that. I want to talk to mom. Does she know I'm here?"

Jamil's grandmother is happy to be of help. She tells Jamil she will call his mother, who is at work, and let her know her son is in the emergency department. The nurse leaves to get the pain medication. When she returns, she finds Jamil talking to his mother on the telephone, with his grandmother at his side.

In report, one nurse states: "Jamil's back—can you believe it? Same pain. Is he making it up? Why doesn't he do what we tell him to? He wouldn't have all these problems. He's failing school, he stays home all the time and just lies around. We'll get him stabilized and send him home with a prescription for pain medication. He'll probably sell the pain meds on the street. Might even be taking some street drugs. Who knows? No wonder he ends up back here so often."

Chris Brown speaks up: "You know, sickle cell disease is very complicated. I don't understand it all, but I think we might be missing something with Jamil and with other patients who come to us. What do you think about scheduling an inservice on it? And for Jamil, I'd really like social service to see him. We need to make sure he sees his doctor after he goes home, and gets other kinds of follow-up."

---

ate family members, and families often oversee and make decisions about the care.

When responses are shared with family members but not with health care professionals, conflicts may arise. In this situation, Mrs. Abdullah has discussed her pain with her family but not with her nurse. To provide culturally competent care, Ms. Smith needs to take the following actions:

- Assess pain level at frequent intervals
- Ask the client to describe how she usually copes with pain
- Clarify with the client and family how pain will be reported and managed
- Provide interventions as appropriate to the situation
- Discuss with family members their role in assisting Mrs. Abdullah

CASE STUDY 13–2

Mrs. Abdullah is a 45-year-old woman admitted to the hospital with multiple injuries after an automobile accident. Mrs. Abdullah was born in Lebanon, moved to the United States in her early 20s, and is a U.S. citizen. She speaks English fluently.

Ms. Smith, the nurse assigned to provide care to Mrs. Abdullah, arrives in the room to perform her admission assessment. Mrs. Abdullah lies quietly in the bed, providing monosyllabic responses to Ms. Smith's questions and failing to make eye contact. Ms. Smith knows that Mrs. Abdullah received strong pain medication in the emergency department, and she hopes that Mrs. Abdullah will rest after her trauma. When questioned, Mrs. Abdullah neither confirms nor denies pain, but she does moan and cry as soon as the nurse leaves the room. A few hours later, Mrs. Abdullah's husband and sister arrive to visit. Ms. Smith is surprised when she is confronted in the hall by Mr. Abdullah, who shouts: "How can you let my wife lie there without giving her something for pain? What kind of inhumane place is this?"

- Recognize that Mrs. Abdullah may always feel most comfortable discussing her pain with her family. Making the family a part of care is an excellent way to deal with this situation. In addition, the nurse should be aware that Arab Americans often use metaphors and analogies to describe their pain. The nurse can encourage this type of communication. Last, the nurse should be aware that different pain episodes result in different responses. Some pain, such as labor pain, induces loud moans, groans, and screams. These responses are part of the coping strategies for pain. The nurse should provide privacy as required.

Culturally Competent Nursing Care of a German-American Man with Cancer Pain

This final scenario of a German-American man with cancer pain further illustrates the principles of pain management through culturally competent nursing actions (Case Study 13-3).

This case demonstrates the positive impact of a culturally competent nurse. The nurse collected data about the pain experience from a variety of sources, including the patient and family members. In addition, the nurse understood the pathophysiology of both stomach cancer and postherpetic neuralgia. She intervened on the part of the patient, obtained the necessary order, educated the patient and family members on what to expect, and involved them in decision making about Mr. Schwartz's care.

Unfortunately, there is still a tendency to undermedicate for pain, even within the hospice program. This tendency exists both in the United States and in other countries. Studies show that 75 to 90% of cancer pain in terminally ill patients is well controlled when the World Health Organization

CASE STUDY	13–3

Mr. Schwartz is an 82-year-old man of German-American descent who received a diagnosis of stomach cancer 2 years ago. He has multiple physical problems, including postherpetic neuralgia and acute pain that remained after the herpes zoster ("shingles") that occurred 10 years ago. Mr. Schwartz underwent a partial gastrectomy when the cancer was diagnosed and received chemotherapy for 18 months. He has been losing weight despite the high-calorie meals and frequent snacks prepared for him by his wife.

Mr. Schwartz has decided that he wants no further medical interventions for his cancer. With the support of his family and his physician, Mr. Schwartz has enrolled in a hospice program, with care provided by his wife and family in his home. Mrs. Berry, the hospice nurse, finds Mr. Schwartz to be cooperative and pleasant. He makes jokes with hospice staff and answers their questions in a jovial way. When asked about pain, he changes the subject, although he winces when touched, grits his teeth, and disengages when pain is discussed. Mrs. Schwartz tells the nurses that she knows when her husband is in pain because he snaps at her.

Mrs. Berry is a gentle, compassionate, and knowledgeable nurse. She understands that Mr. Schwartz is a private individual and doesn't wish to discuss his pain. She tells him that she understands and respects his feelings and that her job is to make him as comfortable as possible. She discusses the situation with the doctor and obtains an order for a strong pain medication. She talks with Mr. and Mrs. Schwartz about the intended effects of the medication, and also alerts them to the side effects of the medicine. She helps them determine the best timing for the medicine.

After several doses, Mr. Schwartz confesses, "This is the first time I haven't had pain in 10 years." He dies 3 months after beginning hospice, at peace and in no pain.

approach is used: mean medication doses are as high as 30 milligrams of morphine every 4 hours. However, appropriate doses are often not used.

The barriers to effective palliative care appear to be similar worldwide (Rhymes, 1996). A German-language study of treatment of cancer pain (cited in Rhymes, 1996) found that only 322 of 16,630 cancer patients received strong opiates, that adjuvant therapy was rarely used, and that treatment for breakthrough pain was rarely given. Health care professionals may be concerned about addiction and respiratory depression or may think that morphine is a drug only for those actively dying. Similar beliefs exist among patients and family members. For example, a study in Poland (cited in Rhymes, 1996) identified common lay myths, including the belief that morphine is to be given only in the very last stages of disease, that it will cause addiction, and that if it is used too early there will be nothing stronger to use for pain relief.

• COMPLEMENTARY AND ALTERNATIVE PRACTICES FOR PAIN

Many practices have been used for centuries in the management of pain. However, the predominant biomedical system has adapted very few of these techniques, resulting in the growth of complementary and alternative medicine (CAM). Research indicates that alternative therapies were used by 42% of persons in both the United States and Canada in 1997 (Eisenberg et al., 2000; National Council for Reliable Health Information, 1998). Patients are turning to CAM for several reasons, which include the following:

- Frustration with conventional medicine
- Increasing evidence of the influence of lifestyle, nutrition, and emotions on disease
- Expectations of wellness rather than just the absence of symptoms
- The desire to take less medication and decrease health costs
- Increasing awareness of other cultures and their practices

Physicians and nurses are being encouraged to consider CAM therapies as they manage care (Novey, 2000; Ang-Lee, Moss, & Yuan, 2001). In addition, 25% of the hospitals in major metropolitan areas offer some complementary and alternative medicine (*Vitality Notes,* 2001). Many of these hospitals use relaxation, hypnosis, acupuncture, and acupressure to help patients reduce their need for pain medication.

This section is not designed to prepare the nurse to deliver the alternative practices described. Instead, it is meant to sensitize the nurse to the many options available to clients. In addition, the nurse and the client may choose together to use some of the techniques described below and summarized in Table 13-4, including **relaxation techniques**, **transcendental meditation**, **autogenic training**, **hypnosis**, **yoga**, **distraction**, **imagery**, **cutaneous stimulation**, **herbal remedies** (Figure 13-2), **religious rituals**, **biofeedback**, **acupuncture** (Figure 13-3), and **acupressure**.

In CAM therapies, the connection between mind, body, and spirit is emphasized. The culturally competent nurse must talk with patients about their use of CAM therapies. To begin dialogue, the nurse might simply ask what the patient is doing to reduce pain or improve health. As the patient identifies the use of CAM therapies, the nurse can explore areas such as these:

- The safety and effectiveness of the therapy
- The experience of the practitioner
- The cost of therapy (most patients must pay for CAM therapies themselves because they are typically not covered by insurance)
- The benefits and risks of therapy
- Other activities, therapies, or medications to be avoided during the CAM therapy

As seen in this brief overview, several alternative practices may be used to assist clients in the management of pain. Some practices involve only the nurse and the client. Other techniques involve different types of healers, family members, and significant others. Nurses who are familiar with these techniques will feel more comfortable suggesting, observing, participating in, or performing a variety of healing practices.

TABLE 13–4	COMPLEMENTARY AND ALTERNATIVE METHODS OF PAIN CONTROL
Relaxation techniques	Many relaxation techniques result in physiologic changes that reduce the damaging effects of stress and promote a sense of physical, mental, and spiritual well-being. All these techniques result in an altered state of consciousness and produce a decrease in sympathetic nervous system activity. Each technique requires a calm and quiet environment, a comfortable position, a mental device or image, and a willingness to let relaxation happen
Benson's relaxation response	Relaxation is achieved through six basic steps: sit quietly, close eyes, deeply relax all muscles, breathe through nose, continue for 20 minutes, allow relaxation to occur at its own pace. (For further information, see Benson, 1976.)
Transcendental meditation	This type of meditation is taught individually, involves the use of a specific mantra during the meditation, and was originally developed by the Maharishi Mahesh Yogi, an Indian scholar and teacher.
Autogenic training	This emphasizes passive attention to the body. The training, which was first recognized within the biomedical model in 1910, incorporates elements of hypnotism, spiritualism, and various yogic disciplines. (See Luthe and Schultz, 1970, for specific meditative exercises.)
Progressive relaxation	Originated by Jacobson (1964), this is probably the most widely used relaxation technique today. The method teaches the client to concentrate on various gross muscle groups in the body by first tensing and then relaxing each group.
Hypnosis	This technique was introduced into Western medical practice in the 18th century by Franz Anton Mesmer. A hypnotic state may be induced either by a hypnotist or by the client (autohypnosis). Hypnosis is based on the power of suggestion and the process of focusing attention. It has been used as an adjunct to other pain-relieving therapies and has been found to be helpful in dentistry, surgery, and childbirth as well as malignancies.
Yoga	Yoga techniques have been used within the Hindu culture for thousands of years. Yoga involves the practice of both physical exercise (hatha yoga) and meditation (raja yoga). The correct performance of yoga results in deep relaxation without drowsiness or sleep.
Distraction	Distraction from pain is a kind of sensory shielding in which one is protected from the pain sensation by focusing on and increasing the clarity of sensations unrelated to the pain. Research suggests that distraction techniques, like pain, may be a cultural phenomenon. Clinical and research findings suggest that distraction

(continued)

TABLE 13–4	COMPLEMENTARY AND ALTERNATIVE METHODS OF PAIN CONTROL (Continued)
	may be a potent method of pain relief, usually by increasing the client's tolerance for pain by placing pain at the periphery of awareness. Distraction techniques include watching television, listening to music, reading, telling jokes, walking, playing with pets, crocheting, doing housework, interacting with children, and getting out of the house. Distraction appears to place the pain at the periphery of awareness. (For further information, see McCaffery, 1990; Miller, Hickman, & Lemasters, 1992; and Zadinsky & Boyle, 1996.)
Imagery	Imagery techniques for physical healing date back hundreds of years. Guided imagery involves using one's imagination to develop sensory images that decrease the intensity of pain or that become a nonpainful or pleasant substitute for pain. During guided imagery the client is alert, concentrating intensely and imagining sensory images. Research suggests that pleasant imagery can effectively reduce the perception of post-surgical pain. Music therapy is being used with increased frequency to augment imagery and other relaxation techniques. (For further information, see McCaffery & Pasero, 1999; and Novey 2000.)
Cutaneous stimulation	This reduces the intensity of pain or makes the pain more bearable. Types of cutaneous stimulation for pain relief include massage/pressure, vibration, heat or cold application, topical application, and transcutaneous electrical nerve stimulation (TENS). Stimulation need not be applied directly to the painful site to be effective (McCaffery, 1990).
Herbal remedies	Herbal treatments have been used in many cultures for centuries. Although adherence to herbalism diminished in the West, interest is currently increasing, as exemplified by the popularity of herbal teas. Many of the herbs used have a physiologic effect and must be understood by the health care professional. (For additional details, see Novey, 2000.)
Religious rituals	Clients should be encouraged to use their religious practices as they desire, to help in pain management. Privacy should be provided as needed. Various amulets and charms should also be respected and incorporated into the care provided. Christianity has included the notion of healing through divine intervention since its inception. Roman Catholic clients in pain may wish to pray the rosary or attend mass. Clients of many Christian denominations may actively seek healing through prayer and other rituals. Jewish clients

(continued)

TABLE 13–4	COMPLEMENTARY AND ALTERNATIVE METHODS OF PAIN CONTROL *(Continued)*
	experiencing pain may ask to speak to a rabbi. In other faith traditions, a shaman may conduct a religious ritual for the purpose of healing or pain relief. In this context, the illness or pain is viewed as a disorder of the total person, involving all parts of the individual as well as relationships to others. Working with client, family members, and others, the shaman focuses on strengthening or stimulating the client's own natural healing powers.
Biofeedback	Biofeedback techniques use instrumentation to provide a client with information about changes in bodily functions of which the person is usually unaware. Clients are taught to manipulate and control their degree of relaxation and tension by way of biofeedback training using electroencephalography (EEG) or electromyogram muscle potential (EMG).
Acupuncture	Acupuncture, practiced for at least 3,000 years, is a method of preventing, diagnosing, and treating pain and disease by the skilled insertion of special needles into the body at designated locations and at various depths and angles. According to Chinese thought, life energy, or *ch'i,* constantly flows and energizes humans through a pattern known as meridians. *Ch'i* may be intercepted at various acupoints throughout the body. Acupuncture has been used as an alternative to other forms of analgesia for many minor surgical procedures in China. It has also been used in the treatment of pain in a variety of other countries. There are no simple explanations for the mechanisms that underlie the analgesia-producing effects of acupuncture. However, research has documented the release of endorphins into the vascular system during acupuncture, contributing to pain relief (Novey, 2000).
Accupressure	Acupressure involves a deep-pressure massage of the appropriate acupoints. Shiatsu is the most widely known form of acupressure, used in Japan for over 1,000 years to treat pain and illness and maintain general health. (For more information, see Novey, 2000.)
Other therapies	
Alexander technique	This is based on the belief that tension restricts movement and tightens the body. An Alexander technique teacher works to restore freedom of movement and enhance body awareness by applying subtle adjustments in posture and alignment. (See Novey, 2000.)
Aromatherapy	Aromatherapy may take a variety of forms, including esthetic (aromas used for pleasure), holistic (aromatherapy used for general stress), environmental fragrancing

(continued)

TABLE 13–4	**COMPLEMENTARY AND ALTERNATIVE METHODS OF PAIN CONTROL** *(Continued)*
	(aromas used to manipulate mood), and clinical (essential oils used for specific measurable outcomes). Aromatherapy has been used in pain management to enhance strong analgesics. The specific essential oils used are based on the type of pain. (See Novey, 2000.)
Craniosacral therapy	This manual procedure is used to remedy distortions in the structure and function of the brain, spinal cord, skull and sacrum. It is used to treat chronic pain and migraine headaches. (See Novey, 2000.)
Trager	Practitioners move the client's trunk and limbs in a gently rhythmic way. These noninvasive movements help to release physical and mental patterns, allowing the recipient to experience new sensations of freedom and lightness. (See Novey, 2000.)

Figure 13–2. Above are the ten herbs named in the prescription in Table 13-4. The client brews the herbs into a tea and then drinks it on an empty stomach. (Reprinted by permission of William Arnold, MD, Advocate Medical Group and Advocate Lutheran General Hospital, Park Ridge, IL)

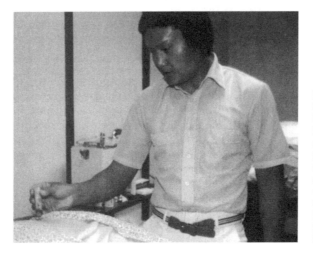

Figure 13–3. Traditionally a Chinese practice, acupuncture has gained acceptance in the United States and Canada. Research reveals that the procedure produces an analgesic effect because it causes the release of enkephalin, a naturally occurring endorphin that has opiate-like effects. The practitioner shown here is using moxibustion (heat) to enhance the therapeutic effects of acupuncture.

Summary

Pain has been experienced throughout the ages. Sophisticated pharmacologic interventions do not necessarily relieve pain, which people define, express, cope with, and manage in a variety of ways. Culture is a major influence in this process. Culture helps determine the innermost feelings of the individual. According to Mead, the behavior of an individual may be understood only in terms of the behavior of the whole social group of which he or she is a member (Mead, 1934). To examine the phenomenon of pain in its entirety, a model of pain is needed. This model incorporates physical, psychologic, social, and cultural factors, which interact and define the pain experience for individuals.

Nurses practicing in the United States and Canada come in contact with people from a variety of cultural backgrounds. In addition, nurses encounter clients experiencing pain in virtually every clinical setting. Recognizing cultural differences in beliefs about pain and suffering, and cultural views about appropriate responses to pain, can prevent misunderstanding and lead to the delivery of culturally competent care.

Review Questions

1. How is pain defined?
2. How does the expression of pain vary by culture? By gender? By type of pain?
3. How does the nursing subculture view pain? What are nurses' typical expectations for expressions of pain by others?
4. What techniques may appropriately be used for assessing pain?
5. How may the nurse demonstrate his or her competence to clients and families?
6. What alternative practices may be used by clients experiencing pain? How may nurses support these practices?

C R I T I C A L   T H I N K I N G   A C T I V I T I E S

1. Think about the last time you experienced pain. Describe it. How intense was the pain? What do you think caused the pain? Did you want others to know about it? How did you respond to the pain? Did you want to be alone or with other people? What treatments did you use for the pain? Did you worry about the pain?

2. Ask five of your friends or relatives what treatments they use when they have a headache. Be sure to ask about folk remedies, and who taught them to use a particular treatment. Identify similarities and differences compared with the treatments you use.

3. Think about one of the clients in pain for whom you have provided care. How did that client respond to pain? How did you help the client? How would you modify your practice based on what you have learned in this chapter?

4. Identify three times when you have encouraged (or have seen others encourage) a client to accept more pain. What words were used? How were family members involved? What was the ultimate outcome? Did you realize you were applying principles of encouraging tolerance to pain?

5. Select several clients with different cultural backgrounds. Assess their pain, using several different techniques. Which technique is most helpful? Are your clients able to use numbers to describe their pain? Can they draw pictures or use colors to describe their pain? What words do they use to describe their pain?

• References

Acheson, E. S. (1988). *Nurses' inferences of pain and the decision to intervene for culturally different patients.* Unpublished dissertation, University of Texas at Austin, Austin, Texas.

Alternative therapies come to America's hospitals (August 2001). *Vitality Notes, 3.*

Ang-Lee, M. K., Moss, J, and Yuan, C.-S. (2001). Herbal medicines and perioperative care. *Journal of the American Medical Association, 286*(2), 208–216.

Baer, E., Davitz, L. J. and Lieb, R. (1970). Inferences of physical pain and psychological distress in relation to verbal and nonverbal patient communication. *Nursing Research, 19*:388.

Ballas, S. K. (1998). *Sickle cell pain: Progress in pain research and management* (Vol. 11, pp. 51–89). Seattle: IASP Press.

Benoliel, J. Q., & Crowley, D. M. (1974). *The patient in pain: New concepts.* New York: American Cancer Society.

Benson, H. (1976). *The relaxation response.* New York: Avon Books.

Beyer, J. E. (2000). Judging the effectiveness of analgesia for children and adolescents during vaso-occlusive events of sickle cell disease. *Journal of Pain and Symptom Management, 19*(1), 63–72.

Beyer, J. E., & Kuott, C. B. (1998). Construct validity estimation for the African-American and Hispanic versions of the oucher scale. *Journal of Pediatric Nursing, 13*(1), 20–31.

Beyer, J., Platt, A. F., Kinney, T. R., & Treadwell, M (1999). Practice guidelines for the assessment of children with sickle cell pain. *Journal of the Society of Pediatric Nurses, 4*(2), 61–73.

Cohen, F. L. (1980). Postsurgical pain relief: Patients' status and nurses' medication choices. *Pain, 9*(1), 265–274.

Conner-Warren, R. L. (1996). Pain intensity and home pain management of children with sickle dell disease. *Issues in Comprehensive Pediatric Nursing, 19,* 183–195.

Crook, J., Rideout, E., & Brown, G. (1984). The prevalence of pain complaints in a general population. *Pain, 18,* 299–314.

Davitz, L. J. & Davitz, J. R. (1975). How do nurses feel when patients suffer? *American Journal of Nursing, 75,* 1505.

Davitz, J. R., & Davitz, L.J. (1981). *Influences of patients' pain and psychological distress.* New York: Springer-Verlag.

Davitz, L. J., Sameshima, Y., & Davitz, J. (1976). Suffering as viewed in six different cultures. *American Journal of Nursing, 76,* 1296.

Dudley, S. R., & Holm, K. (1984). Assessment of the pain experience in relation to selected nurse characteristics. *Pain, 18*(2), 179–186.

Eaton, M. L., Haye, J. S., Armstrong, F. D., Pegelow, C. H., & Thomas, M. (1995). Hospitalizations for painful episodes: Association with school absenteeism and academic performance in children and adolescents with sickle cell anemia. *Issues in Comprehensive Pediatrics, 18*(1), 1–9.

Eisenberg, D. M., Davis, R. B., Ettner, S. L., Appel, S., Wilkey, S., Van Rompay, M., & Kessler, R. C. (2000). Trends in alternative medicine use in the United States, 1990–1997: Results of a follow-up national survey. *Journal of the American Medical Association, 283*(7), 884–446.

Encandela, J. A. (1993). Social science and the study of pain since Zborowski: A need for a new agenda. *Social Science Medicine, 36*(6), 783–791.

Ferrell, B. R., & Ferrell, B. A. (1990). Easing the pain. *Geriatric Nursing, 11,* 175–178.

Ferrell, B., Virani, R., Grant, M., Vallerand, A., & McCaffery, M. (2000). Analysis of pain content in nursing textbooks. *Journal of Pain and Symptom Management, 19*(2), 216–228.

Herr, K. A., & Mobily, P. R. (1991). Complexities of pain assessment in the elderly: Clinical considerations. *Journal of Gerontological Nursing, 17,* 12–19, 44–45.

Hofland, S. L. (1992). Elder beliefs: Blocks to pain management. *Journal of Gerontological Nursing, 18,* 19–24, 39–40.

Howell, D., Butler, L., Vincent, L., Watt-Watson, J., & Stearns, N. (2000). Influencing nurses' knowledge, attitudes, and practice in cancer pain management. *Cancer Nursing, 23*(1), 55–63.

Jacobson, E. (1964). *Self-operations control: A manual of tension control.* Chicago: National Foundation for Progressive Relaxation.

Kleinman, A. (1988). *The illness narratives.* New York: Basic Books.

Kotarba, J. (1983). *Chronic pain: Its social dimension.* Beverly Hills, CA: Sage.

Lang, S., & Pratt, R. (1994). *You don't have to suffer: A complete guide to relieving cancer pain for patients and their families.* Oxford University Press.

Lawlis, G. G., Achterberg, J., Kenner, L., & Kopetz, K. (1984). Ethnic and sex differences in response to clinical and induced pain in chronic spinal pain patients. *Spine, 9,* 751–754.

Leininger, M. M. (1991). *Cultural care diversity and universality: A theory of nursing.* New York: National League for Nursing.

Luthe, W., & Schultz, J. H. (1970). *Autogenic therapy: Medical applications.* New York: Grune & Stratton.

McCaffery, M., Ferrell, B. R., and Pasero, C. (2000). Nurses' personal opinions about patients' pain and their effect on recorded assessments and titration of opioid doses. *Pain Management Nursing, 1*(3), 79–87.

McCaffery, M., & Pasero, C. (1999). *Pain: A clinical manual for nursing practice* (2nd ed.). St. Louis, MO: Mosby.

McCaffery, M. (1990). Nursing approaches to nonpharmacological pain control. *International Journal of Nursing Studies, 27*(1), 1–5.

McLeod-Fletcher, C. (1996). Appraisal and coping with vaso-occlusive crisis in adolescents with sickle cell disease. Unpublished doctoral dissertation, University of Miami, Miami, Florida.

Mead, G. (1934). *Mind, self and society.* Chicago: University of Chicago Press.

Melding, P. S. (1991). Is there such a thing as geriatric pain? *Pain, 46,* 119–121.

Melzack, R., & Wall, P. D. (1983). *The challenge of pain.* New York: Basic Books.

Miller, A. C., Hickman, L. C., & Lemasters, G. K. (1992). A distraction technique for control of burn pain. *Journal of Burn Care and Rehabilitation, 13*(5), 576–580.

National Council for Reliable Health Information (1998, January/February). Canadians increase use of alternative medicine. *NCAHF Newsletter, 21*(1), ¶1. Available at Health Source: Nursing/Academic Edition database. http://www.ncahf.ovg/nl/1998/index.html. Accessed January 10, 2002.

National Institute of Health (1987). The integrated approach to the management of pain. *Journal of Pain and Symptom Management, 2,* 35–44.

Novey, D. W. (2000). *Clinician's complete reference to complementary and alternative medicine.* St. Louis; Mosby.

Reizian, A., & Meleis, A. I (1986). Arab-Americans' perceptions of and responses to pain. *Critical Care Nurse, 6*(6), 30–37.

Rhymes, J. A. (1996). Barriers to effective palliative care of terminal patients. *Clinics in Geriatric Medicine, 12*(2), 407–416.

Roy, R., & Thomas, M. (1986). A survey of chronic pain in an elderly population. *Canadian Family Physician, 32,* 513–516.

Shapiro, B. S., Benjamin, L. J., Payne, R., & Heidrich, G. (1997). Sickle cell–related pain: Perceptions of medical practitioners. *Journal of Pain and Symptom Management, 14*(3), 168–174.

Sorkin, B. A., Rudy, T. E., Hanlon, R. B., Turk, D. C., & Steig, R. L. (1990). Chronic pain in older and younger patients: Differences are less important than similarities. *Journal of Gerontology, 45,* 64–68.

Streltzer, J., & Wade, T. C. (1981). The influence of cultural group on the undertreatment of postoperative pain. *Psychosomatic Medicine, 43*(5), 397–403.

Teske, K., Daut, R. L., & Cleeland, C. S. (1983). Relationship between nurses' observation and patients' self-reports of pain. *Pain, 16,* 289–296.

Todd, K. H., Samaroo, N., & Hoffman, J. R. (1993). Ethnicity as a risk factor for inadequate emergency department analgesia. *Journal of the American Medical Association, 269*(12), 1537–1539.

U.S. Department of Health and Human Services (February, 1992). *Acute pain management: Operative or medical procedures and trauma.* Rockville, MD: Agency for Health Care Policy and Research, Public Health Service, U.S. Department of Health and Human Services.

Villarruel, A., & Denyes, M. (1991). Pain assessment in children: Theoretical and empirical validity. *Advances in Nursing Science, 14,* 32–41.

Waldrop, R. D., & Mandy, C. (1995). Health professional perceptions of opioid dependence among patients with pain. *American Journal of Emergency Medicine, 13*(5), 529–531.

Witte, M. (1989). Pain control. *Journal of Gerontological Nursing, 15,* 32–37, 40–41.

Wolff, B. B., & Langley, S. (1977). Cultural factors and the response to pain. *Culture, disease, and healing.* New York: Macmillan.

Yates, P., Dewar, A., & Fentiman, B. (1995). Pain: The view of elderly people living in long-term residential care settings. *Journal of Advanced Nursing, 21,* 667–674.

Zadinsky, J. K., & Boyle, J. S. (1996). Experiences of women with chronic pelvic pain. *Health Care for Women International, 17,* 223–232.

Zborowski, M. (1952). Cultural components in response to pain. *Journal of Social Issues, 8,* 16–30.

Zborowski, M. (1969). *People in pain.* San Francisco: Jossey-Bass.

CHAPTER 14

Religion, Culture, and Nursing

Margaret M. Andrews

Patricia A. Hanson

KEY TERMS

Allah
Amish
Bad death
Baha'i International Community
Bereavement
Brahman
Brit milah
Buddha
Buddhism
Caste system
Catholic Charities
Catholicism
Christian Science
The Church of Jesus Christ of
   Latter-Day Saints
   (Mormonism)
Curandero
Eucharist
Faith healing
Fasting
Five core characteristics of the
   Amish
Five major dimensions of religion
Four Noble Truths

Friendscraft
Funeral
Garment
Good death
Grief
Hadith
Halal
The Health Ministries
Hindu
Islam
Jehovah
Jehovah's Witnesses (Watch
   Tower Bible and Tract Society)
Judaism
Karma
Kosher
Mennonites
Mohel
Moslem/Muslim
Mourning
Native American Church (Peyote
   Religion)
Nirvana
Noble Eightfold Way

Ordinances
Pillars of Faith
Principle of totality
Protestantism
Qur'an (Koran)
Reincarnation
The Relief Society
Religion
Sacrament of the Sick
Seventh-Day Adventists
Shema
Shiva
Spiritual assessment
Spiritual concerns
Spiritual distress
Spiritual health
Spirituality
Spiritual nursing care
Talmud
Torah
Unitarian Universalist
Vedas
Wake (viewing, calling hours)
Word of Wisdom

OBJECTIVES

1. Explore the meaning of spirituality and religion in the lives of clients across the life span.
2. Identify the components of a spiritual needs assessment for clients from diverse cultural backgrounds.
3. Examine the ways in which spiritual and religious beliefs can be incorporated into the nursing care of clients from diverse cultures.
4. Discuss cultural considerations in the nursing care of dying or bereaved clients and families.
5. Describe the health-related beliefs and practices of selected religious groups in North America.

As an integral component of culture, religious beliefs may influence a client's explanation of the cause(s) of illness, perception of its severity, and choice of healer(s). In times of crisis, such as serious illness and impending death, religion may be a source of consolation for the client and family and may influence the course of action believed to be appropriate.

The first half of this chapter discusses dimensions of religion, religion and spiritual nursing care, religious trends in the United States and Canada, and contributions of religious groups to the health care delivery system. The second half highlights the health-related beliefs and practices of selected religions, which are presented in alphabetic order.

• DIMENSIONS OF RELIGION

Religion is complex and multifaceted in both form and function. Religious faith and the institutions derived from that faith become a central focus in meeting the human needs of those who believe. "Not a single faith fails to address the issues of illness and wellness, of disease and healing, of caring and curing. Stated more positively, most faiths were born as, at least in part, efforts to heal" (Marty, 1990, p. 14; Scherer, 1996; Woods & Ironson, 1999). Consequently, the influence of religion on health-related matters requires a few preliminary remarks.

Religious Factors Influencing Human Behavior

First, it is necessary to identify specific religious factors that may influence human behavior. No single religious factor operates in isolation but rather exists in combination with other religious factors. Faulkner and DeJong (1966) have proposed **five major dimensions of religion**: experiential, ritualistic, ideologic, intellectual, and consequential.

Experiential Dimension

The experiential dimension recognizes that all religions have expectations of members and that the religious person will at some point in life achieve direct knowledge of ultimate reality or will experience religious emotion. Every religion recognizes this subjective religious experience as a sign of religiosity.

Ritualistic Dimension

The ritualistic dimension pertains to religious practices expected of the followers and may include worship, prayer, participation in sacraments, and fasting.

Ideologic Dimension

The ideologic dimension refers to the set of beliefs to which its followers must adhere in order to call themselves members. Commitment to the group or movement as a social process results, and members experience a sense of belonging or affiliation.

Intellectual Dimension

The intellectual dimension refers to specific sets of beliefs or explanations or to the cognitive structuring of meaning. Members are expected to be informed about the basic tenets of the religion and to be familiar with sacred writings or scriptures. The intellectual and the ideologic are closely related because acceptance of a dimension presupposes knowledge of it.

Consequential Dimension

The consequential dimension refers to religiously defined standards of conduct and to prescriptions that specify what followers' attitudes and behaviors should be as a consequence of their religion. The consequential dimension governs people's relationships with others.

Religious Dimensions in Relation to Health and Illness

Obviously, each religious dimension has a different significance when related to matters of health and illness. Different religious cultures may emphasize one of the five dimensions to the relative exclusion of the others. Similarly, individuals may develop their own priorities related to the dimension of religion. This affects the nurse providing care to clients with different religious beliefs in several ways. First, it is the nurse's role to determine from the client, or from significant others, the dimension or combinations of dimensions that are important so that the client and nurse can have mutual goals and priorities.

Second, it is important to determine what a given member of a specific religious affiliation believes to be important. The only way to do this is to ask either the client or, if the client is unable to communicate this information personally, a close family member.

Third, the nurse's information must be accurate. Making assumptions about clients' religious belief systems on the basis of their cultural, or even religious, affiliation is imprudent and may lead to erroneous inferences. The following case example illustrates the importance of verifying assumptions with the client.

Observing that a patient was wearing a Star of David on a chain around his neck and had been accompanied by a rabbi upon admission, a nurse inquired whether he would like to order a kosher diet. The patient replied, "Oh, no. I'm a Christian. My father is a rabbi, and I know it would upset him to find out that I have converted. Even though I'm 40 years old, I hide it from him. This has been going on for 15 years now."

The key point in this anecdote is that the nurse validated an assumption with the patient before acting. Furthermore, not all Jewish persons follow a kosher diet or wear a Star of David.

Fourth, even when individuals identify with a particular religion, they may accept the "official" beliefs and practices in varying degrees. It is not the nurse's role to judge the religious virtues of clients but rather to understand those aspects related to religion that are important to the client and family members. When religious beliefs are translated into practice, they may be manipulated by individuals in certain situations to serve particular ends; that is, traditional beliefs and practices are altered. Thus, it is possible for a Jewish person to eat pork or for a Catholic to take contraceptives to prevent pregnancy.

Although some find it necessary to label such occurrences as exceptional or accidental, such a point of view tends to ignore the fact that change can and does occur within individuals and within groups. Homogeneity among members of any religion cannot be assumed. Perhaps the individual once embraced the beliefs and practices of the religion but has since changed his or her views, or perhaps the individual never accepted the religious beliefs completely in the first place. It is important for the nurse to be open to variations in religious beliefs and practices and to allow for the possibility of change. Individual choices frequently arise from new situations, changing values and mores, and exposure to new ideas and beliefs. Few people live in total social isolation, surrounded by only those with similar religious backgrounds.

Fifth, ideal norms of conduct and actual behavior are not necessarily the same. The nurse is frequently faced with the challenge of understanding and helping clients cope with conflicting norms. Sometimes conflicting norms are manifested by guilt or by efforts to minimize or rationalize inconsistencies.

Sometimes norms are vaguely formulated and filled with discrepancies that allow for a variety of interpretations. In religions having a lay organization and structure, moral decision making may be left to the individual without the assistance of members of a church hierarchy. In religions having a clerical hierarchy, moral positions may be more clearly formulated and articulated for members. Individuals retain their right to choose regardless of official church-related guidelines, suggestions, or even religious laws; however, the individual who chooses to violate the norms may experience the consequences of that violation, including social ostracism, public removal from membership rolls, or other forms of censure.

•RELIGION AND SPIRITUAL NURSING CARE

For many years, nursing has emphasized a holistic approach to care in which the needs of the total person are recognized. Most nursing textbooks emphasize the physical and psychosocial needs of clients rather than ways to address spiritual needs. Little has been written about guidelines for providing spiritual care to culturally diverse clients. Because the nurse provides holistic health care, addressing spiritual needs becomes essential.

Religious concerns evolve from and respond to the mysteries of life and death, good and evil, and pain and suffering. Although the religions of the world offer various interpretations of these phenomena, most people seek a personal understanding and interpretation at some time in their lives. Ultimately, this personal search becomes a pursuit to discover a God, or some unifying truth, that will give meaning, purpose, and integrity to existence (Ebersole & Hess, 2000).

Before spiritual care for culturally diverse clients is discussed, an important distinction needs to be made between religion and spirituality. **Religion** refers to an organized system of beliefs concerning the cause, nature, and purpose of the universe, especially belief in or the worship of God or gods. **Spirituality** is born out of each person's unique life experience and his or her personal effort to find purpose and meaning in life.

The goal of **spiritual nursing care** is to assist clients in integrating their own religious beliefs about God or a unifying truth into the ultimate reality that gives meaning to their lives in relationship to the health crisis that has precipitated the need for nursing care. Spiritual nursing care promotes clients' physical and emotional health as well as their **spiritual health**. When providing care, the nurse must remember that the goal of spiritual intervention is not, and should not be, to impose his or her religious beliefs and convictions on the client.

Although spiritual needs are recognized by many nurses, spiritual care is often neglected. Among the reasons why nurses fail to provide spiritual care are the following: (1) they view religious and spiritual needs as a private matter concerning only an individual and his or her Creator; (2) they are uncomfortable about their own religious beliefs or deny having spiritual needs; (3) they lack knowledge about spirituality and the religious beliefs of others; (4) they mistake spiritual needs for psychosocial needs; and (5) they view meeting the spiritual needs of clients as a family or pastoral responsibility, not a nursing responsibility.

Spiritual intervention is as appropriate as any other form of nursing intervention and recognizes that the balance of physical, psychosocial, and spiritual is essential to overall good health. Nursing is an intimate profession, and nurses routinely inquire without hesitation about very personal matters such as hygiene and sexual habits. The spiritual realm also requires a personal, intimate type of nursing intervention.

In the United States and Canada, efforts to integrate spiritual care and nursing have been under way for several decades. For example, in 1971 at the White House Conference on Aging, the spiritual dimension of care was defined as those aspects of individuals pertaining to their inner resources, especially their ultimate concern, the basic value around which all other values are focused, the central philosophy of life that guides their conduct, and the supernatural and nonmaterial dimensions of human nature. The spiritual dimension encompasses the person's need to find satisfactory answers to questions about the meaning of life, illness, or death (Ebersole & Hess, 2000; Moberg, 1971).

In 1978, the Third National Conference on the Classification of Nursing Diagnoses recognized the importance of spirituality by including "spiritual concerns," "spiritual distress," and "spiritual despair" in the list of approved diagnoses. Because of practical difficulties, these three categories were combined at the 1980 National Conference into one category, **spiritual distress**, which is defined as disruption in the life principle that pervades a person's entire being and that integrates and transcends the person's biologic and psychosocial nature. Moberg (1981) acknowledges the multidimensional nature of **spiritual concerns** and defines them as the human need to deal with sociocultural deprivations, anxieties and fears, death and dying, personality integration, self-image, personal dignity, social alienation, and philosophy of life.

Cultural Assessment of Religious and Spiritual Issues

As discussed in Chapter 3, cultural assessment includes assessment of the relationship between religious and spiritual issues as they relate to the health care status of the client. In the integration of health care and religious/spiritual beliefs, the focus of nursing intervention is to help the client maintain his or her own beliefs in the face of the health crisis and to use those beliefs to strengthen individual coping patterns. If the religious beliefs are contributing to the overall health problem (e.g. guilt, remorse, expectations), you can conduct a **spiritual assessment**. To be therapeutic, begin by asking questions that clarify the problem, and nonjudgmentally support the client's problem solving.

Summarized in Box 14–1 are guidelines for assessing spiritual needs in clients from diverse cultural backgrounds (Figure 14–1).

Spiritual Nursing Care for Ill Children and Their Families

Religion is especially important to clients during periods of crisis. In a broad sense, any hospitalization or serious illness can be viewed as stressful and therefore has the potential to develop into a crisis. You may find that religion plays an especially significant role when a child is seriously ill and in circumstances that include dying, death, or bereavement.

Illness during childhood may be an especially difficult clinical situation. Children as well as adults have spiritual needs that vary according to their developmental level and the religious climate in the family. Parental perceptions about the illness of their child may be partially influenced by religious beliefs. For example, some parents may believe that a transgression against a religious law has caused a congenital anomaly in their offspring. Other parents may delay seeking medical care because they believe that prayer should be tried first.

The nurse should be respectful of parents' preferences regarding the care of their child. When parental beliefs or practices threaten the child's well-

BOX 14–1	**ASSESSING SPIRITUAL NEEDS IN CULTURALLY DIVERSE CLIENTS**

Environment

- Does the client have religious objects, such as a Bible, prayer book, devotional literature, religious medals, rosary or other type of beads, photographs of historic religious persons or contemporary church leaders (e.g., Pope, church president), paintings of religious events or persons, religious sculptures, crucifixes, objects of religious significance at entrances to rooms (e.g., holy water founts, a mezuzah, or small parchment scroll inscribed with an excerpt from the Bible), candles of religious significance (e.g., Paschal candle, menorah), shrine, or other?
- Does the client wear clothing that has religious significance (e.g., head covering, undergarment, uniform)?
- Are get well greeting cards religious in nature or from a representative of the client's church?
- Does the client receive flowers or bulletins from his or her church?

Behavior

- Does the client appear to pray at certain times of the day or before meals?
- Does the client make special dietary requests (e.g., kosher diet, vegetarian diet, or diet free from caffeine, pork, shellfish, or other specific food items)?
- Does the client read religious magazines or books?

Verbalization

- Does the client mention God (Allah, Buddha, Yahweh), prayer, faith, church, or religious topics?
- Does the client ask for a visit by a clergy member or other religious representative?
- Does the client express anxiety or fear about pain, suffering, or death?

Interpersonal Relationships

- Who visits? How does the client respond to visitors?
- Does a priest, rabbi, minister, elder, or other church representative visit?
- How does the client relate to the nursing staff? To his or her roommate(s)?
- Does the client prefer to interact with others or to remain alone?

Spiritual Care: The Nurse's Role, 3d Ed., by Judith Allen Shelly and Sharon Fish. © 1998 by InterVarsity Press, Christian Fellowship of the USA. Used by permission of InterVarsity Press, P.O. Box 1400, Downers Grove, IL 60515.

being and health (from your perspective), you are obligated to discuss the matter with the parents. It may be possible to reach a compromise in which parental beliefs are respected and necessary care is provided. On rare occasions, it may become a legal matter. Religion may be a source of consolation and support to parents, especially those facing the unanswerable questions associated with life-threatening illness in their children.

Figure 14–1. This statue commemorates the Roman Catholic saint Martin De Porres. Born in Peru during the 16th century to a Spanish father and a Black mother, Martin De Porres studied medicine, which he later, as a member of the Dominican Order, put to use in helping the poor. He is honored by some Catholics as the patron saint of African Americans. When assessing the needs of clients from diverse backgrounds, nurses can observe for the presence of religious objects in the client's home or yard.

Spiritual Nursing Care for the Dying or Bereaved Client and Family

"All Americans do not mourn alike. Mourning is cultural behavior and we live in a multicultural society. But the way we are raised dictates patterns we regard as proper or natural. Just as we celebrate holidays or marriages differently, we also mourn differently. The mourning customs of others may seem unusual when compared to your tradition, but like yours, they help people cope with death" (*Memory and Mourning: American Expressions of Grief,* 1994. Rochester, NY: Strong Museum).

Nurses inevitably focus on restoring health or on fostering environments in which the client returns to a previous state of health or adapts to physical, psychologic, or emotional changes. However, one aspect of care that is often avoided or ignored, though every bit as crucial to clients and their families, is death and the accompanying dying and grieving processes.

Death is indeed a universal experience, but one that is highly individual and personal. Although each person must ultimately face death alone, rarely does one person's death fail to affect others. There are many rituals, serving many purposes, that people use to help them cope with death. These rituals are often determined by cultural and religious orientation. Situational factors, competing demands, and individual differences are also important in determining the dying, bereavement, and grieving behaviors that are considered socially acceptable.

The role of the nurse in dealing with dying clients and their families varies according to the needs and preferences of both the nurse and client, as well as the clinical setting in which the interaction occurs. By understanding some of the cultural and religious variations related to death, dying, and bereavement, the nurse can individualize the care given to clients and their families.

Nurses are often with the client through various stages of the dying process and at the actual moment of death, particularly when death occurs in a hospital, nursing home, extended care facility, or hospice. The nurse often determines when and whom to call as the impending death draws near. Knowing the religious, cultural, and familial heritage of a particular client as well as his or her devotion to the associated traditions and practices may help the nurse determine whom to call when the need arises.

Religious Beliefs Associated with Dying

Universally, people want to die with dignity. Historically this was not a problem when individuals died at home in the presence of their friends and families. Now, when more and more people are dying in institutions (hospitals, nursing homes, and extended care facilities) ensuring dignity throughout the dying process is more complex. Once death is seen as a problem for professional management, the hospital displaces the home, and specialists with different kinds and degrees of expertise take over for the family.

The way in which people commemorate death tells us much about their attitude and philosophy of life and death. Although it is beyond the scope of this book to explore the philosophic and psychologic aspects of death in detail, some points will be made that relate to nursing care.

Preparation of the Body

A nurse may or may not actually participate in the rituals associated with death. When people die in the United States and Canada, they are usually transported to a mortuary, where the preparation for burial occurs.

In many cultural groups, preparation of the body has traditionally been very important. Whereas members of many cultural groups have now adopted the practice of letting the mortician prepare the body, there are some, particularly new immigrants, who want to retain their native and/or religious customs. For example, for certain Asian immigrants it is customary for family and friends of the same sex to wash and prepare the body for burial or cremation. In other situations, the family or religious representatives may go to the funeral home to prepare the body for burial by dressing the person in special religious clothing.

If a person dies in an institution, it is common for the nursing staff to "prepare" the body according to standard procedure. Depending on the ethnoreligious practices of the family, this may be objectionable—the family members may view this washing as an infringement on a special task that belongs to them alone. If the family is present, you should ask family members about their preference. If ritual washings will eventually take place at the mortuary, you may carry out the routine procedures and reassure the family that the mortician will comply with their requests, if that has in fact been verified.

North American funeral customs have been the topic of lively discussion. The initial preparation of the body has been described in the following way:

"After delivery to the undertaker, the corpse is in short order sprayed, sliced, pierced, pickled, trussed, trimmed, creamed, waxed, painted, rouged and neatly dressed...transformed from a common corpse into a beautiful memory picture. This process is known in the trades as embalming and restorative art, and is so universally employed in the U.S. and Canada that the funeral director does it routinely without consulting the corpse's family. He regards as eccentric those few who are hardy enough to suggest it might be dispensed with. Yet no law requires it, no religious doctrine commends it, nor is it dictated by considerations of health, sanitation or even personal daintiness. In no part of the world but in North America is it widely used. The purpose of embalming is to make the corpse presentable for viewing in a suitably costly container, and here too the funeral director routinely without first consulting the family prepares the body for public display" (Kalish & Reynolds, 1981, p. 65).

This extensive preparation and attempt to make the body look "alive," "just as he used to" or "just as if she were asleep" may reflect the fact that Anglo North Americans have come into contact with death and dying less than have other cultural groups. Anglo North Americans constitute a culture-bound ethnic group, and the avoidance of death may reflect cultural and religious differences. For example, if a patient has died and a family member does not want to see the body until the mortician has "fixed it up," this request needs to be respected, regardless of your personal beliefs.

Funeral Practices

By their very nature, people are social beings who need to develop social attachments. When these social attachments are broken by death, people need to bring closure to the relationships. The **funeral** is an appropriate and socially acceptable time for the expression of sorrow and grief. Although there are some mores that dictate acceptable behaviors associated with the expression of grief, such as crying and sobbing, the wake and funeral are generally viewed as times when members of the living social network can observe and comfort the grieving survivors in their mourning, and say a last goodbye to the dead person. It is important to keep in mind that even the terms used for the wake and the funeral may vary according to religious and cultural beliefs. What is called a **wake** in many North American religions may be called a **viewing** or **calling hours** by others.

Customs for disposal of the body after death vary widely. Muslims have specific rituals for washing, dressing, and positioning the body. In traditional Judaism, cosmetic restoration is discouraged, as is any attempt to hasten or retard decomposition by artificial means. As part of their lifelong preparation for death, Amish women sew white burial garments for themselves and for their family members (Wenger, 1991). For the viewing and burial, faithful Mormons are dressed in white temple garments. Burial clothes and other religious or cultural symbols may be important items for the funeral ritual. If such items are present, you should ensure that they are taken by the family or sent to the funeral home.

Believing that the spirit or ghost of the deceased person is contaminated, some Navajos are afraid to touch the body after death. In preparation for burial, the body is dressed in fine apparel, adorned with expensive jewelry and money, and wrapped in new blankets. After death, some Navajos believe that the structure in which the person died must be burned. There are specific members of the culture whose role is to prepare the body and who must be ritually cleansed after contact with the dead.

Funeral arrangements vary from short, simple rituals to long, elaborate displays. Among the Amish, family members, neighbors, and friends are relied on for a short, quiet ceremony. Many Jewish families use unadorned coffins and stress simplicity in burial services. Some Jews fly the body to Jerusalem for burial in ground considered to be holy. Regardless of economic considerations, some groups believe in lavish and costly funerals.

Attitudes Toward Death

TABOOS

In some cultures, people believe that particular omens, such as the appearance of an owl or a message in a dream, warn of approaching death. Breaking a taboo may be believed to cause death, and the nurse may be seen as the responsible agent! The literature contains numerous reports of incidents in which nurses have removed objects of religious and spiritual significance that are believed to have healing powers from clients and patients of all ages—rosaries from the cribs of infants, necklaces worn by elderly Native Americans, and so forth. In some cases, the intention of the nurse was benevolent, as when the nurse indicated that the item was removed to be kept in a safe place with other valuables.

Voodoo beliefs and practices are known to exist in North America. Incidents of sudden death or minor injuries after hexing have been attributed to the power of suggestion and to total social isolation, which have been thought to trigger fatal physiologic responses and sensitization of the autonomic nervous system.

AWARENESS OF DYING

Whether individuals should be made aware of their impending death has been debated extensively by physicians, nurses, and others. In the Kalish and Reynolds (1981) study, 71% of Anglos, 60% of African Americans, 49% of Japanese Americans, and 37% of Mexican Americans favored telling clients that they were dying (Stolley & Koenig, 1997). Each cultural group believed that the physician was the most appropriate person to communicate the information, whereas a family member was the second most appropriate choice. However, individual preferences should be respected. In some cultures, not telling the dying individual of his or her impending death is a way for that person to be allowed to "save face."

UNEXPECTED DEATH, VIOLENT DEATH, AND SUICIDE

Acceptance of sudden, violent death is difficult for family members in most societies. For example, suicide is strictly forbidden under Islamic law. In the

Filipino culture, suicide brings shame to the individual and to the entire family. Many Christian religions prohibit suicide and may impose sanctions even after death for the "sin." For example, a Roman Catholic who commits suicide may be denied burial in blessed ground or in a Catholic cemetery. In some religions, a church funeral is not permitted for a suicide victim, requiring the family to make alternative arrangements. This imposition of religious law can further add to the grief of surviving family members and friends.

The Northern Cheyenne believe that suicide, or any death resulting from a violent accident, disturbs the individual's spiritual balance. This disharmony is termed **bad death** and is believed to render the spirit earthbound in its wanderings, thus preventing it from entering the spirit world. A **good death** among the Tohono O'odham comes at the end of a full life, when a person is prepared for death. A bad death, by contrast, occurs unexpectedly and violently, leaving the victim without a chance to settle affairs or to say good-bye.

"A 'bad death' is 'bad' because evil caused it, which leaves the soul of the dead unrestful, unfulfilled, and desirous of returning to the living out of a longing for what has been taken away. The soul returns to the living, although not out of malevolence, to visit loved ones. It is on these visits, that the dead can bring a form of *ka:cim mumkidag* (staying–Indian–sickness), to the living—hence their dangerousness" (Kozak, 1991, p. 214).

In addition to exploring Tohono O'odham (Papago) categories of death, Kozak looks at the larger causes of the increase in violent deaths, arguing "that shifting mortality trends indicate shifts in other aspects of society" (Kozak, 1991, p. 211). Increased deaths are tied to declining economic conditions on the reservation, where jobs have disappeared.

"...the O'odham's economic transition has meant either migrating away from family and friends to find work or remaining on the reservation at home usually to confront extreme unemployment and welfare dependency. Neither option is considered satisfactory or desirable. The social and psychologic side effects of these economic transformations are highlighted, in an inverse relationship in alcohol and drug abuse, violence, and a general increase in dependency" (Kozak, 1991, p. 213).

The categories of "good" and "bad" deaths among the Tohono O'odham have implications for research on excess deaths. Accidents, homicide, and suicide produce bad deaths; in Tohono O'odham eyes, these are deaths that should not occur, deaths that should be avoided if possible. "Bad" deaths are excess deaths. If the medical community's concern is with eliminating excess deaths, it must also be concerned with the larger cultural, social, and economic context in which these deaths occur. Other causes of death, while still important, may affect a people to a much lesser degree. Diabetes mellitus, for example, most often affects people of more advanced years and, because of its slow progress, allows them to prepare for death. This is still an excess death by Western medical standards, but it is not a "bad" death (Hickey & Hall, 1993; Huttlinger et al., 1992).

Death memorials provide a place for the dead to go without bringing harm to the living, and a place for the living to go to help the dead to a proper afterlife. Among the Tohono O'odham, there has been a notable increase in violent deaths, particularly for young males, since 1955. The majority of these violent deaths are the result of motor vehicle accidents and are marked by the Tohono O'odham people with roadside death memorials or shrines. Suicides and homicides are also sometimes commemorated with death memorials.

Deaths resulting from nonviolent but untimely causes can be equally difficult for the patient, family, and friends. Cancers and chronic diseases may give the patient and family time to "prepare" for the death, but the death still occurs and must receive attention.

HOLISM

Buddhism has a holistic approach to death. To the Buddhist way of thinking, illness is inevitable and is a consequence of events and actions taken, not necessarily in this life but also in previous lives. The Buddhist belief is in the cause and effect of events in this life as well as in previous lives. There is an acceptance of death, which means that the choice has been made to anticipate the grief and accept the inevitability of death. This does not mean resignation or the denial of conventional medicine. It does mean moving peacefully from the presence of loving family and friends into the next existence.

The Death of a Child

Although a great deal has been written about children's conceptions of death, cross-cultural studies have not yet been reported. Children develop a concept of death through innate cognitive development, which has significant cultural variations, and through acquired notions conveyed by the family, which vary according to the family's cultural beliefs. Thus, it is unsafe to assume that all children, regardless of family culture, will develop parallel concepts of and reactions to death.

Most children's initial experiences with death occur with the loss of a pet rather than a person. Because of reduced childhood mortality and delayed adult mortality, Western children are much less exposed to death in family than they used to be, and they tend to be sheltered from the experience. The current lack of direct exposure of children to death is both a class phenomenon and a cultural phenomenon.

In many societies of the Western world, children are considered precious, valued, and vulnerable; they are protected and often the first to be saved in emergencies. In less developed societies, by contrast, parents are less likely to see most of their children grow into adulthood because of a very high infant mortality rate. As a result, a child's life may be viewed as less valued and precious than an adult's, but it is still viewed as valuable to the parents and other loved ones. Regardless of the sociocultural situation, each society has a special view of the significance of children and their death as it affects the bereaved family.

Bereavement, Grief, and Mourning

Bereavement is a sociologic term indicating the status and role of the survivors of a death. **Grief** is an affective response to a loss, whereas **mourning** is the culturally patterned behavioral response to a death. What differs between races and cultural groups is not so much the feelings of grief but their forms of expression or mourning.

Different family systems may alleviate or intensify the pain experienced by bereaved persons. In the typical nuclear Anglo North American family, the death of a member leaves a great void because the same few individuals fill most of the roles. By contrast, cultural groups in which several generations and extended family members commonly reside within a household may find that the acute trauma of bereavement is softened by the fact that the familial role of the deceased is easily filled by other relatives. It should be noted, however, that the loss is experienced and mourned irrespective of the person's cultural background.

Although nurses frequently encourage clients and their families to express their grief openly, many people are reluctant to do so in the institutional setting. The nurse often sees family members when they are still in shock over the death and are responding to the situation as a crisis rather than expressing their grief. Three fourths of Blacks, Japanese, and Anglos stated that they would try hard to maintain control of their emotions in public, whereas less than two thirds of Mexican Americans were concerned with the public expression of grief. When asked about crying, either publicly or privately, 88% of Mexican American, 71% of Japanese, 70% of Anglos, and 60% of Blacks indicated that this was acceptable, particularly in private (Kalish & Reynolds, 1981).

When asked who would be sought for comfort and support in a time of bereavement, these groups most frequently named a family member or a member of the clergy. In an institutional setting, a nurse who has been with the patient and family throughout the dying process may be surprised at the time of death when the grieving persons turn to other family, and the nurse is "left out."

Although the experience of grief is a universal phenomenon, a nurse should recognize that the expression of grief is strongly influenced by cultural factors. For example, mourning may vary according to the lines of emotional attachment. In matrilineal societies, a woman may be expected to grieve for male members of her maternal family, such as fathers and brothers, but not for her spouse.

It is not uncommon for a surviving spouse to have a serious illness within a year or two after the death. Although the exact reasons for this are unknown, the stress of losing a spouse seems to render the surviving partner more vulnerable to illness. Caring for a person who is seriously ill but who is also mourning a recent death requires added sensitivity by the nurse to the patient's emotional needs.

Some mourning rituals are highly structured and lengthy, whereas others are relatively simple and short. In the Jewish tradition, there are five successive stages of mourning, which extend for a year and include practices that influence virtually every aspect of life.

Summary of Beliefs Related to Death and Dying

Contemporary bereavement practices of various cultural and religious groups demonstrate the wide range of expressions of bereavement. Each group reflects practices that best meet its members' needs. Once you understand this, you can better appreciate their role in promoting a culturally appropriate grieving process, and to realize that hindering or interfering with practices that the client and family find meaningful can disrupt the grieving process. Bereaved people can experience physical and psychologic symptoms, and they may succumb to serious physical illnesses, leading even to death. Although bereavement is regarded as a universal stressor, the magnitude of the stress and its meaning to the individual vary significantly cross-culturally. For example, one Western misconception is that it is more stressful to mourn the death of a child than the death of an older or more distant relative. Yet, cross-cultural studies show that emotional attachments to relatives vary significantly and are not based on Western concepts of kinship (Eisenbruch, 1984b).

Although traditional funeral and post-funeral rituals have benefited both bereaved persons and their social groups in their original settings, the influence of the contemporary Western urban setting is unknown. It is likely that in North America, most individuals have assimilated United States and Canadian practices in varying degrees. You should obtain information from individual clients in a caring manner, explaining that you wish to provide culturally appropriate nursing care.

• RELIGIOUS TRENDS IN THE UNITED STATES AND CANADA

The United States and Canada are cosmopolitan nations to which all of the major and many of the minor faiths of Europe and other parts of the globe have been transplanted. Religious identification among people from different racial and ethnic groups is important because religion and culture are interwoven. In a recent survey, 64% of Latino and 50% of Black congregations in the United States regard their churches as a means of preserving their cultural heritage, whereas fewer than one third of White congregations link their religious denomination with the preservation of cultural heritage (Broadway, August 23, 2001), *The Washington Post*, p. C15. During the past two decades, there has been an unusually large group of immigrants from Asia and Latin America. The changing composition of the Asian population has resulted in fewer Christians (63% in 1990 compared with 43% in 2001), and those professing Asian religions (e.g. Buddhism, Hinduism, Islam) has risen from 15% to 43%. These immigration patterns have resulted in significant shifts. For example, there are three times as many Hindus in the United States today as there were in 1990. Most of the Latin American immigrants, on the other hand, are Roman Catholic, although the numbers are not large enough to make a significant statistical shift overall.

With such a complex mosaic of religions, no one has succeeded in enumerating all the denominations. Table 14–1 details the statistical breakdown of major religious affiliations of the United States and Canada (Figure 14–2). Religious bodies with 60,000 or more members in the United States and Canada are identified in Table 14–2.

TABLE 14–1	MAJOR RELIGIOUS AFFILIATIONS OF U.S. AND CANADA (%)	
	USA	CANADA
Christianity	85	83.3
Atheism, Agnosticism, no affiliation	9.1	13
Judaism	1.7	1.2
Islam	1.2	0.9
Major Christian Faith Groups		
Roman Catholic	23	46
Protestant	60	36
Eastern Orthodox	2.0	1.4

Source: www.religioustolerance.org, April 9, 2002

As discussed, a wide range of beliefs frequently exists within religions—a factor that adds complexity. Some religions have a designated spokesperson or leader who articulates, interprets, and applies theological tenets to daily life experiences, including those of health and illness. These leaders include Jewish rabbis, Catholic priests, and Lutheran ministers. Some churches rely more heavily on individual conscience, whereas others entrust decisions to a group of individuals, or to a single person vested with ultimate authority within their church.

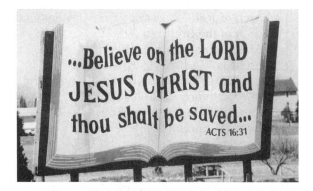

Figure 14–2. Eighty-five percent of North Americans report religious affiliation with a Christian church. Of the 60% affiliated with protestant groups in the United States, Baptists account for 21%; Methodists, 9%; Lutherans, 7%; Presbyterians, 5%; and Episcopalians, 2%. Catholics comprise 3%. Those belonging to non-Christian religions total 6% of the population, whereas those reporting no religious affiliation account for 9%.

TABLE 14–2	MEMBERSHIP FOR SELECTED RELIGIOUS BODIES IN THE UNITED STATES AND CANADA

RELIGIOUS BODY (YEAR REPORTED)	MEMBERSHIP
African Methodist Episcopal Church (1999)	2,500,000
African Methodist Episcopal Zion Church (1996)	1,252,000
American Baptist Association (1996)	275,000
American Baptist Churches in the U.S.A. (1996)	1,507,000
Antiochian Orthodox Christian Archdiocese of North America (1996)	65,000
Armenian Apostolic Church of America (1998)	200,000
Assemblies of God (1998)	2,526,000
Baha'i International Community	161,000
Baptist Bible Fellowship International (1997)	1,200,000
Baptist General Conference (1998)	141,000
Baptist Missionary Association of America (1999)	235,000
Buddhist (1990)	780,000
Christian and Missionary Alliance (1998)	346,000
Christian Brethren (Plymouth Brethren) (1997)	100,000
Christian Church (Disciples of Christ) (1997)	879,000
Christian Churches and Churches of Christ (1996)	1,072,000
Christian Congregations, Inc. (1996)	117,000
Christian Methodist Episcopal Church (1983)	719,000
Christian Reformed Church in North America (1996)	199,000
Church of God (Anderson, IN) (1996)	234,000
Church of God (Cleveland, TN) (1995)	753,000
Church of God in Christ (1991)	5,500,000
Church of God of Prophecy (1997)	77,000
Church of Jesus Christ of Latter-Day Saints (1997)	8,000,000
Church of the Brethren (1997)	141,000
Church of the Nazarene (1996)	867,000
Churches of Christ (1999)	1,500,000
Conservative Baptist Association of America (1998)	200,000
Coptic Orthodox Church (1992)	180,000
Cumberland Presbyterian Church (1998)	87,000
Episcopal Church (1996)	2,365,000
Evangelical Covenant Church (1996)	97,000
Evangelical Free Church of America (1995)	243,000
Evangelical Lutheran Church of America (1998)	5,178,000
Evangelical Presbyterian Church (1998)	61,000
Free Methodist Church of North America (1998)	73,000
Full Gospel Fellowship of Churches and Ministers (1999)	275,000
General Baptists (General Association of) (1997)	72,000
General Association of Regular Baptist Churches (1998)	102,000
General Conference of Mennonite Brethren (1996)	82,000

(continued)

TABLE 14–2	*(Continued)*

RELIGIOUS BODY (YEAR REPORTED)	MEMBERSHIP
Grace Gospel Fellowship (1992)	60,000
Greek Orthodox Diocese America (1998)	1,955,000
Hindu (1990)	227,000
Independent Fundamental Churches of America (1999)	62,000
International Church of the Foursquare Gospel (1998)	238,000
International Council of Community Churches (1998)	250,000
International Pentecostal Holiness Church (1998)	177,000
Jehovah's Witnesses (1999)	1,099,644
Jewish (1998)	7,320,000
Lutheran Church—Missouri Synod (1998)	2,594,000
Mennonite Church (1998)	330,515
Muslim/Islamic (1990)	3,600,000
National Association of Congregational Christian Churches (1998)	67,000
National Association of Free Will Baptists (1998)	210,000
National Baptist Convention of America, Inc. (1987)	3,500,000
National Baptist Convention, U.S.A., Inc. (1992)	8,200,000
National Missionary Baptist Convention, U.S.A., Inc. (1992)	2,500,000
Old Order Amish Church (1993)	81,000
Orthodox Church in America (1998)	1,000,000
Pentecostal Assemblies of the World, Inc. (1998)	1,500,000
Pentecostal Church of God (1998)	104,000
Presbyterian Church in America (1997)	280,000
Presbyterian Church (U.S.A.) (1998)	3,575,000
Progressive National Baptist Convention, Inc. (1995)	2,500,000
Reformed Church in North America (1998)	296,000
Religious Society of Friends (conservative) (1994)	104,000
Reorganized Church of Jesus Christ of Latter-Day Saints (1998)	140,000
Roman Catholic Church (1998)	96,000,000
Romanian Orthodox Episcopate of America (1996)	65,000
Salvation Army (1998)	471,000
Serbian Orthodox Church in the U.S.A. and Canada (1986)	67,000
Seventh-Day Adventist Church (1998)	946,962
Southern Baptist Convention (1998)	15,729,000
Unitarian Universalist (1990)	221,760
United Church of Christ (1998)	1,421,000
United Methodist Church (1998)	8,400,000
Wesleyan Church (USA) (1998)	177,000
Wisconsin Evangelical Lutheran Synod (1997)	411,000

Data from U.S. Bureau of the Census (1996). *Statistical Abstracts of the United States: 1996* (116th ed.). Washington, DC: U.S. Government Printing Office; and *Yearbook of American and Canadian Churches,* 1999.

Although it is impossible to address the health-related beliefs and practices of any religion adequately, this chapter offers a brief overview of some groups. Some of the world's religions fall into major branches or divisions, such as Vaishnavite and Shaivite Hinduism; Theravada and Mahayana Buddhism; Orthodox, Reform, and Conservative Judaism; Roman Catholic, Orthodox, and Protestant Christianity, and Sunnite and Shi'ite Islam. There also are subdivisions into what are often called denominations, sects, or schools of thought and practice.

• CONTRIBUTIONS OF RELIGIOUS GROUPS TO THE HEALTH CARE DELIVERY SYSTEM

In the United States, many denominations own and operate health care institutions and make significant fiscal contributions that help control health care costs. For example, the Roman Catholic Church, the largest single denomination in the United States, is also a major stakeholder in the health care field. According to the *Catholic Almanac* (2000), the nation's nearly 600 Catholic hospitals treat 17.2 million patients annually and account for approximately 10% of all hospital beds. In addition, the Catholic Church is responsible for treating 5.2 million patients at its 529 health centers and 134,000 individuals at its 1,378 day care and extended day care centers. Moreover, there are under direct Catholic auspices 84 nonresidential schools for the handicapped, 14 facilities for the deaf and hearing impaired, 4 centers for the blind and visually impaired, 517 facilities for the aged, 72 facilities for abused, abandoned, neglected, and emotionally disturbed children, 116 centers for those with developmental disabilities, 2 residences for the orthopedically and physically handicapped, 8 cancer hospitals, and 11 substance abuse centers. Catholic Charities U.S.A., an umbrella agency that oversees nonhospital work, reports that its agencies serve more than 10 million people each year, often functioning as a centralized referral source for clients ultimately treated in non-Catholic agencies (Catholic Almanac, 2000).

Similarly, there are many Jewish hospitals, day care centers, extended care facilities, and organizations to meet the health care needs of Jewish and non-Jewish persons in need. For example, the National Jewish Center for Immunology and Respiratory Medicine is a research and treatment center for respiratory, immunologic, allergic and infectious diseases, whereas the Council for Jewish Elderly provides a full range of social and health care services for seniors, including adult day care, care/case management, counseling, transportation, and advocacy.

Many other denominations, including the Lutheran, Mennonite, Methodist, Muslim, and Seventh-Day Adventist groups, own and operate hospitals and health care organizations similar to those described previously.

In Canada, hospital care, outpatient care, extended care, and medical services have been publicly funded and administered since the Medical Care Act of 1966. However, before the Medical Care Act and into the present, religious organizations have made important contributions to the health and well-being of Canadians at individual, community, and societal levels. For example, countless church-run agencies, charities, and facilities offer care and social support to individuals and families coping with such conditions as chronic illness, disability, poverty, and homelessness. At the national level, church-run organizations, such as the Catholic Health Association of Canada, are committed to addressing social justice issues that affect the health system and offer leadership through research and policy development regarding health care ethics, spiritual and religious care, and social justice.

• AMISH

The term **Amish** refers to members of several ethnoreligious groups who choose to live separately from the modern world through manner of dress, language, family life, and selective use of technology. There are four major orders or affiliating groups of Amish: (1) *Old Order Amish,* the largest group, whose name is often used synonymously with "the Amish"; (2) the ultraconservative *Swartzentruber* and *Andy Weaver Amish*, both more conservative than the Old Order Amish in their restrictive use of technology and shunning of members who have dropped out or committed serious violations of the faith; (3) the less conservative *New Order Amish,* which emerged in the 1960s with more liberal views of technology but with an emphasis on high moral standards in restricting alcohol and tobacco use and in courtship practices; and (4) the *Liberal Beachy Amish.*

The total population of Amish is estimated at 160,000, spread throughout more than 220 settlements in 21 states and one Canadian province (about 1/20th of 1% of the total populations of the United States and Canada). In 1900, there were approximately 5,000 Amish, representing the number who immigrated to the United States during the 18th and 19th centuries. During the 20th century, however, the population grew as the Amish became less frequent targets for conversion and growing numbers of children (80% to 85%) chose, as adults, to be baptized Amish. As a result, the population grew to 85,000 by 1979 and has nearly doubled that number today. More than half are younger than age 18 (Donnermeyer, 1997).

General Beliefs and Religious Practices

The imperative to remain separate is the common theme of the nearly 500-year history of the Amish and is based on the following scripture passages:

> "Be not conformed to this world, but be ye transformed by the renewing of your mind"

> (Romans 12:2)

> "Be ye not unequally yoked together with unbelievers; for what fellowship hath righteousness with unrighteousness? and what communion hath light with darkness?"

> (II Corinthians 6:14)

The Amish are direct descendants of a branch of *Anabaptists* (which means "to be rebaptized") that emerged during the Protestant Reformation and resided in Switzerland, The Netherlands, Austria, France, and Germany. Anabaptists stressed adult baptism, separation from and nonassimilation with the dominant culture, conformity in dress and appearance, marriage to others within the group, nonproselytization, nonparticipation in military service, and a disciplined lifestyle with an emphasis on simple living. These basic tenets remain today.

A former Catholic priest from The Netherlands named Menno Simmons (1496–1561) wrote down the beliefs and practices of the Anabaptists, who became known as **Mennonites**. In 1693, under the leadership of a church elder named Jacob Ammann (1656–1730), a more conservative group broke away and formed the group currently known as the Amish.

Core Characteristics

According to Donnermeyer (1997), there are **five core characteristics of the Amish**.

SUBCULTURE

First, the Amish are a subculture: a group with beliefs, values, and behaviors that are distinct from the greater culture of which the group is a part. The Amish maintain their separateness and distinctiveness from United States and Canadian societies in a variety of ways. Geographically, the Amish live close together in areas referred to as settlements and rely primarily on the horse and buggy for transportation.

The Amish continue to practice their faith in the tradition of Anabaptism, which includes small church districts of a few dozen families led by a bishop, church services that rotate from house to house of each family (no church building), the practice of adult baptism, communion twice a year, and shunning. Church leaders are chosen through a process of nomination and drawing by lot, and they serve for life. All but a few Amish marry, extended family remains important, and divorce is rare. The Amish dress in distinctive clothing (plain colors and mostly without buttons and zippers). They speak a form of German among themselves known as Pennsylvania Dutch or High German, and they sometimes refer to non-Amish as the "English."

ORDUNG

The second core feature of the Amish is the *ordung*, which is used for passing on religious values and way of life from one generation to the next. Parts of the *ordung* are based on specific biblical passages, but much of it consists of rules for living the Amish way.

MEIDUNG/SHUNNING

The third characteristic of the Amish is *meidung*, the practice of shunning members who have violated the *ordung*. After all members of the church district have discussed the case and agreed to impose *meidung*, the individual is separated from the rest of his or her community. It is the church's method of enforcing the *ordung*. *Meidung* is an important way of maintaining both a sense of community among Amish and a sense of separation from the rest of the world. Sanctions for violations against important values, beliefs, and behaviors that define distinctiveness from the majority culture enable the Amish to retain their religious and cultural identity. In most cases, when *meidung* is applied, it is for a limited time. *Meidung* applies only to Amish adults who have been baptized, not to their unbaptized children. Children of Amish who choose not to be baptized often become members of neighboring Mennonite congregations and maintain contact with their Amish relatives.

With less serious violations of the *ordung,* a member is visited privately by the deacon and a minister, and the matter is resolved quietly. For more serious offenses, the punishment is carried out publicly during a church service. A few offenses, such as adultery and divorce, are automatically conditions of excommunication. By displaying deep sorrow and repentance for an offense, excommunicated members can be allowed back, but this is not easily accomplished.

SELECTIVE USE OF TECHNOLOGY

The fourth core characteristic is the selective use of technology. The Amish selectively use many modern technologies, but only if they do not threaten their ability to maintain a community of believers. Technologically, the Amish restrict the use of electricity in their homes and farms, and they limit their use of telephones. Although they ride in automobiles, trains, and airplanes, they do not operate them. Tractors for farm field work might reduce the opportunity for sons and daughters to help parents with farm chores, and the farm would become larger, reducing the number available for future generations. Thus, technology is not inherently bad, but when its consequences result in destruction of family and community life, it is avoided (Figure 14–3).

GELASSENHEIT

The fifth and final core characteristic of the Amish is *gelassenheit.* This term means "submission," or yielding to a higher authority, and it represents a general guide for behavior among Amish members. *Gelassenheit* represents the

Figure 14–3. Although the Amish restrict their use of technology for reasons that are, in part, health-related, they ironically find themselves at a high risk for accidents that frequently result from the careless use of technologic developments by non-Amish neighbors.

high value that the Amish place on maintaining a sense of community, which is accomplished by not drawing too much attention to one's self. Amish cite *gelassenheit* as the reason they avoid having their photographs taken and prohibit mirrors in their homes.

Holy Days and Sacraments

Amish hold church services every other Sunday on a rotating basis in the homes or barns of church district members. The church services last several hours with hymns, scriptures, and services in High German or Pennsylvania Dutch. The family hosting the services is expected to provide a meal for all in attendance. Christmas celebrations include family dinners and exchanges of gifts. Weddings last all day and include eating and singing. An important part of Amish life is informal visiting. Families often visit one another without advance notice, and it is common for unexpected visitors to stay for a meal. Amish observe adult baptism and communion twice a year.

Social Activities (Dating, Dancing)

The Amish strive for high standards of conduct in both their private and public lives. This includes chastity before marriage and humility in dress, language, and behavior. The function of dating is to afford individuals an opportunity to become acquainted with each other's character. Couples contemplating marriage may engage in a practice called bundling, in which they lie together in bed, fully clothed, without having sexual contact.

Substance Use

Alcoholic beverages and drugs are forbidden unless prescribed by a physician. Tobacco use is prohibited.

Health Care Practices

Illness is seen as the inability to perform daily chores; physical and mental illness are equally accepted. Health care practices within the Amish culture are varied and include folk, herbal, homeopathic, and Western biomedicine. Unlike the use of episodic biomedicine, however, preventive medicine may be seen as against God's will. The use of the Western biomedical health care system is largely episodic and crisis oriented. If Western biomedicine fails, there is no hesitancy in visiting an herb doctor, pow-wow doctor (a practitioner of a folk healing art, known as *brauche*, in which touch is used to heal) or a chiropractor. Folk, professional, and alternative care are often used simultaneously. Cost, access, transportation, and advice from family and friends are the major factors that influence healing choices (Wenger, 1990).

Medical and Surgical Interventions

The use of narcotic drugs is prohibited. There are no restrictions against the use of blood, blood products, or vaccines if advised by health care providers.

Practices Related to Reproduction

The Amish believe that the fundamental purpose of marriage is the procreation of children, and couples are encouraged to have large families. Children are an economic asset to the family because they assist their parents with housework, farm chores, gardening, and family business. Women are expected to have children until menopause. If situations arise that justify sterilization (e.g., removal of cancerous reproductive organs), those called upon to make the decisions would rely on the best medical advice available and the council of the church leaders. Although the Amish family structure is patriarchal, the grandmother is often a key decision maker concerning reproductive and other health-related issues.

Abortion is inconsistent with Amish values and beliefs. Artificial insemination, genetics, eugenics, and stem cell research are also inconsistent with Amish values and beliefs.

Religious Support System for the Sick

VISITORS

Individual members of local and surrounding communities assist and support one another in time of need. From cradle to grave, each person knows that he or she will be cared for by those in the community. **Friendscraft** is a unique three-generational extended family support network inherent in the Amish community that provides informal support, emotional and financial assistance, and advice. The extended family consists of aunts, uncles, cousins, and grandparents, who usually live only a few miles away and can be counted on to assist in times of illness.

TITLE OF RELIGIOUS REPRESENTATIVE

The Amish do not use religious titles. There are approximately 1,100 Amish church districts in the United States and Canada, each representing about 20 to 35 families, and a minimal hierarchy of church leaders (a bishop, deacon, and two ministers). The bishop is the spiritual head; the deacon assists the bishop and is responsible for donations to help members with medical bills and other expenses; and the ministers help the bishop with preaching at church services and providing spiritual direction for the church district and its members. Although bishops meet periodically, there is no church hierarchy above the level of the church district. Because the Amish are surrounded by American and Canadian societies, which continuously exert strong economic and cultural pressures that are incompatible with Amish values, the Amish represent a subculture that is among the most "self-consciously engineered of all societies" (Donnermeyer, 1997, p. 9).

CHURCH ORGANIZATIONS TO ASSIST THE SICK

Individual members of local church districts look after the needs of the sick person and his or her family.

Practices Related to Death and Dying

Prolongation of life (right to die) and euthanasia are personal matters that may be discussed with the bishop, ministers, and/or family members. Autopsy is acceptable in the case of medical necessity or legal requirement but is seldom performed on the Amish. Although there is no specific prohibition, the Amish usually prefer to bury the intact body and generally do not donate body parts for medical research. Bodies are buried in small cemeteries in Amish communities on private property.

Addendum: Meeting Health Expenses

The Amish beliefs in self-sufficiency, separation from the world, and mutual aid have resulted in their rejection of formal assistance that comes from outside the Amish community. For example, the Amish obtained exemption for self-employed workers from Social Security, including Medicare, in 1965 on religious grounds and received exemption for all Amish workers from these programs in 1988. Amish seldom purchase commercial health insurance; instead, they have traditionally relied on personal savings and various methods of mutual assistance within the immediate and larger Amish community to meet their medical expenses. It is expected that each family has planned for future health care needs (e.g., childbirth and minor illness), but it is recognized that catastrophic illnesses resulting in extensive medical expenses do sometimes occur. In these instances, the Amish community provides assistance, usually through participation in one of the Amish Hospital Aid plans.

As indicated in Evidence-Based Practice 14–1, changing occupational patterns among the Amish have resulted in shifting views toward commercial health insurance. According to Donnermeyer (1997), in Holmes County, Ohio, only 32.9% of Amish breadwinners earn their living as farmers: 24.5% are active farmers, 4% are retired farmers, and 3.4% hold dual occupations (both farm and nonfarm). Similar trends have been reported among other Amish settlements, where 30% to 80% of adult men work in nonfarm wage labor jobs in construction, factories, and home-based shops (e.g., cabinetmaking, harness making, blacksmithing, and so forth). The underlying reasons for the change are attributed to two factors: population growth and difficulty finding sufficient farmland for the growing numbers of Amish.

• BAHA'I INTERNATIONAL COMMUNITY

The Baha'i Faith is an independent world religion. It has members in approximately 340 countries and localities and represents 1,900 ethnic groups and tribes. North American membership is 161,366, and worldwide membership is 7,666,000.

General Beliefs and Religious Practices

The writings that guide the life of the **Baha'i International Community** comprise numerous works by Baha'u'llah, prophet-founder of the Baha'i Faith.

EVIDENCE-BASED PRACTICE 14–1
Old Order Amish and Commercial Health Insurance

Although Old Order Amish families have in the past been prohibited from using commercial health insurance on religious grounds, the increasing cost of hospitalization, combined with changing occupational patterns by the Amish, has resulted in a change in health care use patterns. The data for the study were obtained through observation of participants and informal open-ended interviews with Old Order Amish families residing in Geauga County, Ohio. The findings indicate that there is an increasing tendency for Old Order Amish families in this county to use health insurance provided by non-Amish employers. The pattern is associated with increased use of biomedical health services, which is related to the availability of extensive health services and facilities in neighboring Cleveland.

CLINICAL APPLICATION

The Old Order Amish is a dynamic group that has managed to survive at least partially because they have selectively incorporated new components into their cultural system. One important change over the past few generations involves the transition from an agrarian way of life to one based on wage labor and the accompanying increased use of employer-provided commercial health insurance. The researchers also noted that an additional cost for Amish seeking biomedical health care is transportation—a sum that may equal or exceed that paid to the health care provider. Perhaps the most important consideration for nurses is to understand is that Old Order Amish society is dynamic and that there is greater heterogeneity between and within congregations than might be expected from the outward manifestations of conformity in dress and selective use of technology.

Greksa, L. P., & Korbin, J. E. (1997). Influence of changing occupational patterns on the use of commercial health insurance by the Old Order Amish. *Journal of Multicultural Nursing & Health, 3*(2), 13–18.

Central teachings are the oneness of God, the oneness of religion, and the oneness of humanity. Baha'u'llah proclaimed that religious truth is not absolute but relative, that Divine Revelation is a continuous and progressive process, that all the great religions of the world are divine in origin, and that their missions represent successive stages in the spiritual evolution of human society.

For Baha'is, the basic purpose of human life is to know and worship God and to carry forward an ever-advancing civilization. To achieve these goals, they strive to fulfill certain principles:

1. Fostering of good character and the development of spiritual qualities, such as honesty, trustworthiness, compassion, and justice.
2. Eradication of prejudices of race, creed, class, nationality, and sex.
3. Elimination of all forms of superstitions that hamper human progress, and achievement of a balance between the material and spiritual aspects of life. An unfettered search for truth, and belief in the essential harmony of science and religion, are two aspects of this principle.

4. Development of the unique talents and abilities of every individual through the pursuit of knowledge and the acquisition of skills for the practice of a trade or profession.
5. Full participation of both sexes in all aspects of community life, including the elective, administrative, and decision making processes, along with equality of opportunities, rights, and privileges of men and women.
6. Fostering of the principle of universal compulsory education.

Baha'is may not be members of any political party, but they may accept nonpartisan government posts and appointments. They are enjoined to obey the government in their respective countries and, without political affiliation, may vote in general elections and participate in the civic life of their communities.

The Baha'i administrative order has neither priesthood nor ritual; it relies on a pattern of local, national, and international governance, created by Baha'u'llah. Institutions and programs are supported exclusively by voluntary contributions from members.

The Baha'i International Community has consultative status with the United Nations Economic and Social Council and with the United Nations Children's Fund. It is also affiliated with the United Nations Environment Program and with the United Nations Office of Public Information.

The World Center of the Baha'i Faith is in Israel, established in the two cities of Haifa and 'Akka. The affairs of the Baha'i world community are administered by the Universal House of Justice, the supreme elected council, in Haifa.

Holy Days and Sacraments

Extending from sunset to sunset are Baha'i holy days, feast days, and days of fasting. These holy days are not contraindications to medical care or surgery.

Although the Baha'i Faith does not have sacraments in the same sense that Christian churches do, it does have practices that have similar meanings to members. These practices include the recitation of obligatory prayers and participation in the observance of holy days and the Nineteen-Day Fast, which is mandatory for all Baha'is between the ages of 15 and 70 years. Exceptions are made for illness, travel away from home, and pregnancy. **Fasting** occurs from sunrise to sunset for an entire Baha'i month, which consists of 19 days.

Social Activities (Dating, Dancing)

Baha'is strive for high standards of conduct in both their private and public lives; this includes chastity before marriage; moderation in dress, language, and amusements; and complete freedom from prejudice in their dealings with peoples of different races, classes, creeds, and orders.

The Baha'i Faith forbids monastic celibacy, noting that marriage is fundamental to the growth and continuation of civilization. The function of dating is to afford individuals an opportunity to become acquainted with each other's character. Those contemplating marriage are encouraged to engage in some form of work and service together—a practice intended to promote assessment of their own maturity and readiness for marriage as well as to improve their knowledge of the character and values of the prospective marriage partner.

Substance Use

Alcoholic beverages and drugs are forbidden unless prescribed by a physician. Tobacco use is strongly discouraged.

Health Care Practices

With an attitude of harmony between religion and science, Baha'is are encouraged to seek out competent medical care, to follow the advice of those in whom they have confidence, and to pray.

Medical and Surgical Interventions

The use of narcotic drugs is prohibited except by prescription. There are no restrictions against the use of blood, blood products, or vaccines if advised by health care providers. Amputations, organ transplantation, biopsies, and circumcision are permitted if advised by health care providers.

Practices Related to Reproduction

BIRTH CONTROL

Baha'is believe that the fundamental purpose of marriage is the procreation of children. Individuals are encouraged to exercise their discretion in choosing a method of family planning. Baha'u'llah taught that to beget children is the highest physical fruit of man's existence. The Baha'i teachings imply that birth control constitutes a real danger to the foundations of social life. It is against the spirit of Baha'i law, which defines the primary purpose of marriage to be the rearing of children and their spiritual training. It is left to each husband and wife to decide how many children they will have. Baha'i teachings state that the soul appears at conception. Therefore, it is improper to use a method that produces an abortion after conception has taken place (e.g., intrauterine device). Methods that result in permanent sterility are not permissible under normal circumstances. If situations arise that justify sterilization (e.g., removal of cancerous reproductive organs), those called upon to make the decision would rely on the best medical advice available and their own consciences.

AMNIOCENTESIS

Amniocentesis is permitted if advised by health care providers.

ABORTION

Members are discouraged from using methods of contraception that produce abortion after conception has taken place (e.g., intrauterine device). A surgical operation for the purpose of preventing the birth of an unwanted child is strictly forbidden.

Baha'i teachings state that the human soul comes into being at conception. Abortion and surgical operations for the purpose of preventing the birth of unwanted children are forbidden unless circumstances justify such actions on medical grounds. In this case, the decision is left to the consciences of those concerned, who must carefully weigh the medical advice they receive in the light of the general guidance given in the Baha'i writings.

ARTIFICIAL INSEMINATION

Although there are no specific Baha'i writings on artificial insemination, Baha'is are guided by the understanding that marriage is the proper spiritual and physical context in which the bearing of children must occur. Couples who are unable to bear children are not excluded from marriage, because marriage has other purposes besides the bearing of children. The adoption of children is encouraged.

EUGENICS AND GENETICS

The Baha'is view scientific advancement as a noble and praiseworthy endeavor of humankind. Baha'i writings do not specifically address these two branches of science.

Religious Support System for the Sick

Individual members of local and surrounding communities assist and support one another in time of need. Religious titles are not used. Individual members of local communities look after the needs of the sick.

Practices Related to Death and Dying

Because human life is the vehicle for the development of the soul, Baha'is believe that life is unique and precious. The destruction of a human life at any stage, from conception to natural death, is rarely permissible. The question of when natural death has occurred is considered in the light of current medical science and legal rulings on the matter.

Autopsy is acceptable in the case of medical necessity or legal requirement. Baha'is are permitted to donate their bodies for medical research and for restorative purposes. Local burial laws are followed. Unless required by state law, Baha'i law states that the body is not to be embalmed. Cremation is forbidden. The place of burial must be within 1 hour's travel from the place of death. This regulation is always carried out in consultation with the family, and exceptions are possible.

•BUDDHIST CHURCHES OF AMERICA

Buddhism is a general term that indicates a belief in Buddha and encompasses many individual churches. In 1999, there were approximately 780,000 Buddhists in North America, and the worldwide membership was greater than 500 million.

The Buddhist Churches of America is the largest Buddhist organization in mainland United States. This group belongs to the largest subsect of Jodo Shinshu Buddhism (Shin Buddhism), Honpa Hongwanji, which is the largest traditional sect of Buddhism in Japan. The Jodo Shinshu sect was started by Shinran (1173–1263) in Japan; its headquarters are in Kyoto, Japan. The group of churches in Hawaii is a different organization of Shin Buddhism, called Honpa Hongwanji Mission of Hawaii. There are numerous Buddhist sects in the United States and Canada, including Indian, Sri Lankan, Vietnamese, Thai, Chinese, Japanese, Tibetan, and so on.

Buddhism was founded in the 6th century B.C. in northern India by Gautama Buddha. In the 3rd century B.C., Buddhism became the state religion of India and spread from there to most of the other Eastern nations. The term **Buddha** means "enlightened one."

At the beginning of the Christian era, Buddhism split into two main groups: Hinayana, or southern Buddhism, and Mahayana, or northern Buddhism. Hinayana retained more of the original teachings of Buddha and survived in Sri Lanka (formerly Ceylon) and southern Asia. Mahayana, a more social and polytheistic Buddhism, is strong in the Himalayas, Tibet, Mongolia, China, Korea, and Japan.

General Beliefs and Religious Practices

Buddha's original teachings included **Four Noble Truths** and the **Noble Eightfold Way**, the philosophies of which affect Buddhist responses to health and illness. The Four Noble Truths expound on suffering and constitute the foundation of Buddhism. The truths consist of (1) the truth of suffering, (2) the truth of the origin of suffering, (3) the truth that suffering can be destroyed, and (4) the way that leads to the cessation of pain.

The Noble Eightfold Way gives the rule of practical Buddhism, which consists of (1) right views, (2) right intention, (3) right speech, (4) right action, (5) right livelihood, (6) right effort, (7) right mindfulness, and (8) right concentration. **Nirvana**, a state of greater inner freedom and spontaneity, is the goal of all existence. When one achieves Nirvana, the mind has supreme tranquility, purity, and stability (Hinnell, 1984).

Although the ultimate goals of Buddhism are clear, the means of obtaining those goals are not religiously prescribed. Buddhism is not a dogmatic religion, nor does it dictate any specific practices. Individual differences are expected, acknowledged, and respected. Each individual is responsible for finding his or her own answers through awareness of the total situation.

Holy Days

In 2002, special holy days occur on January 1 (Temple day), February 12 (New Year 4700), March 20 (Spring Ohigon), March 31 (Kwan Yin Day), April 13–14 (Saka New Year), May 26 (Wesak), July 26 (Wassana), August 12 (Dharma Day), September 2 (Ullambana), September 22 (Fall Ohigon), October 2 (Parvarana and Founder's Day), and November 1 (Kathina) (Figure 14–4). Although there is no religious restriction for therapy on those days, they can be highly emotional, and a Buddhist patient should be consulted about his or her desires for medical or surgical intervention.

Figure 14–4. A Buddhist woman lights incense in remembrance of deceased ancestors during the Chinese New Year celebration

Sacraments

Buddhism does not have any sacraments. A ritual that symbolizes one's entry into the Buddhist faith is the expression of faith in the Three Treasures (Buddha, Dharma, and Sangha).

Diet

Moderation in diet is encouraged. Specific dietary practices are usually interconnected with ethnic practices.

Health Care Practices

Buddhists do not believe in healing through a faith or through faith itself. However, Buddhists do believe that spiritual peace, and liberation from anxiety by adherence to and achievement of awakening to Buddha's wisdom, can be important factors in promoting healing and recovery.

Medical and Surgical Interventions

There are no prescriptions in Buddhism for nutritional therapies, medications, vaccines, and other therapeutic interventions. Buddha's teaching on the Middle Path may apply here; he taught that extremes should be avoided. What may be medicine to one may be poison to another, so generalizations are to be avoided. Medications should be used in accordance with the nature of the illness and the capacity of the individual. Whatever will contribute to the attainment of Enlightenment is encouraged. Treatments such as amputations, organ transplants, biopsies, and other procedures that may prolong life and allow the individual to attain Enlightenment are encouraged.

Practices Related to Reproduction

The immediate emphasis is on the person living now and the attainment of Enlightenment. If practicing birth control or having an amniocentesis or sterility test will help the individual attain Enlightenment, it is acceptable.

Buddhism does not condone the taking of a life. The first of Buddha's Five Precepts is abstention from taking lives. Life in all forms is to be respected. Existence by itself often contradicts this principle (e.g., drugs that kill bacteria are given to spare a patient's life). With this in mind, it is the conditions and circumstances surrounding the patient that determine whether abortion, therapeutic or on demand, may be undertaken.

Religious Support System for the Sick

Buddhist priests often offer support to the ill client. Support of the sick is more of an individual practice in keeping with the philosophy of Buddhism.

Practices Related to Death and Dying

If there is hope for recovery and continuation of the pursuit of Enlightenment, all available means of support are encouraged. If life cannot be prolonged so that the person can continue to search for Enlightenment, conditions might permit euthanasia. If the donation of a body part will help another continue the quest for Enlightenment, it might be an act of mercy and is encouraged. The body is considered but a shell; therefore, autopsy and disposal of the body are matters of individual practice rather than of religious prescription. Burials are usually a brief graveside service after a funeral at the temple. Cremations are common (Chapman, 1991).

Addendum

The headquarters of the Buddhist Churches of America are at 1710 Octavia Street, San Francisco, California 94109 (Telephone: [415] 776-5600). Additional material is available at the Buddhist Bookstore of the Buddhist Churches of America Headquarters. Information on Buddhism and temple locations in Canada can be found at http://buddhismcanada.com/

• CATHOLICISM (ACCORDING TO THE ROMAN RITE)

With a North American membership of approximately 96 million and a worldwide membership of more than 1 billion, some 32 rites exist within **Catholicism**. Of these, the Roman Rite is the major body.

General Beliefs and Religious Practices

The Roman Catholic Church traces its beginnings to about A.D. 30, when Jesus Christ is believed to have founded the church. Catholic teachings, based on the Bible, are found in declarations of church councils and Popes and in short statements of faith called creeds. The oldest and most authoritative of these creeds are the Apostle's Creed and the Nicene Creed, the latter being recited during the central act of worship, called the **Eucharistic Liturgy**, or Mass. The creeds summarize Catholic beliefs concerning the Trinity and creation, sin and salvation, the nature of the church, and life after death.

Holy Days

Catholics are expected to observe all Sundays (including Easter Sunday) as holy days. Sunday or holy day worship services may be conducted any time from 4:00 PM on Saturday until Sunday evening. Other days are set aside for special liturgical observance are: Christmas (December 25th), Solemnity of Mary, Mother of God (January 1st), Ascension Thursday (the Lord's ascension bodily into Heaven, observed 40 days after Easter), Feast of the Assumption (August 15th), All Saints Day (November 1st), and the Feast of the Immaculate Conception (December 8th).

Sacraments

The Roman Catholic Church recognizes seven sacraments: Baptism, Reconciliation (formerly Penance or Confession), Holy Communion or the Eucharist (Figure 14–5), Confirmation, Matrimony, Holy Orders, and Anointing of the Sick (formerly Extreme Unction).

Figure 14–5. In the Roman Catholic tradition, when children reach the age of reason (about 7 years), they continue the ongoing initiation into their religion by making their First Communion. In addition to the religious ritual, there are sometimes cultural traditions surronding this event, many of which involve a family celebration after the religious services have concluded.

Diet (Foods and Beverages)

The goods of the world have been given for use and benefit. The primary obligation people have toward foods and beverages is to use them in moderation and in such a way that they are not injurious to health. **Fasting** in moderation is recommended as a valued discipline. There are a few days of the year when Catholics have an obligation to fast, which means to abstain from meat and meat products. Catholics fast and abstain on Ash Wednesday and Good Friday, and abstinence is required on all of the Fridays of Lent. The sick are never bound by this prescription of the law. Healthy persons between the ages of 18 and 62 are encouraged to engage in fasting and abstinence as described.

Social Activities (Dating, Dancing)

The major principle is that Sunday is a day of rest; therefore, only unnecessary servile work is prohibited. The 7 holy days are also considered days of rest, although many persons must engage in routine work-related activities on some of these days.

Substance Use

Alcohol and tobacco are not evil per se. They are to be used in moderation and not in a way that would be injurious to one's health or that of another party. The misuse of any substance is not only harmful to the body but also sinful.

Health Care Practices

In time of illness, the basic rite is the **Sacrament of the Sick**, which includes anointing of the sick, communion if possible, and a blessing by a priest. Prayers are frequently offered for the sick person and for members of the family. The Eucharistic wafer (a small unleavened wafer made of flour and water) is often given to the sick as the food of healing and health. Other family members may participate if they wish to do so.

Medical and Surgical Interventions

As long as the benefits outweigh the risk to the individuals, judicious use of medications is permissible and morally acceptable. A major concern is the risk of mutilation. The Church has traditionally cited the **principle of totality**, which states that medications are allowed as long as they are used for the good of the whole person. Blood, blood products, and amputations are acceptable if consistent with the principle of totality. Biopsies and circumcision are also permissible.

The transplantation of organs from living donors is morally permissible when the anticipated benefit to the recipient is proportionate to the harm done to the donor, provided that the loss of such an organ does not deprive the donor of life itself or of the functional integrity of his or her body.

Practices Related to Reproduction

BIRTH CONTROL

The basic principle is that the conjugal act should be one that is love-giving and potentially life-giving. Only natural means of contraception, such as abstinence, the temperature method, and the ovulation method are acceptable. Ordinarily, artificial aids and procedures for permanent sterilization are forbidden. Birth control (anovulants) may be used therapeutically to assist in regulating the menstrual cycle.

AMNIOCENTESIS

The procedure in and of itself is not objectionable. However, it is morally objectionable if the findings of the amniocentesis are used to lead the couple to decide on termination of the pregnancy or if the procedure injures the fetus.

ABORTION

Direct abortion is always morally wrong. Indirect abortion may be morally justified by some circumstances (e.g., treatment of a cancerous uterus in a pregnant woman). Abortion on demand is prohibited. The Roman Catholic Church teaches the sanctity of all human life, even of the unborn, from the time of conception.

STERILITY TESTS AND ARTIFICIAL INSEMINATION

The use of sterility tests for the purpose of promoting conception, not misusing sexuality, is permitted. Although artificial insemination has been debated heavily, traditionally it has been looked on as illicit, even between husband and wife.

EUGENICS, GENETICS, AND STEM CELL RESEARCH

Research in the fields of eugenics and genetics is objectionable. This violates the moral right of the individual to be free from experimentation and also interferes with God's right as master of life and human beings' stewardship of their lives. Some genetic investigations to help determine genetic diseases may be used, depending on their ends and means. There is support for research using adult stem cells, but opposition for the use of embryonic stem cells.

Religious Support System for the Sick

VISITORS

Although a priest, deacon, or lay minister usually visits a sick person alone, the family or other significant people may be invited to join in prayer. In fact, that is most desirable, since they too need support.

The priest, deacon, or lay minister will usually bring the necessary supplies for administration of the Eucharist or administration of the Sacrament of the Sick (in the case of a priest). The nursing staff can facilitate these rites by ensuring an atmosphere of prayer and quiet and by having a glass of water on hand (in case the patient is unable to swallow the small wafer-like host). Consecrated wine can be made available but is usually not given in the hospital or home. The nurse may wish to join in the prayer. Candles may be used if the patient is not receiving oxygen. The priest, deacon, or lay minister will usually appreciate any information pertaining to the patient's ability to swallow. Any other information the nurse believes may help the priest or deacon respond to the patient with more care and effectiveness would be appreciated.

Catholic lay persons of either sex may visit hospitalized or homebound elderly or sick persons. Although they may not administer the Sacrament of the Sick or the Sacrament of Reconciliation, they may bring Holy Communion (the Eucharist).

TITLE OF RELIGIOUS REPRESENTATIVE

The titles of religious representatives include Father (priest), Mr. or Deacon (deacon), Sister (Catholic woman who has taken religious vows), and Brother (Catholic man who has taken religious vows).

ENVIRONMENT DURING VISIT BY RELIGIOUS REPRESENTATIVE

Privacy is most conducive to prayer and to the administration of the sacraments. In emergencies, such as cardiac or respiratory arrest, medical personnel will need to be present. The priest will use an abbreviated form of the rite and will not interfere with the activities of the health care team.

CHURCH ORGANIZATIONS TO ASSIST THE SICK

Most major cities have outreach programs for the sick, handicapped, and elderly. More serious needs are usually handled by **Catholic Charities** and other agencies in the community or on the local parish level. Organizations such as the St. Vincent DePaul Society may provide material support for the poor and needy as well as some counseling services, depending on the location. In the United States, the Catholic Church owns and operates hospitals, extended care facilities, orphanages, maternity homes, hospices, and other health care facilities. Although the majority of tertiary care facilities in Canada are publicly owned, many such institutions are strongly influenced by the leadership of the Catholic Church and its members. It is usually best to consult the pastor or chaplain in specific cases for local resources.

Practices Related to Death and Dying

PROLONGATION OF LIFE (RIGHT TO DIE)

Members are obligated to take ordinary means of preserving life (e.g., intravenous medication) but are not obligated to take extraordinary means. What constitutes extraordinary means may vary with biomedical and technologic advances and with the availability of these advances to the average citizen. Other factors that must be considered include the degree of pain associated with the procedure, the potential outcome, the condition of the patient, economic factors, and the patient's or family's preferences.

EUTHANASIA

Direct action to end the life of patients is not permitted. Extraordinary means may be withheld, allowing the patient to die of natural causes.

AUTOPSY AND DONATION OF BODY

This is permissible as long as the corpse is shown proper respect and there is sufficient reason for doing the autopsy. The principle of totality suggests that this is justifiable, being for the betterment of the person who does the giving.

DISPOSAL OF BODY AND BURIAL

Ordinarily, bodies are buried. Cremation is acceptable in certain circumstances, such as to avoid spreading a contagious disease. Because life is considered sacred, the body should be treated with respect. Any disposal of the body should be done in a respectful and honorable way.

• CHRISTIAN SCIENCE (CHURCH OF CHRIST, SCIENTIST)

Christian Science accepts physical and moral healing as a natural part of the Christian experience. Members believe that God acts through universal, immutable, spiritual law. They hold that genuine spiritual or Christian healing through prayer differs radically from the use of suggestion, willpower, and all forms of psychotherapy, which are based on the use of the human mind as a curative agent. In emphasizing the practical importance of a fuller understanding of Jesus' works and teachings, Christian Science believes healing to be a natural result of drawing closer to God in one's thinking and living. The church does not keep membership data; there are 3,000 congregations worldwide.

General Beliefs and Religious Practices

Holy Days

Besides the usual weekly day of worship (Sunday), other traditional Christian holidays are observed on an individual basis. Worldwide, Wednesday evenings are observed as times for members to gather for testimony meetings.

Sacraments

Although sacraments in a strictly spiritual sense have deep meaning for Christian Scientists, there are no outward observances or ceremonies. Baptism and holy communion are not outward observances but deeply meaningful inner experiences. Baptism is the daily purification and spiritualization of thought, and communion is finding one's conscious unity with God through prayer (Christian Science Publishing Society, 1994).

Social Activities (Dating, Dancing) and Substance Use

Members are encouraged to be honest, truthful, and moral in their behavior. Although every effort is made to preserve marriages, divorce is recognized. The Christian Science Sunday School teaches young people how to make their religion practical in daily life as related to school studies, social life, sports, and family relationships. Members abstain from alcohol and tobacco; some abstain from tea and coffee.

Health Care Practices

Viewed as a by-product of drawing closer to God, healing is considered proof of God's care and one element in the full salvation at which Christianity aims. Christian Science teaches that faith must rest not on blind belief but on an understanding of the present perfection of God's spiritual creation. This is one of the crucial differences between Christian Science and **faith healing** (Christian Science Publishing Society, 1994).

The practice of Christian Science healing starts from the Biblical basis that God created the universe and human beings "and made them perfect." Christian Science holds that human imperfection, including physical illness and sin, reflects a fundamental misunderstanding of creation and is therefore subject to healing through prayer and spiritual regeneration.

An individual who is seeking healing may turn to Christian Science practitioners, members of the denomination who devote their full time to the healing ministry in the broadest sense. In cases requiring continued care, nurses grounded in the Christian Science faith provide care in facilities accredited by the mother church, the First Church of Christ, Scientist, in Boston, Massachusetts. Individuals may also receive such care in their own homes. Christian Science nurses are trained to perform the practical duties a patient may need while also providing an atmosphere of warmth and love that supports the healing process. No medication is given, and physical application is limited to the normal measures associated with hygiene. *The Christian Science Journal,* a monthly publication, contains a directory of qualified Christian Science practitioners and nurses throughout the world.

Before they can be recognized and advertised in *The Christian Science Journal,* practitioners must have instruction from an authorized teacher of Christian Science and provide substantial evidence of their experience in healing. There are some 4,000 Christian Science practitioners throughout the world. Practitioners who speak other languages may also be listed in appropriate editions of *The Herald of Christian Science,* which is published in 12 languages.

The denomination has no clergy. Practitioners are thus lay members of the Church of Christ, Scientist, and do not conduct public worship services or rituals. Their ministry is not an office within the church structure but is carried out on an individual basis with those who seek their help through prayer. Both members and nonmembers are welcome to contact practitioners by telephone, by letter, or in person for help or for information.

Christian Science practitioners are supported not by the church but by payments from their patients. Their ministry is not restricted to local congregations but extends worldwide. Many insurance companies include coverage of payments to practitioners and Christian Science nursing facilities in their policies. In spite of such superficial resemblances to the health care professions, the work of Christian Science practitioners involves a deeply religious vocation, not simply alternative health care. Practitioners do not use medical or psychologic techniques.

The term *healing* applies to the entire spectrum of human fears, griefs, wants, and sin as well as to physical ills. Practitioners are called upon to give

Christian Science treatment not only in cases of physical disease and emotional disturbance but also in family and financial difficulties, business problems, questions of employment, schooling problems, theological confusion, and so forth. The purpose of prayer, or Christian Science treatment, is to deal with these interrelated and complex problems of establishing God's law of harmony in every aspect of life. When healings are accomplished through perception and living of spiritual truth, they are effective and permanent. Physical healing is often the manifestation of a moral and spiritual change (Christian Science Publishing Society, 1978, 1994).

Ordinarily, a Christian Science practitioner and a physician are not employed in the same case, because the two approaches to healing differ so radically. During childbirth, however, an obstetrician or qualified midwife is involved. Since bone setting may be accomplished without medication, a physician is also employed for repair of fractures if the patient requests this medical intervention. In cases of contagious or infectious disease, Christian Scientists observe the legal requirements for reporting and quarantining affected individuals. The denomination recognizes public health concerns and has a long history of responsible cooperation with public health officials.

Christian Scientists are not arbitrarily opposed to doctors. They are always free to make their own decisions regarding treatment in any given situation. They generally choose to rely on spiritual healing because they have seen its effectiveness in the experience of their own families and fellow church members—experience that goes back over 100 years and in many families for three or four generations. Where medical treatment for minor children is required by law, Christian Scientists strictly adhere to the requirement. At the same time, they maintain that their substantial healing record needs to be seriously considered in determining the rights of Christian Scientists to rely on spiritual healing for themselves and their children. They do not ignore or neglect disease, but they seek to heal it by the means they believe to be most efficacious.

Medical and Surgical Procedures

Christian Scientists ordinarily do not use medications. Immunizations and vaccines are acceptable only when required by law. Ordinarily, members do not use blood or blood components. A Christian Scientist who has lost a limb might seek to have it replaced with a prosthesis. Christian Scientists are unlikely to seek transplants and are unlikely to act as donors. Christian Scientists do not normally seek biopsies or any sort of physical examination. Circumcision is considered an individual matter.

Practices Related to Reproduction

Matters of family planning (i.e., birth control) are left to individual judgment. Because abortion involves medication and surgical intervention, it is normally considered incompatible with Christian Science. Artificial insemination is unusual among Christian Scientists. Christian Scientists are opposed to programs in the field of eugenics and genetics.

Religious Support System for the Sick

As discussed previously, Christian Scientists have their own nurses and practitioners. No special religious titles are used. Although each branch church elects two Readers for Sunday and Wednesday services, Christian Scientists are a church of laymen and laywomen. Organizations to assist the sick include Benevolent Homes staffed by Christian Science nurses, and visiting home nurse services.

Practices Related to Death and Dying

A Christian Science family is unlikely to seek medical means to prolong life indefinitely. Family members pray earnestly for the recovery of a person as long as the person remains alive.

Euthanasia is contrary to the teachings of Christian Science. Most Christian Scientists believe that they can make their particular contribution to the health of society and of their loved ones in ways other than donation of the body. Disposal of the body is left to the individual family to decide. The individual family decides the form of burial and burial service.

Addendum

A wide variety of books and journals are published by the Christian Science Publishing Society, Boston, Massachusetts. Most major cities have Christian Science Reading Rooms, which carry these publications and which are staffed by church members, who are available to provide additional information.

• THE CHURCH OF JESUS CHRIST OF LATTER-DAY SAINTS (MORMONISM)

The Church of Jesus Christ of Latter-Day Saints, commonly known as Mormonism, is a Christian religion established in the United States in the early 1800s. North American membership in 2001 was approximately 8 million, and the worldwide membership was 11.1 million.

General Beliefs and Religious Practices

Holy Days/Special Days

Sunday is the day observed as the Sabbath in the United States. In other parts of the world the Sabbath may be observed on a different day; in Israel, for example, Mormons observe the Sabbath on Saturday.

Sacraments

Sacraments are commonly called **ordinances**.

Ordinances of Salvation

1. Baptism at the age of accountability (8 years or after); never performed in infancy or at death; always by immersion
2. Confirmation at the time of baptism to receive the gift of the Holy Ghost

3. Partaking of the sacrament of the Lord's Supper at weekly Sunday sacrament meetings
4. Endowments*
5. Celestial Marriage*
6. Vicarious ordinances*

Ordinances of Comfort, Consolation, and Encouragement

1. Blessing of babies
2. Blessing of the sick
3. Consecration of oil for use in blessing of the sick
4. Patriarchal blessings
5. Dedication of graves

After being deemed worthy to go to a temple, a Mormon will wear a special type of underclothing, called a **garment**. In a health care setting, the garment may be removed to facilitate care. As soon as the individual is well, he or she is likely to want to wear the garment again. An elderly person may not wish to part with the garment in the hospital. The garment has special significance to the person, symbolizing covenants or promises the person has made to God.

Diet

Mormons have a strict dietary code called the **Word of Wisdom**. This code prohibits all alcoholic beverages (including beer and wine), hot drinks (i.e., tea and coffee, although not herbal tea), tobacco in any form, and any illegal or recreational drugs.

Fasting to a Mormon means no food or drink (including water), usually for 24 hours. Fasting is required once a month on the designated fast Sunday. Pregnant women, the very young, the very old, and the ill are not required to fast. The purpose of fasting is to bring oneself closer to God by controlling physical needs. The person is expected to donate the price of what has not been eaten to the church to be used to care for the poor.

Social Activities (Dating, Dancing)

The Mormon Church has a wide variety of activities for its youth and encourages group activities until young people are at least 16. Young men are highly encouraged to perform missions for the church for 2 years at their own expense, beginning at the age of 19 years. Women may go on missions when they are 21, but marriage is more strongly emphasized for them.

Substance Use

Alcohol, caffeinated beverages (such as tea, coffee, and soda), and tobacco are forbidden. In recent years, "recreational drugs" and nonmedically indicated sedatives and narcotics have also been considered forbidden substances.

*These ordinances occur in temples. Temples are sacred places of worship that are accessible only to observant Mormons, who are "worthy" to enter them as deemed by their local religious leaders.

Health Care Practices

Mormons believe that the power of God can be exercised on their behalf to bring about healing at a time of illness. The ritual of blessing the sick consists of one member (Elder) of the priesthood (male) anointing the ill person with oil and a second Elder "sealing the anointing with a prayer and a blessing." Commonly, both Elders place their hands on the individual's head. Faith in Jesus Christ and in the power of the priesthood to heal, requisite to the healing use of priesthood, does not preclude medical intervention but is seen as an adjunct to it. Mormons believe that medical intervention is one of God's ways of using humans in the healing process.

Medical and Surgical Procedures

There is no restriction on the use of medications or vaccines in Mormon Church doctrine. It is not uncommon to find many members of the Mormon Church using herbal folk remedies, and it is wise to explore in detail what an individual may already have done or taken. There is no restriction on the use of blood or blood components.

Surgical intervention is a matter of individual decision in cases of amputations, transplants, and organ donations (of both donor and recipient). Biopsies and resultant surgical procedures are also a matter of individual choice. The circumcision of infants is viewed as a medical health promotion measure and is not a religious ritual.

Practices Related to Reproduction

BIRTH CONTROL

According to Mormon belief, one of the major purposes of life is procreation; therefore, any form of prevention of the birth of children is contrary to church teachings. Exceptions to this policy include ill health of the mother or father and genetic defects that could be passed on to offspring.

AMNIOCENTESIS

Amniocentesis is a matter of individual choice. However, even if the fetus is found to be deformed, abortion is not an option unless the mother's life is in danger.

ABORTION

Abortion is forbidden in all cases except when the mother's life is in danger. Even in these circumstances, abortion is looked upon favorably only if the local priesthood authorities, after fasting and prayer, receive divine confirmation that the abortion is acceptable.

In the event of pregnancy resulting from rape, the church position is that the child should be born and put up for adoption if necessary, rather than be aborted. The final decision rests with the mother. No official church sanction is used if she chooses to abort the child. Abortion on demand is strictly forbidden.

STERILITY/FERTILITY TESTING AND ARTIFICIAL INSEMINATION

Because bearing children is so important, all measures that can be taken to promote having children are acceptable. Artificial insemination is acceptable if the semen is from the husband.

Religious Support System for the Sick

VISITORS

Mormonism has a highly organized network, and many church representatives are likely to visit a hospitalized member, including the bishop and two counselors (leaders of the local congregation), home teachers (two men assigned to visit the family each month), and visiting teachers (two women assigned to visit the female head of household each month). Friends within the local congregation can also be expected to visit.

TITLE OF RELIGIOUS REPRESENTATIVE

Various titles are used for members of the Mormon hierarchy. The term *Elder* is generally acceptable regardless of a man's position, and the term *Sister* is acceptable for women.

ENVIRONMENT NEEDED FOR HEALTH-RELATED RITUALS

To perform a blessing of the sick, the Elders performing the blessing need privacy and, if possible, quiet. They generally bring a vial of consecrated oil with which to anoint the person. If they plan to perform a Sacrament of the Lord's Supper, they usually bring what they need with them. Bread and water are used for this ordinance.

CHURCH ORGANIZATIONS TO ASSIST THE SICK

The Relief Society is the Mormon organization for helping members. It is organized by the women of the church, who work closely with priesthood leaders to determine the general needs of members, including use of the church-run welfare organization. Church members who are in need may receive local help, such as child care when parents are ill or hospitalized and money for medical expenses.

Practices Related to Death and Dying

Whenever possible, medical science and faith healing are used to reverse conditions that threaten life. When death is inevitable, the effort is to promote a peaceful and dignified death. Mormons firmly believe that life continues beyond death and that the dead are reunited with loved ones; therefore, the belief is that death is another step in eternal progression (Green, 1992a; 1992b).

Euthanasia is not acceptable because Mormons believe that life and death are in the hands of God, and humans must not interfere in any way. Autopsy is permitted with the consent of the next of kin and within local laws. Organ donation is permitted; it is an individual decision. Cremation is discouraged but not forbidden; burial is customary. A local priesthood member dedicates the graves.

• HINDUISM

The **Hindu** religion may be the oldest religion in the world. There are over 1.4 billion Hindus worldwide, with a North American following of approximately 1.3 million members.

General Beliefs and Religious Practices

No common creed or doctrine binds Hindus together. There is complete freedom of belief. One may be monotheistic, polytheistic, or atheistic. The major distinguishing characteristic is the social caste system.

The religion of Hinduism is founded on sacred, written scripture called the **Vedas**. **Brahman** is the principle and source of the universe and the center from which all things proceed and to which all things return. **Reincarnation** is a central belief in Hinduism. The law of **karma** determines life. According to karma, rebirth is dependent on moral behavior in a previous stage of existence. Life on earth is transient and a burden. The goal of existence is liberation from the cycle of rebirth and redeath and entrance into what in Buddhism is called nirvana (a state of extinction of passion).

The practice of Hinduism consists of roles and ceremonies performed within the framework of the **caste system**. These rituals focus on the main socioreligious events of birth, marriage, and death. Hindu temples are dwelling places for deities to which people bring offerings. There are numerous places for religious pilgrimage.

Holy Days (based on a lunar calendar)

1. Purnima (day of full moon)
2. Janamasthtmi (birthday of Lord Krishna)
3. Ramnavmi (birthday of Rama)
4. Shivratri (birth of Lord Shiva)
5. Naurate (nine holy days occurring twice a year; in about April and October)
6. Dussehra
7. Diwali
8. Holi

Diet, Social Activities (Dating, Dancing), and Substance Use

The eating of meat is forbidden because it involves harming a living creature. Social activities are strictly limited by the caste system. Substance use is not restricted.

Health Care Practices

Some Hindus believe in faith healing; others believe illness is God's way of punishing people for their sins.

Medical and Surgical Procedures

The use of medications, blood, and blood components is acceptable. Persons who lose a limb are not outcasts from society. Loss of a limb is considered to be caused by "sins of a previous life." Organ transplantations are acceptable for both donors and recipients.

Practices Related to Reproduction

All types of birth control are acceptable. Amniocentesis is acceptable, although not often available. No Hindu policy exists on abortion, either therapeutic or on demand. Artificial insemination is not restricted, but it is not often practiced because of lack of availability.

Religious Support System for the Sick

Religious representatives use the title of priest. Church organizations to assist the sick do not exist; family and friends within the caste provide help.

Practices Related to Death and Dying

No religious customs or restrictions related to the prolongation of life exist. Life is seen as a perpetual cycle, and death is considered as just one more step toward nirvana. Euthanasia is not practiced. Autopsy is acceptable. The donation of body or parts is also acceptable.

Cremation is the most common form of body disposal. Ashes are collected and disposed of in holy rivers. The fetus or newborn is sometimes buried.

• ISLAM

Islam is a monotheistic religion founded between 610 and 632 A.D. by the prophet Muhammad. Derived from an Arabic word meaning "submission," *Islam* literally translated means "submission to the will of God." A follower of Islam is called **Moslem** or **Muslim**, which means "one who submits." The current North American membership is 3.6 million, and the worldwide membership is 1.78 billion.

Muhammad, revered as the prophet of **Allah** (God), is seen as succeeding and completing both Judaism and Christianity. Good deeds will be rewarded at the last Judgment, whereas evil deeds will be punished in hell.

General Beliefs and Religious Practices

Pillars of Faith

Islam has five essential practices, or **Pillars of Faith**. These are (1) the profession of faith (*shahada*), which requires bearing witness to one true God and acknowledging Muhammad as his messenger; (2) ritual prayer five times daily at dawn, noon, afternoon, sunset, and night, facing Mecca, Saudi Arabia, Islam's holiest city (*salat*); (3) almsgiving (*zakat*) to the needy, reflecting the Koran's admonition to share what one has with those less fortunate, including widows, orphans, homeless persons, and the poor; (4) **fasting** from dawn until sunset throughout Ramadan during the ninth month of the Islamic lunar calendar; and (5) making a pilgrimage to Mecca at least once during one's lifetime (*hajj*).

Sources of Faith

The sources of the Islamic faith are the **Qur'an** (Koran), which is regarded as the uncreated and eternal Word of God, and **Hadith** (tradition), regarded as sayings and deeds of the prophet Muhammad. All Muslims recognize the existence of the sharia and the five categories into which it divides human conduct: required, encouraged, permissible, discouraged, and prohibited.

Sects of Islam

Various sects of Islam have developed. When Muhammad died, a dispute arose over the leadership of the Muslim community. One faction, the *Sunni,* derived from the Arabic word for "tradition," felt that the caliph, or successor of Muhammad, should be chosen as Arab chiefs customarily are: by election. Therefore, they supported the succession of the first four (the "rightly guided") caliphs who had been Muhammad's companions. The other group maintained that Muhammad chose his cousin and son-in-law, Ali, as his spiritual and secular heir and that succession should be through his bloodline. In 680 A.D., one of Ali's sons, Hussein, led a band of rebels against the ruling caliph. In the course of the battle Hussein was killed, and with his death began the *Shi'a,* sometimes called the Shi'ite movement, whose name comes from the word meaning "partisans of Ali." The Shi'a and the Sunni are the two major branches of Muslims; the Sunni constitute about 85% of the total. The Sunni are found in Lebanon, the West Bank, Jordan, and throughout Africa, whereas the Shi'a are in Iran, Iraq, Yemen, Afghanistan, and Pakistan. The Shi'a and the Sunni also have different rituals, practices, and structural and political orientations.

Holidays, Special Observances, and Sacraments

Days of observance in Islam are not "holy" days but days of celebration or observance. The Muslims follow a lunar calendar, so the days of observance change yearly.

Each Muslim observance has its own significance. They are listed here in the same order in which they occur in the Muslim lunar calendar, and their standard Arabic names are used. However, the Arabic spellings for the names of the holidays may vary, or local names may be used.

Muharam 1 Rasal-Sana (or New Year): The first day of the first month, celebrated much the same as the first day of the year is celebrated throughout the world.

Muharam 10 Ashura (the 10th of the first month): A religious holiday through which pious Muslims may fast from dawn to sunset. For Shi'ite Muslims, this is a special day of sorrow commemorating the assassination of the prophet's grandson, Hussein.

Rabi'i 12 Maulid al-Nabi: The birthday of the prophet Muhammad. In some regions this holiday goes on for many days; it is a time of festivities and exchanging of gifts.

Rajab 27 Lailat al-Isra wa al Miraj (literally, "The Night of the Journey and Ascent"): Commemorates Muhammad's night journey from Mecca to the al-Aqsa mosque in Jerusalem and his ascent to heaven and return on the same night.

Sh'ban 14: This is the 14th night of the 8th month of Sh'ban. It is widely celebrated by pious Muslims and is sometimes called the Night of Repentance. It is treated in many parts of the Muslim world as a New Year's celebration.

Ramadan (the ninth month of the Muslim year): This entire month is devoted to meditation and spiritual purification through self-discipline. It is a period of abstinence from eating, drinking, smoking, and sexual relations. The fast is an obligation practiced by Muslims throughout the world unless they are old, infirm, traveling, or pregnant. The fast is from sunup to sundown, at which time a meal (*iftar*) is taken.

Ramadan 27 Lailat al-Qadir (next to the last night of the fasting month): This is simply called the Night of Power and Greatness, and it is by custom a very special holy time. It commemorates the time when revelation was first given to Muhammad.

Shawwal 1 "Id ad-Fitr": This is called the Lesser Feast because it begins immediately after the month-long Ramadan feast. It is perhaps Islam's most joyous festival, marking as it does the month of abstinence and the cleansing of the believer. It usually lasts for 2 or 3 days. Families and friends visit one another's homes, new clothes and presents are exchanged, and sweet pastries are a favorite treat.

Dhu al-Hijjah 1–10: Muslims, if they are able, are obliged to undertake a pilgrimage to Mecca at least once in their lifetime. This journey, called the Hajj, is performed during the last month of the Muslim calendar, Dhu al-Hijjah.

Dhu al-Hijjah 10: All Muslims, whether they are on the pilgrimage or at home, participate in the feast of the sacrifice, Id al-Adha, which marks the end of the Hajj on the tenth of Dhu al-Hijjah. The feast is the Feast of the Sacrifice, called the Greater Feast, and is observed by the slaughtering of animals and distribution of the meat. In some places this is done individually. The meat is shared equally among the family and the poor. Sometimes the slaughtering takes place in public areas, and the meat is then distributed.

Sacraments are not observed.

Diet and Substance Use

Eating pork and drinking alcoholic or other intoxicating beverages are strictly prohibited. In all cases, moderation in one's life is expected. Some Muslims consume meat that has been ritually slaughtered by the process called **halal**, which means "the lawful or that which is permitted by Allah."

Fasting during the month of Ramadan is one of the pillars of Islam. Children (boys 7 years old, girls 9 years old) and adults are required to fast. Pregnant women, nursing mothers, the elderly, and anyone whose physical condition is so fragile that a physician recommends not fasting, are exempt from fasting but are expected to fast later in the year or to feed a poor person to make up for the unfasted Ramadan days.

Health Care Practices

Faith healing is not acceptable unless the psychologic health and morale of the patient are deteriorating. At that time, faith healing may be used to supplement the physician's efforts.

Medical and Surgical Procedures

There are no restrictions on medications. Even items normally forbidden (e.g., pork derivatives) are permitted if prescribed as medicine. The use of blood and blood components is not restricted. Amputations are not restricted. Organ transplantations are acceptable for both donor and recipient. Biopsies are acceptable. No age limit is fixed, but circumcision is practiced on boys at an early age. For adult converts, it is not obligatory, although it is sometimes practiced.

Practices Related to Reproduction

BIRTH CONTROL

All types of birth control are generally acceptable in accordance with the law of "what is harmful to the body is prohibited." The family physician's advice on method of contraception is required. The husband and wife should agree on the method.

AMNIOCENTESIS

Amniocentesis is available in many Islamic countries. "Progressive" doctors and expectant parents use amniocentesis only to determine the status of the fetus, not the sex of the child; this is left in the hands of God.

ABORTION

No official policy on abortion, either therapeutic or on demand, exists. There is a strong religious objection to abortion, which is based on Muhammad's condemnation of the ancient Arabian practice of burying unwanted newborn girls alive.

ARTIFICIAL INSEMINATION, EUGENICS, AND GENETICS

Artificial insemination is permitted only if from the husband to his own wife. No official policy exists on practices in the fields of eugenics and genetics. Different Islamic schools of thought accept differing opinions.

Religious Support System for the Sick

In Islam, care of the physical body is not regarded highly. In many wealthy, oil-rich Middle Eastern nations, expatriates are hired to staff hospitals and provide for health care. Even in the United States, care of the sick does not resemble the Catholic corporal work of mercy or the Jewish mitzvah. Islamic clerics, called *imams,* may provide guidance that could be helpful for emotional and psychologic disorders. Formal, organized support systems to assist the sick do not exist; family and friends provide emotional and financial support.

Practices Related to Death and Dying

The right to die is not recognized in Islam. Any attempt to shorten one's life or terminate it (suicide or otherwise) is prohibited. Euthanasia is thus not acceptable. Autopsy is permitted only for medical and legal purposes. The donation of body parts or body is acceptable, without restrictions.

Burial of the dead, including fetuses, is compulsory. It is important in Islam to follow prescribed burial procedures. Under conditions that cause fragmentation of the body, sections of the burial ritual may be omitted. The burial procedure consists of five steps:

1. Ghasl El Mayyet: Rinsing and washing of the dead body according to Muslim tradition. Muslim women cleanse a woman's body; Muslim men, a man's body.
2. Muslin: After being washed three times, the body is wrapped in three pieces of clean white cloth. The Muslim word for "coffin" is the same as that for "muslin."
3. Salat El Mayyet: Special prayers for the dead are required.
4. The body should be processed and buried as soon as possible. The body should always be buried so that the head faces toward Mecca.
5. Burial of a fetus: Before a gestational age of 130 days, a fetus is treated like any other discarded tissue. After 130 days, the fetus is considered a fully developed human being and must be treated as such.

• JEHOVAH'S WITNESSES

North American membership of the **Jehovah's Witnesses** is 1,099,644; worldwide membership is 6,035,564.

General Beliefs and Religious Practices

Many North Americans have at one time or another encountered ministers of the **Watch Tower Bible and Tract Society**, known as Jehovah's Witnesses. The name Jehovah's Witnesses (the name that members prefer) is derived from the Hebrew name for God (**Jehovah**) according to the King James Bible. Thus, Jehovah's Witnesses is a descriptive name, indicating that members profess to bear witness concerning Jehovah, his Godship, and his purposes. Every Bible student devotes approximately 10 hours or more each month to proselytizing activities.

Holy Days and Sacraments

Although Witnesses do not celebrate Christmas, Easter, or other traditional Christian holy days, a special observance of the Lord's Supper is held.

Witnesses and others may attend this important meeting, but only those numbered among the 144,000 chosen members (Revelation 7:4) may partake of the bread and wine as a symbol of the death of Christ and the dedication to God. This memorial of Christ's death should take place on the day corresponding to Nisa 14 of the Jewish calendar, which occurs some time in March or April. These elite members will be raised with spiritual bodies (without flesh, bones, or blood) and will assist Christ in ruling the universe. Others who benefit from Christ's ransom will be resurrected with healthy, perfected physical bodies (bodies of flesh, bones, and blood) and will inhabit this earth after the world has been restored to a paradisiacal state. Sacraments are not observed.

Social Activities (Dating, Dancing) and Substance Use

Youth are encouraged to socialize with members of their own religious background. Members abstain from the use of tobacco and hold that drunkenness is a serious sin. Alcohol used in moderation, however, is acceptable.

Health Care Practices

The practice of faith healing is forbidden. However, it is believed that reading the scriptures can comfort the individual and lead to mental and spiritual healing.

Medical and Surgical Procedures

MEDICATIONS

To the extent that they are necessary, medications are acceptable.

BLOOD AND BLOOD PRODUCTS

Blood in any form, and agents in which blood is an ingredient, are not acceptable. Blood volume expanders are acceptable if they are not derivatives of blood. Mechanical devices for circulating the blood are acceptable as long as they are not primed with blood initially. In some cases, children have been made wards of the court so they could receive blood when a medical condition mandating blood transfusion was life threatening. This can threaten the standing of the child in the community and must be approached with great care.

The determination of Jehovah's Witnesses to abstain from blood is based on scriptural references and precedents in the history of Christianity. Courts of justice have often upheld the principle that each individual has a right to bodily integrity, yet some physicians and hospital administrators have turned to the courts for legal authorization to force blood to be used as a medical treatment for an individual whose religious convictions prohibit the use of blood (Sugarman, Churchill, Moore, & Waugh, 1991).

SURGICAL PROCEDURES

Although surgical procedures are not in and of themselves opposed, the administration of blood during surgery is strictly prohibited (Smith, 1986).

There is no church rule pertaining to the loss of limbs or the amputation of body parts. If they are a violation of the principle of bodily mutilation, transplants are forbidden. However, this is usually an individual decision. Blood may not be used in this or any surgical procedure. Biopsies are acceptable. Circumcision is an individual decision.

Practices Related to Reproduction

Sterilization is prohibited because it is viewed as a form of bodily mutilation. Other forms of birth control are left to the individual. Amniocentesis is acceptable. Both therapeutic and on-demand abortions are forbidden. Sterility testing is an individual decision. Artificial insemination is forbidden both for donors and for recipients. Jehovah's Witnesses do not condone any activities in the areas of eugenics and genetics; they are considered to interfere with nature and therefore are unacceptable.

Religious Support System for the Sick

Individual members of congregation, including elders, visit the ill. Visitors pray with the sick person and read scriptures. Because members do not smoke, it is preferred that patients be placed in rooms where no smoking is allowed. If a man, the religious representative is referred to as "Mr." or "Elder"; if female, as "Ms." or "Mrs." Religious titles are not generally used. Individuals and members of the congregation look after the needs of the sick.

Practices Related to Death and Dying

The right to die or the use of extraordinary methods to prolong life is a matter of individual conscience. Euthanasia is forbidden. An autopsy is acceptable only if it is required by law. No parts are to be removed from the body. The human spirit and the body are never separated. The donation of a body is forbidden. Disposal of the body is a matter of individual preference. Burial practices are determined by local custom. Cremation is permitted if the individual chooses it.

Addendum

Jehovah's Witnesses are opposed to saluting the flag, serving in the armed forces, voting in civil elections, and holding public office. These prohibitions are related to belief in a theocracy that is in harmony with New Testament Christianity. Governed by a body of individuals, members united with the theocracy are to dissociate themselves from all activities of the political state and give full allegiance to "Jehovah's organization." This practice is related to the belief that Jesus Christ is King and Priest and that there is no need to hold citizenship in more than one kingdom. Members also refrain from gambling.

A pamphlet entitled *Jehovah's Witnesses and the Question of Blood* may be obtained free of charge from the World Headquarters for the Jehovah's Witnesses at 117 Adams Street, Brooklyn, NY, 11201.

• JUDAISM

Judaism is an Old Testament religion that dates back to the time of the prophet Abraham. Worldwide, there are approximately 18 million Jews. Membership includes approximately 7 million members in the United States and 320,000 members in Canada.

General Beliefs and Religious Practices

Judaism is a monotheistic religion. Jewish life historically has been based on interpretation of the laws of God as contained in the **Torah** and explained in the **Talmud** and in oral tradition. Ancient Jewish law prescribed most of the daily actions of the people. Diet, clothing, activities, occupation, and ceremonial activities throughout the life cycle are all part of Jewish daily life.

Today there are at least three schools of theological thought and social practice in Judaism. The three main divisions include Orthodox, Conservative, and Reform. There is also a fundamentalist sect, called Hasidism. Hasidic Jews cluster in metropolitan areas and live and work only within their Jewish communities.

Any person born of a Jewish mother or anyone converted to Judaism is considered a Jew. All Jews are united by the core theme of Judaism, which is expressed in the **Shema**, a prayer that professes a single God.

Holy Days

The Sabbath is the holiest of all holy days. The Sabbath begins each Friday 18 minutes before sunset and ends on Saturday, 42 minutes after sunset, or when three stars can be seen in the sky with the naked eye.

Other Holy Days are as follows:

1. Rosh Hashanah (Jewish New Year)
2. Yom Kippur (Day of Atonement, a fast day)
3. Succot (Feast of Tabernacles)
4. Shmini Atzeret (8th Day of Assembly)
5. Simchat Torah
6. Chanukah (Festival of Lights, or Rededication of the Temple in Jerusalem)
7. Asara B'Tevet (Fast of the 10th of Tevet)**
8. Fast of Esther
9. Purim
10. Passover
11. Shavuot (Festival of the Giving of the Torah)
12. Fast of the 17th of Tammuz
13. Fast of the 9th of Ave (Commemoration of the Destruction of the Temple)

Holy days are very special to practicing Jews. If a condition is not life-threatening, medical and surgical procedures should not be performed on the Sabbath or on holy days. Preservation of life is of greatest priority and is the

---

**Not observed by liberal or Reform Jews.

major criterion for determining activity on holy days and the Sabbath. If a Jewish patient is hesitant to receive urgent and necessary treatment because of religious restrictions, a rabbi should be consulted.

Sacraments/Rituals

Brit milah, the covenant of circumcision, is performed on all Jewish male children on the 8th day after birth (Figure 14–6). Although circumcision is a surgical procedure, for Jews it is a fundamental religious obligation. Circumcision is usually performed by a **mohel**, a pious Jew with special training, or by the child's father. Because the severing of the foreskin constitutes the essence of the ritual, the practice of having a non-Jewish or nonobservant physician perform the circumcision in the presence of a rabbi or other person who pronounces the blessing is not acceptable according to Jewish law. Circumcision may be delayed if medically contraindicated. For example, if the child has hypospadias, a congenital defect of the urethral wall for which surgical repair usually occurs at age 3 years and requires the use of the foreskin in reconstructive plastic surgery, the circumcision may be delayed. At times, Jewish law requires postponement of circumcision, though contemporary medical science recognizes no potential threat to the health of the baby (e.g., for physiologic jaundice). As soon as the jaundice disappears, the brit milah may be performed. In Reform and Conservative traditions, girls mark the eighth day

Figure 14–6. The *brit milah*, or covenant of circumcision, is being performed in the home of this 8-day-old Jewish infant by two mohels, one of whom is a Jewish pediatrician.

of life with a dedication ceremony in which prayers and blessings are invoked on her behalf.

The bar mitzvah (meaning "son of the commandment") is a confirmation ceremony for boys at age 13 that has been preceded by extensive religious study, including mastery of key Torah passages in Hebrew. In Reform and Conservative traditions, the bas (or ba*t*) mitzvah (meaning "daughter of the commandment") is the equivalent ceremony for girls.

Diet

The dietary laws of Judaism are very strict; the degree to which they are observed varies according to the individual. Strictly observant Jews never eat pork, never eat predatory fowl, and never mix milk dishes and meat dishes. Only fish with fins and scales are permissible; shellfish and other water creatures are prohibited.

The word **kosher** comes from a Hebrew word that means "proper" All animals must be ritually slaughtered to be kosher. This means that the animal is to be killed by a specially qualified person, quickly, with the least possible pain. More colloquially, many people think that "kosher" refers to a type of food. If a patient asks for kosher food, it is important to determine what he or she means.

Social Activities (Dating, Dancing)

Like all ethnic groups, Jews tend toward endogamy. Social activities that might lead to marriage outside the faith are discouraged. However, it is recognized that a significant number of individuals in Jewish society will seek partners outside. When this occurs, every effort is made to bring the non-Jewish partner into Judaism and to keep the Jewish partner a member and part of Jewish society.

Substance Use

The guideline is moderation. Wine is a part of religious observance and used as such. Drunkenness is not a sign of a good Jew. Historically, Jews well connected with their faith have had a low incidence of alcoholism.

Health Care Practices

Medical care from a physician in the case of illness is expected according to Jewish law. There are many prayers for the sick in Jewish liturgy. Such prayers and hope for recovery are encouraged.

Medical and Surgical Procedures

There are no restrictions when medications are used as part of a therapeutic process. There is a prohibition in Judaism against ingesting blood (e.g., blood sausage, raw meat). However, this does not apply to receiving blood transfusions. Beliefs and practices related to body mutilation (e.g., organ transplantation, amputations) vary widely among Jews. Individual beliefs should be explored with the client before any procedure that involves body mutilation.

Practices Related to Reproduction

BIRTH CONTROL

It is said in the Torah that Jews should be fruitful and multiply; therefore, it is a *mitzvah* (a good deed) to have at least two children. Since the Holocaust of World War II, it has been increasingly acceptable to have more children to replace those that were lost. It is permissible to practice birth control in traditional and liberal homes (Forsythe, 1991).

In the past, contraception was limited to the woman; vasectomy was prohibited. Currently, Judaism permits contraception by either partner, although Hasidic and Orthodox Jews rarely use vasectomy.

ABORTION

Although therapeutic abortion is always permitted if the health of the mother is jeopardized, traditional Judaism regards the killing of an unborn child to be a serious moral offense, whereas liberal Judaism permits it with strong moral admonitions (i.e., it is not to be used as a means of birth control). The fetus, although not imbued with the full sanctity of life, is a potential human being and is acknowledged as such.

STERILITY TESTING AND ARTIFICIAL INSEMINATION

Sterility testing is permissible when the goal is to enable the couple to have children. Artificial insemination is permitted under certain circumstances. A rabbi should be consulted in each individual case.

EUGENICS AND GENETICS

Jews have an understandable aversion to genetic engineering because of the experimentation carried on during the Nazi era. At the same time, eugenic practices are permitted under a limited range of circumstances. The Jewish belief in the sanctity of life is a guiding factor in rabbinical counseling.

Religious Support System for the Sick

VISITORS

The most likely visitors will be family and friends from the synagogue. To visit the sick is a *mitzvah* of service (an obligation, a responsibility, and a blessing). There are often many Jewish social service agencies to help those in need. The Jewish Federation and Jewish Community Service are two large organizations that provide services to fulfill a variety of needs.

TITLE OF RELIGIOUS REPRESENTATIVE

The formal religious representative from a synagogue is the rabbi. A visit from the rabbi may be spent talking, or the rabbi may pray with the person alone or in a minyan, a group of 10 adults 13 years or older. If the patient is male and strictly observant, he may wish to have a prayer shawl (tallit), a cap (kippah), and tefillin (special symbols tied onto the arms and forehead). If the patient's own materials are not at the hospital, it may be necessary to ask that they be brought. Prayers are often chanted. If possible, privacy should be provided.

Practices Related to Death and Dying

PROLONGATION OF LIFE (RIGHT TO DIE)

A person has the right to die with dignity. If a physician sees that death is inevitable, no new therapeutic measures that would artificially extend life need to be initiated. It is important to know the precise time of death for the purpose of honoring the deceased after the first year has passed.

EUTHANASIA

Euthanasia is prohibited under any circumstances. It is regarded as murder. However, in the administration of palliative medications that carry the calculated risk of overdose, the amelioration of pain is paramount.

AUTOPSY

Any unjustified alteration in a corpse is considered a desecration of the dead, to be avoided in normal circumstances. When postmortem examinations are justified, they must be limited to essential organs or systems. Needle biopsy is preferred. All body parts must be returned for burial. Jewish family members may ask to consult with a rabbinical authority before signing an autopsy consent form.

DONATION OF BODY PARTS

This is a complex matter according to Jewish law. If it seems necessary, consultation with a rabbi should be encouraged (Weiss, 1988).

BURIAL

The body is ritually washed at a funeral home after death, if possible by members of the Chevra Kadisha (Ritual Burial Society). The body is then clothed in a simple white burial shroud. Embalming, a process wherein the blood of the deceased is replaced by an embalming fluid, and cosmetic treatment of the body are forbidden. Public viewing of the body is considered a humiliation of the dead. Relatives are forbidden to touch or embrace the deceased, except when involved in preparation for interment. The exact time of burial is significant for sitting **shiva**, the mourning period. After death in an institution, a nurse may wash the body for transport to the funeral home. Ritual washing then occurs later. Human remains, including a fetus at any stage of gestation, are to be buried as soon as possible. Cremation is not in keeping with Jewish law.

Addendum

Additional information can be obtained from Synagogue Council of America, 432 Park Avenue South, New York, NY 10016; phone (212) 686-8670; or the Canadian Jewish Congress, 100 Sparks Street Suite 650, Ottawa, Ontario, K1P

5B7, phone (613) 233-8703, fax (613) 233-8748, e-mail canadianjewish-congress@cjc.ca

• MENNONITE CHURCH

Membership in the United States is 122,545; in Canada: 207,970; and worldwide: 1,250,000.

Mennonites take their name from Menno Simons, an Anabaptist bishop who united a fragmented group of Anabaptists in the early 1500s. Menno had been a Catholic priest in Holland but left the church over theological differences after his brother was killed as an Anabaptist. The word "Anabaptist" comes from the doctrine that baptism to be valid must be upon confessed faith.

General Beliefs and Religious Practices

Mennonites believe that each person is responsible before God to make decisions based on his or her understanding of the Bible. For this reason, there are a minimum of official statements or regulations. Even when these are to be found, e.g., the Mennonite Confession of Faith, they are perceived by members as guidelines rather than proclamations to supplant individual responsibility. It should also be noted that the Mennonite faith encompasses a wide spectrum of cultural circumstances, which are more responsible for variations among individual Mennonites than is the basic theology, which is relatively uniform. It is therefore necessary to ascertain individual preferences and to work with patients on a one-to-one basis rather than stereotyping according to religious affiliation.

Holy Days and Sacraments

Mennonites observe the religious days of the traditional Christian churches. Observance places no restrictions on health-related procedures on these days. Mennonites observe Baptism and Holy Communion as official church sacraments. Patients will request sacraments as necessary. Neither sacrament is believed necessary for salvation.

Social Activities (Dating, Dancing)

No restrictions are placed on social activities.

Health Care Practices

Healing is believed to be a part of God's work in the human body through whatever means he chooses to use, whether medical science or healing that comes in answer to specific prayer. There is no religious ritual to be applied unless the patient asks for one in whatever way is personally meaningful. Sometimes anointing of oil is practiced.

Medical and Surgical Procedures

No specific guidelines or restrictions exist for the administration of medications, blood and blood components, or surgical procedures.

Practices Related to Reproduction

BIRTH CONTROL

All types of contraception are acceptable. The choice is left to the individual.

ABORTION

Therapeutic abortions are acceptable. Mennonites generally believe that on-demand abortion must be decided according to the specifics of individual cases. The church has chosen to avoid making a ruling that must be followed unquestionably. The individual must follow her own conscience and learn to live with the consequences. Some parts of the Mennonite Church have adopted statements opposing abortion on demand.

ARTIFICIAL INSEMINATION

The church does not have regulations regarding artificial insemination. The individual conscience and point of view of the patient need to be respected. Usually, artificial insemination is sought only if husband and wife are donor and recipient, respectively.

EUGENICS AND GENETICS

The church accepts scientific endeavor as a valid activity that needs to respect all of God's creation. The concerns of eugenics and genetics in its future potential have not been fully confronted. Mennonites believe that God and human beings work together in caring for and improving the world.

Practices Related to Death and Dying

The church does not believe that life must be continued at all cost. Health care professionals should decide whether to take heroic measures on the basis of the patient's individual circumstances and the emotional condition of the family. When life has lost its purpose and meaning beyond hope of meaningful recovery, most Mennonites feel that relatives should not be censured for allowing life-sustaining measures to be withheld.

Euthanasia as the termination of life by an overt act of the physician is not condoned. Autopsy and the donation of the body are acceptable, without restrictions. Procedures for disposal of body and burial follow local customs and legal requirements.

• NATIVE NORTH AMERICAN CHURCHES

Differentiating Native North American health care practices from their religious and cultural beliefs is much more difficult than with the other religions presented in this chapter. Native North Americans represent 2 million people and more than 300 tribal units within North America. Each group has individual beliefs and practices, yet they maintain a similar nonprescriptive attitude toward health care.

There is in the United States and Canada today a specific religion called the **Native American Church** or **Peyote Religion**. Encompassing members of many tribes, its focus is on the revival of Native North American culture, beliefs and spirituality.

When trying to support a Native American in physical or psychologic crisis, the nurse needs to remember several seemingly unrelated facts. First, the non-Westernized Native North American belief about disease is not necessarily based on symptoms. Disease may be attributed to intrusive objects, soul loss, spirit intrusion, breach of taboo, or sorcery. Disease may also be attributed to natural or supernatural causes (Vogel, 1970). Second, the Native North American may embrace an organized, usually Christian religion and still be a member of a particular Native North American tribe. Native North Americans also balance "modern theories of disease" with long-standing tribal beliefs or customs. Therefore, during illness and particularly hospitalization, Native North Americans may ask to see a priest or minister as well as a tribal "medicine man" or *curandero*. Visits from these persons will likely be spiritually supportive, although the form of the support may vary greatly.

The spiritual basis for much of Native North American belief and action is symbolized by the number four. This number, which pervades much North American Indian thought, is seen in the extended hand, which means life, unity, equality, and eternity. The clasped hand symbolizes unity, the spiritual law that binds the universe.

It is this unity on which decisions should be made. Questions about abortion, the use of drugs, giving and receiving blood, the right to life, euthanasia, and so on do not have dogmatic "yes" or "no" answers; rather, answers are based on the situation and the ultimate unity or disunity that a decision would produce.

To the Native North American, everything is cyclical. Communication is the key to learning and understanding; understanding brings peace of mind; peace of mind leads to happiness; and happiness is communicating. Other guidelines also function in groups of four (Steiger, 1975).

Four guidelines toward self-development are

1. Am I happy with what I am doing?
2. What am I doing to add to the confusion?
3. What am I doing to bring about peace and contentment?
4. How will I be remembered when I am gone, in absence and in death?

The four requirements of good health are

1. Food
2. Sleep
3. Cleanliness
4. Good thoughts

The four divisions of nature are

1. Spirit
2. Mind
3. Body
4. Life

The four divisions of goals are

1. Faith
2. Love
3. Work
4. Pleasure

The four ages of development are the

1. Learning age
2. Age of adoption
3. Age of improvement
4. Age of wisdom

The four expressions of sharing are

1. Making others feel you care
2. An expression of interest
3. An expression of friendship
4. An expression of belonging

Unity, the great spiritual law, also can be expressed in four parts

1. Going into the silence in spirit, mind, and body
2. The union through which all spirituality flows
3. A goal toward communicating with all things in nature
4. Recognized through sense, emotions, and impressions.

In concert with the belief in the interconnectedness of all things, natural remedies in the form of herbal medicine are often used. (It is interesting to note that Native North American folk medicine and herbal remedies provided the forerunners of many of today's pharmaceutical remedies.) Herbal treatments are still used today and may be requested by Native North American patients in a Western medical setting.

A nurse caring for a Native North American client should be careful to obtain a careful and complete history, including a list of whatever native remedies have been tried. The patient may not know the names of herbs used in treatment, and the tribal medicine man or woman may need to be consulted.

Respecting the concept that religion, medicine, and healing are insepa-rable to the Native North American, one must be sensitive to the fact that asking for the names of native medicines or descriptions of healing prac-tices tried in an attempt to cure the person before his or her entrance into the Western medical system is not just simply obtaining a history, but also entering into the realm of what might be not only private but also very sacred. The nurse must use care and sensitivity and show deep respect for the information received.

• PROTESTANTISM

In its broadest meaning, **Protestantism** denotes the whole movement within Christianity that originated in the 16th century with Martin Luther and the Protestant Reformation. Historically and traditionally, the chief characteris-tics of Protestantism are the acceptance of the Bible as the only source of infal-lible revealed truth, the belief in the universal priesthood of believers, and the doctrine that Christians are justified in their relationship to God by faith alone, not by good works or dispensations of the church.

It is difficult to accurately categorize Protestant churches and impossible to mention them all, because there are more than 30,000 denominations. Protestantism is basically non-Roman Western Christianity, and it can be divided into four major forms: Lutheran, Anglican, Reformed, and free (or independent) church (Johnson, Kurian, Kurian & Barett, 2001).

Lutheranism

The oldest and second largest Protestant religion, Lutheranism began in 1517 with Martin Luther's split from the Roman Catholic Church. Lutherans empha-size theological doctrine and spirituality. Many North American Lutherans are of German or Scandinavian heritage.

Anglicanism

Anglicanism is represented by the established Church of England and similar churches. Unlike most other Protestant churches, they have an episcopal sys-tem of government in which each church or parish is served by a priest who is supervised by a bishop. A bishop supervises a group of churches called a diocese. A bishop, in turn, is responsible to a council of bishops. Anglican churches allow their clergy to marry. The Methodist church was established by followers of John Wesley, an 18th-century Anglican who sought to bring reform to the Church of England. Wesley's movement spread to the United States and Canada in the 18th century.

Reformed Denominations

The Reformed denominations include Presbyterianism and are based on the teachings of John Calvin and his followers. These churches are distinguished from Lutheranism and Anglicanism, which maintain symbolic and sacramental traditions that originated before the Protestant Reformation.

Free or Independent Churches

Free or independent churches, including the Baptists, Congregationalists, Adventists, and Churches of Christ exercise congregational government. Each local denomination is an independent autonomous unit and there is no official doctrine.

With 27 million members, the Baptist church makes up more than 10% of the population of the United States. Black and White Baptist church denominations exist separately. The largely White Southern Baptist Convention has about 12 million members, whereas 9 million Blacks (30% of all Blacks in the United States) are members of the National Baptist Conventions.

Health Care Practices

Given the wide diversity that exists within Protestant denominations, it is beyond the scope of this text to identify health-related beliefs and practices for each group. Selected Protestant denominations (e.g., Adventists, Jehovah's Witnesses) have been included in this section largely because they have significant health-related practices. For further information about specific Protestant churches, you are encouraged to visit www.adherents.com or the official web pages of the various groups for a synopsis of their beliefs.

• SEVENTH-DAY ADVENTISTS

North American membership of **Seventh-Day Adventists** is 946,962; worldwide membership is 10.65 million.

Doctrinally, Seventh-Day Adventists are heirs of the interfaith Millerite movement of the late 1840s, although the movement officially adopted the name Seventh-Day Adventist in 1863. Between 1831 and 1844, William Miller, a Baptist preacher and former army captain in the War of 1812, launched the "great second advent awakening," which eventually spread throughout most of the Christian world. At first, the work was largely confined to North America, but it quickly spread to Switzerland, Africa, Italy, Egypt, and many other nations.

General Beliefs and Religious Practices

Seventh-Day Adventists accept the Bible as their only creed and hold certain fundamental beliefs to be the teaching of the Holy Scriptures. The official statements by the General Conference of the Seventh-Day Adventists concerning the scriptures, the trinity, creation, nature of man, the great controversy (Christ versus Satan), life, death, resurrection, and other topics may be found at www.adventist.org

Holy Days

The seventh day (Saturday) is observed as the Sabbath, from Friday sundown to Saturday sundown. The Sabbath is the day that God blessed and sanctified. It is a sacred day of worship and rest. Saturday worship services are held, as are weekly evening prayer meetings (usually midweek).

Sacraments/Rituals

There are three church ordinances: (1) baptism by immersion, (2) the Ordinance of Humility, and (3) the Lord's Supper or Communion. There are no rituals at the time of birth. There is no requirement for a final sacrament at death. If requested by individual or family member, the dying person might be anointed with oil.

Diet

Seventh-Day Adventists believe that because the body is the temple of God, it is appropriate to abstain from any food or beverage that could prove harmful to the body. Because the first human diet consisted of fruits and grains, the Church encourages a vegetarian diet. Nevertheless, some members prefer to eat meat and poultry. Based on a passage in Leviticus 11:3, nonvegetarian members refrain from eating foods derived from any animal having a cloven hoof that chews its cud (e.g., meat derived from pigs, rabbits, or similar animals). Although fish with fins and scales are acceptable (e.g., salmon), shellfish are prohibited. Consumption of some birds is prohibited, but common poultry such as chicken and turkey are acceptable. Fermented beverages are prohibited. **Fasting** is practiced, but only when members of a specific church elect to do so. Practiced in degrees, fasting may involve abstention from food or liquids. Fasting is not encouraged if it is likely to have adverse effects on the individual.

Social Activities (Dating, Dancing) and Substance Use

Dancing is not encouraged as a form of recreation or social activity. Members are encouraged to date other members or persons holding similar beliefs and values. Members should abstain from the use of fermented beverages and tobacco products.

Health Care Practices

The church believes in divine healing and practices anointing with oil and prayer. This is in addition to healing brought about by medical intervention. Since 1865, the church has maintained chaplains and physicians as inseparable in its institutions.

Medical and Surgical Procedures

Adventists operate one of the world's largest religiously operated health systems, including a medical school. **The Health Ministries** include 166 hospitals and sanitariums, 117 nursing homes and retirement centers, 371 clinics and dispensaries, 30 orphanages and children's homes, and 12 airplanes and medical launches. Physical medicine and rehabilitation are emphasized and recommended, along with therapeutic diets. There are no restrictions on the use of vaccines. Similarly, there are no restrictions on the use of blood and blood products, amputations, organ transplants, donation of organs, biopsies, and circumcisions.

Practices Related to Reproduction

The use of birth control is an individual decision; the church prohibits cohabitation except between husband and wife. There are no restrictions on amniocentesis. Therapeutic abortion is acceptable if the mother's life is in danger and in cases of rape and incest. On-demand abortion is unacceptable because Adventists believe in the sanctity of life. Artificial insemination between husband and wife is acceptable. Although the church views practices in the fields of eugenics and genetics as an individual decision, it upholds the principle of responsibility in dealing with children.

Religious Support System for the Sick

At the request of the sick person or the family, the pastor and elders of the church will come together to pray and anoint the sick person with oil. The religious representative is referred to as Doctor, Pastor, or Elder. There is a worldwide Seventh-Day Adventist health system, which includes hospitals and clinics.

Practices Related to Death and Dying

Although there is no official position, the church has traditionally followed the medical ethics of prolonging life and euthanasia. Autopsy and the donation of the entire body or parts are acceptable. No directives or recommendations exist regarding disposal of the body. No specific directives concerning burial exist; this is an individual decision.

ADDENDUM

The Seventh-Day Adventist church is opposed to the use of hypnotism in the practice of medicine or under any other circumstance.

•UNITARIAN UNIVERSALIST CHURCH

Worldwide, **Unitarian Universalist** membership is 600,000, with a North American membership of 221,760.

General Beliefs and Religious Practices

Unitarianism was officially organized in 1774 in England. This organization occurred after a long history of debate and dissension regarding the nature of God, particularly regarding the Trinitarian concept, which existed in various forms in the Catholic and Protestant religions. The Unitarian Universalist Association is the modern institutional embodiment of two separate denominations that grew out of movements and faith traditions extending back to the Christian Reformation era (14–16th century C.E.). Universalist convictions include the belief that all creation will ultimately be drawn back to its divine source and that no person or thing would be ultimately and forever excluded. The Unitarian conviction is reflected in the belief that God is ultimately and absolutely one.

Holy Days and Sacraments

No religious holy days are celebrated. Members come from various cultural and religious backgrounds and observe special days according to their own heritage and desire.

Normal milestones of life (birth, marriage, death) may be celebrated religiously. Although it is uncommon, puberty and divorce may include religious observances.

Unitarian Universalism does not believe in a need for sacraments. Baptism of infants and occasionally of adults is sometimes performed as a symbolic act of dedication. The Lord's Supper is administered in some congregations.

Diet and Substance Use

No restrictions on diet exist. Substances should be used according to reason.

Health Care Practices

Faith healing is considered largely superstitious and wishful thinking. Members believe in use of the empirical method, reason, and science to facilitate healing.

Medical and Surgical Procedures

The use of medications is not restricted. The use of blood and blood products is similarly not restricted. Amputations, organ transplants, biopsies are not restricted. Circumcision is viewed as a health practice, not a religious one.

Practices Related to Reproduction

Unitarian Universalists strongly favor all types of birth control as a human right. Both therapeutic and on-demand abortion are acceptable. Members strongly favor the right of the mother to decide. Amniocentesis is not restricted and is encouraged if medical evaluation deems it necessary. Sterility testing is acceptable; in fact, more research is encouraged. Both donation and receipt of artificial insemination are acceptable and strongly favored as a human right.

Practices Related to Death and Dying

Members favor the right to die with dignity. Personhood is sacred, not the spark of life. Members tend to favor nonaction, including withdrawal of technical aids when death is imminent or when the patient has made a written request in advance. Autopsy is recommended. The donation of the body is acceptable. Cremation is most common. Donation to a medical school for study is not uncommon. Burial of a fetus is rare. A memorial service in the church or at home without the body present is customary.

SUMMARY

Religious and cultural beliefs are interwoven and influence a client's understanding of illness and health care practices. In times of serious illness and death, religion may be a source of consolation for the client. Five dimensions of religion influence human behavior, including health-related practices. The goal of spiritual nursing care is to assist clients in integrating their own religious beliefs about God or a unifying truth into the ultimate reality that gives meaning to their lives in relationship to the health care crisis that has precipitated the need for nursing care. For the nurse providing spiritual nursing care, issues related to death and dying are of particular importance. Health-related beliefs and practices of select religions are important to understand,, especially considering the diverse religious groups in the United States and Canada. Evidence-Based Practice 14–2 provides information regarding other research done on this topic, and Box 14–2 summarizes some of the religious and nonreligious holidays covered in this chapter.

REVIEW QUESTIONS

1. When assessing the spiritual needs of clients from diverse cultural backgrounds, what key components should you consider?
2. In providing nursing care for the dying or bereaved client and family, what cultural considerations should the nurse include in the plan?
3. Compare and contrast the religious beliefs and practices concerning diet, medications, and procedures for five of the religious groups discussed in this chapter.
4. Analyze the contributions of religious bodies to the United States (or Canadian) health care delivery system.
5. What effect do health care facilities that are owned and operated by religious groups have on the overall cost and quality of health care in the United States and Canada?
6. What religious rituals mark significant developmental milestones for chil-

EVIDENCE-BASED PRACTICE 14-2
Do Religious Beliefs Have a Positive Effect on the Health of Practicing Members?

A question that may be asked in relationship to religious beliefs and health is: Do religious beliefs have a positive effect on the health of practicing members? There is a body of research, mostly experimental or quasiexperimental in design, that seems to document a salutary effect of some force, energy, or field considerably more subtle than Western bio-medicine is able to demonstrate within three-dimensional physical reality. This effect has been demonstrated in more than 150 published empirical studies of these types of healing in human beings. Included in this section is a review of selected studies that examine the health-promoting and healing aspects of religious beliefs and practices, including prayer.

Woods, T. E. & Ironson, G. H. (1999). Religion and spirituality in the face of illness. *Journal of Health Psychology*, 4(3), 393-412.

This study reported the qualitative and quantitative results of semistructured interviews with 60 medically ill people with the intent of uncovering the meaning of the terms *religion* and *spiritual* as they applied in the face of serious illness. Many similarities were discovered between spirituality and religion, as well as qualitative and quantitatively significant differences. Differences included variations in "overall belief systems and interpretation of the mechanisms whereby subjects' beliefs impacted their health and their recovery."

Participants who identified themselves as spiritual indicated that they believed their recovery and healing occurred through themselves, whereas those identifying themselves as religious described a belief that healing was something that "happened to them."

Scherer, R. P. (1996). Hospital caregivers' own religion in relation to their perceptions of psychosocial inputs into health and healing. *Review of Religious Research, 37*(4), 302–323.

A survey of 1,237 health care providers, including physicians, nurses, and others, was conducted regarding their openness to psychosocial and mind–body inputs into health and healing. Chaplains, social workers, psychologists, and occupational and physical therapists were the most favorable to psychosocial and mind–body inputs into healing. Nurses were slightly more favorable than were physicians, and those physicians who had very little interaction with patients were the least favorable. Statistical significance was not shown between a caregivers' own religion and religiosity and his or her openness to psychosocial and mind–body input into health and healing.

Simpson, M. R. & King, M. G. (1999). "God brought all these churches together": Issues in developing religion-health partnerships in an Appalachian community. *Public Health Nursing, 16*(1), 41–49.

This ethnographic study explored the health-related and organizational religious activities in a central Appalachian community and attempted to identify cultural issues in the development of religion-health partnerships. Thirteen religious sites constituted the sample, and data were collected by attendance at organizational activities through both structured interviews and artifact review. Results to the question "what are health-related activities found in religious services" included prayer requests, anointing, and testimonials. Organizational activities that influenced religion and health partnerships included interdenominational cooperation, community outreach services, association, and local church governance.

Simpson, M. R. & King, M. G. (1999). "God brought all these churches together": Issues in developing religion-health partnerships in an Appalachian community. *Public Health Nursing, 16*(1), 41–49.

BOX 14–2	**RELIGIOUS AND NONRELIGIOUS HOLIDAYS IN THE UNITED STATES AND CANADA**

This calendar is a guide to religious and nonreligious holidays that are celebrated in the United States and Canada. The list is not exhaustive but is given to encourage the reader to be aware of the many holidays and festivals that are reflective of the great mixture of religious and ethnic groups in North America.

B = Buddhist	J = Jewish	P = Protestant
Ba = Baha'i	Ja = Jain	RC = Roman Catholic
C = Christian (general)	M = Mormon	S = Sikh
Ci = Civic holiday	O = Eastern Orthodox	
H = Hindu	Christian	
I = Islam		

JANUARY

1 New Year's Day Ci
1 Feast of St. Basil O
6 Epiphany C
7 Nativity of Jesus Christ O
3rd Monday Martin Luther King, Jr.
  Birthday Observance Ci

FEBRUARY

Black History Month (U.S.)
8 Scout Day Ci
14 Valentine's Day Ci
Mid-month President's Day (U.S.) Ci

Other holidays that often fall in February according to the lunar calendar

Chinese New Year
Ramadan (30 days) I
Nehan-e (Death of Buddha) B
Vasant Panchami (Advent of Spring)
  H, Ja
Ash Wednesday RC, P
Purim J

MARCH

Women's History Month (U.S.)
17 St. Patrick's Day C
25 Annunciation C

Other holidays that often occur in March according to the lunar calendar

Eastern Orthodox Lent begins O
Higan-e (First Day of Spring) B

Naw-Ruz (Baha'i and Iranian New Year)
Palm Sunday RC, P
First Day of Passover (8 days) J
Holi (Spring Festival) H, Ja
Maundy Thursday RC, P
Good Friday RC, P
Easter C, RC, P, M
Mahavir Jayanti (Birth of Mahavir) Ja

APRIL

16 Yom Ha'atzmaut (Israel
  Independence Day) J

Holidays that often occur in April according to the lunar calendar

Hanamatsuri (Birth of Buddha) B
Yom Hashoah (Holocaust
  Remembrance Day) J, Ci
Baisakhi (Brotherhood) S
Huguenot Day P
Ramavani (Birth of Rama) H
Palm Sunday O
Holy Friday O
Easter O

MAY

5 Cinco de Mayo Ci
23 Victoria Day (Canada)
30 Memorial Day Ci

Holidays that often occur in May according to the lunar calendar

(continued)

| BOX 14–2 | **RELIGIOUS AND NONRELIGIOUS HOLIDAYS IN THE UNITED STATES AND CANADA (Continued)** |

Shavuot J
Idul-Adha (Day of Sacrifice) I
Ascension Day RC, P
Pentecost RC, P

JUNE

12 Anne Frank Day
14 Flag Day (U.S.) Ci
24 Nativity of St. John the Baptist RC, P, O

Holidays that often occur in June according to the lunar calendar

Ratha-yatra
Ascension Day O
Muharam (I)
Pentecost O
Islamic New Year I
Hindu New Year H

JULY

1 Canada Day (Canada) Ci
4 Independence Day (U.S.) Ci
24 Pioneer Day M

Holidays that often occur in July according to the lunar calendar

Obon-e B

AUGUST

6 Transfiguration C
15 Feast of the Blessed Virgin Mary RC, O

SEPTEMBER

1st Monday Labor Day (U.S.) Ci
15 National Hispanic Heritage Month (30 days) Ci
17 Citizenship (U.S. Constitution) Ci
19 San Gennaro Day RC
25 Native American Day Ci

Holidays that often occur in September according to the lunar calendar

Higan-e (First Day of Fall) B

Rosh Hashanah (Jewish New Year: 2 days) J

OCTOBER

12 Columbus Day (U.S.) Ci
Thanksgiving Day (Canada) Ci
24 United Nations Day Ci
31 Reformation Day P
31 Halloween RC, P, Ci

Holidays that often occur in October according to the lunar calendar

Dusserah (Good over Evil) H, JA
Yom Kippur (Atonement) J
Sukkot (Tabernacles) J
Shemini 'Azeret (end of Sukkot)
Diwali, or Dipavali (Festival of Lights) H, Ja

NOVEMBER

1 All Saints Day RC, P
11 Veterans Day Ci
25 Religious Liberty Day Ci
1st Tuesday Election Day (U.S.) Ci
4th Thursday Thanksgiving Day (U.S.) Ci

Holidays that often occur in November according to the lunar calendar

Baha'u'llah Birthday Ba
Guru Nanak Birthday S

DECEMBER

6 St. Nicholas Day C
8 Feast of the Immaculate Conception RC
10 Human Rights Day Ci
12 Festival of Our Lady of Guadalupe (Mexico-Hispanic)
25 Christmas C, RC, P, M, Ci

Holidays that often occur in December according to the lunar calendar

Bodhi Day (Enlightenment) B
Hanukkah (Jewish Festival of Lights: 8 days) J
Kwanzaa (7 days)

dren and adolescents? Identify the ritual or ceremony, the approximate age at which the child or adolescent participates in it, and the name of the religion(s) associated with it.

CRITICAL THINKING ACTIVITIES

1. Visit a church or worship center not of your own belief system and interview a member of the clergy or an official representative about the health-related beliefs of that religion. Discuss with him or her the implications of those beliefs for someone hospitalized for an acute illness or a chronic illness. Inquire about the ways in which nurses can be of most help to hospitalized members of this religion.
2. Interview members of various religions about their beliefs about health and illness. Compare these interviews with the published beliefs or official statements from these religions. Discuss the implications of the differences (if any) that you found.
3. Interview fellow students, classmates, or coworkers (if you are employed) about what they know of the health beliefs of various religions, especially those religions most often encountered among the patients with whom you work. Make a poster or prepare a presentation comparing the results of your interviews with the official beliefs of those religions. Share this information with your classmates.
4. Interview four or more members of the same religious group who are of various ages (i.e., children, teenagers, young adults, middle-aged and elderly). Ask them about their religious beliefs and how they affect their health. Compare the results, commenting on similarities and differences.
5. If you have thought about the above exercises in terms of physical health, consider each of the questions from the perspective of mental health and spiritual health.

• References

Chapman, A. (1991). The Buddhist way of dying. *Nursing Praxis in New Zealand, 6*(2), 23–26.

Christian Science Publishing Society (1978). *What is a Christian Science practitioner?* Boston: Christian Science Publishing Society.

Christian Science Publishing Society (1994). *Science and health.* Boston: Christian Science Publishing Society.

Donnermeyer, J. F. (1997). Amish society: An overview. *The Journal of Multicultural Nursing & Health, 3*(2), 6–12.

Ebersole, P., & Hess, P. (2000) *Toward healthy aging.* St. Louis, MO: C. V. Mosby.

Faulkner, J. E., & DeJong, C. F. (1966). Religiosity in 5 D: An empirical analysis. *Social Forces, 45,* 246–254.

Forsythe, E. (1991). Religious and cultural aspects of family planning. *Journal of the Royal Society of Medicine, 84*(3), 177–178.

Green, J. (1992a). Death with dignity: Christianity. *Nursing Times, 88*(3), 25–29.

Green, J. (1992b). Death with dignity: Jehovah's Witnesses. *Nursing Times, 88*(5), 36–37.

Greksa, L. P., & Korbin, J. E. (1997). Influence of changing occupational patterns on the use of commercial health insurance by the Old Order Amish. *The Journal of Multicultural Nursing & Health, 3*(2), 13–18.

Hickey, M. E., & Hall, T. R. (1993). Insulin therapy and weight change in Native American NIDDM patients. *Diabetes Care, 16*(1), 364–368.

Hinnell, J. R. (1984). *The Penguin dictionary of religions.* New York: Penguin Books.

Huttlinger, K., Krefting, L., Drevdahl, D., Tree, P., Bacca, E., & Benally, A. (1992). Doing battle: A metaphorical analysis of diabetes mellitus among Navajo people. *American Journal of Occupational Therapy, 46*(8), 706–712.

Kalish, R. A., & Reynolds, D. K. (1981). *Death and ethnicity: A psychocultural study.* New York: Baywood.

Marty, M. M. (1990). *Health, medicine, and the faith traditions. Healthy people 2000: A role for America's religious communities.* Atlanta, GA: Emory University, The Carter Center, and the Park Ridge Center.

Moberg, D. (1971). *Spiritual well-being.* Washington, DC: White House Conference on Aging.

Moberg, D. (1981). Religion and the aging family. In P. Ebersole & P. Hess (Eds.). *Toward healthy aging (pp. 349–351).* St. Louis, MO: C.V. Mosby.

Scherer, R. P. (1996). Hospital caregivers' own religion in relation to their perceptions of psychological inputs into health and healing. *Review of Religious Research, 37*(4), 302–324.

Smith, E. B. (1986). Surgery in Jehovah's Witnesses. *Journal of National Medical Association, 78*(7), 668–669.

Steiger, B. (1975). *Medicine talk.* New York: Doubleday.

Stolley, J. M. & Koenig, H. (1997). Religion/spirituality and health among elderly African Americans and Hispanics. *Journal of Psychosocial Nursing, 35*(11), 32–38.

Sugarman, J., Churchill, L. R., Moore, J. K., & Waugh, R. A. (1991). Medical, ethical, and legal issues regarding thrombolytic therapy in the Jehovah's Witnesses. *American Journal of Cardiology, 68*(15), 1525–1529.

Vogel, V. J. (1970). *American Indian medicine.* Norman, OK: University of Oklahoma Press.

Weiss, D. W. (1988). Organ transplantation, medical ethics and Jewish law. *Transplantation Proceedings, 20*(1), 1071–1075.

Wenger, A. F. (1990). The culture care theory and the Old Order Amish. In M. M. Leininger (Ed.). *Culture care diversity and universality: A theory of nursing.* New York: National League for Nursing Press, 147–178.

Wenger, A. F. (1991, April/May). Culture specific care and the Old Order Amish. *IMPRINT,* 80–85.

Woods, T. E., & Ironson, G. H. (1999). Religion and spirituality in the face of illness. *Journal of Health Psychology, 4*(3) 393–412.

Yearbook of American and Canadian Churches, Annual. (2001). New York: National Council of the Churches of Christ in the United States of America.

2000 census of the population and housing data paper listing (CPH-L-133). Washington, DC: U.S. Government Printing Office.

CHAPTER 15

Cultural Competence in Ethical Decision-Making

Dula F. Pacquiao

KEY TERMS

Advance directives	Deontological theories of	Moral philosophy
Autonomy	ethics	Naturalism
Beneficence	Duty-based ethics	Nonmaleficence
Categorical imperative	Emic	Patient Self-Determination Act
Community-based theory of	Ethic of care	Rationalism
ethics	Ethics	Teleological theories of
Consequential theories of ethics	Etic	ethics
Culturally competent decision-	Fidelity	Utilitarianism
making	Justice	Veracity

OBJECTIVES

1. Compare moral beliefs and assumptions in Western and non-Western societies.
2. Describe how moral philosophies are socially and culturally constituted.
3. Define ethical concepts, principles, and theories.
4. Discuss cultural variability in ethical decision-making.
5. Describe the culturally competent model of ethical decision-making.
6. Use research findings relevant to ethical decision-making.
7. Explain the significance of transcultural nursing in ethical care.

"The tie between the social and personal worlds is mediated by language, symbols, value hierarchies, and aesthetic forms that are the pervasive cultural apparatus, which orders social life" (Kleinman, 1988, p. 3).

The evolution of nursing as a profession has been intimately linked with society's moral philosophy, because the work of caring for and treating the sick, and comforting and protecting the suffering, are themselves morally worthy work (Jameton, 1984). Religion and spirituality have profoundly influenced the development of nursing. Many individuals engaged in caring and healing have traditionally been motivated by practical, moral, and spiritual beliefs (Donahue, 1996). Nursing deals with very personal and private aspects of life, involving ethical decision-making that draws on the moral philosophies of various participants in the situation.

The current environment of nursing practice is fraught with potential conflicts from differing values and philosophies. Increasing cultural diversity in the population of health care workers and patients creates ambiguity and lack of agreement in decision-making about many issues, including folk versus biomedical healing, and individual patient autonomy versus family harmony. Technologic advancements and computerization have opened a whole new group of ethical dilemmas regarding patient confidentiality, quality of life versus sanctity of life, and biomedical versus lay definition of death. The current debate on stem cell research pits science and the pursuit of cures for human diseases made possible by technologic advancement against the sanctity of embryonic life. Cost containment and the infusion of business practices into health care have been associated with problems in the distribution of resources, professional versus managerial autonomy, and patient safety. Indeed, nurses deal with situations that invoke moral and ethical beliefs from the perspective of different persons and entities: patients, their families and communities, multidisciplinary and multicultural practitioners and care providers, institutional, and societal norms.

• SOCIAL CONSTRUCTION OF MORALITY

A **moral philosophy** consists of beliefs and assumptions about what is right and wrong. This is the basis of **ethics**, which prescribes the proper action to take in a given situation. Ethics translates moral philosophies into action. The American Nurses Association Code of Ethics and the Canadian Nurses Association Code of Ethics are sets of principles or standards guiding professional nursing practice. They reflect the norms of valued beliefs and ideals in mainstream American and Canadian societies.

Morals and philosophic beliefs are constituted within the social, historical, and cultural experiences of a society. These beliefs evolve as normative patterns or sets of assumptions and beliefs that serve as an implicit framework to guide the actions and thoughts of group members. These normative patterns or sets of assumptions and beliefs may or may not be shared by persons outside the cultural group. Whereas filial piety and respect for the authority of one's elders are the guiding principles among traditional Chinese in making decisions about a family member's surgery, this may not be acceptable to Western health care providers, who value the individual patient's autonomy in decision-making. Highly influenced by the teachings of Confucius, Chinese culture upholds the necessity of ordered inequality among group members to achieve collective harmony. By contrast, the Western value of instrumental individualism prizes the ability of individuals to make choices and to rely upon themselves to achieve their purpose in life. In contrast to an adult Chinese patient who relies upon the experts and his or her family to make decisions, a typical American or Canadian adult will make a decision and expects experts and family members to provide him or her with information.

Western Moral Philosophic Theories

Articulated by philosophers such as Voltaire, Diderot, and Condorcet, a new awareness swept the Western world during the Enlightenment of the 17th and 18th centuries. These new ideas or assumptions postulated that the human mind is "intendedly rational and scientific, that the dictates of reason are equally binding for all regardless of time, place, culture, race, personal desire or individual endowment, and that in reason can be found a universally applicable standard for judging validity and truth" (Lovejoy, 1974, pp. 288–314). This Western moral philosophy respects the authority of reason and evidence and assumes that people universally value reason. It further believes that human beings around the world have similar lifeways and beliefs about right and wrong.

Naturalism versus Rationalism

Two philosophic theories of ethics, naturalism and rationalism, stemmed from the era of Enlightenment. **Naturalism** holds that all people have similar psychologic tendencies and capacities. Divergence in moral codes is attributed to differences in social conditions such as poverty or lack of education. Once social conditions are ameliorated, it is presumed that uniform morality can be achieved. By contrast, **Rationalism** emphasizes the existence of universal moral truths independent of human nature, known through reason and not by feeling or sensing (Raphael, 1994). Rationalism denies variability in moral truths across cultures because reason is presumed to be universal and the common pathway to achieve the truth.

Teleogical Theories of Ethics

Teleological theories of ethics are derived from naturalism and grounded in the belief that an action is judged by its consequence or outcome. **Consequential theories** such as **utilitarianism** are teleological in perspective. Utilitarianism believes in the idea of the greatest good for the greatest number. Proponents of utilitarianism such as Jeremy Bentham and John Stuart Mill argued that no action should be judged by itself but rather by its usefulness or end results (Quinn & Smith, 1987). Consequentialism believes in the idea that the utility or consequence of an action is the only relevant consideration in judging behaviors (Beauchamp & Childress, 1994). Utilitarianism can be viewed as a form of consequentialism, although not all consequentialists are utilitarians (Beauchamp & Steinbock, 1999). Decisions about distributive justice (the fair allocation of resources) can be justified by a teleological theory, which would support the allocation of resources that may favor some groups over others because it accomplishes good results, such as the health of the population. Allocation of resources to disadvantaged ethnic minority groups, for example, is believed to achieve equity in access to health services and health outcomes across population groups.

Deontological Theories of Ethics

Deontological theories of ethics are based on the rationalist view that the rightness or wrongness of an act depends on the nature of an act itself rather than on its consequence. According to Immanuel Kant's formulation of this theory, humans, because they are rational beings, are subject to universal rules, which have no exceptions and which are discovered by reasoning. The most general of these rules is the **categorical imperative**, which states that every human being has a moral obligation to act in such a way that his or her actions could become a moral law for everyone (Paton, 1961). This theory is the basis of **duty-based ethics**, according to which the morality of an action is judged by its good will and intention. Based on the deontological theory of ethics, a professional code of ethics serves as a guide to actions by members of the nursing profession (Burkhardt & Nathaniel, 1998). Insuring patient confidentiality, for example, is a practice standard for all nurses.

Ethical Principles

Ethical principles are basic moral truths that are taken for granted and guide deliberations and actions. Each of these principles is an application of both deontological and teleological theories of ethics. Central to these principles is respect for the person.

Autonomy

The principle of **autonomy** is closely linked with respect for an individual's free will and includes the right to make choices about issues affecting one's being. Autonomous persons should be allowed to determine their own actions or delegate decision-making to others when they become incapable of making such decisions. The **Patient Self-Determination Act** of 1991 is a legal protection of a person's autonomy or self-determination in these situations through advance directives (Blackhall, Murphy, Frank, Michel, & Azen, 1995). An individual patient's autonomy is assured when a nurse provides appropriate information that could enhance the patient's ability to make a decision about the surgery or treatment.

Beneficence and Nonmaleficence

The principle of **beneficence** is the obligation to do good. The principle of **nonmaleficence** is the obligation to prevent harm. The principles of beneficence and nonmaleficence require that care providers act in ways that benefit and cause no harm to consumers of their care. The decision to give larger doses of morphine to relieve the pain of a terminally ill patient with cancer is weighed carefully for its intended benefits against the possible harm it may cause, such as addiction, respiratory depression, and death. In most cases, promoting the patient's comfort and peaceful death is judged more beneficial over prolonging life and suffering. To do the latter is to create more harm than good to the patient.

Justice

The principle of **justice** relates to the fair, equitable, and appropriate treatment or use of resources in light of what a person needs, weighed against the needs of others. The documents *Healthy People 2010* (U.S. Public Health Service, 2000) and *Achieving Health for All: A Framework for Health Promotion* (Health Canada, 2001) describe existing disparities in access to health care services and health outcomes among population groups in the United States and Canada, respectively. The allocation of resources to combat increasing infant mortality among Blacks, for example, applies the principle of distributive justice. Resources are allocated to achieve the desired health outcome by providing accessible and culture-specific maternal and child health services to this group.

Fidelity and Veracity

The principle of **fidelity** is the obligation to remain faithful to one's commitments (Fry, 1994). Nurses have an obligation to maintain standards of professional practice as a condition of continuing licensure. The principle of **veracity** upholds the virtue of honesty and telling the truth. Truth telling is recognized as a prerequisite to a trusting relationship (Fry, 1994; Norton, 1999). For example, informed consent requires veracity of information presented to the patient and fidelity of practitioners to professional standards.

Individualism as the Context for Ethical Decisions in Western Society

The philosophic traditions of universalism and rationalism have shaped the Western concept of the person as the focus of moral reasoning. The person is the basic unit imbued with universal capacity for reason and action. Differences are attributed to deficits in cognitive skills, motivation, information, and/or linguistic tools (Shweder & Bourne, 1997). Approaches to ethical dilemmas, therefore, are based on the belief that by compensating for these deficits, a person can be expected to make a rational decision that is universally regarded as logical and morally acceptable. Furthermore, a person is viewed as a separate entity, independent of his or her social roles and relationships (Geertz, 1975). A person's existence is distinct from that of his or her significant others.

As noted by many authors, respect for patient autonomy has become the focal context for health care decisions in the United States and Canada (Beauchamp & Childress, 1994; DeWolf Bosek, Savage, Anderson Shaw, & Renella, 2001; Hoffmaster, 1999; Ruhnke, 2000). Ethical principles are applied to ensure and maximize individual autonomy. The autonomy paradigm, which has been institutionalized in health care, underlines the interactions of practitioners, patients, and their families and their expectations of one another, and has become the framework for decisions about their care (Detmar, Muller, Wever, Shornagel, & Aaronson, 2001; Koenig & Gates-Williams, 1995; Orona, Koenig, & Davis, 1994). Patient autonomy is supported by such legal mandates as the 1991 Patient Self-Determination Act (DeWolf Bosek et al., 2001). The debate that surrounded the Patients' Bill of Rights in the U.S. Congress is an example of the tension between protecting individual rights and preserving scarce resources for the benefit of the many. The right of every patient to seek protection under the law from managed care companies is perceived as a major factor driving up the costs of health care. Government initiatives to combat skyrocketing health care costs are often in conflict with the dominant societal value of the individual's right to choose and decide what is best for his or her well-being. In contrast to the Western value of individualism, members of the Xhosa tribe in South Africa emphasize collective decisions about individual member's care. Elders in the tribe make major decisions about the distribution of human and material resources to provide care for their members (Figure 15–1).

Figure 15–1. Women of the South African Xhosa tribe at a wedding of a family member *(Courtesy of Beatrice Mabutho)*.

• ETHICS AND CULTURAL DIVERSITY

Richard Shweder (1997) has argued that not all human behaviors can be classified as simply rational or irrational. Culture, according to Shweder, is primarily concerned with nonrational ideas, whose expression speaks of how reality is constructed by groups of people. Social order is ultimately nonrational, and many of the customary practices of a society, from table manners and dress codes to child training, are symbolic expressions of these nonrational choices. Culture is the realm of the arbitrary, where human beings create their own distinctive, symbolic universe. Schweder states:

"There are cases where canons of rationality, validity, truth and efficiency are simply beside the point—irrelevant! ...There is the possibility ...that there's something more to thinking than reason and evidence—culture, the arbitrary, the symbolic, the expressive, the semiotic—that many of our ideas and practices are beyond logic and experience" (p. 38).

This is illustrated by the members of Jehovah's Witnesses, who disregard the scientifically based treatment of blood transfusion as a life-saving measure and violate the logic of biomedical reasoning. Similarly, Christian Scientists may prefer their own religious and spiritually based practices of healing to those of scientific medicine. To professional practitioners, their resistance to valid and scientifically proven measures belie common sense, yet the traditions of these groups hold that what is morally good transcends physical life. Indeed, common sense is not common after all; it is uniquely constructed within the social and cultural life contexts of human groups.

Cultural diversity requires us to switch our frames of understanding, recognizing the coequality of fundamentally different perspectives and the ability of each of several persistent yet incompatible frames to handle any and all new evidence (Shweder, 1997). Frame switching permits us to accept variances in common sense and to recognize that logic and science are limited in understanding differences. Belief in the universality of reason prevents us from considering other ways of life and appreciating other systems of meanings. Bracketing our own values and beliefs allows us to discover the emic ways of people from other cultures. There are two perspectives in any given situation: the **emic** (insider's) view and the **etic** (outsider's) view. For example, the husband of a terminally ill patient (both are Filipino) was distressed by the nurse's suggestion that his wife be given a clear liquid diet until her nausea, vomiting, and diarrhea were relieved. From his emic perspective, providing food such as *arroz caldo* (rice and chicken soup) would promote health and signify caring, but the nurse's etic interpretation of his behavior was that he lacked knowledge about the proper care of the patient.

Indeed, contrary to the Western emphasis on self-determination, many societies value collective harmony and relationships of individuals with one another. Group-centeredness recognizes the importance of solidarity and cohesiveness with members of the collective over individualistic motives and achievements (Dahrendorf, 1979; Hsu, 1963; Parsons, 1951). The valued person is one who promotes group welfare over self-centered goals and manifests such attributes as loyalty, generosity, and warmth. Maintaining the integrity of the collective motivates decisions, and mutual dependence characterizes interactions among group members (Pacquiao, 1996). Family and kinship patterns delineate the different roles, status, and power assigned to members of the group. The social hierarchy governs decision-making and the social interactions, roles, and obligations of members. For example, among traditional Japanese, the elder man is generally accorded higher status and authority. His decisions are respected and accepted by the group. His position carries a sense of responsibility for the entire group; conversely, members are expected to honor and obey him.

In some groups, religious and spiritual dimensions highly influence behaviors. Among such ethnoreligious groups as devout Muslims, Hindus, and Jews, religion is embedded in everyday life. Decisions about euthanasia, for example, may not be acceptable to an Orthodox Jew whose beliefs uphold the sanctity of life. Religion increases the awareness of the power and benevolence of God over humans; hence, earthly decisions are left to God, and the attitude is one of acceptance of fate rather than control over one's destiny.

In contrast to the autonomy paradigm, the social framework paradigm plays a greater role in other countries as well as in many cultural groups in the United States and Canada (Kagawa-Singer, 1994; Koenig & Gates-Williams, 1995; Pacquiao, 2001). Patient autonomy is a lower priority than beneficence, nonmaleficence, and distributive justice among Blacks, Chinese, Koreans, and Mexicans (Hopp & Duffy, 2000; Ip, Gilligan, Koenig, & Raffin, 1998; Valle, 2001). Communitarian groups such as Koreans and Chinese use a family-centered approach. They also lean toward less assertive decision-making and defer more to the physician's judgment (Post, Blustein, Gordon, & Dubler, 1996; Valle, 2001). See Evidence-Based Practice 15–1 for a discussion of Korean American female caregivers.

A **community-based theory of ethics** emphasizes communal values, the common good, and social goals based on the members' shared assumptions and beliefs about morality that is rooted in a common sense and tradition (Beauchamp & Childress, 1994). Pluralistic conceptions of right and wrong, and orientation toward relationship with others, are the tenets of this theory. This perspective is embedded in the **ethic of care** originated by feminist authors such as Carol Gilligan (1982). This philosophy recognizes the importance of actions promoting positive relationships (Beauchamp & Childress, 1994; Ray, 1994).

• CULTURAL CONFLICT IN ETHICAL DECISION-MAKING

This section presents selected case studies in health care and nursing relevant to cultural diversity. Each is discussed by use of a bifocal analysis, comparing the Western and culture-specific perspectives. Although these case studies are based on real events, caution should be exercised in generalizing the cultural characteristics presented. Readers should be cognizant of the intercultural and intracultural differences among people.

> ## EVIDENCE-BASED PRACTICE 15–1
> ### *Korean Caregivers*
>
> A descriptive study using interviews of 30 Korean American female caregivers found that they were the elderly wives of elderly husbands who maintained separate households from their adult children. They were unemployed, with low income and educational attainment, and isolated from social connections. The norm of filial obligation remained strong among the older caregivers, who saw their role as their final duty as a spouse and resisted putting their husbands in nursing homes. Many of them saw their sons' lack of filial obligation as part of the changes that had come with living in the United States. The traditional Korean norm for women to be tolerant of hardships and suppress their emotions prevented these caregivers from sharing their hardships with others. The study findings suggested that practitioners go beyond the traditional Korean cultural norms to discover real-life situations among these women.
>
> ### CLINICAL APPLICATION
>
> 1. Describe the appropriate assessment needed to define the problem of Korean women caregivers.
> 2. Discuss how practitioners can preserve traditional cultural norms while providing for the needs of the Korean female caregivers.
>
> Kim, J. H., & Theis, S. L. (2000). Korean caregivers: Who are they? *Journal of Transcultural Nursing*, 11(4), 264–273.

Compliance with Professionally Prescribed Regimen: A Hmong Family

Fadiman's (1997) story about a Hmong family's experience with health care in Merced, California, portrays two contrasting explanatory models for illness (epileptic seizures). The family members attributed their daughter's seizures to spirits in their universe that needed to be appeased by ritual offerings. Taking the biomedical approach, her physicians attributed her seizures to pathologic changes in the neuronal pathway.

The Hmong people, who have traditionally lived in the mountainous and remote areas of Laos in Southeast Asia, share a worldview that the environment is vast, imbued with power, and beyond their control. Hence, rituals to appease the spirits that dwell in these forests are needed to promote and restore health. Human beings are seen as an integral part of the universe, with an inseparable body and soul. Such beliefs are in direct confrontation with the biomedical worldview of the human body as a separate entity from the soul, and of humans as independent of their universe and capable of controlling their environment.

The situation was compounded by communication barriers. Both parents were illiterate, as is common among Hmong adults who grew up in a culture of purely oral traditions. Hmong interpreters are neither easily accessible nor available, and using young children to interpret is an affront to the established family hierarchy, which recognizes the father as the primary authority and decision maker.

Although both the family and the medical community had the best interest of the child in mind, this clash of two cultures reached a predictable end: the victory and superiority of the dominant biomedical worldview, entrenched in health care and supported by societal legal mandates. In this case, the child was removed from her family and placed in a home with a foster mother, to be followed up by a social worker. Equipped with knowledge of the language and culture of the dominant and professional cultures, the foster mother and social worker were deemed credible by the medical community. Their observations and a culturally congruent interpretation of the family's care eventually convinced the medical community to return the child to her family.

The physicians applied the principles of beneficence, nonmaleficence, and justice within the context of the biologic welfare of the child. The child's personal autonomy was the prime consideration, even to the extent of separating her from her loving family, who were viewed as incapable of performing the prescribed medical regimen. By contrast, the parents applied the ethical principles of beneficence, nonmaleficence, and distributive justice within the context of the holistic beliefs and family obligations to their child. Their daughter's life was inseparable from their own, and her well-being was assured by the family's performance of rituals in addition to the medical regimen. In fact, they sacrificed much of their resources to obtain a spiritual folk healer for the child.

Clearly, a different paradigm for decision-making was needed that promoted the welfare of the child and the integrity of the family, which is so valued by the collective-oriented Hmongs. Knowledge of their lifeway would have prevented the unwarranted separation of the child from her parents by accommodating their beliefs and practices, which, for the most part, were not harmful to the child. This situation demonstrates the need to understand the different ways in which groups of people express caring on the basis of their learned way of life. Although caring is a universal human characteristic, assuming that it is carried out the same way across groups can be very damaging for the intended recipients.

Visiting Rules in Health Care Organizations: A Gypsy Family

In hospitals, space is a prime commodity and is allocated on the basis of the staff members' care-giving activities for patients. In critical care areas, where constant surveillance of patients occurs, the continued presence of several family members is generally viewed as interfering with care-giving activities by staff members and may make the institution vulnerable to liability. Family members can indeed be emotional and demanding, and this may be perceived as an additional burden for practitioners, who are focused on the individual patient's physical well-being. Whereas limiting the number of visitors and visiting hours per patient is considered essential for efficient and safe care giving by staff, the physical presence of visitors is considered by many cultures to be the essence of caring.

A Gypsy boy was admitted to a pediatric intensive care unit, accompanied by a large group of relatives and non–family members. Several women in addition to his mother insisted on staying at the bedside, and the men requested that they stay in a separate room adjacent to the unit. Caring among the Gypsies involves close surveillance and physical presence by members of the social organization. Gypsy social organization extends beyond kin to include groups of extended families that travel and reside together and maintain allegiance to a group of male leaders, or *kumpania* (Bodnar & Leininger, 1995). The societal norm of nuclear family that has guided visiting policies in acute care settings, specifically intensive care units, is in conflict with the Gypsy kinship and social structure. Professional health care generally recognizes the child's parents as the primary caregiver of the child; yet, among the Gypsies the authority of the male leaders of their community supersedes parental authority. Gender-based roles in caregiving delegate caretaking to the mother and female members and decision-making to the adult male leaders.

Practitioners should negotiate with adult male leaders rather than giving instructions to the mother and expecting her to speak to her husband for important decisions. Visiting hours and requests that visitors take turns to visit the unit are better negotiated with the leader, who has the status and power within the group. Beneficence and nonmaleficence should be implemented within the context of the established social hierarchy of the collective rather than based solely on patient autonomy. Distributive justice requires accommodation of their lifeway and the contextual definition of caring by the group, independent of the professional worldview. Gypsies are committed to maintaining their cultural identity separate from outsiders (gadje), and there are strong sanctions against members who violate this rule (Sutherland, 1986; Sway, 1988). Evidence-Based Practice 15–2 discusses some of the difficulties encountered by nurses when they care for people from different cultures than their own.

Truth-Telling about Diagnosis and Prognosis: The Pakistani Culture

Veracity and fidelity are ethical principles guiding the interactions of practitioners with patients and families. These principles are supportive of individual autonomy and are assumed to benefit and minimize harm to the patient, who needs truthful information to make a sound decision. However, in other cultures where the family is the fundamental unit of society, inextricable social bonds between members are the source of vital decisions. This is especially true when an illness is terminal. The family generally protects the patient from the anxiety and distress associated with the knowledge of impending death.

After training and practicing as a physician in the United States, Moazam (2000) accepted a position at a medical university in Pakistan. Moazam noted that when illness struck a family member, it was the family and the doctor rather than the patient who took center stage. Family members generally avoided disclosing terminal illness to patients. This was believed to prevent further burden on the patient and allow the patient to die in peace. Family-centered decision-making worked with the active, directive role assumed by

EVIDENCE-BASED PRACTICE 15-2
Caring for People from Other Cultures

Using a hermeneutic approach, the study focused on the experience and reflections of 17 registered nurses in Auckland, New Zealand, in caring for people from cultures other than their own. A total of 39 interviews and four written anecdotal records were analyzed. The study found that nurses' reflective thinking was action oriented and primarily focused on the immediate situation. These reflections did not recognize the historical and cultural influences on their practice, such as the power differentials inherent in the delivery of service. In dealing with conflicts, nurses tended to use the same assumptions and values intrinsic to their practice rather than reexamine these implicit beliefs for new understanding. The findings suggest the need for education and mentoring of nurses in fostering environments of care that foster egalitarian and pluralistic interactions, and implementing processes rather than solutions, to uncover prejudices and paradoxes in existing assumptions.

CLINICAL APPLICATION

1. Cite an example of a problem or conflict in your practice.
2. Identify components of the problem that relate to professional and organizational values.
3. Identify the values that need to be modified to achieve culturally congruent ethical care.

Spence, D. G. (2001). Prejudice, paradox, and possibility: Nursing people from cultures other than one's own. *Journal of Transcultural Nursing, 12*(2), 100–106.

the physician, emphasizing the principles of beneficence and nonmaleficence rather than patient autonomy.

Studies done in Africa, Hungary, Japan, Portugal, Italy, and Spain show that fewer than 40% of oncologists avoid using the word "cancer " or "terminal" when talking to patients (Holland, Geary, Marchum, & Tross, 1987). Valle (2001) also notes that among communitarian groups such as Mexicans, Chinese, and Koreans, patient autonomy and truth telling are secondary to beneficence and nonmaleficence in ethical decisions.

Pakistani medical decision-making is deeply rooted in the moral philosophy shared by many Eastern cultures that recognize the religious obligation of the family and the physician to the patient. This moral philosophy is not based on the secular, reason-based philosophy, dominant in Western societies, which emphasizes the legal rights of individuals. The Muslim religion defines the role of the individual, the family, and the physician in life transitions such as illness and death (Moazam, 2000). The physician is viewed as a trusted family member and an instrument of God, who is part of the extended family. Likewise, Koreans and Chinese tend to accept the physician's decision rather than assume an assertive role in decision-making (Valle, 2001).

Decisions regarding full disclosure about an illness or prognosis need to take into account the religious and moral contexts of people's lives. Accommodating their system of meanings can prevent divisions within a family unit. Practitioners should not assume that the principles of veracity and fidelity are universally defined and expressed, and should realize that the ethical principles of nonmaleficence and beneficence can be applied differentially across cultures. Understanding the different life context of families and groups is the starting point for meaningful decision-making. Working with the families' own moral philosophies can assure culturally congruent applications of the principles of beneficence and nonmaleficence.

Advance Directives: The Filipino Family

Health care practitioners are mandated to provide patients with information about advance directives. **Advance directives** are intended to assure patients' autonomy in situations when they can no longer make a decision. Individuals' choices are presumably carried out on their behalf in the event that they cannot consciously and competently represent their own will. Although the intent of advance directives is laudable within the Western ethos of self-determination, other cultures subscribe to the belief that the fate of human beings is beyond their control.

Among traditional Filipinos, a sense of fatalism that is deeply rooted in their religious and supernatural beliefs conditions an individual to attribute either positive or negative events to God's will (Miranda, McBride, & Spangler, 1998). Planning for one's illness or death—events considered beyond one's control—is viewed as tempting fate and will likely bring the potential event into reality. Therefore, discussions of a living will are avoided even with family members (Pacquiao, 2001). Asking a Filipino patient if he or she has a living will is likely to produce a negative answer, which can have different meanings: the subject is to be avoided, the patient does not want a living will, or the patient does not have one. Discussing advance directives is likely to be perceived as an uncomfortable cultural imposition by the individual and the family. Conversely, Filipino and Chinese nurses express discomfort in discussing advance directives with hospitalized patients because they see their role as caregivers to patients. They would much prefer to refer patients to the clergy and pastoral care services for discussions about advance directives (Pacquiao, 2001).

Measures intended to expand patients' autonomy, such as advance directives, may transgress cultural taboos in certain cultures, creating more anxiety and discomfort in patients and families. Many Blacks equate advance directives as legitimizing abandonment by practitioners, stemming from their experience with the health care system in the Tuskegee experiment (Dupree, 2000). As with many Filipinos, the patient's welfare is entrusted to family members, who will act according to his or her best interests. Family members are bound by the ethos of caring for one another and are trusted to act on behalf of one another. Consequently, the patient with strong family ties does not find it necessary to execute a living will. In fact, Dupree (2000) has found that family members expect to be the decision-makers for family members who are ill.

Advance directives represent a conflict between patient autonomy and family solidarity. Individual autonomy is not a priority in cultures where strong social bonds exist among family members and the individual's best interest is taken for granted as the inherent responsibility of the group. Cohesiveness and mutuality among members removes the necessity for an individual to worry about his or her future, because the individual's goals and aspirations are deeply embedded in the group.

Informed Consent: The Mexican Family

The Western presumption that a competent adult can be relied on to make decisions and is willing to take that responsibility is not universal. Cultures emphasizing collective solidarity have an established social structure that governs the actions of members based on their positions within the hierarchy. Individuals in positions of authority are called on to make decisions for other members. Such privilege is associated with a sense of responsibility and accountability for the group members.

Because of pain in her toes, a Mexican widow was taken to the hospital by her adult daughter. On examination, the physician determined that her toes were gangrenous and needed immediate surgery. When the surgical consent needed to be signed, however, the patient and her daughter refused to sign. They insisted on speaking with the patient's oldest son, residing in another state, who in turn refused to give consent until he consulted his uncle in Mexico. The surgeon was angered by the family's lack of understanding of the emergency nature of the surgery. The uncle eventually consented after several weeks when he witnessed the patient (his sister) suffering from much pain.

The ethos of machismo in Mexican culture upholds the role of the older man in decision-making for the family. Family hierarchy within the male-dominated structure significantly influences decisions about other members (Purnell, 1998). The Western assumption about individual autonomy is not equally valued and becomes less significant as a consideration in family decision-making.

In the previous example of the Mexican family, understanding the social structure dimension and negotiating with the adult men would have shortened the waiting period for the surgical consent to be signed. No doubt, both family members and the physicians cared about the patient's well-being. In contrast to the physicians who used the context of pathophysiology in deciding the urgency of the surgery, family members based their decision on their collective interpretation of the patient's comfort. The patient's surgery was a family decision, congruent with the gender-based hierarchy of their social organization rather than an individual decision. The act of obtaining an informed consent needed to accommodate family hierarchy and family involvement (Stasiak, 1991; Villaruel & Leininger, 1995).

Concepts of the Human Body: The Muslim Patient

Religious beliefs often color the perceptions of different cultures regarding such procedures as amputation and organ donation. Members of Islamic groups generally hesitate to submit to autopsies or organ donations for fear of disrespecting the integrity of the human body. Devout Muslims prefer to bury the body whole so the individual can meet his or her creator with integrity (Meleis, 1996). Muslim scholars have deduced from the Qur'anic text that it may be possible for the deceased to feel pain and that breaking the bone of the dead is like breaking the bone of the living (Gatrad & Sheikh, 2001). Orthodox Jews also value the integrity of the human body. Respect and the provision of privacy for the deceased during ritual cleansing are closely observed (Bonura, Fender, Roesler, & Pacquiao, 2001).

After a motor vehicle accident, a Muslim teenager was brought to the hospital emergency room. The medical team recommended that his right leg be amputated. The family refused to give consent to the emergency surgery until an imam could be present to bless the amputated leg. An imam is a Muslim priest, who is generally called after death (Meleis, 1996). Fortunately, the imam contacted by the family was available and rushed to the operating room where the amputation was done. He supervised the ritual of washing, and he blessed the amputated leg before it was removed from the operating room.

The Western concept of dualism, which reduces the human body into distinct parts with separate body and soul, is not shared by many cultures that subscribe to a holistic and integrated view of human beings, rooted in the religious belief that the human being is a unified entity composed of body, soul, and spirit. In the case of this family, biophysical trauma and possibly death were secondary to maintaining the wholeness of the individual, for without the soul, the body cannot exist. Hence, the spirit and soul should not be disrespected for the sake of corporeal survival. Integrity of the human being is to be promoted even in death. Evidence-Based Practice 15–3 discusses one study that examined the beliefs of a group of Blacks regarding organ donation.

The ethical principles of beneficence and nonmaleficence are not limited to biophysical goals. For this Muslim family, these principles were meaningless without the context of the spiritual dimension. Accommodating this belief through culturally congruent practice rendered biomedical interventions meaningful in the emic views of the family. Measures to promote survival are inadequate and harmful when religious beliefs are ignored.

Quality versus Sanctity of Life: The Orthodox Jewish Family

The inherent conflict between the quality of life and sanctity of life underlines the pros and cons of physician-assisted suicide. American and Canadian medicine is thought to be leaning toward a utilitarian practice model in which patients are deemed as discardable when quality of life is not possible (Booth, 2001; Burgess, Stephenson, Ratanakul, & Suwonnakote, 1999; McCain, 2001). Quality of life is ideally determined by the patient in collaboration with the physician. This concept, though congruent with the ethos of self-determination, is incompatible with the values and beliefs of many cultures.

EVIDENCE-BASED PRACTICE 15–3
Organ Donation Beliefs
of Rural African American Women

Using the ethnonursing method, in-depth interviews of 10 key and 22 general informants were conducted during community visits to discover culture care beliefs, meanings, and practices regarding organ donation. The key informants consisted of mostly Baptist African American women between 26 and 66 years of age, residing in a small, rural town in Mississippi. The study found that decisions regarding organ donation were strongly influenced by their religious beliefs and kinship ties. Informants shared the belief that God will take care of the needs of the "righteous" and that the "bad" ones deserve to suffer. All participants who were willing to donate their organs expressed a strong preference for giving their organs to family members. Although the study found a lack of knowledge about the process involved in organ donation, the findings suggest the strong social and cultural influences on participants' decisions that have implications on the decreased rate and long waiting period for organ donation among ethnic minority groups.

CLINICAL APPLICATION

1. Identify culturally congruent actions that promote cultural preservation and accommodation for this group.
2. Describe cultural repatterning strategies needed in ethical decision making.

Wittig, D. R. (2001). Organ donation beliefs of African American women residing in a small southern community. *Journal of Transcultural Nursing, 12*(3), 203–210.

An 80-year-old Orthodox Jewish woman, with an earlier diagnosis of terminal breast cancer, was admitted to the hospital while her family was away on vacation. Her condition, which had remained stable for the past 6 months, deteriorated to the point where she could no longer eat or sleep because of pain. Feeding tubes and intravenous fluids were started when she was admitted, and she was given round-the-clock pain medication. Her family came to visit her within 48 hours of her admission. Throughout her hospitalization, groups of visitors from her community took turns visiting and praying at her bedside. Because the patient was never left alone, the hospital administrator decided to transfer her to a private room. The rabbi from the patient's synagogue came often and prayed with her. The family consulted him before any major decision about the patient's care was made. When physicians recommended withdrawal of the feeding tube and intravenous fluids, the family requested that the physicians speak to their rabbi. After consulting with the family, the rabbi communicated agreement in removing the feeding tube but requested that the intravenous line be kept for pain medication. Until the day the patient died, the family members were vigilant in monitoring her care, emphasizing her comfort and spiritual care.

In Judaism, death is seen as a natural ending of the cycle of life and all living things. It is a transition from this life to the life that is yet to come. Because life is not forever, one is taught to value life and to live one's potential. When death is imminent, the person is faced with anxiety—not about dying but about how he or she will be judged after death. One's life is measured by one's deeds and by whether one has lived up to his or her potential, so the dying patient spends most of the remaining time in reviewing his or her life (Levine, 1997; Ponet, 1996).

In Jewish tradition, because life is God given, human beings cannot take it away. Because human beings were created in the image of God, the body and the soul must not be altered nor disrespected. Every life, even as it ebbs, is to be respected and revered. Death must not be hastened, but one may pray for the death of another as a release from insufferable pain. Jewish law permits praying for mercy for a very sick person. Although the dying must be made as comfortable as possible, nothing must keep the soul from leaving the body. This provision in the Talmud has been interpreted to allow for acceptance of "do not resuscitate" orders or withdrawal of life support (Levine, 1997; Selekman, 1998).

Judaism also mandates the obligation to visit and pray for the sick and to be with the dying and the grieving to dispel the loneliness that comes with death and bereavement (Bonura et al., 2001). This obligation is true for both the family and members of the community, and religious beliefs are embedded in the rituals that must be carried out with and for the sick.

For decisions to be meaningful, they must recognize those inherent beliefs and social bonds that extend beyond the immediate family. The role of the rabbi is particularly significant in bridging the realms of biomedicine and religion. Collective presence at the bedside manifests communal obligations congruent with meanings of caring from the social, cultural, and religious dimensions. Decisions that are deemed beneficial and meaningful are not defined within the context of the patient's autonomy but rather are made within the multifaceted framework of religion and community. The religious leader, who guides decisions relevant to mortality, mediates many decisions and is guided by religious laws governing immortality. The Judaic tenet of life created by and in the image of God emphasizes sanctity of life over biomedical definitions of quality of life (see Figure 15-2).

The Meaning of Life in the Context of Hinduism

The biomedical definition of life and death is not shared across cultures. In the Western worldview, death connotes finality, and only the legacy of the deceased lives on in the minds of those left behind. When death is imminent, promoting the comfort of the dying is the paramount concern. In contrast to this Western worldview, death is viewed by Hindus and Buddhists as a step to another life, and birth, life, and death are part of a never-ending cycle. Buddhism's pervasive belief in impermanence underlies the concept of ceaseless transmutation of all existing beings and forces; the endless cycle of birth, death, and rebirth; and the suffering that inevitably accompanies impermanence. The ultimate goal of existence is to attain a state of timeless, deathless, blissful nirvana (Gielen, 1997).

An older Hindu man was hospitalized with terminal pancreatic cancer. He did not describe having pain, and he refused pain medication. For two days, family members remained at his bedside, praying and sometimes singing aloud. Although he was in a private room, the praying and singing disturbed other patients and caused concern among the staff members. The staff also noted that family members lifted the patient out of bed and placed him on the floor.

The Hindu belief in reincarnation or transmigration of life is rooted in the cosmologic concept of samsara. Whereas the material body is mortal, the soul is eternal. The ultimate goal of the soul is to escape the cycle of death and rebirth and to attain moksha, liberation from this cycle and reabsorption into the oneness of the Universal Soul (Madan, 1988). A devout Hindu who senses impending death prepares for a "good death." A good death is a death in which the dying person is in full possession of his or her mental and physical faculties, is fully cognizant of what is to come, and is not overtaken by death but "lets go of life" deliberately and willingly (Parry, 1982). Hence, a dying Hindu may refuse nourishment and pain medication. Family members remain at the bedside and pray or may sing devotional songs to help the dying fix his or her mind on the Divine. They may also request to have the patient lifted from the bed to a purified spot on the ground (Vatuk, 1996).

The rituals performed by the family for the dying member demonstrate the salience of religious and spiritual beliefs in caring. Their practices negate the importance of the biomedical interventions that practitioners generally provide for a dying patient. In fact, interventions such as pain medication are in direct conflict with the goals of maintaining awareness and experiencing what is to come that are central to preparing for a good death. Whereas practitioners may view such practices as prolonging suffering, the family views these practices as actions that carve a pathway to a better life in the next cycle. Hence, the application of beneficence and nonmaleficence need to fit the religious context of the patient and family rather than biomedical goals.

Figure 15–2. The rabbi visits this resident of a geriatric center.

• CULTURALLY COMPETENT MODEL FOR ETHICAL DECISION-MAKING

Assumptions of the Model

In her theory of culture care diversity and universality, Leininger (1991) identified the centrality of culturally congruent approaches in humanistic caring. Caring that is meaningful or beneficial occurs when a culture's care values, expressions, or patterns are known and used appropriately by care providers. Knowledge of culture-specific and universal phenomena enables practitioners to make care decisions that fit people's lifeways. This knowledge is grounded in the emic perspectives of individuals, families, groups, and communities about caring that is inductively generated from the people themselves.

Leininger makes a distinction between generic care and professional care. Any care situation involves both emic (insider) and etic (outsider) perspectives. Professional caregivers and health care organizations may have very different sets of values and assumptions about caring from those of people who use their services. Cultural conflicts arise from competing worldviews and moral assumptions, which lead to ethical dilemmas. Leininger (1991) identifies three action strategies that are grounded in cultural knowledge of the care recipients and in coparticipation of practitioners and consumers in decision-making:

1. Cultural care preservation or maintenance—assistive, supportive, facilitative, or enabling professional actions and decisions that help people of a particular culture to retain and/or preserve relevant care values so that they can maintain their well-being, recover from illness, or face handicaps and/or death.
2. Cultural care accommodation or negotiation—assistive, supportive, facilitative, or enabling professional actions and decisions that help people of a designated culture adapt to, or negotiate with, others for beneficial or satisfying health outcomes with professional care providers.
3. Cultural care repatterning or restructuring—assistive, supportive, facilitative, or enabling professional actions and decisions that help a client reorder, change, or greatly modify his or her lifeways for a new, different, and beneficial health care pattern, and maintenance of respect for the client's cultural values and beliefs while still providing a beneficial or healthier lifeway than before the changes were coestablished with the client (Leininger, 1991, pp. 48–49).

Components of the Model

Jonathan Mann proposed the human rights framework as the new template for public health (Mann & Burris, 1998). Promoting and protecting human rights is inextricably linked with promoting and protecting health. Human rights must be respected, not only for their instrumental value in contributing to public health goals but as a societal good of preeminent importance. According to Mann, the modern human rights framework, which arises outside the health domain and seeks to articulate preconditions for human well-being at the societal level, may provide a useful framework, vocabulary, and template for public health (Mann & Burris, 1998, p. 3).

Drawn from Mann's insight and Leininger's theory, this model adopts the human rights framework for ethical decision-making. It affirms the fundamental right of individuals, families, groups, and populations to health care that is meaningful, supportive, and beneficial. It is predicated on the basic human right of respect for diversity of values and assumptions about life transitions and events. It is based on the principle that caring preserves human rights and dignity.

Within the context of human rights and culturally congruent care, ethical principles such as beneficence, nonmaleficence, and justice are reconceptualized within the values and assumptions of the client(s). The model mandates that practitioners learn about the cultural lifeways of their client(s) and work with them to resolve issues in a way that client(s) can find satisfying and meaningful (Case Study 15–1). The ethical principle of autonomy is excluded

CASE STUDY	15–1

A 70-year-old Pakistani man with a diagnosis of terminal pancreatic cancer was referred by his physician for home care services after hospitalization. The nurse made a home visit to admit the patient. She met the patient in the dining room alone while his wife and daughter stayed in the kitchen. Before retirement, the patient had worked for the Consulate of Pakistan in New York City. He had been living with his wife, daughter, son-in-law, and two young granddaughters. The patient spoke English well and interacted without difficulty with the nurse. The nurse noted that the physician had prescribed multivitamins and no pain medication. When asked about his main problem, the patient responded that he had difficulty sleeping. Expecting to hear him describe having pain, the nurse asked the patient four times if he had pain. He responded negatively. The nurse also noted that the patient appeared comfortable throughout the assessment interview. When the nurse rephrased the question and asked the patient if he was in any discomfort, he replied, "Yes." At this point, the nurse attempted to find out the intensity and duration of his discomfort. The patient, however, continued to assert that the discomfort was not much. The nurse then asked if the discomfort went away, and the patient replied, "Only when I'm sleeping."

Using the culturally competent model of ethical decision making:

- Assess cultural factors influencing the patient's behavior.
- Explain how the nurse's approach was effective in eliciting information about the symptom.
- Define the patient's needs.
- Suggest ways of communicating his needs to the physician and other visiting nurses.
- In validating your assessment, how would you communicate your diagnosis to the patient? Should you use the principle of veracity?
- Identify interventions congruent with cultural preservation, negotiation, and repatterning.
- Describe new insights the model has generated.

from the model to prevent the interpretation of advocacy, commonly assumed in the Western world, as being limited to the individual client. A human rights framework subsumes the Western concept of individual autonomy as well as the non-Western value of collectivity. It provides a continuum for accommodating different values, assumptions, and morals across culture groups. It presupposes human rights for individuals, families, groups, and populations. Within this framework, an individualistic Westerner's values of self-autonomy is recognized as equal to a non-Westerner's value of family solidarity.

The action strategies suggested by Leininger are adopted in this model. These actions are based on the following prerequisites: (1) cultural knowledge of the client(s), (2) the prime importance of the emic perspectives of the client(s), and (3) care providers' roles as learners of the consumers' culture and coparticipants in decision-making. Culturally congruent decisions are ethical because they respect and protect the inherent values and assumptions of people that have provided a context of meanings to their lives. Ethical principles are rendered meaningful when any of these actions are taken. These principles gain importance only when the intended recipients find them congruent with their valued ways of being. Culturally congruent actions force care providers to protect human rights to achieve meaning and comfort in caring. Culturally congruent actions are the processes by which ethical principles are applied and human rights are preserved.

All three components—human rights, ethical principles, and culturally congruent actions—are the necessary ingredients for **culturally competent decision-making**. Figure 15–3 depicts the relationship of the components of

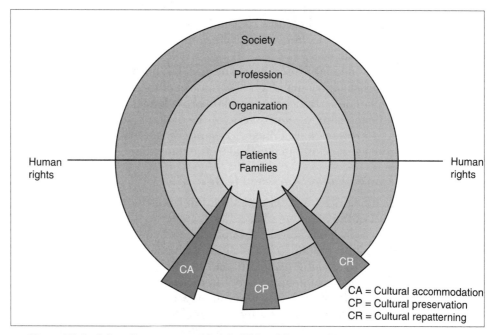

Figure 15–3. Culturally competent Model of Ethical Decision-Making.

the model. Cultural competence is achieved when ethical decisions preserve a patient's human right to meaningful and satisfying care that is grounded in the patient's culturally constituted values and lifeways. This cultural context is paramount in achieving care that is judged moral and ethical by consumers themselves.

Using the Model

Table 15–1 provides a schema for using the model within the paradigm of the nursing process.

Assessment

The three component parts of assessment are (1) assessment of clients and families, (2) assessment of organizational culture, and (3) assessment of dominant professional and societal norms. Client/family assessment is focused on determining the cultural variables that influence their thoughts and behaviors. Data are collected to gain knowledge of their cultural values, beliefs, and practices that can provide insight into their thoughts and behaviors about their care. Philosophic beliefs about life transitions such as birth, illness, and death can often be determined by assessing religious and spiritual traditions. Assessment includes ethnohistory, premigration and postmigration patterns, social organization and hierarchy, patterns of interaction, and family and community resources.

Assessment of staff and organizational cultures, organizational resources and flexibility, and staff members' knowledge and skills in dealing with the client(s) culture will yield valuable information on the ability of the organization and care providers to handle the situation. Most conflicts stem from inherent differences between the cultures of the client(s) and the organization/staff (Figure 15-4).

Dominant professional and societal norms are embedded in legal, ethical, and regulatory mandates. Awareness of these parameters will facilitate realistic collaboration between care providers and consumers that protects the human rights of consumers, other patients, and staff. Assessing the societal and professional contexts promotes realistic decision-making by addressing the needs of others external to the immediate situation.

Planning and Outcome Identification

Defining the problem and situation from the viewpoint of the client(s) is the goal of the planning phase. Understanding the emic worldview of clients facilitates problem solving that preserve their human rights and cultural sets of meanings. Building relationships with clients, families, and groups is a prerequisite to forming respectful and trusting copartnerships that enhance understanding a problem from multiple perspectives.

Transcultural nursing is integrated in the Master of Nursing program at Kean University in New Jersey. Graduates of the program are expected to have the knowledge and skills to design and implement culturally congruent care for diverse clients and to manage a cultural diverse workforce (Figure 15–4).

TABLE 15–1	GUIDE FOR USING THE CULTURALLY COMPETENT MODEL

Assessment

Client/families	Ethnohistory
	Concepts of the human body and soul
	Meaning of life, pain, suffering, and death
	Caring values, patterns, and expressions
	Social organization
	Established social hierarchy
	Roles and obligation of family members and kin
	Differential acculturation of family/group members
	Family and community resources
	Cultural gatekeepers and brokers in the community
	Communication norms and linguistic patterns
	Experience with professional health care
Organizational cultural variables	Staff cultural knowledge and skills
	Conflicting values between staff and patient/family/group
	Conflicting values among care providers
	Cultural expertise available
	Policies and procedures
	Flexibility in accommodating cultural differences
	Material resources available
Determination of professional and societal variables	Legal mandates
	Regulatory requirements
	Impact of decisions on other patients and staff
	Professional code of ethics

Planning

Establish relationship with client(s)/families/communities
Define problems and priorities that reflect the emic perspectives of client(s)
Determine material and personnel resources needed
Determine aspects of action plans that need to be negotiated with participants

Intervention

Cultural care preservation or maintenance
Cultural care accommodation or negotiation
Cultural care repatterning or restructuring

Evaluation

Allow clients/families to identify outcomes and indices for achievement
Differentiate culturally meaningful from biomedical outcomes
Validate outcomes achievement with clients/families

Intervention

During the intervention phase, culturally congruent actions are implemented. All three strategies of preservation, negotiation, and repatterning may be used simultaneously. Using these nursing actions requires a relative perspective about the application of ethical principles of beneficence, nonmaleficence,

Figure 15–4. Assessment of the staff and organizational culture is a beginning step toward culturally congruent decision making.

and justice based on the contexts of people's way of life. These principles may be given different levels of priority across cultural groups. Understanding the cultural variables and the emic worldviews of clients is salient to the selection and implementation of actions. Culturally congruent actions are predicated on trusting relationships between consumers and practitioners, and on interactions that integrate the cultural norms and language patterns of clients.

Outcome Evaluation

In evaluation, outcomes of care are not limited to the achievement of biomedical goals. Holistic indices inclusive of physical, psychologic, social, cultural, and spiritual being are evaluated and monitored. The meanings and indices of outcomes of care may be different across cultural groups. Biomedical outcomes of care that define the effectiveness of professional health care may be secondary to other outcomes, such as the observance of religious and spiritual beliefs. The client's subjective, personal definition of, and affirmation of outcomes are paramount. Many meaningful outcomes may be variably expressed and may not be visible to outsiders to the culture. Validation from clients and an understanding of their context of meanings will provide valuable information in identifying appropriate outcomes and indices of achievement.

Application of the Culturally Competent Model of Ethical Decision-Making

A teenager was rushed to the emergency room in critical condition after a motor vehicle accident. He was rushed to the critical care unit, and ventilatory assistance and fluid therapy were given on admission. A diagnosis of massive and irreversible brain injury was made, and the physicians informed the family of imminent brain death. As soon as brain death was established, the parents were informed by the physician, who suggested discontinuing life support and encouraged them to consider donating their son's organs. The parents reacted with anger and flatly refused the physician's recommendations. Furthermore, they threatened to bring legal action if the recommended actions were taken. Several problems occurred within the unit as a consequence of the parents' refusal: (1) the financial implications of continuing critical care for the patient, whose condition no longer warranted this level of service; (2) the constant presence of family and community members praying at the bedside, which disturbed other patients and interfered with staff activities; (3) the staff member's negative reaction to what they perceived as lack of cooperation by parents. The patient stayed in the critical care unit for 2 weeks before he died.

Using the model, an appropriate assessment would have generated information about the family's religious and moral beliefs. Identifying themselves as born-again Christians, the parents believed in the sanctity of life over quality of life. Although the parents accepted the inevitability of their son's death, their definition of life was based on a holistic conception of body and soul. Hence, brain death was an unacceptable marker of death. The family belonged to a close-knit congregation whose members believed that prayers are needed for the soul's redemption. They also believed that the dying person should never be left alone to allow the soul to leave the body in peace.

Cultural repatterning of the hospital's staff is needed to permit understanding of diverse beliefs and practices. Copartnering with families in discovering their emic worldviews and planning culturally congruent interventions requires that practitioners develop openness to differences in people. Cultural preservation of the family's moral assumptions will facilitate the most meaningful actions. The principles of beneficence and nonmaleficence are applied when the family's context of meanings is used in interpreting actions. The spiritual dimension becomes a priority as life ebbs. Sanctity of life, however, requires that the integrity of the individual's body and soul should be respected by not hastening death.

A comparative knowledge of similarities and differences across cultures is fundamental to transcultural nursing practice. Representation of diverse communities in health care is essential to facilitate intercultural and intracultural interactions that foster increased understanding and sensitivity. In a transcultural nursing course, students from different cultures are encouraged to share their heritage with their peers (Figure 5–5).

An organization will have realistic constraints that must be considered when culture-specific aspects of care are addressed. The application of distributive justice becomes problematic in many situations. When conflict arises between organizational policies and allocation of resources and the patient's need to have valued traditions accommodated, a decision that supports one side and disregards the other results in dissatisfaction and resentment. Cultural negotiation becomes a necessity when preservation of cultural beliefs and practices is not fully possible. In the previous case study, working with the religious leader to negotiate between the family's concerns and the limitations within an acute care organization could have facilitated the accommodation of

Figure 15–5. Transcultural nurses who attended Leininger's seminar at Kean University (left to right: Yoruba, Igbo, Haitian and Filipino nurses).

mutual goals. The religious leader is a trusted insider, who is knowledgeable about the family's beliefs and moral philosophies. Practitioners need to restructure their thinking and recognize that in cultural conflicts, they may not take center stage. Practitioners should be committed to the skill of switching roles and frames of reference when dealing with ethical issues related to cultural diversity.

SUMMARY

As health care becomes progressively multicultural, a different framework for decision-making is needed—one built on an understanding of differences and similarities across population groups. In ethical decision-making, universal principles are differentially applied within the context of meanings of the clients and consumers. Although the ethical principle of patient autonomy is given top priority in the Western world, it creates cultural dissonance and pain when used as the primary framework for decisions in non-Western cultures. Human rights offers a paradigm for accommodating both Western and non-Western cultures' inherent desire for culturally congruent care. Cultural assessment and understanding of the emic worldview of consumers relevant to ethical issues is a prerequisite to achieving culturally congruent decisions. Cultural competence in ethical decision-making incorporates the human rights principle and culturally congruent care.

REVIEW QUESTIONS

1. Describe ethical dilemmas associated with the current state of health care and nursing.
2. Contrast the values that form the basis for moral philosophies of dominant and diverse groups in the United States and Canada.
3. Give examples of actions or decisions that demonstrate the ethical theories and principles.
4. Explain why the application of the principles of veracity and autonomy may be problematic in some cultural groups.

CRITICAL THINKING ACTIVITIES

Identify an example of an ethical dilemma that you have encountered at work. Note that ethical dilemmas occur more frequently in clinical situations. For some of them, you may need some time to think before making a decision on your own, whereas other decisions are more complex and need referral to the ethics committee of the organization.

Identify the particulars of the situation:

1. What people are involved?
2. What is the setting?
3. How do different individuals or groups perceive the problem?
4. Identify conflicting values and beliefs at the individual, organizational, and societal levels that influence perceptions.
5. What assessment data about the situation are missing?
6. How can additional information be obtained?
7. Using the culturally competent model of ethical decision-making, how would you redefine the problem?
8. What culturally congruent strategies do you recommend?

• ETHICS RESOURCES

Center for Medical Ethics and Health Policy
Baylor College of Medicine
One Baylor Plaza
Houston, TX 77030-3498
Tel. (713)798-6290
Fax (713) 798-5678
www.bcm.tmc.edu/ethnics

Center for Bioethics
University of Pennsylvania Medical Center
3401 Market Street, Suite 320
Philadelphia, PA 19104-3308
Tel. (215) 898-7136
Fax (215) 573-3036
www.med.upenn.edu.bioethic

The Hastings Center
21 Malcolm Gordon Road
Garrison, NY 10524-5555
Tel. (845) 424-4040
Fax (845) 424-4545
www.thehastingscenter.org

Kennedy Institute for Ethics
Georgetown University
Box 571212
Washington, DC 20057-1212
Tel. (202) 687-8099
Fax (202) 687-8089
www.georgetown.edu/kie

Maclean Center for Clinical Medical Ethics
University of Chicago
Chicago, IL 60637-14
Tel. (773) 702-1453
Fax (773) 702-0090
www.ethics.bsd.uchicago.edu

Center for the Study of Bioethics
8701 Watertown Plank Road
Milwaukee, WI 53226
www.mcw.edu/bioethics

Midwest Bioethics Center
1021-1025 Jefferson Street
Kansas City, MO 64105
Tel. (800) 344-3829 or (816) 221-1100
Fax (816) 221-2002
www.midbio.org

The National Catholic Bioethics Center
159 Washington Street
Boston, MA 02135
Tel. (617) 787-1900
Fax (617) 787-4900
www.ncbcenter.org

• References

Beauchamp, T. L., & Childress, J. F. (1994). *Principles of biomedical ethics* (3rd. ed.). New York: Oxford University Press.

Beauchamp, D. E., & Steinbock, B. (1999). *New ethics for the public's health.* New York: Oxford University Press.

Blackhall, L. J., Murphy, S. T., Frank, G., Michel, V., & Azen, S,. (1995). Ethnicity and attitudes toward patient autonomy. *Journal of the American Medical Association, 274*(10), 820–825.

Bodnar, A., & Leininger, M. (1995). Transcultural nursing care of American Gypsies. In M. Leininger (Ed.). *Transcultural nursing concepts, theories, research and practice (pp. 445–470).* New York: McGraw-Hill.

Bonura, D., Fender, M., Roesler, M., & Pacquiao, D. (2001). Culturally congruent end-of-life care for Jewish patients and families. *Journal of Transcultural Nursing, 12*(3), 211–220.

Booth, B. (2001). Time to die. *American Medical News, 44*(19), 19.

Burgess, M., Stephenson, P., Ratanakul, P., & Suwonnakote, K. (1999). End-of-life decisions: Clinical decisions about dying and perspectives on life and death. In H. Coward & P. Ratanakul (Eds.), *A cross-cultural dialogue on healthcare ethics (pp. 190–206).* Waterloo, ON: Wilfrid Laurier University Press.

Burkhardt, M. A., & Nathaniel, A. K. (1998). *Ethics and issues in contemporary nursing.* Albany, NY: Delmar Publishers.

Dahrendorf, R. (1979). *Life chances: Approaches to social and political theory.* IL: University of Chicago Press.

Detmar, S. B., Muller, M. J., Wever, L. D. V., Shornagel, J. H., & Aaronson, N. K. (2001). Patient–physician communication during outpatient palliative treatment visits: An observational study. *Journal of the American Medical Association, 285*(10), 1351–1357.

DeWolf Bosek, M. S., Savage, T., Anderson Shaw, L., & Renella, C. (2001). When surrogate decision making is not straightforward. *JONA's Healthcare Law, Ethics, and Regulation, 3*(2), 47–57.

Donahue, M. P. (1996). *Nursing: The finest art.* St. Louis, MO: C. V. Mosby.

Dupree, C.Y. (2000). The attitudes of Black Americans toward advance directives. *Journal of Transcultural Nursing, 11*(1), 12–18.

Fadiman, A. (1997). The spirit catches you and you fall down. New York: Farrar, Straus & Giroux.

Fry, S. T. (1994). *Ethics in nursing practice: A guide to ethical decision making.* Geneva: International Council of Nursing.

Gatrad, A. R., & Sheikh, A. (2001). Medical ethics and Islam: Principles and practice. *Archives of Diseases in Childhood, 84*(1), 72–75.

Geertz, C. (1973). *Interpretation of cultures.* New York: Basic Books.

Gielen, U. P. (1997). A death on the roof of the world: The perspective of Tibetan Buddhism. In C. M. Parkes, P. Laungani, & B. Young (Eds.), *Death and bereavement across cultures (pp. 73–97).* London: Routledge.

Gilligan, C. (1982). *In a different voice: Psychological theory and women's development.* Cambridge, MA: Harvard University Press.

Health Canada (2001, October 11). Achieving health for all: A framework for health promotion. Available at: http://www.hc-sc.gc.ca/english/care/achieving_health.html. Accessed November 23, 2001.

Hoffmaster, B. (1999). Secular healthcare ethics. In H. Coward & P. Ratanakul (Eds.), *A cross-cultural dialogue on healthcare ethics (pp. 139–145).* Waterloo, ON: Wilfrid Laurier University Press.

Holland, J. C., Geary, N., Marchum, A., & Tross, S. (1987). An international survey of physician's attitudes and practice in regard to revealing the diagnosis of cancer. *Cancer Investigation, 5,* 151–54.

Hopp, F., & Duffy, S. A. (2000). Racial variations in end-of-life care. *Journal of the American Geriatrics Society, 48,* 658–663.

Hsu, F. L. (1963). *Clan, caste and club.* Princeton, NJ: Van Nostrand.

Ip, M., Gilligan, T., Koenig, B., & Raffin, T. A. (1998). Ethical decision making in critical care in Hongkong. *Critical Care Medicine, 26,* 447–451.

Jameton, A. (1984). *Nursing practice. The ethical issues.* Englewood Cliffs, NJ: Prentice-Hall.

Kagawa-Singer, M. (1994). Diverse cultural beliefs and practices about death and dying in the elderly. In D. Weland (Ed.), *Cultural diversity and geriatric care: Challenges to the health professions (pp. 101–116).* New York: Haworth Press.

Kleinman, A. (1988). *Rethinking psychiatry: From cultural category to personal experience.* New York: The Free Press.

Koenig, B. A., & Gates-Williams, J. (1995). Understanding cultural differences in caring for dying patients. *Western Journal of Medicine, 163,* 244–249.

Leininger, M. (Ed.). (1991). Culture care diversity and universality: A theory of nursing. New York: NLN Press. Reprinted in 2001.

Levine, E. (1997). Jewish views and customs on death. In C. M. Parkes, P. Laungani, & B. Young (Eds.), *Death and bereavement across cultures (pp. 98–130).* London: Routledge.

Lovejoy, A. O. (1974). *The great chain of being.* Cambridge, MA: Harvard University Press.

Madan, T. N. (1988). *Non-renunciation: Themes and interpretations of Hindu culture.* Delhi, India: Oxford University Press.

Mann, J. M., & Burris, S. (1998). Public health and human rights. *Human Rights, 25*(4), 2–5.

McCain, R. S. (2001, May 20). Insight on the news. *Washington Times* (http://library.kean.edu:2068/pqdwe, 6/1/01).

Meleis, A. (1996). Arab-Americans. In J. Lipson, S. Dibble, & P. Minarik (eds.), *Culture and nursing care: A pocket guide (pp. 23–36)*. San Francisco: University of California in San Francisco Press.

Miranda, B. F., McBride, M. R., & Spangler, Z. (1998). Filipino-Americans. In L. Purnell & B. Paulanka, *Transcultural health care (pp. 245–272)*. Philadelphia: F. A. Davis.

Moazam, F. (2000). Families, patients, and physicians in medical decision making: A Pakistani perspective. *The Hastings Center Report, 30*(6), 28–37.

Muller, J. H., & Desmond, B. (1992). Ethical dilemmas in cross-cultural context: A Chinese example. *Western Journal of Medicine, 157(3)* 323–327.

Norton, M. (1999). Ethics and culture: Contemporary challenges. In M. Andrews and J. Boyle, Transcultural concepts in nursing care (3rd ed., pp. 444–470). Philadelphia: Lippincott Williams & Wilkins.

Orona, C. J., Koenig, B. A., & Davis, A. J. (1994), Cultural aspects of non-disclosure. *Cambridge Quarterly of Health Care Ethics, 3,* 338–346.

Pacquiao, D. F. (1996). Infusing philosophical thought into transcultural nursing understanding. In V. Fitzsimons & M. E. Kelley, *The culture of learning (pp. 23–32)*. New York: NLN Press.

Pacquiao, D. F. (2001). Addressing cultural incongruities of advance directives. *Boethics Forum, 17*(1), 27–31.

Parry, J. (1982). Sacrificial death and the necrophagous ascetic. In M. Bloch and J. Parry (Eds.), *Death and regeneration of life*. UK: Cambridge University Press.

Parsons, T. (1951). *The social system*. New York: Free Press.

Paton, H. J. (1961). *The moral law.* London: Hutchinson & Co.

Ponet, J. E. (1996). Reflections on mortality from a Jewish perspective. In H. M. Spiro, G. McCrea Curnen, & L. P. Wandel (Eds.), *Facing death (pp. 129–136)*. New Haven, CT: Yale University Press.

Post, L. F., Blustein, J., Gordon, E., & Dubler, N. (1996). Pain, ethics, culture, and informed consent to relief. *Journal of Law, Medicine, and Ethics, 24,* 348–359.

Purnell, L. (1998). Mexican-Americans. In L. Purnell & B. Paulanka, *Transcultural health care (pp. 397–422)*. Philadelphia: F. A. Davis.

Quinn, C. A. , & Smith, M. D. (1987). *The professional commitment: Issues and ethics in nursing*. Philadelphia: W. B. Saunders.

Raphael, D. D. (1994). *Moral philosophy* (2nd. ed). New York: Oxford University Press.

Ray, M. A. (1994). A framework and model for transcultural ethical analysis. *Journal of Holistic Nursing, 12*(3), 251–264.

Ruhnke, G. W. (2000). Ethical decision making and patient autonomy: Comparison between the United States and Japan. *Chest, 118,* 1172–1182.

Selekman, J. (1998). Jewish-Americans. In L. Purnell & B. Paulanka, *Transcultural health care (pp. 371–396)*. Philadelphia: F. A. Davis.

Shweder, R. A. (1997). Anthropology's romantic rebellion against the enlightenment, or there's more to thinking than reason and evidence. In R. A. Shweder & R. A. LeVine (Eds.), *Culture theory: Essays on mind, self and emotion (pp. 27–66)*. UK: Cambridge University Press.

Shweder, R. A., & Bourne, E. J. (1997). Does the concept of the person vary crossculturally? In R. A. Shweder & R. A. LeVine (Eds.), *Culture theory: Essays on mind, self and emotion (pp. 158–199)*. UK: Cambridge University Press.

Stasiak, D. B. (1991). Culture care theory with Mexican-Americans in an urban context. In M. Leininger (Ed.), *Culture care diversity and universality: A theory of nursing (pp. 179–202)*. New York: NLN Press. (Reprinted by Jones and Bartlett in 2001).

Sutherland, A. (1986). *Gypsies: The hidden Americans.* Prospect Heights, IL: Waveland Press.

Sway, M. (1988). *Familiar strangers.* Urbana, IL: University of Illinois Press.

U.S. Public Health Service. (2000). *Healthy people 2010.* Washington, DC: U.S. Government Printing Office.

Valle, R. (2001). Cultural assessment in bioethical advocacy: Toward cultural competency and bioethical practice. *Bioethics Forum, 17*(1), 15–31.

Vatuk, S. (1996). The art of dying in Hindu India. In H. M. Spiro, M. G. McCrea Curnen, & L. P. Wandel (Eds), *Facing death (pp. 121–128)*. New Haven, CT: Yale University Press.

Villaruel, A., & Leininger, M. (1995). Culture care of Mexican-Americans. In M. Leininger, *Transcultural nursing concepts, theories, research and practice (pp. 365–382)*. New York: McGraw-Hill.

Andrews/Boyle Transcultural Nursing Assessment Guide

- ## BIOCULTURAL VARIATIONS AND CULTURAL ASPECTS OF THE INCIDENCE OF DISEASE

Are there any specific genetic or acquired conditions that are more prevalent for a specific cultural group (e.g., hypertension, cardiovascular disease, sickle cell anemia, Tay Sachs, G6PD, lactose intolerance)?

Are there socioenvironmental diseases more prevalent among a specific cultural group (e.g., lead poisoning, alcoholism, HIV/AIDS, drug abuse, ear infections, family violence)?

Are there diseases against which the client has an increased resistance (e.g., skin cancer in darkly pigmented individuals, malaria for those with sickle cell anemia)?

Does the client have distinctive features characteristic of a particular ethnic or cultural group (e.g., skin color, hair texture)? Does the client have any variations in anatomy characteristic of a particular ethnic or cultural group (e.g., body structure, height, weight, facial shape and structure, [nose, eye shape, facial contour], upper and lower extremities)?

How do anatomic, racial, and ethnic variations affect the physical examination?

- ## COMMUNICATION

What language does the client speak at home? In what language would the client prefer to communicate with you? What other languages do the client and his/her family members speak or read?

What is the fluency level of the client in English—both written and spoken?

Does the client need an interpreter? Does the health care setting provide interpreters? Who would the client prefer to assist with interpretation? Is there anyone whom the client would prefer did not serve as an interpreter (e.g., member of the opposite sex, person younger/older than the client, member of a rival tribe or nationality)?

What are the rules and modes (style) of communication? How does the client prefer to be addressed and/or what are the preferred terms for greeting?

How is it necessary to vary the technique and style of communication during the interview and/or relationship with the client to accommodate his/her cultural background (eg., tempo of conversation, eye contact, sensitivity to topical taboos, norms of confidentiality, and style of explanation)?

What are the styles of nonverbal communication?

How does the client's nonverbal communication compare with that of individuals from other cultural groups? From the health care provider? How does it affect the client's relationship with you and with other members of the health care team?

How does the client feel about health care providers who are not of the same cultural background (e.g., Black, middle-class nurse; Hispanic of a different social class)? Does the client prefer to receive care from a nurse of the same cultural background, gender, and/or age?

• CULTURAL AFFILIATIONS

With what cultural group(s) does the client report affiliation (e.g. American, Hispanic, Irish, Black, Navajo, or combination). It is becoming increasingly common for Americans to identify with two or more groups, such as Native North American and Black. Tiger Woods, for example, has identified himself as being of Thai and African-American heritage. Equally important, to what degree does the client identify with the cultural group (e.g., "we" concept of solidarity or as a fringe member)?

What is the preferred term by the cultural group?

Where was the client born?

Where has the client lived (country, city, or area within a country) and when (during what years of his/her life)? If the client has recently immigrated to the United States, knowledge of prevalent diseases in country of origin as well as sociopolitical history may be helpful. Current residence? Occupation?

• CULTURAL SANCTIONS AND RESTRICTIONS

How does the client's cultural group regard expression of emotion and feelings, spirituality, and religious beliefs? How are dying, death, and grieving expressed in a culturally appropriate manner?

How is modesty expressed by men and women? Are there culturally defined expectations about male–female relationships, including the nurse–client relationship?

Does the client have any restrictions related to sexuality, exposure of various parts of the body, certain types of surgery (e.g., vasectomy, hysterectomy)?

Are there restrictions against discussion of dead relatives or fears related to the unknown?

• DEVELOPMENTAL CONSIDERATIONS

Are there any distinct growth and development characteristics that vary with the client's cultural background (e.g., bone density, psychomotor patterns of development, fat-folds)?

What factors are significant in assessing children of various ages from the newborn period through adolescence (e.g., male and female circumcision, expected growth on standard grid, culturally acceptable age for toilet training, duration of breast feeding, introduction of various types of foods, gender differences, discipline, socialization to adult roles)?

What are the beliefs and practices associated with developmental life events such as pregnancy, birth, and death?

What is the cultural perception of aging (e.g., is youthfulness or the wisdom of old age more highly valued)?

How are elderly persons cared for within the cultural group (e.g., cared for in the home of adult children, placed in institutions for care)? What are culturally accepted roles for the elderly?

• EDUCATIONAL BACKGROUND

What is the client's highest educational level obtained?

Does the client's educational level affect his or her knowledge level concerning the health care delivery system, how to obtain the needed care, teaching-learning, and any written material that he or she is given in the health care setting (e.g., insurance forms, educational literature, information about diagnostic procedures and laboratory tests, admissions forms, etc.)? Does the client's educational level affect health behavior? As an example, cigarette smoking and obesity have been linked to economic levels.

Can the client read and write English, or is another language preferred? If English is the client's second language, are health-related materials available in the client's primary language?

What learning style is most comfortable and familiar? Does the client prefer to learn through written materials, oral explanations, videos, and/or demonstrations?

• HEALTH-RELATED BELIEFS AND PRACTICES

To what cause does the client attribute illness and disease or what factors influence the acquisition of illness and disease (e.g., divine wrath, imbalance in hot/cold, yin/yang, punishment for moral transgressions, hex, soul loss, pathogenic organism, past behavior)?

What are the client's cultural beliefs about ideal body size and shape? What is the client's self image in relation to the ideal?

How does the client describe his or her health-related condition? What names or terms are used? How does the client express pain?

What does the client believe promotes health (eating certain foods; wearing amulets to bring good luck; sleep; rest; good nutrition; reducing stress; exercise; prayer or rituals to ancestors, saints, or intermediate deities)?

What is the client's religious affiliation? How is the client actively involved in the practice of this religion?

Does the client rely on cultural healers (e.g., curandero, shaman, spiritualist, priest, minister)? Who determines when the client is sick and when he or she is healthy? Who influences the choice/type of healer and treatment that should be sought?

In what types of cultural healing or health promoting practices does the client engage (use of herbal remedies, potions, massage; wearing of talismans, copper bracelets or chains to discourage evil spirits; healing rituals; incantations; prayers)?

How are biomedical/scientific health care providers perceived? How do the client and his or her family perceive nurses? What are the expectations of nurses and nursing care?

Who will care for the client at home? What accommodations will be made by family members to provide care giving?

How does the client's cultural group view mental disorders? Are there differences in acceptable behaviors for physical versus psychological illnesses?

• KINSHIP AND SOCIAL NETWORKS

Who comprises the client's social network (family, friends, peers, cultural healer)? How do they influence the client's health or illness status? What is the composition of a "typical" family?

How do members of the client's social support network define caring or caregiving? What is the role of various family members during health and illness? Who makes decisions about health and health care?

How does the client's family participate in the promotion of health (e.g., lifestyle changes in diet, activity level, etc.) and nursing care (e.g., bathing, feeding, touching, being present) of the client?

Does the cultural family structure influence the client's response to health or illness (e.g., beliefs, strengths, weaknesses, and social class)? Who is the principle wage earner in the client's family and what is the income level? Is there more than one wage earner? Are there other sources of financial support? (Note: these may be potentially sensitive questions.)

What insurance coverage (health, dental, vision, pregnancy, cancer, or special conditions) does the client have?

What impact does the economic status have on the client's lifestyle and living conditions?

What influence do ethnic/cultural organizations have on the lifestyle and quality of life of the client (e.g., the National Association for the Advancement of Colored People [NAACP], churches [such as African American, Muslim, Jewish, Catholic, and others] that may provide schools, classes, and/or community-based health care programs and clinics.

Are there special gender issues within this cultural group? Does the client conform to traditional roles (e.g., women may be viewed as the caretakers of home and children while men work outside the home and have primary decision-making responsibilities)?

• NUTRITION

What nutritional factors are influenced by the client's cultural background? What is the meaning of food and eating to the client?

With whom does the client usually eat? What types of foods are eaten? What is the timing and sequencing of meals? What are the usual meal patterns?

What does the client define as food? What does the client believe comprises a "healthy" versus an "unhealthy" diet? Are these beliefs congruent with what the client actually eats?

Who shops for and chooses food? Where are the foodstuffs purchased? Who prepares the actual meals?

How are the foods prepared at home (type of food preparation, cooking oil[s] used, length of time foods are cooked [especially vegetables], amount and type of seasoning added to various foods during preparation)?

Has the client chosen a particular nutritional practice such as vegetarianism or abstinence from red meat or from alcoholic or fermented beverages?

Do religious beliefs and practices influence the client's diet (e.g., amount, type, preparation, or delineation of acceptable food combinations, [e.g., kosher diets])? Does the client abstain from certain foods at regular intervals, on specific dates determined by the religious calendar, or at other times? Are there other food prohibitions or prescriptions?

If the client's religion mandates or encourages tasting, what does the term fast mean (e.g., refraining from certain types of quantities of foods, eating only during certain times of the day)? For what period of time is the client expected to fast?

Are special utensils used (e.g., chopsticks, cookware)?

Does the client use home and folk remedies to treat illnesses (e.g., herbal remedies, acupuncture, cupping, other healing rituals often involving eggs, lemons, candles)?

• RELIGIOUS AFFILIATION

How does the client's religious affiliation affect health and illness (e.g., life events such as death, chronic illness, body image alteration, cause and effect of illness)?

What is the role of religious beliefs and practices during health and illness? Are there special rites or blessings for those with serious or terminal illnesses?

Are there healing rituals or practices that the client believes can promote well-being or hasten recovery from illness? If so, who performs these? What materials or arrangements are necessary for the nurse to have available for the practice of these rituals?

What is the role of significant religious representatives during health and illness? Are there recognized religious healers (e.g., Islamic imams, Christian Scientist practitioners or nurses, Catholic priests, Mormon elders, Buddhist monks)?

• VALUES ORIENTATION

What are the client's attitudes, values, and beliefs about his/her health and or illness status?

How do these influence behavior in terms of promotion of health and treatment of disease? What are the client's attitudes, values, and beliefs about health care providers?

Does culture affect the manner in which the client relates to body image change resulting from illness or surgery (e.g. importance of appearance, beauty, strength, and roles in cultural group)? Is there a cultural stigma associated with the client's illness (i.e., how is the illness or the manner in which it was contracted viewed by the larger culture)?

How does the client view work, leisure, education?

How does the client perceive and react to change?

How does the client perceive changes in lifestyle related to current illness or surgery?

How does the client view biomedical/scientific health care (e.g., suspiciously, fearfully, acceptingly, unquestioningly, with awe)?

How does the client value privacy, courtesy, touch, and relationships with others?

How does the client relate to persons outside of his or her cultural group (e.g., withdrawal, suspicion, curiosity)?

Key to page references:

b refers to material located in a box
c refers to a case study
e refers to evidence-based practice
f refers to illustrative material
t refers to tabular material